The Routledge Handbook of Translation and Health

The Routledge Handbook of Translation and Health provides a bridge between translation studies and the burgeoning field of health humanities, which seeks novel ways of understanding health and illness. As discourses around health and illness are dependent on languages for their transmission, impact, spread, acceptance and rejection in local settings, translation studies offers a wealth of data, theoretical approaches and methods for studying health and illness globally.

Translation and health intersect in a multitude of settings, historical moments, genres, media and users. This volume brings together topics ranging from interpreting in healthcare settings to translation within medical sciences, from historical and contemporary travels of medicine through translation to areas such as global epidemics, disaster situations, interpreting for children, mental health, women's health, disability, maternal health, queer feminisms and sexual health, and nutrition. Contributors come from a wide range of disciplines, not only from various branches of translation and interpreting studies, but also from disciplines such as psychotherapy, informatics, health communication, interdisciplinary health science and classical Islamic studies.

Divided into four sections and each contribution written by leading international authorities, this timely *Handbook* is an indispensable resource for all students and researchers of translation and health within translation and interpreting studies, as well as medical and health humanities.

Şebnem Susam-Saraeva is a Senior Lecturer in Translation Studies at the University of Edinburgh, Scotland. Her research interests have included gender and translation, retranslations, translation of literary and cultural theories, research methodology in translation studies, internationalisation of the discipline, translation and popular music, and translation and maternal and neonatal health.

Eva Spišiaková is REWIRE Research Fellow at the University of Vienna, Austria. Her project is positioned at the intersection of translation studies and critical disability studies, where she focuses on the changing depiction of disabled characters in translated literature in the former Eastern Bloc. Her interests also include the intersection of translation with LGBTQ issues and medical humanities.

Routledge Handbooks in Translation and Interpreting Studies

Routledge Handbooks in Translation and Interpreting Studies provide comprehensive overviews of the key topics in translation and interpreting studies. All entries for the handbooks are specially commissioned and written by leading scholars in the field. Clear, accessible and carefully edited, Routledge Handbooks in Translation and Interpreting Studies are the ideal resource for both advanced undergraduates and postgraduate students.

The Routledge Handbook of Translation and Education
Edited by Sara Laviosa and Maria González-Davies

The Routledge Handbook of Translation and Cognition
Edited by Fabio Alves and Arnt Lykke Jakobsen

The Routledge Handbook of Translation and Activism
Edited by Rebecca Ruth Gould and Kayvan Tahmasebian

The Routledge Handbook of Translation, Feminism and Gender
Edited by Luise von Flotow and Hala Kamal

The Routledge Handbook of Translation and Globalization
Edited by Esperança Bielsa and Dionysios Kapsaskis

The Routledge Handbook of Translation and Ethics
Edited by Kaisa Koskinen and Nike K. Pokorn

The Routledge Handbook of Translation and Health
Edited by Şebnem Susam-Saraeva and Eva Spišiaková

For a full list of titles in this series, please visit www.routledge.com/Routledge-Handbooks-in-Translation-and-Interpreting-Studies/book-series/RHTI.

The Routledge Handbook of Translation and Health

Edited by Şebnem Susam-Saraeva and Eva Spišiaková

Routledge
Taylor & Francis Group
LONDON AND NEW YORK

First published 2021
by Routledge
2 Park Square, Milton Park, Abingdon, Oxon OX14 4RN

and by Routledge
605 Third Avenue, New York, NY 10158

Routledge is an imprint of the Taylor & Francis Group, an informa business

British Library Cataloguing-in-Publication Data
A catalogue record for this book is available from the British Library

Library of Congress Cataloging-in-Publication Data
Names: Susam-Saraeva, Şebnem, editor. | Spišiaková, Eva, editor.
Title: The Routledge handbook of translation and health /
edited by Şebnem Susam-Saraeva and Eva Spišiaková.
Description: Abingdon, Oxon; New York, NY: Routledge, 2021. |
Series: Routledge handbooks in translation and interpreting studies |
Includes bibliographical references and index.
Identifiers: LCCN 2020051528
Subjects: LCSH: Medicine–Translating. |
Health facilities–Translating services. | Communication in medicine. |
Translating and interpreting–Social aspects.
Classification: LCC R119.5 .R68 2021 | DDC 610.1/4–dc23
LC record available at https://lccn.loc.gov/2020051528

ISBN: 978-1-138-33534-9 (hbk)
ISBN: 978-0-367-76667-2 (pbk)
ISBN: 978-1-003-16798-3 (ebk)

DOI: 10.4324/9781003167983

Typeset in Times New Roman
by Newgen Publishing UK

The Open Access version of Introduction and Chapter 18 was funded by The University of Vienna (as part of the European Union's Horizon 2020 Research and Innovation Programme under the Marie Skłodowska-Curie grant).

This project was completed with the support of the University of Vienna and has received funding from the European Union's Horizon 2020 research and innovation programme under the Marie Skłodowska-Curie grant agreement No 847693.

Contents

Acknowledgements

The fact that this volume came into being in the midst of a pandemic, despite the unprecedented changes to the personal and professional lives of everyone involved, makes us all the more grateful for the support we have received. First of all, we would like to thank our contributors for sharing their expertise with us and for responding to our numerous emails with patience and efficiency, regardless of their ever-changing circumstances. The editorial team at Routledge – Louisa Semlyen, Hannah Rowe and Eleni Steck – accompanied the handbook at every stage of its production. Our advisory board members, Eivind Engebretsen, Karen Korning Zethsen, Vicent Montalt, Jemina Napier and Sharon O'Brien, as well as two anonymous reviewers, helped us shape the scope of the volume in its preparatory stages.

Şebnem Susam-Saraeva would like to thank The Institute of Feminist and Gender Studies, University of Ottawa, for hosting her as the Bank of Montreal Visiting Scholar in Women's Studies during the initial stages of this volume in 2018. She is grateful for the comments received from colleagues and students at the Institute, as well as those at the School of Translation and Interpretation, University of Ottawa; School of Translation, Glendon College, York University, Toronto; and, Department of Linguistics and Translation, University of Montreal.

Eva Spišiaková would like to thank Miro Griffiths for his generous comments on her contribution to the volume, and her former colleagues at the University of Liverpool and University of Exeter for their support during her time there as an AHRC Postdoctoral Research Associate.

Figure 2.1 illustrating Japanese translations of Western works in Chapter 2 is used with the kind permission of Cambridge University Press, and Bertha M. Gutiérrez Rodilla granted us the permission to use Figure 3.2 in Chapter 3, detailing the interlingual and intercultural movements in the history of medicine.

Contributors

Rachele Antonini is an Associate Professor at the Department of Interpreting and Translation of the University of Bologna at Forlì. Her research interests include child language brokering, audiovisual translation, non-professional interpreting and translation, and humour studies.

Michela Baldo is an independent researcher and freelance translator. Her research revolves around the written and audiovisual translation of Italian-Canadian works into Italian and the role of translation in Italian queer transfeminist activism. She published various articles, edited *Il re Nudo. Per un archivio drag king in Italia* (2014) and is coediting a special issue on translation and LGBTQ+ activism.

Nesrine Bessaïh holds a masters in anthropology and PhD in translation studies. Her research interests bring together translation studies, gender studies and linguistic anthropology. She is co-founder and co-ordinator of *La CORPS féministe (La collective pour un ouvrage de référence participatif sur la santé féministe)*, the association that leads the translation and adaptation of *Our Bodies, Ourselves* in Quebec.

Alexandra Birch is currently an Innovation Fellow at Informatics at the University of Edinburgh. Her recent interests have focused on neural machine translation where advances using sub-word units and monolingual data have beaten state-of-the-art baselines. She is the co-ordinator of the H2020 EU project called GoURMET which investigates low-resource machine translation, and she is a co-founder of Aveni.ai.

Hanneke Bot worked till she retired in 2016 as a psychotherapist and programme leader in a clinic for the treatment of asylum seekers and refugees with severe mental illnesses where she cooperated daily with interpreters. Her PhD (Utrecht, 2005) is about the theory and practice of interpreter mediated mental healthcare.

Matilde Nisbeth Brøgger is Associate Professor of International Business Communication and Health Communication at Aarhus University. She has published on various aspects of medical translation, including comprehensibility and back translation, and health communication in journals such as *Meta*, *Linguistica Antverpiensia*, *Communication & Medicine*, *Patient Education & Counseling* and *Health Expectations*.

Joost Buysschaert is an Emeritus Professor at Ghent University, Belgium. He is active in the Terminology Centre of the Department of Translation, Interpreting and Communication (www.cvt.ugent.be). His research focuses on terminology and medical translation.

Patrick Cadwell is an Assistant Professor of Translation Studies in the School of Applied Language and Intercultural Studies at Dublin City University (DCU). He teaches specialised translation, terminology, and translation theory, among other subjects. His current research centres on translation in crisis settings and translation communities of practice.

Luciana Carvalho Fonseca is an experienced interpreter and translator. She is an Assistant Professor in the Department of Modern Languages at the University of São Paulo, where she teaches English and translation at graduate and undergraduate levels. Her research interests include translation, power and activism, women translators in history and feminist translation.

Robyn K. Dean has been a certified signed language interpreter for over thirty years with particular service in healthcare. Her scholarship in ethics and reflective practices in community interpreting is recognised internationally. She is currently an Assistant Professor at the Rochester Institute of Technology, where she leads the institute's postgraduate degree in healthcare interpretation.

Renée Desjardins is an Associate Professor at the School of Translation at the Université de Saint-Boniface, Winnipeg, Canada. She has been involved with *CuiZine: The Journal of Canadian Food Cultures* in various roles including social media lead and editor-in-chief. She has published on the subject of menu translation, Canada's Food Guide, and the intersections between food studies and translation studies.

Bruce T. Downing is an Associate Professor Emeritus at the University of Minnesota, USA, where he has served as chair of the Department of Linguistics and director of the Program in Translation and Interpreting. His research areas include English linguistics, refugee bilingualism, and healthcare interpreting.

Eivind Engebretsen is Full Professor of Interdisciplinary Health Science at the University of Oslo. He studies the interfaces of political ideologies and knowledge production in healthcare, drawing on political philosophy and discourse analysis. He is the Vice-Dean for Postgraduate Studies at the Faculty of Medicine.

Barry Haddow is a Senior Researcher at the School of Informatics at the University of Edinburgh. He has worked mainly on machine translation since 2008, participating in several EU-funded projects, and coordinated the Horizon 2020 'Health in my Language' project from 2012–2015.

Kenneth Heafield is a Reader at the University of Edinburgh working to improve the quality and efficiency of machine translation. He coordinates European Union projects on private browser-based translation, parallel corpus mining, and computational efficiency. He holds a PhD from Carnegie Mellon and a BSc from Caltech.

Gina Fraas Henrichsen is researcher at the Centre for Health Sciences Education at the Faculty of Medicine, University of Oslo, Norway. Her research interests are knowledge translation in healthcare, the introduction of mindfulness into healthcare, and science studies.

Ji-Hae Kang is Professor of Translation Studies at Ajou University, South Korea. Her research focuses on translation in institutional settings and issues of power and discourse in the transnational production of knowledge. She is the guest-editor of the special issue *Translation in Institutions* (2014) and co-editor of *Translating and Interpreting in Korean Contexts: Engaging with Asian and Western Others* (2019).

Wioleta Karwacka is a translator and Assistant Professor at the Division of Translation Studies, University of Gdańsk, Poland. Her work centres on translation and translation studies. Her research focuses on medical translation and eco-translation. She has authored publications on various aspects of medical translation, medical terminology and anthropomorphism in translation.

Raquel Lázaro Gutiérrez is an Associate Professor at the University of Alcalá and teaches on the Modern Languages and Translation degree course and the MA in Intercultural Communication and Public Service Interpreting and Translation. She is a member of FITISPos-UAH research group, and ENPSIT, European Network of PSIT.

Vicent Montalt teaches and researches at the Department of Translation and Communication Studies, Universitat Jaume I (UJI), Spain. He is director of the Master's Programme in Medical and Health Translation and the research institute López Piñero (IILP), both at UJI. He is a regular visiting professor at CenTraS, University College London.

Christopher J. Moreland, MD MPH, is Associate Professor of Internal Medicine, and Associate Residency Program Director, at Dell Medical School at the University of Texas at Austin. His education and research interests include addressing healthcare disparities impacting deaf and hard of hearing populations, and healthcare workforce diversity.

Anne Birgitta Nilsen is a Professor of Interpreting Studies at Oslo Metropolitan University. Her research includes interpreting in the public sector services, sight translation and interpreting for children.

John Ødemark is Professor of Cultural History and Cultural Encounters at the Faculty of Humanities, University of Oslo. His research interests are the theory and history of translation and the human sciences. He is principal researcher for the project The Body in Translation – Historicising and Reinventing Knowledge Translation.

Carmen Quijada Diez is a Lecturer at the University of Oviedo, after having taught at the University of Salamanca. She teaches German and German-Spanish translation and her research focuses on specialised translation, mainly in the medical field, science reception in 19th century Spain and the use of translation as a didactic tool in second-language learning.

Tony Joakim Sandset is a Research Fellow at the Centre for Sustainable Healthcare Education, Faculty of Medicine, University of Oslo. Research areas include HIV/AIDS prevention, global pandemics, evidence-based medicine, the role of knowledge translation in medical discourses and how knowledge is transferred and adopted through various forms of translation.

Eva Spišiaková received her PhD in translation studies from the University of Edinburgh and presently holds the post of a REWIRE Research Fellow at the University of Vienna, Austria. Her project is positioned at the intersection of Translation Studies and Critical Disability Studies, and she focuses on the changing depiction of disabled characters in translated literature of the former Eastern Bloc.

Şebnem Susam-Saraeva is a Senior Lecturer in Translation Studies at the University of Edinburgh, Scotland. Her research interests have included gender and translation, retranslations, translation of literary and cultural theories, research methodology in translation studies, internationalisation of the discipline, translation and popular music, and translation and maternal and neonatal health.

Laurie Swabey is Professor of Interpreting at St Catherine University in St Paul, Minnesota, USA. She holds a PhD from the University of Minnesota in Linguistics and her research interests include interpreting pedagogy and healthcare interpreting.

Ira Torresi is Associate Professor at the Department of Interpreting and Translation of the University of Bologna at Forlì. Her research interests include child language brokering, promotional translation, gender studies, visual semiotics, and James Joyce.

Elaine van Dalen is Assistant Professor of Classical Islamic Studies at Columbia University. Her research focuses on the history of medicine and the translation of Greek scholarly works into Arabic and their subsequent reception in Classical Islamic medical scholarship. She obtained her PhD in Classics and Ancient History from the University of Manchester in 2017.

Karen Korning Zethsen is Professor of Translation Studies at Aarhus University. Her primary research interests include translation studies (in particular intralingual translation) and health communication. She has published in journals such as *Target*, *the Translator*, *TTR*, *Meta*, *Across*, *Jostrans*, *Text & Talk*, *Communication & Medicine* and *the Journal of Pragmatics*.

Beyond translation and medicine

Initiating exchanges between translation studies and health humanities

Şebnem Susam-Saraeva and Eva Spišiaková

1 Introduction

This volume was born out of curiosity. As translation studies[1] scholars focusing on maternal and neonatal health (Susam-Saraeva) and disability (Spišiaková), and coming from descriptive and sociological perspectives on translation, we were familiar with a small portion of the field of translation and medicine and aware that both interpreting within healthcare settings and translation of medical texts had been growing areas of research. The linguistic, social and ethical aspects of community interpreting that takes place in hospitals and general practices have been studied extensively; literature on the specificities of medical texts, terminology and translation has been flourishing. Invaluable as these studies are in making the process of translation and interpreting in medicine visible, emphasising their crucial impact on patient/healthcare provider interactions as well as on health literacy and knowledge transfer, they inevitably look at a small part of what goes on in relation to translation and human health.

The overriding question for us was this: what would happen if we changed the focus from translation in healthcare settings, or more generally, translation and medicine, to translation and health? Medicine is but one component of health and wellbeing, which signify more than the absence of disease or illness. The more we looked into translation and health, the more it has become apparent to us that they intersect in a multitude of settings, historical moments, genres, and users. With the increasing emphasis on person-centred healthcare, which recognises the initiative, responsibility and empowerment of 'the patient', and on the promotion of health across populations, interesting avenues of research open up to scholars working on translation and interpreting in relation to health, beyond the diagnosis and treatment of diseases.

This line of thought, novel as it may be for translation studies, is of course not entirely new. Since the early 21st century, the discipline of health humanities has gradually emerged, encompassing the slightly older and arguably narrower discipline of medical humanities. Health humanities suggests that health matters are too important to be entrusted solely to doctors and other healthcare professionals, and that health is an issue all academic disciplines may approach, examine, sustain and enhance. It seeks novel ways of understanding

DOI: 10.4324/9781003167983-1

health and illness, borrowing methods and frameworks from the humanities and social sciences to bear on biomedicine, clinical practice, and the politics of healthcare. To this end, several disciplines in the humanities, such as literary studies, film studies and cultural studies, have so far been used to shed light on health matters.

Considering that discourses around health and illness are dependent on languages for their transmission, impact, spread, acceptance and rejection in local settings, one can begin to appreciate the wealth of data, theoretical approaches and methods translation studies can offer in studying health and illness globally. Conversely, translation studies can learn from the developments in health humanities regarding the expansion of topics for research, recent frameworks and debates shaping areas of health. Therefore, while this handbook ensures that well-established research areas in translation and medicine are covered, it also intends to open up new avenues of exchange between translation studies and health humanities by initiating research into previously neglected areas.

Compared to medical humanities, interdisciplinarity and interprofessionality are much more emphasised and encouraged in health humanities, bringing in contributions from groups previously marginalised in the former, such as allied health professionals, nurses, patients and carers (Jones *et al.* 2017). The implications of such a broadening of the field for translators and interpreters cannot be underestimated; it would mean more interaction and cooperation between the different professions, as translators and interpreters become an organic part of care-giving, involved in the developments and decision-making processes in healthcare settings.

It is increasingly recognised that 'medicine is only a minor determinant of health in human populations alongside other social factors' (Jones *et al.* 2017: 933), such as class, education, occupation, religion, environment, race, disability, sexuality and gender. Given these overlapping determinants – and the influence of other disciplines such as women's studies, disability studies, postcolonial studies, and queer studies starting to have a bearing on medical education – courses 'far more concerned with individual and cultural experiences of illness and disability and with the social/structural/political impediments to health and healing' have begun to be offered as part of medical education (*ibid.*). This shift is in line with an emphasis on intersectionality, another key concept borrowed by health humanities, which highlights the health-related discrimination and disadvantages caused by the interconnected nature of social categorisations as they apply to a given individual or group. In this volume, we endeavoured to reflect the impact of intersectionality on translation and health-related concerns, in chapters focusing on women's health, disability and health in LGBTQ communities.

In translation studies, the focus has traditionally remained on translation and interpreting within biomedicine, 'owing to its economic and political power and prestige' (Montalt in this volume, p. 134). Examining translation and interpreting both in relation to biomedicine and outside its boundaries, several contributions in this volume underline the links between translation, medicine and power (e.g. Baldo, Bessaih, Kang, Moreland and Swabey, Sandset, Spišiaková, Susam-Saraeva and Carvalho Fonseca). The power in question goes beyond ethical considerations surrounding the interpreter/healthcare provider/patient triad, and encompasses a range of issues, such as patient autonomy, informed consent, empowerment of oppressed and/or marginalised groups, challenging institutional attitudes and practices, and the connection between the adoption of 'Western' medical knowledge and nationalism, including the processes of modernisation. Other contributions on enhancing health literacy through improving accessibility and readability, on recent projects in medical terminology and machine translation, and on knowledge translation between science in laboratories and clinical application reveal further implications regarding the positioning of the 'patient' vis-à-vis biomedicine.

2 Healthcare-focused research in translation studies

While the topics covered in this handbook are, in many cases, well-established areas of research either within or outside translation studies, there has been, to our knowledge, no single volume that brought together such a range of topics on human health and well-being as seen through the prism of inter- (and intra-)lingual transfer. The following brief overview outlines some of the most prominent general works on the subject of health in translation, in order to complement the highly specialised information included in the contributions to this handbook.

The first volume bringing together research on a range of topics related to translation in medical settings was Henry Fischbach's *Translation and Medicine* (1998). The volume explores topics such as the historical and cultural aspects of medical translation, the training of translators in healthcare settings, and the translation of medical terminology, and as such, could be considered an early precursor to the current volume. With the rise of translation studies as an academic discipline in the early 2000s came the increasing specialisation of its subfields, and research on subjects related to translation and health have gradually become more subject-specific. Out of these subjects, the most comprehensively covered one relates to interpreting in healthcare settings, reflecting the growing need to ensure equal access to medical care in increasingly multilingual societies. The first volume bringing together research articles on the subject was Franz Pöchhacker and Miriam Shlesinger's *Healthcare Interpreting: Discourse and Interaction* (2007), which focuses on cross-cultural communication, the role played by interpreters in healthcare settings, and the discursive patterns of interaction involving a medical interpreter. A later volume by Brenda Nicodemus and Melanie Metzger, *Investigations in Healthcare Interpreting* (2014), centres on the communicative aspects of interpreter-mediated encounters in healthcare, and explores the different methods for improving accuracy in these encounters. The bilingual volume (Spanish and English) *Translating and Interpreting Healthcare Discourses/Traducir e interpretar en el ámbito sanitario*, edited by María-José Varela Salinas and Bernd Meyer (2015), comprises both interpreting and translation, and touches upon subjects such as sign language interpreting, quality assurance in the translation process, and translation of specialised medical texts and terminology. The most recent addition to the field is the *Handbook of Research on Medical Interpreting*, by Izabel de V. Souza and Effrossyni Fragkou (2020), which covers areas such as healthcare administration and education, patient care and safety, and interpreting for victims of violence, amongst others.

Another area frequently explored in studies on medical translation and interpreting is the question of intercultural communication. Claudia Angelelli's volume *Medical Interpreting and Cross-Cultural Communication* (2004) has an ethnographic study of a bilingual hospital at its core, and uses interviews with interpreters to highlight their agency in situations where they are required to bridge cultural as well as linguistic divides. *Health, Communication and Multicultural Communities: Topics on Intercultural Communication for Healthcare Professionals* by Carmen Valero-Garces (2014) places an emphasis on the communicative element of interpreted encounters, and offers reflections and experiences from the author's long career in training mediators and translators in multicultural medical settings. Elaine Hsieh's *Bilingual Health Communication: Working with Interpreters in Cross-Cultural Care* (2016) likewise uses interviews with both interpreters and healthcare providers to explore the phenomenon of bilingual healthcare in a wide range of language combinations. Finally, *Multicultural Health Translation, Interpreting and Communication* by Meng Ji, Mustapha Taibi and Ineke Crezee (2019) brings together a range of research topics in empirical health translation, and covers both macro questions concerning national healthcare systems and micro studies of areas such as mental health interpreting.

Several other volumes in the field of medical translation are aimed specifically at professional translators and interpreters with no formal training in interpreting within healthcare settings. These volumes are particularly important, as not all institutions teaching translation and interpreting offer specialised courses on the topic. Ineke Crezee's *Introduction to Healthcare for Interpreters and Translators* (2013) serves as a comprehensive guidebook for those with no prior experience in healthcare interpreting, and provides a well-organised overview of the terminology, concepts and systems they are likely to encounter. The handbook has generated versions for specific languages, including Spanish (Crezee, Mikkelson and Monzon-Storey 2015), Japanese (Crezee and Asano 2016), Chinese (Crezee and Ng 2016) and Arabic (Crezee, Gailani and Gailani 2016). Claudia Angelelli's recent volume *Healthcare Interpreting Explained* (2019) is likewise a guidebook for students and practising interpreters, and teaches problem-solving strategies through real-life examples, alongside chapters on ethics, protocol and professionalisation. Vicent Montalt and Maria González Davies' volume *Medical Translation Step by Step* (2007) turns towards the problem of translation in the medical sphere and offers a comprehensive overview, including detailed instructions on the writing and improving of drafts, and large-scale issues related to the role and responsibilities of translators specialising in medical texts.

It is on the basis of this existing body of research that this handbook intends to propel studies on translation and health into areas beyond healthcare interpreting and medical translation. Crucial though the emphasis on the interpreter/translator working in/on medical encounters/texts has been, we hope that contributions in this volume will demonstrate the significance of other agents translating and interpreting in relation to health, as well as of the various contexts that sustain or hinder translation and interpreting.

3 Editing a handbook on translation and health during a pandemic

The final stages of the editing process of this handbook were completed in the midst of the COVID-19 pandemic. When we exchanged emails with our contributors, we sent greetings from one lockdown to another, often starting 'Hope this email finds you and yours well, under the circumstances'. While the situation is still unfolding and scholarly studies on translating and interpreting within this pandemic are only in their initial stages, we feel we need to mention some pointers here for future research.

Translation has been used as a trope in medicine for the last 20 years or so, in terms such as translational research and knowledge translation; however, it has rarely been applied as a critical concept, unlike its use in the humanities (Engebretsen 2 July 2020).[2] This trope tends to suggest a linear production of knowledge, produced in laboratories and medical institutions, which is then supposedly disseminated intact to healthcare providers, clinical practitioners, and ultimately, lay people. The COVID-19 pandemic, however, laid bare the messiness of this process, as well as its cultural-embeddedness, as opposed to the 'timeless' and 'universal' aspects of scientific knowledge. Which type of mask is most effective against the virus? Would face coverings as opposed to medical-grade masks suffice? How much social distancing is required: two metres, one and a half, or one? At the time of writing this introduction, debates range from the anti-malarial drug trials to the widening use of remdesivir. In short, there has not been sufficient time to establish the truth of scientific knowledge in the case of this particular pandemic. As one of our contributors, Eivind Engebretsen, aptly notes in an interview, during the COVID-19 pandemic 'the distinction between the moment of production and the moment of translation of knowledge is fundamentally blurred' (*ibid.*). The pandemic has forced us to act without relying on an established body of evidence-based knowledge (based on e.g. randomised controlled trials) that is temporally associated with the past – in translation studies terms, a solid 'source text' – and to 'translate' what little knowledge we have on the virus and possible treatments into global clinical practice.

Arguably, at no other time in recent history were we forced to make sense of disease and illness on such a global scale and so rapidly as we have been since the start of the pandemic. Lay people had to 'translate' the languages of science, politicians and statistics on a daily basis in order to make sense of the situation (cf. Gardini 15 May 2020),[3] as well as rely on various forms of interlingual translation in order to supplement the frequently insufficient information provided in their local languages. They had to adjust their daily lives to the changing narratives and guidelines in accordance with these 'translations'. The changes were not limited to behavioural ones; language was also implicated. New terms emerged almost overnight (mostly in Anglophone countries), such as 'lockdown', 'social distancing', 'contact tracing', 'flattening the curve', 'self-isolation/self-quarantine' and 'herd immunity'. Through international health organisations which rely on English as a lingua franca, these terms spread worldwide, and were translated into – or simply borrowed and transliterated in – a multitude of languages, with varying degrees of success. While the speed and spread of the virus necessitate that we 'speak the same language', preferably that of science, it is becoming increasingly clear that the vastly different responses to the pandemic in each country also reflect the languages of politics, culture, infrastructure, and, most importantly, socio-economic power or the lack thereof. As one senior health advisor at BBC Media Action puts it:

> Many organizations are promoting concepts that are alien to our audiences, no matter how they are described [...]. Social distancing and self-isolation present particular problems if you live in a two-room house with 10 others, and then even more so if that house is in a slum with thousands of other people. Another issue is advice around hand-washing, if people don't have access to enough water or don't have the money for soap or hand sanitizer.[4]

As widely discussed in the media, the pandemic has made certain existing inequalities starkly visible. These inequalities and their impact on translating and interpreting are not restricted to countries with limited economic means. One debate, for instance, revolved around the provision of sign language interpreting during the UK government's daily briefings on the pandemic. British Sign Language users and activists argued that they have been discriminated against, because critical information was not being conveyed to them; they accordingly initiated legal proceedings against the government.[5] Elsewhere, previously neglected areas of translation and interpreting were brought to the fore. Over the course of the pandemic, the Slovak sign language interpreter of COVID-19 press briefings, Barbara Randušková, has become a national celebrity due to her nearly constant on-screen presence, providing much-needed visibility to the practice of sign language interpreting amongst the wider population in Slovakia.[6]

The pandemic impacted not only on the people at the receiving end of translation and interpreting services, but also on translators and interpreters themselves. Owing to shortage of interpreters, cancellation of short-term and long-term interpreting contracts and the exponential increase in remotely-held meetings, EU officials were unable to express themselves in their mother tongues in parliamentary meetings and had to revert to English.[7] In US medical settings, a sudden decline in on-site interpreting (up to 40%) and a corresponding, and seemingly long-term, increase in the use of telephone/video interpreters were noted (Heilweil 2020). Beyond the damage to their livelihood and the transformation of the way they worked, (remote) interpreters have found themselves

> in the middle of some of the pandemic's most sensitive, stressful, and heartbreaking moments. They're frequently called upon to share the results of a COVID-19 test, and if it's positive, the interpreter must communicate the next steps, including the rules of social isolation. Interpreters can be asked to help patients in tough times, like being admitted to the hospital or discussing the scenario of going onto a ventilator. More rarely, they can be called upon to interpret the news from a doctor that a family member has died of COVID-19.
>
> *Heilweil 2020*

The situation has been further complicated by the fact that healthcare providers at the other end of remote interpreting devices wear protective masks which render them hard to understand and that the patients themselves may be on ventilators (*ibid.*).[8]

The pandemic has been labelled as 'history's biggest translation challenge'.[9] To cope with the amount of material that needed to be translated in such a short period of time, some volunteer organisations have introduced unprecedented initiatives. Translators without Borders (TWB), for instance, launched the COVID-19 Community Translation Program, 'providing community organizations with free and open access to TWB's online translation environment'[10] so that they can connect and collaborate directly with 'TWB's community of over 30,000 translators, many of whom are generously donating their time to help people access COVID-19 information in their language'.[11] The translations requested have included 'translating travel ban information for refugees and immigrants into Chinese and Korean; translating what social distancing means into Spanish; and translating infection prevention and control information into Spanish, Chinese, French and Portuguese'.[12]

We anticipate that the COVID-19 crisis under which this volume is edited will shift the discourse on health, translation and interpreting into entirely new directions, and bring about questions and research areas we are, as yet, unable to foresee.

4 Future directions

When we first put together the proposal for this handbook, we had a rather ambitious wish-list for the topics we wanted to cover. Soon, however, we found out that very few researchers focused on areas that we thought would have been particularly noteworthy. The following overview sketches out some of the directions we were not able to pursue in this volume, signalling potential directions for research at the intersection of translation and health.

Our section on the travels of health-related translations focuses overwhelmingly on the transfer of Western sources, with scholarship largely based on the writings of Galen and harking back to Ancient Greece. Translation and transfer of medical knowledge from other parts of the world, including Ayurvedic texts, ancient Egyptian medicine and Chinese medicine, remain underexplored. Translations related to particular events in human history – e.g. doctors' testimonies during the Holocaust, the dissemination of scientific findings such as the germ theory of disease or the invention of penicillin – represent further avenues of research. The role of colonial structures in the spread of biomedical knowledge through translation remains largely untouched, as does the historical and present-day production and transfer of healthcare information in the southern hemisphere. Another area we hope to see further research in is the medical knowledge of indigenous peoples around the world and how this knowledge has been translated. Last but not least, while several chapters in this volume touch upon the subject of translations and interpreting for refugees, translation and health as part of the so-called European migrant crisis is yet to be explored in full.

Another significant area in which we anticipate seeing rapid progress is the use of technology and corpus-based approaches in supporting and improving medical translations. The chapter by Haddow, Birch and Heafield on machine translation in this volume represents an insight into these possibilities; many other areas, such as the role of translation technologies and localisation in the distribution of medical information, or the challenges presented by the interlingual transfer of digital medical records, will likely become the focus of extensive future research.

Recent years have also seen a boom in the publication of narratives penned by healthcare professionals for a general public, from Oliver Sacks' now iconic *The Man Who Mistook His Wife for a Hat* (1985) to more recent bestsellers, such as Paul Kalanithi's *When Breath Becomes Air* (2016). The translations of these works, requiring considerable technical knowledge as well as expertise in literary translation, present a number of challenges worth exploring. Such studies will particularly address the interdisciplinary nature of both health humanities and translation studies, not only by bringing together these two disciplines, but also literary studies and different medical fields, such as neurology and oncology.

As we have deliberately chosen the title translation and health, as opposed to medicine, we also wanted to explore other areas that contribute to human wellbeing than just those that treat illness and disease. We hoped to complement the chapter on translation and nutrition in this volume with others, for instance, on translation, sports and exercise; there is large research potential in the growing interest in self-help publications aiming to improve overall physical wellbeing. Books, blogs, websites and social media apps aiming to enhance people's health, many of which require translation and localisation in order to match their rapid global spread, all represent a gap in current scholarship.

Spiritual, emotional and mental health is another direction we hoped to pursue in more depth. While the chapter on mental health in this volume by Bot provides an illuminating insight into the process of interpreting during therapy sessions, there are many other areas where translation and mental health intersect, including clinical care for mental health patients and global campaigns raising awareness about anxiety or depression. Other areas such as translation of meditation, yoga or mindfulness apps, books or videos will also need to be covered in future publications. Lastly, we hope to see future research exploring the occupational health of translators and interpreters themselves; as many contributions in this volume demonstrate, their work is frequently associated with high levels of stress and pressure, and perhaps never more so than when their work has a direct effect on human lives and wellbeing.

5 Structure of this handbook

The handbook is divided into four sections that reflect the key thematic clusters of present-day research on translation and health. The first part focuses on journeys of medical texts from ancient to modern times, following informational flows in different eras and geographic locations. The contributions unpick the spread of Western medical knowledge from Ancient Greece through Arab empires to medieval Europe, and later through the invention of the printing press, into other regions including East Asia in the 19th and early 20th centuries. The section also considers the role of the various lingua francas of medical knowledge, from Arabic through Latin, to the present-day prevalence of English.

The second section is dedicated to the role of translation in medicine and the medical sciences. The chapters explore challenges posed by medical terminology, international standards of patient information leaflets, and questions of intralingual and interlingual medical translation. Other contributions in this section highlight the growing applicability of machine translation to medical contexts, consider the dual meaning of the word translation in relation to medicine (interlingual translation and knowledge translation), and investigate how the field of translation studies intersects with medical humanities.

The third section turns towards the role of interpreting in healthcare. The contributions explore not only the challenges of interpreting delivered by trained professionals, both in-person or remotely via telephone and videoconferencing, but also the role of non-professional interpreters in healthcare settings, such as child language brokers. Other chapters in this section consider the ethical aspects of interpreting in healthcare settings and the role of language concordance between deaf healthcare professionals and deaf patients.

The final section of the handbook presents insights into and case studies in a range of areas where health and translation intersect. The contributions attest to the specific challenges in providing language access in emergencies, such as disaster situations and pandemics, as well as in everyday life: the health of minoritised groups, such as the disabled and LGBTQ+ communities; women's health, including maternal and neonatal care; the highly sensitive issues related to interpreter-mediated communication with children and in mental health; and, the ever-growing importance of nutrition and health.

We hope that the handbook will be an invaluable resource for students and researchers in translation studies interested in health-related issues, as well as those in health humanities interested in language and communication. Healthcare practitioners who work in multilingual and multicultural environments, as well as translators and interpreters working in healthcare settings will also undoubtedly benefit from the contributions.

Notes

This project was completed with the support of the University of Vienna and has received funding from the European Union's Horizon 2020 research and innovation programme under the Marie Skłodowska-Curie grant agreement No 847693.

1 Throughout the handbook, we have used translation studies as an umbrella term covering translation and interpreting studies, except in contributions which specifically focus on interpreting.
2 https://podcasts.ox.ac.uk/masks-vaccine-and-cure-translating-medical-evidence-during-and-after-pandemic. Podcast with Eivind Engebretsen, by Marta Arnaldi, 2 July 2020. Also available at www.youtube.com/watch?v=to49m8TcfbI (Accessed: 8 July 2020).
3 https://podcasts.ox.ac.uk/translating-illness-case-COVID-19. Podcast with Nicola Gardini, by Marta Arnaldi, 15 May 2020. Also available at www.youtube.com/watch?v=gujukayRJ28 (Accessed: 8 July 2020).
4 www.devex.com/news/how-do-you-say-social-distancing-in-swahili-96856 (Accessed: 8 July 2020).
5 www.bbc.co.uk/news/disability-52323854 (Accessed: 8 July 2020).
6 See e.g. www1.pluska.sk/spravy/z-domova/exkluzivne-vdaka-matovicovi-ju-pozna-cele-slovensko-minulost-sexi-tlmocnicky-vas-dostane (Accessed: 10 November 2020).
7 www.politico.eu/article/coronavirus-COVID-19-confinement-restrictions-create-havoc-in-the-secret-world-of-eu-interprets/ (Accessed: 8 July 2020).
8 The compulsory use of masks and other facial coverings in public spaces also significantly affected the lives of deaf or hard-of-hearing persons who partially or mainly rely on lipreading for communication.
9 www.wired.com/story/covid-language-translation-problem/ (Accessed: 9 November 2020).
10 https://translatorswithoutborders.org/translations-COVID-19/ (Accessed: 9 November 2020).
11 https://translatorswithoutborders.org/COVID-19-application (Accessed: 9 November 2020).
12 *Ibid.*

References

Angelelli, C. V. (2004) *Medical Interpreting and Cross-Cultural Communication.* Cambridge: Cambridge University Press.

Angelelli, C. V. (2019) *Healthcare Interpreting Explained.* London and New York: Routledge.

Crezee, I. H. M. (2013) *Introduction to Healthcare for Interpreters and Translators.* Amsterdam and Philadelphia: John Benjamins.

Crezee, I. H. M. and Asano, T. (2016) *Introduction to Healthcare for Japanese-speaking Interpreters and Translators.* Amsterdam and Philadelphia: John Benjamins.

Crezee, I. H. M., Gailani, N. and Gailani, A. N. (2016) *Introduction to Healthcare for Arabic-speaking Interpreters and Translators.* Amsterdam and Philadelphia: John Benjamins.

Crezee, I. H. M., Mikkelson, H. and Monzon-Storey, L. (2015) *Introduction to Healthcare for Spanish-speaking Interpreters and Translators.* Amsterdam and Philadelphia: John Benjamins. DOI:10.1075/z.193.

Crezee, I. H. M. and Ng, E. N. S. (2016) *Introduction to Healthcare for Chinese-speaking Interpreters and Translators.* Amsterdam and Philadelphia: John Benjamins. DOI: 10.1075/z.205.

de V. Souza, I. E. T. and Fragkou, E. (2020) *Handbook of Research on Medical Interpreting.* Hershey, PA: IGI Global.

Fischbach, H. (1998) *Translation and Medicine.* Amsterdam and Philadelphia: John Benjamins.

Heilweil, R. (2020) 'What It's Like to Interpret for Coronavirus Patients Remotely', *Vox.* Available at: www.vox.com/recode/2020/5/16/21250477/medical-interpreters-remote-certified-languages-telelanguage-COVID-19 (Accessed: 16 May 2020).

Hsieh, E. (2016) *Bilingual Health Communication: Working with Interpreters in Cross-Cultural Care.* London and New York: Routledge.

Ji, M., Taibi, M. and Crezee, I. H. M. (2019) *Multicultural Health Translation, Interpreting and Communication.* London and New York: Routledge.

Jones, T., Blackie, M., Garden, R., and Wear, D. (2017) 'The Almost Right Word: The Move From Medical to Health Humanities', *Academic Medicine*, 92(7), pp. 932–935. Available at: https://journals.lww.com/academicmedicine/fulltext/2017/07000/the_almost_right_word__the_move_from_medical_to.31.aspx (Accessed: 15 December 2020).

Kalanithi, P. (2016) *When Breath Becomes Air.* New York: Random House.

Montalt, V. and González Davies, M. (2007), *Medical Translation Step by Step: Learning by Drafting.* London and New York: Routledge. DOI:10.4324/9781315760377.

Nicodemus, B. and Metzger, M. (2014) *Investigations in Healthcare Interpreting*. Washington, DC: Gallaudet University Press.
Pöchhacker, F. and Shlesinger, M. (2007) *Healthcare Interpreting: Discourse and Interaction*. Amsterdam and Philadelphia: John Benjamins.
Sacks, O. (1985) *The Man Who Mistook His Wife for a Hat*. New York: Summit Books.
Valero-Garces, C. (2014) *Health, Communication and Multicultural Communities: Topics on Intercultural Communication for Healthcare Professionals*. Newcastle upon Tyne: Cambridge Scholars Publishing.
Varela Salinas, M.-J. and Meyer, B. (2015) *Translating and Interpreting Healthcare Discourses/ Traducir e interpretar en el ámbito sanitario*. Berlin: Frank & Timme.

Part I

Travels of medicine from ancient to modern times

1
Medical translations from Greek into Arabic and Hebrew

Elaine van Dalen

This chapter will consider a wave of Greco-Arabic translations that experienced their peak in the ninth century CE, and the Arabic-Hebrew translations that took place in the 12th and 14th centuries. The two movements had wide-ranging implications for medical research and practice both during their own era and subsequent ones. The chapter will briefly discuss the methods and techniques of pioneer translators such as al-Biṭrīq (active around 800), as well as those of the prolific translator Ḥunayn ibn Isḥāq (809–873) and his colleagues, including his son Isḥāq ibn Ḥunayn (*c.*830–*c.*910) and nephew Ḥubaysh ibn al-Ḥasan (died in late ninth century). In addition, the chapter will introduce leading views on the increased demand and production of medical translations between the 8th and 10th centuries, highlighting practices of patronage that involved both wealthy families and the caliphs. It will also explain patrons' and translators' preferences for particular Greek medical texts, and the influence of translations on medical education and scholarship. Lastly, the chapter will look at the practices of Hebrew translation in Italy and Southern France, including the work of the Tibbonide family, Shem Tov ben Isaac (born in 1196) and Nathan ha-Me'ati (1279–1283), and discuss the role of medical translations in Jewish communities in Southern Europe.

1 Greco-Arabic translations: beginnings

The majority of translations from Greek into Arabic in the Middle East were conducted in the 7th to 10th centuries CE, in an era characterised by wide-ranging political and linguistic reconfigurations. The Arabs, arriving from the Arabian Peninsula, established vast empires that stretched from Southern Europe and North Africa to the Middle East and South East Asia, regions previously ruled by the Byzantines and the Persian Sassanid dynasty. The scholarly languages in these regions had been predominantly Syriac, Greek and Persian, and this did not change immediately. Syriac, a dialect of Aramaic, was an important language among Christian intellectual communities in late antiquity. In the centuries prior to the Muslim conquests, Syriac scholars translated Greek works into Syriac and produced Syriac scholarship (Tannous 2010). Such activities continued, as will

DOI: 10.4324/9781003167983-3

be illustrated below, after the conquests. Gradually, the use of Arabic spread; it officially replaced Greek as an administrative language in the 7th century, and increasingly took the place of Syriac and other languages as the main scholarly language in the 9th and 10th centuries. With this Arabisation came the demand for Arabic translations of scholarly texts written in Greek, Syriac, Persian and other languages.

The first of these Arab empires, the Umayyad Empire, lasted from 661 until 750 and had its capital in Damascus in modern day Syria. Not many translations into Arabic were produced during this time, possibly because Greek and Syriac continued to be used by intellectuals even though Arabic had been made the official administrative language. The main translations from this era that are alluded to in Classical Islamic records are alchemical texts. According to the bookseller Ibn al-Nadīm (died *c.*995 CE), the first Umayyad caliph Muʿāwiya, who ruled between 661–680, asked a group of Egyptian scholars to translate alchemical works from Coptic and classical Greek (Ibn al-Nadīm 1970: 581; Saliba 2007: 45). Medical books seem to have been sporadic among these Umayyad translations. According to the Islamic scholars Ibn Juljul and Ibn al-Qiftī, an 8th-century Jewish scholar called Māsarjawayh translated a Syriac medical compendium, written by the Christian Ahrun ibn Aʿyun, into Arabic during the reign of the Umayyad caliph ʿUmar ibn ʿAbd al-ʿAzīz (ruled 717–720) (quoted in Van Koningsveld 1998: 351–352). Most Greco-Arabic translations however took place in later eras, after the ʿAbbasids took over from the Umayyads in the 750s.

2 Medical translations in the ʿAbbasid Empire

In the 750s, a revolution brought a new family into power in the Middle East, the ʿAbbasids. They founded a new capital, called Baghdad, in what is today's Iraq, which had a more central location than the previous capital Damascus. The early ʿAbbasid Empire flourished politically and economically, and brought together Persians, Syrians, Copts, Arabs and others. Although each of these groups had their own language, Arabic became increasingly important as a unifying political and scholarly language, much more so than during the Umayyad Empire. This era was characterised by a large-scale translation effort originating in Baghdad, and the most commonly translated languages were Persian, Syriac, and Greek. Translators from Greek first focused on medicine and applied sciences such as astrology and geometry, later followed by philosophy. By the end of the 10th century, translators had rendered nearly all available Greek works of science, medicine, and philosophy into Arabic.

The need for translations can be seen as a sign of flourishing scholarship at the time. The medical translations were often made by scholars who were themselves trained physicians and therefore familiar with many of the concepts in the texts. A prolific translator at this time was Ḥunayn ibn Isḥāq (died around 873), a Syriac speaking Nestorian Christian who learnt Greek. He was himself a physician who practised medicine and translated Greek medical texts into Syriac and Arabic with his son Isḥāq ibn Ḥunayn (died 910), nephew Ḥubaysh ibn al-Ḥasan (active around 860), and other colleagues.

According to a legend, the activities of these translators began after caliph al-Maʾmūn (ruled 813–833) had a dream about Aristotle. The historians Ibn al-Nadīm (died 990 CE) and Ibn Abī Uṣaybiʿa describe how, in his dream, al-Maʾmūn asked Aristotle what the ultimate good was, to which Aristotle replied, 'that which is considered good to reason'. He explained this as meaning 'that which is considered good by law', which in turn means 'that which people consider good'. Ibn al-Nadīm further recounts that this dream led al-Maʾmūn to contact the king of Byzantium and ask permission to send a group of scholars to procure books treasured in Byzantium. After these books were brought back, al-Maʾmūn ordered them to be translated (Dodge 1970; Saliba 1970: 48; Gutas 1998; Van Koningsveld 1998: 356). Another account claims that caliph ʿUmar ordered all the books in Alexandria to be destroyed when he conquered Egypt.[1]

These legends make it appear as if the translation efforts were an attempt to import books to an empire which was alien to these scholarly traditions. In fact, however, many of the medical books that were present in the region before the conquests could still be found there under Umayyad and early ʿAbbasid rule, and Alexandrian practices of medical scholarship continued in the early Islamic world. In 6th- and 7th-century Alexandria, scholars such as Palladius, John of Alexandria and Stephen of Athens produced medical commentaries that offered interpretations of earlier Galenic and Hippocratic material. They moreover worked in an academic environment where medicine was taught using a particular collection of Galenic and Hippocratic texts, which became known as the Alexandrian curriculum. These included four works of Hippocrates, four Aristotelian works on logic (the first four of the *Organon*) and the *Sixteen Books* of Galen, including *On Sects*, *On the Art of Medicine* and *On the Pulse for Beginners*. Early translators such as Yaḥyā ibn al-Biṭrīq (died in early 9th century) and his father al-Biṭrīq (died around 800) had started translating some of these books into Arabic already before Maʾmūn's mission to Byzantium. A few decades after this mission, the translator Ḥunayn ibn Isḥāq recounts in a letter[2] addressed to his patron ʿAlī ibn Yaḥyā how he searched widely for copies of Greek manuscripts in the former Byzantine cities which were now part of the Islamic Empire, such as Alexandria and Damascus. Ḥunayn mentions that it was easier to find manuscripts of Galenic texts that were part of the Alexandrian curriculum than of texts that were not; for example, the manuscript of *On the Therapeutic Method* was difficult to locate 'as it was not read in the school of the Alexandrians', according to his comments (Lamoreaux 2016: 48). This illustrates that, rather than having been destroyed with the conquests as the myth of caliph ʿUmar suggests, many of the Greek medical and philosophical books central to late-antique Alexandrian medical scholarship continued to be present and possibly used in the early Islamic world, and they did not all have to be brought from Byzantium. Not only were these works still available in Greek, many of them also circulated in the region in Syriac translations.

Ḥunayn and his colleagues followed in the steps of Syriac scholars who had translated Greek texts into Syriac in previous centuries. An example of these earlier translation activities is the work of Sergius of Resh ʿAyna (died 536), who translated Galen's *Ars Medica* (also known as the *Tegni* or *Microtegni*), the second of Galen's *Sixteen Books*, into Syriac. Such activities continued after the Muslim conquests with the work of Christian scholars such as Jacob of Edessa (died 708) and Ḥunayn himself, who often first translated texts into Syriac and used them as an intermediary to then translate into Arabic. For instance, Ḥunayn retranslated the *Ars Medica* into Syriac three centuries after Sergius' translation and then also rendered the work into Arabic (Tannous 2010). When studying the Greco-Arabic translations, it is important therefore to keep the central role of Syriac in mind.

3 Patronage

Translations produced in this time period were the result of well-organised efforts supported by statesmen and elite families, and executed by highly skilled translators. According to Dimitri Gutas, the ʿAbbasid caliphs supported the translations partly out of ideological concerns, seeking political legitimisation by adopting the intellectual traditions of the Sassanid Empire that they replaced (Gutas 1998). He further demonstrates that members of the elite paid for translations as they could benefit from them practically. A quote from the Andalusian physician Ibn Juljul (*c.*944–*c.*994), where he argues that scholars appear only in states whose kings seek knowledge (Vernet 2008), seems to support this view. On the other hand, George Saliba suggests that it was middle-class administrators competing for governmental positions who were responsible for the increase in translations (Saliba 2007).

We can get an insight into the role of the elite in supporting the translation movement from Ḥunayn's *Epistle*. In this text, Ḥunayn also gives information about his patrons, who were either related to the ʿAbbasid court or were themselves physicians who wished to enhance their medical knowledge, such as the Bukhtīshūʿ dynasty. This prominent family of physicians spanning six generations over 250 years commissioned medical texts such as Galen's *Book on the Method of Healing*. So did the Banū Mūsa, another family with close ties to the caliph. The caliphs themselves also commissioned translations and patrons generally supported multiple translators. Jibrīl Bukhtīshūʿ (died 828), for instance, payed both Ḥunayn and Job of Edessa (died around 835), another translator of Greek into Syriac. Ḥunayn further reports that at least five other patrons supported him, both Christian and Muslim, physician and courtier. Some works he would first translate into Syriac for one patron and then into Arabic for another, as he did for example with Galen's works *Pulse to Teuthras* and *Therapeutics to Glaucon*. This patronage contributed to the large number of translations created in this era.

4 Translation techniques

Different translators adhered to different approaches in their medical translations. The historian al-Ṣafadī describes two main strategies, one he characterises as word-for-word translation (*ad verbum*) and the other as focusing on the meaning of the entire sentence (*ad sensum*) (Rosenthal 2003: 17). Al-Ṣafadī mentions the translator Yaḥyā ibn al-Biṭrīq as an example of the first approach. The reputation of this translator was generally not positive (Ullmann 2002–2007: 28–48). His versions were word-for-word translations that did not always pay enough attention to the meaning of the sentence. Manfred Ullmann identified his father, Abū Yaḥyā al-Biṭrīq, as the translator of an early version of the *Aphorisms*, of which the later translator Ḥunayn disapproved (Ullmann 2002–2007: 52–53). These early translators were nevertheless pioneers who did important work in developing Arabic medical terminology. According to al-Ṣafadī, Ḥunayn ibn Isḥāq translated by first grasping the meaning of a sentence and subsequently rendering it into Arabic (or Syriac). Ḥunayn's translation approach was precise and had a reputation among historical scholars for being 'without error' (Rosenthal 1946: 254), even though he himself thought it necessary to retranslate several of his earlier translations. He would follow particular strategies to render linguistic features such as conjunctions, conditionals, and subjectivity (Vagelpohl 2011; Overwien 2012, 2015; Van Dalen 2017). For instance, when he considered a sentence to be the reflection of Galen's own views, he would clearly mark this subjectivity by using first-person active voice where Galen had used a passive. He was also aware of the fact that the text was written in a Greek cultural context; when Galen used 'we' as a reference to a general subjectivity, Ḥunayn rendered this as 'the Greeks' (Van Dalen 2017). His nephew Ḥubaysh's language has been characterised as 'translation Arabic', a language that demonstrates clear influence of the source language (Rosenthal 1946: 253).

Another issue Arabic translators dealt with was the polytheistic nature of the texts they translated in a predominantly monotheistic culture. This had consequences for instance in translated references to the Greek gods and can be seen in the way the Hippocratic Oath was translated into Arabic. The beginning of the Greek version of this oath reads in English translation as: 'I swear by Apollo the physician, and Asclepius, and Hygieia and Panacea and all the gods and goddesses as my witnesses, that, according to my ability and judgement, I will keep this Oath and this contract' (for the Greek see Littré 1844: 628–633). In the Arabic this has become: 'Hippocrates said: I swear by God, the Lord of Life and Death, Giver of Health and Creator of Cures and Treatments; and by Asclepius, and by all men and women who are close to God and whom I take as witnesses' (Savage-Smith, Swain and Van Gelder 2020: 4.1.3.1). In this translation, the gods and goddesses have become 'men and women close to God', and Apollo, Hygieia and Panacea have disappeared. Instead, the translator has included the monotheistic God, and only Asclepius remained (see also Pormann and Savage-Smith 2007: 33; for more examples see Picken 2018: 104).

In terms of vocabulary, Ḥunayn and his colleagues drew on contemporary medical terms but also had to create new words to translate Greek terms. They sometimes Arabised words by transliterating them in Arabic script, and occasionally added explanations of their meaning to the translation. In other cases, they used Syriac words that we assume were known to contemporary readers. Sometimes Ḥunayn described the meaning of a Greek term with multiple Arabic words (for examples see Picken 2018: 103–104; Overwien 2012: 156–157; Cooper 2016: 12–23). As medical scholarship progressed, some terms were adopted and others were re-interpreted.

5 Translations and scholarship

Medical translations had great impact on medical scholarship in the classical Islamic world. Through the translation efforts that started in Baghdad, all of the Alexandrian curriculum was made available in Arabic and became required reading for medical students (Iskandar 1976). Not only did Islamic physicians follow Alexandrian educational practices, they also adopted late-antique genres such as the medical commentary, and adhered theoretically to what has been described as Galenism[3] more broadly (Temkin 1973). Greek works had competed in the beginning with translated Persian and Sanskrit texts, some of which had themselves adopted the central premises of Greek medical thought. The physician ʿAlī Rabbān al-Ṭabarī (838–870), for instance, draws from Persian texts and translations of Sanskrit texts in his medical encyclopaedia *Paradise of Wisdom*. We also find quotes from Persian and Sanskrit texts in al-Rāzī's *Comprehensive Book of Medicine*, the *Kitāb al-Ḥāwī* (Kahl 2015). Generally, however, interest in medical texts was very much directed at the Greek physicians Hippocrates and Galen. For example, the largest part of Ḥunayn's translations consisted of Galen's texts, and he lists over 100 of Galen's works that he translated in his *Epistle*.

One way to study the impact of the translations on medical scholarship in the classical Islamic world is to analyse Arabic commentaries on Greek works. A good example of such commentaries are those on the *Aphorisms*, one of Hippocrates' most influential medical works. It is a collection originally written in Greek consisting of seven books of short medical verses, the first of which opens with the well-known phrase 'life is short, art is long'.[4] The *Aphorisms* was first translated into Syriac and Arabic, and later into Latin and Hebrew. Its popularity in teaching and research is evidenced by the large amount of surviving manuscripts, which number over 70 in Arabic (Magdelaine 1994: 87), in addition to their transmission in the numerous commentaries on the *Aphorisms* in which they are quoted. These commentaries illustrate the importance of the text for teaching and research. Over 20 Arabic commentaries on the *Aphorisms* written over six centuries are known, at least 15 of which have survived to this day.[5] The commentators, all of them physicians, did not only rely on Ḥunayn's translation of the text, but also on his translation of Galen's commentary of it. Even if direct quotations from that text decrease over centuries (Karimullah 2017), Galen's exegetical format was constitutive of the tradition and his theoretical framework remained influential throughout each commentary. Adopting and occasionally rejecting Galenic theory allowed Islamic physicians to make numerous innovations in the exegesis of the Hippocratic source text (Van Dalen 2020). At the same time, one should keep in mind that the Greco-Arabic scholarship only represents the theoretical medicine at the time. Medical practices were probably not always aligned with what has come down to us in the written traditions (Álvarez-Millán 2010, 2000; Pormann and Savage-Smith 2007: 144–162).

For contemporary scholars, the Arabic translations are valuable witnesses of the Greek texts. For example, Galen's commentary on the Hippocratic *Epidemics*, the largest commentary on a Hippocratic work, is only extant in its Arabic translation (Vagelpohl 2011). In other cases, the Arabic translations offer comparative material to Greek texts which are extant in later or sometimes deficient Greek versions.

6 Translations from Arabic into Hebrew

After the ʿAbbasids took over from the Umayyads, the Umayyads founded an emirate in Andalusia in 756. After this, Arabic scholarship began to diffuse into Islamic Spain, where medical scholarship continued in conversation with research done in the Islamic East over the following centuries. From here, Arabic texts also made their way to Southern France and Italy in the 12th century, where they were translated into Latin and Hebrew. The Arabic-Hebrew translation period lasted approximately 300 years between 1100–1400, with its peak in the 13th century. Although these efforts took place on a much smaller scale than the Greco-Arabic translations in Baghdad, they had a large impact on Hebrew scholarship. Translators first focused on Jewish Arabic works in the fields of grammar and theology, and then moved on to philosophy and medicine, where they translated original Arabic works such as Ibn Sīnā's (*c.*980–1037, known in Latin Europe as Avicenna) *Canon of Medicine* (hereafter *Canon*), and Arabic translations of Greek works, such as Hippocrates' *Aphorisms* and Galen's *Microtegni*. Moritz Steinschneider listed most of these works in his monumental *Die Hebräischen Übersetzungen des Mittelalters und die Juden als Dolmetscher* (The Hebrew Translations of the Middle Ages and the Jews as Interpreters, Steinschneider 1893). Most of these translation activities took place in Southern Europe, especially in Toledo and Barcelona (Christian Spain), cities in Southern France such as Marseille, Lunel and Montpellier, and in Naples (present-day Italy).

In the 12th century, Andalusian Jews fled to Southern France from persecution by the Almohad Caliphate, bringing with them knowledge of Arabic language and scholarship. One of these emigrants was Judah ibn Tibbon (1120–1190), a physician born in Andalusia (Granada), who settled in the French city of Lunel. His descendants, known as the Tibbonides, became a famous family of physician-translators who lived and worked in Southern France and began the Arabic-Hebrew translation movement. They based their translations directly on Arabic sources, including many Arabic translations of Greek medical texts. Judah Ibn Tibbon's son Samuel ibn Tibbon (1150–1232) translated Galen's *Microtegni* in 1199. Gad Freudenthal has confirmed that he also translated the popular commentary on this text by ʿAlī ibn Riḍwān (Freudenthal 2016: 38–41). His son Moses ibn Tibbon, who was active between the years 1240 and 1283, translated medical works by Ḥunayn ibn Isḥāq, al-Rāzī and Ibn Sīnā (Lindberg 1980: 69).

There were multiple reasons for these prolific Arabic-Hebrew and Latin-Hebrew translation activities in Southern Europe, and especially in Southern France. According to scholars such as Friedenwald and Steinschneider, the movement indicates the scientific interest of Jewish physicians who wanted to increase their medical knowledge (Friedenwald 1934: 88). At the end of the 12th century, there were almost no Hebrew medical books in Southern France, as the medical scholarship available at the time was either in Arabic or in Latin translations of Arabic texts. The Jewish communities in Southern France were not proficient in Arabic or Latin, the language of the elite, and aspiring Jewish physicians were generally not allowed into Latin medical schools. The translator Salomon b. Abraham ben Daud (*c.*1110–1180), quoted by Steinschneider, noted that this shortage led him to translate two 'splendid ones', one text by Averroes and one by Ibn Sīnā (Steinschneider 1893: 672; also in Friedenwald 1934: 88; and compare with Ferre 1998). The fact that Jewish scholars did not have access to libraries and books while their Christian colleagues did, gave Christian physicians considerable advantage. The anonymous translator who used the pen name Doeg the Edomite (12th century), as well as Shem Tov of Tartosa (born 1196) explain that they translate in order to give Jewish physicians the opportunity to compete with Christian physicians (see Barkai 1998: 18–22). Both translators observe a tendency among Jewish people to consult Christian doctors, who were ahead of their Jewish counterparts, and therefore ended up taking non-kosher prescriptions (Barkai 1998: 18–22 and Bos 1998: 102–103). Aside from the risk of non-kosher treatment, another motivation was the desire to demonstrate that Hebrew scholarship was not inferior to Latin or Arabic, as the Jewish community was frequently scorned for its lack of literature (Steinschneider 1893: xvi; Friedenwald 1934: 88; Bos 1998: 102; Barkai 1998: 18–22). The translator Nathan ha-Me'ati for instance explains that '[in response to] the contempt in which learnt Christians hold the Jews because the medical works of Solomon and their later writers have been lost, he wished to follow the example of the Tibbonides who had drawn up the books from the marsh and the well of the Arabic language' (Friedenwald 1934: 88).

The translation activities also spread to Italy. Nathan Ben Eliezer ha-Me'ati was a translator who worked in Rome in the last decades of the 13th century, best known for his translation of Ibn Sīnā's *Canon*. He translated medical works from Arabic to Hebrew, but unlike the Tibbonides who were native Arabic speakers, Nathan ha-Me'ati learnt Arabic during his travels in Arab-speaking lands, as he says in his translation of the *Canon* (cf. Bos 2013: 307). He also translated the Hippocratic *Aphorisms* as part of his translation of Maimonides' commentary on this text, and Hippocrates' *On Acute Diseases* and *Airs, Waters, Places*, including Galen's commentary on the latter. This commentary had been translated into Arabic by Ḥubaysh ibn al-Ḥasan.

7 The role of Latin

In addition to the Arabic-Hebrew translations, some of these translators used Latin versions of Arabic originals as their source texts, for example al-Jazzār (*c.*895–979) and Zād al-Musāfir, and of Arabic translations of Greek texts, such as the early translations by Doeg. Between the years 1197–99, Doeg translated 24 medical texts from Latin into Hebrew, which included 17 works on medical practice and seven on theory. These included a Latin translation of Ḥunayn's introduction to Galen's *Ars Medica*, which he called *Sefer*

Ḥaguan (*Book of Ḥunayn*), Galen's *Ars Medica* itself, Hippocrates' *Aphorisms* and the *Prognostics* (Freudenthal 2013).[6] While these works were normally inaccessible to Jews, Doeg was allowed to obtain Latin texts as a convert to Christianity, albeit one who later repented of his conversion. Many of these texts were also translated from their Arabic versions. The Latin texts with which Doeg worked were sometimes abbreviated, which was the main reason why Moses ibn Tibbon decided to retranslate texts from Arabic that Doeg had already translated from Latin (Freudenthal and Fontaine 2016: 17). Doeg also used technical terms in the language of the gentiles, i.e. the Romance vernacular which was not widely understood among the immigrant communities of Jewish refugees from Andalusia in Southern France. When Moses translated the text again, his version exceeded the popularity of Doeg's translation.

8 Major medical works translated into Hebrew

Many texts of Galen's corpus were translated into Hebrew (Lieber 1981). The Galenic work *Ars Medica*, which, as we saw above, was translated into Syriac and Arabic to feature centrally in Islamic medical education and scholarship, was translated into Hebrew three times. Two of these were translated from Latin, first by Doeg and again in the 13th century by Hillel ben Samuel, who used a Latin version by Gerard of Cremona, which in turn was based on an Arabic translation that included Ibn Riḍwān's commentary on the text. The third Hebrew translation from the 12th century was the work by Samuel ibn Tibbon and was based on an Arabic text which had been translated from Greek by Ḥunayn. Galen's *Microtegni* was called *Melaḵah qeṭanah* (*Small Art*) in Hebrew, a translation of the Arabic title *aṣ-Ṣināʿa aṣ-Ṣaġīra* (*The Small Art*), and known in Latin as the *Ars Parva*. Samuel ibn Tibbon's translation of this text survives in nine manuscripts, of which three are incomplete (Freudenthal and Fontaine 2016: 18). Samuel's translation also included Ibn Riḍwān's commentary. In the *Microtegni*, Galen sets out the main principles of the art of medicine, and the text functioned as an introduction for medical students in the Islamic world as well as in later Latin and Jewish communities. The Egyptian physician Ibn Riḍwān (988–1061/8) glossed it passage by passage and his commentary often accompanied the *Ars Medica* in Hebrew translation as was the case in both Samuel ibn Tibbon's and Hillel ben Samuel's later versions, becoming an important element in Jewish medical education.

Ḥunayn, who translated the *Ars Medica* into Syriac and Arabic, added his own introduction to the text known in Arabic under two titles, the *Introduction to Medicine* (*al-mudkhal fī ṭ-ṭibb*) and the *Questions into Medicine* (*al-Masāʾil fī ṭ-ṭibb*), which has led to confusion about whether these were two different texts (Brockelmann 1897: 224) or one and the same work (Iskandar 1978; Ferre 1995: 44; Sezgin 1970: 249–250). Iskandar has shown that shortly after the work was produced, scholars started to use two titles to refer to the same work, the first derived from the work's content and the second from its form (Iskandar 1978). The text was translated into Hebrew multiple times, usually entitled *Sefer mavo le-malakhat ha-refuʾa* (*Book on the Introduction to the Art of Medicine*, Ferre 1995: 42). A shortened version of the work was also translated into Latin and became immensely popular under the name *Isagoge ad tegni Galeni* (*Introduction to Galen's Tegni*). Lola Ferre suggests that the diverse translations and large quantity of manuscripts of Ḥunayn's *Introduction* indicate that the text was popular among Jewish physicians (Ferre 1995: 52).

Ibn Sīnā 's *Canon*, one of the major medical encyclopaedias produced in the classical Islamic world, became widely disseminated among European Jewish and Latin communities. More than 100 manuscripts of the Hebrew translations survive worldwide, which indicates its popularity among Jewish physicians.[7] Nathan ha-Me'ati made the first translation of the complete work into Hebrew in 1279 in Rome, a hundred years after its translation by Gerard of Cremona into Latin.[8] Zerahiah ben Isaac ben Shealtiel Gracian of Barcelona made another translation around 1280, correcting errors in the first two books of Nathan ha-Me'ati's translation. Finally, Joshua Lorki made further corrections of Nathan's translation of these first two books in 1402 (Bos 2013: 310). According to Bos, a Hebrew translation of the *Canon* printed in Naples in 1491 included all three of these translations of the first two books, together with further editions by 15th-century translators (Bos 2013: 310; Singer and Rabin 1946: lxxvi).

As was the case in the Islamic world the *Aphorisms* were of great importance in European medical scholarship. Steinschneider lists multiple translations of the *Aphorisms* into Hebrew under the name *Perakim*, most of which are part of translations of commentaries on the *Aphorisms*, for instance that of Maimonides or that of Galen (in Arabic). Nathan ha-Me'ati translated them as part of Galen's commentary on the *Aphorisms*, using Ḥunayn's Arabic translation of the original Greek text (Steinschneider 1893: 659). Moses ibn Tibbon translated the *Aphorisms* as quoted in Maimonides' commentary on the text. Both Hebrew translations of the Arabic Pseudo-Palladius commentary (see next paragraph) include two separate translations of this Hippocratic collection.

Just as some Arabic translations are important witnesses to Greek texts, the Hebrew translations become witnesses for Greek or Arabic texts. This is the case for instance with the 9th-century Arabic version of Palladius' commentary on the *Aphorisms*, of which only the first two books are extant in an Arabic manuscript. Fortunately, the full seven books survive in a 13th-century Hebrew translation by Shem Tov ben Isaac of Tartosa (on this commentary see Pormann *et al.* 2017). Another example is the translation of Hippocrates' *De superfoetatione* (*On superfetation*), which an anonymous translator rendered into Arabic in a poor-quality translation. A later anonymous Hebrew translation of the Arabic text is a valuable witness that helps us to further understand the extant versions of the Greek source text (Zonta 2003). Some Arabic texts only survive in Hebrew translation. An example of this is ar-Rāzī's Arabic treatise on why many people become medical charlatans, which Nathan ha-Me'ati translated into Hebrew in Rome in the 13th century (Steinschneider 1866; Bos 2013: 308; Pormann 2005).

9 Hebrew translation techniques

Just as Arabic translators before them, Hebrew translators had to develop new Hebrew vocabulary to render medical terminology. They resorted to Biblical and Rabbinical Hebrew terms and used loan translations, employing existing Hebrew terms with a different meaning. They also created neologisms, used transliterations of Arabic and Romance words, or explained terms (see for instance Zonta 2003, Bos 2008 and 2013, and Ferre and Martínez Delgado 2015). Ferre has drawn attention to the fact that not all translators had the necessary language skills, and some were physicians who felt ill prepared for translation (Ferre 1998). This is illustrated by a quote from Samuel Ben Judah, saying 'I have left many places blank and free of one or more words and lines because of my limited knowledge and insufficient grasp of the Arabic language in addition to its uncommon subject matter' (Berman 1967: 305). In turn, both he and his son Samuel 'criticised their rival translators for subordinating meaning to language and style, failing to accurately reproduce difficult philosophical notions in their paraphrastic translations' (Robinson 2005: 822). Shem Tov in the introduction of his translation of the Arabic Pseudo-Palladius commentary (written in 1268) apologises that he translated this text when he was old, which may have led to errors (Pormann *et al.* 2007: 303). This is not to say that the translation is of poor quality; in fact, it follows the Arabic closely. An anonymous translator made a different Hebrew translation of the same Pseudo-Palladius commentary which is preserved in Vatican Library manuscript ebr.567, perhaps because they disliked the first translation, but no evidence for this exists. The medical vocabulary of these two translations differs in some instances.

10 Future directions

Each of the different aspects of medical translation into Arabic and Hebrew introduced in this chapter represent avenues for further research. For instance, we can learn more about how medical translations influenced medical research, and how evolving medical understanding affected the use of medical terms that had entered medical discourse during the translation period. In terms of translation technique, the work that has been done on some Greco-Arabic translators can be expanded further to include more translators and translations, and also to make comparisons with contemporary translations from other languages such as Persian. The same goes for the translation techniques in translations into Hebrew, and the effects of those translations on scholarship. These medical translations offer rich sources for the study of the development of medieval scholarly Hebrew. Some of the work ahead is of a philological nature, as many translations are preserved in manuscripts that have not yet been edited and have unidentified authorship. Here scholars first need to engage in textual criticism before they can continue to address questions of translation techniques and impact, while knowledge of such techniques also aids in the establishing of the text and authorship attribution.

11 Conclusion

The translations discussed in this chapter show the relationship between medical scholarship and translation in the Middle East and Europe throughout history. On the one hand, the presence of committed medical scholars and intellectual activities in both Baghdad and Southern France required translation activity in places where the use of language had changed. On the other hand, these translations also encouraged such activities and stimulated medical scholarship to an unparalleled extent. In Southern Europe, Jewish physicians were able to access Arabic texts in Hebrew translations which their Christian colleagues had already been able to use in Latin translation. This in turn allowed them to provide medical services to Jewish patients who previously may have relied on Christian physicians. Where in the case of Southern France, scholarly works were imported from Andalusia and tended to be new material for the Jewish communities, the situation was different in the classical Islamic world. Here, unlike myths such as those about caliph al-Maʾmūn that made it seem that the medical scholarship was foreign to the new Islamic Empire, the medical texts were already present inside the ʿAbbasid Empire in the ancient centres of learning, such as Alexandria and Damascus, and physicians in the region had already been using them in Greek and Syriac. The Arabic translations thus enabled a continuation of medical practices rather than the import of a new tradition. Greek medical texts, especially those that were part of the so-called Alexandrian curriculum, became of central importance in classical Islamic medical education. Medical students in Baghdad studied the works of Hippocrates and Galen in Arabic with their teachers, and physicians used them as reference works and also contributed to them with new medical findings presented for instance in commentaries, such as those on Hippocrates' *Epidemics* and *Aphorisms*. Greek medical ideas, such as Hippocrates' humoural pathology and Galenic physiology, continued to be influential in the region through the translation of Greek texts and the inclusion of this translated material in new Arabic scholarship. Islamic scholars incorporated this material, sometimes improving on the Galenic theories and at other times rejecting them completely when new empirical evidence turned out to contradict them. The medieval translations of Arabic medical texts and Arabic translations of Greek medical texts into Latin and Hebrew made this scholarship accessible to European students and practitioners of medicine.

Notes

1 According to this myth, which is most completely narrated by the historian al-Qifṭī (died 1248), ʿUmar ordered his commander ʿAmr ibn al-ʿĀṣ to destroy all ancient books found in the libraries of Alexandria. Cf. Van Koningsveld (1998) p. 364.
2 The *Risāla* in Arabic, edited and translated into English in Lamoreaux (2016).
3 Galenism refers to a set of Galenic medical theories, concepts and methods that characterised medicine in late antiquity, the Islamic world, and Europe.
4 For an overview of the Arabic commentaries on this first aphorism, see Rosenthal (1966: 226–245).
5 All of these have been edited by Pormann *et al.*, University of Manchester.
6 See Gad Freudenthal (2013: 118–120).
7 For a list of extant manuscripts of the *Canon* in Hebrew translation see Richler (1981: 145) and Bos (2013: 39).
8 On the history of Hebrew Canon translation see Rabin (1950). On reception of Ibn Sīnā in medieval Jewish communities see Freudenthal and Zonta (2012).

Further reading

Gutas, D. (1998) *Greek Thought, Arabic Culture*. London and New York: Routledge.

Gutas discusses translation activities in classical Baghdad from a social perspective, focusing on translators and patrons, and offers explanations for the surge in translations in this era.

Pormann, P. E. and Savage-Smith, E. (2007) *Medieval Islamic Medicine*. Edinburgh: Edinburgh University Press.

This work provides students with an introduction to Islamic medicine, covering topics such as medical theory, everyday medical practice and prophetic medicine.

Saliba, G. (2007) *Islamic Science and the Making of the European Renaissance*. Cambridge, MA: MIT Press

This book offers different explanations for the beginnings of the translation activities in the classical Islamic world, as well as a discussion of the influence of Islamic astronomy on European scholarship.

Shatzmiller, J. (1994) *Jews, Medicine, and Medieval Society*. Berkeley: University of California Press.

Shatzmiller provides students with an introduction of medical practices among Jewish people in medieval Europe.

Related topics

Dissemination of Academic Medical Research Through Translation, Translations of Western Medical Texts in East Asia, Medical Terminology and Discourse

References

Álvarez-Millán, C. (2000) 'Practice Versus Theory: Tenth-Century Case Histories from the Islamic Middle East', *Social History of Medicine*, 13(2), pp. 293–306.

Álvarez-Millán, C. (2010) 'The Case History in Medieval Islamic Medical Literature: *Tajārib* and *Mujarrabāt* as Source', *Medical History*, 54(2), pp. 195–214.

Barkai, R. (1998) *A History of Jewish Gynaecological Texts in the Middle Ages*. Leiden: Brill.

Berman, L. (1967) 'Greek into Hebrew: Samuel ben Judah of Marseilles, Fourteenth-Century Philosopher and Translator', in Altman, A. (ed.) *Jewish Medieval and Renaissance Studies*. Cambridge, MA: Harvard University Press, pp. 289–320.

Bos, G. (1998) 'On Editing and Translating Medieval Hebrew Medical Texts', *The Jewish Quarterly Review*, 89(1/2), pp. 101–122.

Bos, G. (2008) 'The Creation And Innovation Of Medieval Hebrew Medical Terminology: Shem Tov Ben Isaac, Sefer Ha-Shimmush' in Akasoy, A. and Raven, W. (eds) *Islamic Thought in the Middle Ages*. Leiden: Brill, pp. 195–218.

Bos, G. (2013) 'Medical Terminology in the Hebrew Tradition: Nathan Ben Eliezer ha-Me'ati, Glossary to the Hebrew translation of Ibn Sīnā's K. al-Qānūn fī al-ṭibb', *Revue des études juives*, 173(3–4), pp. 305–321.

Brockelmann, C. (1897) *Geschichte der arabischen Literatur*, vol. 1. Weimar: G. Felber.

Cooper, G. (2016) 'Ḥunayn ibn Isḥāq's Galen Translations and Greco-Arabic Philology: Some Observations from the Crises (De crisibus) and the Critical Days (De diebus decretoriis)', *Oriens*, 44, pp. 1–43.

Gutas, D. (1998) *Greek Thought, Arabic Culture*. London and New York: Routledge.

Ferre, L. (1995) 'The Medical Work of Ḥunayn Ben Isḥaq (Johannitius) in Hebrew Translation', *Korot*, 11, pp. 42–53.

Ferre, L. (1998) 'Hebrew Translations from Medical Treatises of Montpellier', *Korot*, 13, pp. 21–36.

Ferre, L. and Martínez Delgado, J. (2015) 'Arabic into Hebrew, a Case Study: Isaac Israeli's Book on Fevers', *Medieval Encounters*, 21, pp. 50–80.

Freudenthal, G. (2013) 'The Father of the Latin-into-Hebrew Translations: "Doeg the Edomite," the Twelfth-Century Repentant Convert', in Fontaine, R. and Freudenthal, G. (eds) *Latin-into-Hebrew: Texts and Studies*, vol. 1. Leiden: Brill, pp. 105–120.

Freudenthal, G. (2016) 'Samuel ibn Tibbon as the Author of Melaḵah qeṭanah, the Hebrew Translation from Arabic of Galen's Tegni', *Arab Sciences and Philosophy*, 26, pp. 27–43.

Freudenthal, G. and Fontaine, R. (2016) 'Philosophy and Medicine in Jewish Provence, Anno 1199: Samuel ibn Tibbon and Doeg the Edomite translating Galen's Tegni', *Arabic Sciences and Philosophy*, 26(1), pp. 1–26.

Freudenthal, G. and Zonta, M. (2012) 'Ibn Sīnā Among Medieval Jews, The Reception of Ibn Sīnā's Philosophical, Scientific and Medical Writings in Jewish Cultures, East and West', *Arabic Sciences and Philosophy* 22(2), pp. 217–287.

Friedenwald, H. (1934) 'The Use Of The Hebrew Language in Medical Literature', *Bulletin of the Institute of the History of Medicine*, 2(2), pp. 77–111.

Ibn al-Nadīm (1970) *Kitāb. al-Fihrist*. Translated by B. Dodge. New York: Columbia University Press.

Iskandar, A. Z. (1976) 'An Attempted Reconstruction of the Late Alexandrian Medical Curriculum', *Medical History*, 20(3), pp. 235–258.

Iskandar, A. Z. (1978) 'Ḥunayn ibn Isḥāq', in Gillispie, C. C. (ed.) *Dictionary of Scientific Biography*, vol. 15. New York: Charles Scribner's Sons, pp. 230–249.

Kahl, O. (2015) *The Sanskrit, Syriac and Persian sources in the Comprehensive Book of Rhazes*. Leiden: Brill.

Karimullah, K. (2017) 'Transformation of Galen's Textual Legacy from Classical to Post-Classical Islamic Medicine: Commentaries on the Hippocratic Aphorisms', *Intellectual History of the Islamicate World*, 5(3), pp. 311–358.

Lamoreaux, J. C. (ed.) (2016) *Ḥunayn ibn Isḥāq on His Galen Translations: A Parallel English-Arabic Text*. Provo, UT: Brigham Young University Press.

Lieber, E. (1981) 'Galen in Hebrew', in Nutton, V. (ed.) *Galen: Problems and Prospects*. London: Wellcome Institute for the History of Medicine.
Lindberg, D. C. (ed.) (1980) *Science in the Middle Ages*. Chicago: University of Chicago Press.
Littré, É. (1844) *Oeuvres complètes d' Hippocrate*, vol. 4. Paris: J. B. Bailliere.
Magdelaine, C. (1994) *Histoire du Texte et Edition Critique, Traduite et Commentee des Aphorismes d'Hippocrate*. PhD Thesis. Université de Paris-Sorbonne.
Overwien, O. (2012) 'The Art of the Translator, or: How did Ḥunayn ibn ʾIsḥāq and his School Translate?', in Pormann, P. E. (ed.) *Epidemics in Context: Greek Commentaries on Hippocrates in the Arabic Tradition*. Berlin: Walter de Gruyter, pp. 151–169.
Overwien, O. (2015) 'The Paradigmatic Translator and His Method: Ḥunayn ibn Isḥāq's Translation of the Hippocratic Aphorisms from Greek via Syriac into Arabic', *Intellectual History of the Islamic World*, 3(1–2), pp. 158–187.
Picken, G. N. (2018) 'Translation as the Instigator of a new Arabic Discourse in Islamic Intellectual History', in Faiq, S. (ed.) *Discourse in Translation*. London and New York: Routledge, pp. 91–108.
Pormann, P. E. (2005) 'The Physician and the Other: Images of the Charlatan in Medieval Islam', *Bulletin of the History of Medicine*, 79(2), pp. 189–227.
Pormann, P. E. *et al.* (2017) 'The Enigma of the Arabic and Hebrew Palladius', *The Intellectual History of the Islamicate World*, 5(3), pp. 252–310.
Pormann, P. E. and Savage-Smith, E. (2007) *Medieval Islamic Medicine*. Edinburgh: Edinburgh University Press.
Rabim, C. (1950) 'The History of the Translation of the Canon into Hebrew', *Melilah*, 3–4, pp. 132–142.
Richler, B. (1981) 'Manuscripts of Ibn Sīnā's Kanon in Hebrew Translation, a Revised and Up-to-date List', *Korot*, 8(1–2), pp. 145–168.
Robinson, J. (2005) 'Translation, Arabic into Hebrew', in Meri, J. W. (ed.) *Medieval Islamic Civilization: An Encyclopedia*. London and New York: Routledge, pp.821–822.
Rosenthal, F. (1946) 'Galen: On Medical Experience by R Waltzer', *Isis*, 36, pp. 251–255.
Rosenthal, F. (1966) '"Life is Short, the Art is Long": Arabic Commentaries on the First Hippocratic Aphorism', *Bulletin of the History of Medicine*, 40, pp. 226–245.
Rosenthal, F. (2003) *The Classical Heritage in Islam*. London and New York: Routledge.
Saliba, G. (2007) *Islamic Science and the Making of the European Renaissance*. Cambridge, MA: MIT Press.
Savage-Smith, E., Swain, S. and van Gelder, G. J. (eds) (2020) *A Literary History of Medicine*. Leiden: Brill.
Shatzmiller, J. (1994) *Jews, Medicine, and Medieval Society*. Berkeley: University of California Press.
Sezgin, F. (1970) *Geschichte des arabischen Schriftums*, vol. 3. Leiden: Brill.
Singer, C. and Rabin, C. (1946) *Prelude to Modern Science: Being a Discussion of the History Sources and Circumstances of the 'Tabulae Anatomicae Sex' of Vesalius*, Cambridge: Cambridge University Press.
Steinschneider, M. (1866) 'Wissenschaft und Charlatanerie bei den Arabern', *Virchow's Archiv*, 36, pp. 570–586.
Steinschneider, M. (1893) *Die hebräischen Übersetzungen des Mittelalters und die Juden als Dolmetscher: Ein Beitrag zur Literaturgeschichte des Mittelalters, meist nach handschriftlichen Quellen*. Berlin: Kommissionsverlag des Bibliographischen Bureaus.
Tannous, J. (2010) *Syria between Byzantium and Islam: Making Incommensurables Speak*. Princeton: Princeton University.
Temkin, O. (1973) *Galenism: The Rise and Decline of a Medical Philosophy*. Ithaca: Cornell University Press.
Ullmann, M. (2002–2007) *Wörterbuch zu den griechisch-arabischen Übersetzungen des 9. Jahrhunderts*. Wiesbaden: Harrassowitz.
Vagelpohl, U. (2011) 'In the Translator's Workshop', *Arab Sciences and Philosophy*, 21(2), pp. 249–288.
Van Dalen, E. (2017) 'Subjectivity in Translation: Ḥunayn ibn Isḥāq's Ninth-Century Interpretation of Galen's "Ego" in His Commentary on the Hippocratic Aphorisms', *Oriens*, 45(1–2), pp. 53–79.

Van Dalen, E. (2020) 'Pediatrics in Medieval Islamic Theoria', *Journal of the American Oriental Society*, 140(1), pp. 1–16.
Van Koningsveld, P. S. (1998) 'Greek Manuscripts in the Early Abbasid Empire', *Bibliotheca Orientalis*, 55(3–4), pp. 345–372.
Vernet, J. (2008) 'Ibn Juljul, Sulaymān Ibn Ḥasan', in Gillispie, C. C. (ed.) *Complete Dictionary of Scientific Biography*. Detroit: Charles Scribner's Sons.
Zonta, M. (2003) 'A Hebrew Translation of Hippocrates' De superfoetatione: Historical Introduction and Critical Edition', *Aleph: Historical Studies in Science and Judaism*, 3, pp. 97–113.

2

Translations of Western medical texts in East Asia in the second half of the 19th and early 20th centuries

Ji-Hae Kang

1 Introduction

This chapter provides an overview of key issues concerning translations of Western medical texts in East Asia in the second half of the 19th and early 20th centuries. Increased scholarly interest in the history of medicine in Asia and other regions in the last few decades has enhanced our understanding of the ways in which Western medicine has been perceived and disseminated in different geographical contexts (Lewis and Macpherson 2008; Worboys 1997; Kiple 1993; Pols, Thompson and Warner 2017; Bowers 1980). Despite the critical role translation plays in the transmission of thoughts and ideas across national and cultural borders, there has been a notable absence of discussions concerning the intricate connections between translation and the production and circulation of Western medical knowledge in East Asia. The few isolated studies that have touched on this topic (e.g. Hong and Wang 2014; van Hoof 1998) have failed to lead to a sustained engagement.[1] Against this background, this chapter outlines some of the main points and issues central to a discussion on how Western medicine was introduced, adopted, and used by countries in East Asia via translation in the second half of the 19th and early 20th centuries.

In the present chapter, the term 'Western medicine' is used instead of 'biomedicine', 'modern medicine', or 'cosmopolitan medicine', all of which commonly refer to the structured health beliefs and institutionalised therapeutic practices with roots in the 'Western' tradition (cf. Kleinman 1993: 16; Chakrabarti 2013: xiv). It is employed here as a label that encompasses the different terms used to denote the dominant system of medical knowledge in East Asia since the latter half of the 19th century, and highlights the geographical 'starting point' of the medical knowledge that has spread to most parts of the world. It was first in Europe, and then in North America, that this system of medical knowledge developed before it was disseminated to other parts of the world, thereby becoming the overriding system of medical knowledge globally. It should be noted, however, that 'Western medicine' is far from a homogenous category and has changed significantly over time (Andrews 2014). The discussion in this chapter will hopefully make it

DOI: 10.4324/9781003167983-4

clear that 'Western medicine' is neither a single entity nor necessarily a system of knowledge that can be unproblematically connected to 'the West' in the transnational knowledge transmission trajectory.

In this contribution, the geographical region at the centre of inquiry is East Asia, with the focus placed on China, Japan and Korea, where the translation of Western medical knowledge was intricately connected to nationalism and beliefs about and desires towards progress and power. Despite centuries of intraregional exchange within the historical context of Sinocentric world order, where ideas and knowledge were generally transmitted from China to Japan, often via Korea, Japan emerged in the early 20th century as the only non-Western imperialist power with colonies in Asia. Although the three countries all strove to respond to Western intrusions, China found itself in a particularly difficult situation clashing with Western powers, including the Opium Wars (1839–1842, 1856–1860) and other armed conflicts, while it tried to forge its own political direction amid complicated internal power struggles. Meanwhile, Korea was colonised by Japan in 1910 and experienced 35 years of Japanese rule until its independence in 1945. Although by the end of the 20th century the political, economic and cultural circumstances of the three countries changed dramatically, with China emerging as a political superpower, Japan as one of the richest nations in the world, and South Korea as the twelfth global economic power, in the early 20th century the three countries were facing different and extensive internal and external challenges.

The emphasis of this chapter is placed on translations and translators of Western medical knowledge in China, Japan and Korea during this period and their connection to the changing political, social and cultural dynamics in the region. The following sections will shed light upon the translation of Western medicine in terms of the historical, sociopolitical and cultural factors that motivated the translation projects; actors involved in the translation of Western medical knowledge; texts and languages selected for translation; and, the impact of translation on the relevant cultures and societies.[2]

2 Setting the scene

During the second half of the 19th century, intellectuals in East Asia engaged in cultural debates about differences between East and West. Their discourses were dominated by a binary view of the division, shown in such phrases as *Tōyō dōtoku seiyō geijutsu* (Eastern ethics, Western technology) created by the Japanese scholar Satzuma Shozan (1811–1864), *Zhongxue weiti, xixue weiyong* (Chinese learning as essence, Western learning for practical use) devised by the Qing official Zhang Zhidong (1837–1909), and *Tongdosŏgi* (Eastern ways, Western machines) coined by 19th-century Korean reformers espousing *kaehwa*, the 'enlightenment' mind in Korean (Fogel 1996; Kang 2017). East-West dichotomy was used in different ways by politicians and elite groups to instigate nationalist sentiments, but with time, this binary view became much more complicated. Respective countries, and different factions within these countries, adopted positions that best served their interests, as shown in Japan's eventual embracing of the idea of inherent racial differences among Asians, mainly to rationalise its imperialist expansion in Asia. Although there were voices resisting uncritical admiration of a supposedly coherent 'West' (e.g. Chinese writer and translator Lu Xun, 1881–1936), East Asians generally accepted Western material supremacy and the role of Western science in enabling material development from the second half of the 19th century.

The level of interest in Western medicine varied among the three countries during this period, depending on the discourses in circulation concerning Western medicine's role in enabling national development (see the section on 'The translators' below for more details), the reputation of traditional medicine in each country, the levels of hygiene, and the political, religious, and cultural agendas of the actors. Before the transmission of Western medicine, different theories and practices of healing coexisted in the region. Chinese medicine had an extensive influence, despite the existence of a plurality of healing conventions, not all of which could be identified as traditional Chinese medicine. In the case of Korea and Japan, for example, folk remedies, linked to religious rituals, coexisted with Chinese medicine (Motoo, Seki and Tsutani 2011; Kozai 2009).

Initial exposure to Western medicine differed among China, Japan, and Korea. In the case of China, the introduction of Western medicine is mainly related to the activities of the Jesuits who brought European medical knowledge to China in the 17th and 18th centuries (Hanson 2007). However, the number of texts on Western medicine that had been translated by Jesuits at the time was small, especially when compared to their translation of mathematical and Christian texts. The Chinese translation of the French surgeon Ambroise Paré's *Anatomie universelle du corps humain* (Universal Anatomy of the Human Body) by Giacomo Rho, Niccolo Longobardo, and Johann Terrenz Schreck around 1636 is an example of a translated text. Other examples are translations carried out by the French Jesuits Joachim Bouvet and Dominique Parrenin into Manchu, one of the official languages of the Qing dynasty (1636–1911) of China. They include translations of *L'Anatomie de l'homme: suivant la circulation du sang, Et les dernières découvertes, démontrée au Jardin-Royal* (The Anatomy of a Man: Following the Circulation of the Blood and the Latest Discoveries, Demonstrated at the Jardin-Royal; 1690), written by Pierre Dionis, and *Anatome Quartum Renovata* (Anatomy, 4th Edition; 1677), written by Thomas Bartholin (Golvers 2011). These translated texts had limited impact on the spread of Western medicine in China, as their function was largely confined to offering Western anatomical views of the body and Western-style drawing techniques to the Chinese emperors and related officials at the court.

With regard to Korea's first encounter with Western medical knowledge, the texts on Western medicine translated into Chinese by the Jesuits working in China during the 17th and 18th centuries played an important role in shaping Koreans' initial exposure. As Literary Sinitic was commonly used for reading and writing among Korean intellectuals, imported Chinese translations were read without any serious issues in language access (see the section on 'The translations' below for more details on the historical use of Chinese characters in East Asia.). One such example is *Zhuzhi Qunzheng* (Evidence of Divine Providence, 1636), a Chinese translation of *De providentia numinis et animi immortalitate libri duo adversus Atheos et Politicos* (Divine Providence and the Immortality of the Soul against Atheists and Politicians, 1613), originally written by the Jesuit scholar Leonardus Lessius (1554–1623) and translated by the German Jesuit missionary Johann Adam Schall von Bell (1591–1666) (Yeo 2012). The book, which argues the existence of God through natural phenomena, including the human anatomy, influenced such distinguished Korean scholars as Yi Ik (1681–1763) and Yi Kyu-Kyŏng (1788–1856). Yi Ik, for instance, provides a discussion of *Zhuzhi Qunzheng* in an article entitled *Sŏgugŭi* (Medicine in Western countries) released around 1720 (Shin 2009). As the ideas contained in the *Zhuzhi Qunzheng* were significantly different from the existing knowledge of physiology in circulation in Korea, they posed a challenge to the Neo-Confucian view of the body and a traditional understanding of medicine (Yeo 2008). Yet, this initial interest in the concepts and ideas on Western medicine, as well as those on other areas of Western science and Christianity, appeared during the early- and mid-eighteenth century when the country was relatively open to Western knowledge, compared to the period that followed (1790–1876), when Catholicism was officially labelled as an evil religion and banned. During the period of relative openness, Western medicine is mentioned by a small number of Korean thinkers (Shin 2009). Using Literary Sinitic in their writing, scholars such as Yi Ik, Shin Hoo-Dam (1701–1762), Pak Ji-Won (1737–1805), Pak Jae-Ga (1737–1805), An Jeong-Bok (1712–1791), and Yi Ui-Hyeon (1669–1745) discuss their views on the field, albeit based on a partial understanding. A more extensive knowledge of Western medicine appears decades later in the writings of Choe Han-Ki (1803–1877), but the period of initial encounter with Western medicine, which was based on direct readings of Chinese translations as part of *sohak* (Western Learning), did not lead to substantial changes in the approaches to or understanding of healing behaviour in Korea at the time.

In the case of Japan, Western medicine was initially introduced under different circumstances compared to China and Korea. The Japanese were exposed to Western medicine within the context of *rangaku* ('Dutch learning', by extension 'Western learning') during the Edo period (1603–1868). During the 250 years of isolationist foreign policy prior to the official opening of the ports, the Dutch were the only Europeans allowed to enter Japan for commerce, and the Japanese were exposed to scientific developments through texts provided by the Dutch.[3] Western medicine, particularly anatomy, was the focus of interest at the time, and although the translations were limited in number, they functioned as a basis for translation activities that followed in the Meiji era (1868–1912). The first translators of Western works during the Edo period were Nagasaki-based interpreters, who in their official capacity as government officials were responsible for enabling communication between the Japanese and the Dutch, but in their personal capacity, carried out translations from Dutch and related activities that led to the spread of *rangaku* in Japan.

The most widely known translator of Western medicine during this period is Sugita Genpaku, a practitioner of Chinese medicine whose translation of *Ontleedkundige Tafelen* (Dissecting Tables, 1734), a Dutch translation of *Anatomische Tabellen* (*Anatomical Tables,* 1722), a medical text written by the German physician and anatomist Johann Adam Kulmus (1689–1745), became the most representative translation of this period. Convinced that human anatomy was more precisely described in this book than in traditional texts of Chinese medicine, Sugita started the study of *Ranpō* (Dutch medicine) and translated *Ontleedkundige Tafelen* into Japanese, publishing in 1774 what is known today as *Kaitai shinsho* (A New Treatise on Anatomy). The translation work was collaborative, and Sugita and his collaborators carried out the translation with a knowledge of only about 600 Dutch words amongst them (Cunningham 2016).[4]

Translation projects within the *rangaku* scholarship laid the groundwork for Japan's modernisation, enabling the creation of preliminary works that functioned as a framework for Japan's acceptance of Western ideas and knowledge in the following years. Despite the suspicion with which Europe was viewed, Western medical knowledge at the time contributed to casting doubts on the accuracy of Chinese medicine. This was the case even though Chinese medicine still held a crucial position in Japan. Other examples of Japanese translations of Western medical texts within the context of *rangaku* include: a 1706 translation by Narabayashi Chinzan (1643–1711) of a 1649 Dutch translation of the French surgeon Ambroise Paré's work *La methode curative des playes, et fractures de la testes humaine* (Treatment Method for Wounds and Fractures of the Human Head,

1561); Udagawa Genzui's (1755–1797) translation of Johannes de Gorter's *Gezuiverde Geneeskonst* (1744), which appeared for the first time under the title *Naika sen-yo* (Digest of Internal Medicine); and the 1772 Japanese translation, entitled *Yo-I-shin-shô*, from Lorenz Heister's book on surgery in German, carried out by Ôtsuki Gentaku, who in 1811 would take up the position of the director of the Nagasaki Office for the Translation of Foreign Books. During the first half of the 19th century, an increasing number of Japanese physicians studied Dutch medicine under Dutch and German physicians who taught in Nagasaki. As shown in Figure 2.1, translations on Western medicine far outnumbered those in other areas of Western knowledge.

Although the three countries' first contacts with Western medicine have historical significance, these contacts were intermittent and small in scale, compared to the period following the official opening of their ports to Western/foreign powers. Translation during the initial contact phase also occurred irregularly. It was only after the official, and forceful, opening of the ports during the mid- and late-19th century that a consistent, systematic and large-scale transmission of Western medical knowledge took place in East Asia. For China, the official opening of the ports came as a result of the Treaty of Nanking (1842) at the end of the First Opium War against the British, although the port of Macau had been open to Portuguese traders since 1557. Japan's ports were opened by the Treaty of Kanagawa (1853) after American Commodore Matthew Perry led his squadron of US Navy ships into the harbour at Edo Bay (today's Tokyo Bay) and demanded regular trade with Japan. Japan used a similar method to open Korean ports, which involved 'gunboat diplomacy' and led to the Treaty of Ganghwa (1876). Therefore, when Western medicine was practised in the region following the opening of the ports, there was a certain level of

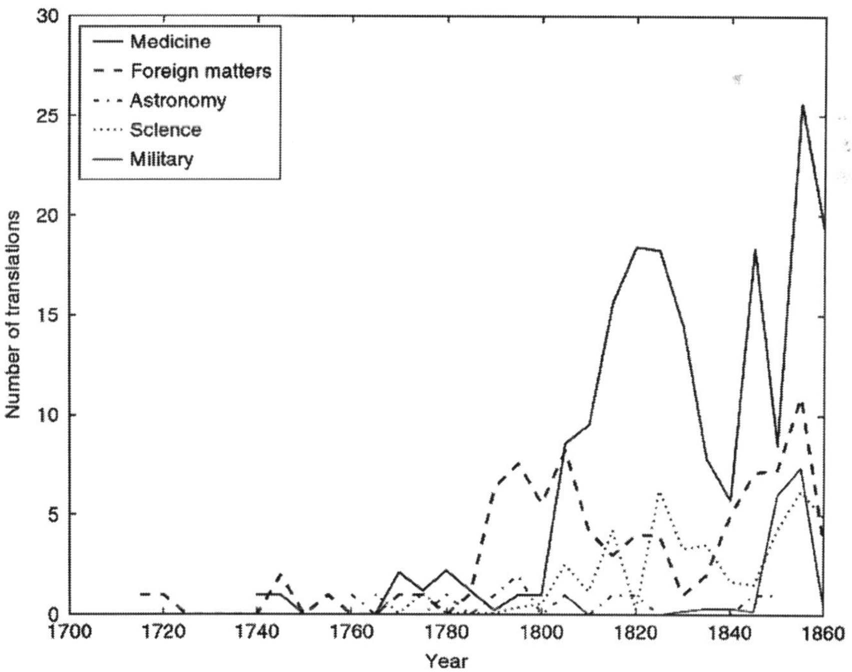

Figure 2.1 Japanese translation of Western works by subjects over time (Clements 2015: 152)

ambivalence among many East Asian intellectuals, as they regarded it as a crucial component of Western/foreign power and as neither 'politically neutral science [n]or benign welfare' (Worboys 1997: 260). However, as it will be shown in the following sections, despite some common aspects in experience among the three counties in relation to external threats and internal conflicts, Western medical knowledge was approached, translated and embraced in different ways during this period.

3 The translators

In the second half of the 19th and early 20th centuries, texts on Western medicine were translated into East Asian languages by both Asians and Westerners. As mentioned in the preceding discussion, the translation of Western medicine before the 19th century was mainly carried out by Japanese translators in Japan and Jesuit translators in China, albeit haphazardly and on a small scale. Chinese translations were read directly in Korea and functioned as the main source of knowledge on Western medicine. Following the opening of the ports, many medical texts were translated in institutional contexts, including missionary hospitals and government bodies. Out of these different sites of institutional translation (Kang 2019), missionary hospitals and medical schools operated by missionaries played a vital role in the transmission of Western medical knowledge, especially in China and Korea, and individuals (doctors, teachers and students) associated with these institutions became crucial actors in translation activities.

The extent to which medical missionaries contributed to the introduction, training, and institutionalisation of Western medicine differed among the three countries. In Japan, for example, the suppression of Christianity beginning in the late 1500s, followed by the expulsion of first the Portuguese, then the Spanish mission from Japan and the exile of Japanese Christians in 1639, led to a situation in which Japan virtually severed its connections with the West and its missionaries. This situation had a negative impact on missionaries' translation activities in the years that followed. Furthermore, there was a growing number of Japanese nationals who had received training in Western medicine and were emerging as medical practitioners and policy makers. Japan had found in Germany a model in which medicine and medical specialists would play a central role in making a nation strong and powerful (Lei 2014). According to one figure, one-fifth of all the Japanese doctors in 1865 were physicians trained in Western medicine, compared with less than 1% of all doctors in China as late as 1921 (Zhao 1991). Thus, Japan was not dependent on missionaries to follow Western medicine, as it had its own doctors being trained within its system or returning from medical training institutions overseas (Nakamura 2013).

In China, Protestant medical missionaries played a key role in carrying out translation activities in the second half of the nineteenth century. Although advocates of China's Self-Strengthening Movement (*Ziqiang yundong*, 1861–1995) focused on adopting Western science, industry, weaponry, and communication, Western medicine was not given as much attention as other branches of science (Lei 2014). Under such conditions, missionaries took up the task of transmitting Western medical knowledge. Out of the eight training institutions teaching Western medicine at the time, seven were run by European or American missionary societies, and only one, the Tianjin Medical School, founded in 1893, was state-run (its predecessor had also been a hospital run by the London Missionary Society). By 1887, a total of 150 medical missionaries had come to China (Choa 1990).

Amongst them, Benjamin Hobson (1816–1873) was a medical missionary who made a major contribution to the practice and teaching of Western medicine in China. As a member of the London Missionary Society during the late Qing dynasty, Hobson published *Quanti xinlun* (A New Treatise on Anatomy) in Guangzhou in 1851, the first text on Western anatomy in Chinese. This book, which he wrote collaboratively with Chen Xiutang, is not a translation of a single source text; instead, it draws on multiple sources, as was often the case for texts on Western medicine originally written in Chinese and Japanese at the time. Hobson also translated *Xiyi lüelun* (First Lines of the Practice of Surgery in the West, 1857), *Neike xinshuo* (Practice of Medicine and Materia Medica, 1858), and *Fuying xinshuo* (Treatise on Midwifery and Diseases of Children, 1858) (Hong and Wang 2014). In the preface of *Neike xinshuo,* Hobson explains that '[m]ethods for disease diagnosis and drug treatments discussed in this book were taken from European medical books. Key points of them were picked up and translated into Chinese' (cited in Hong and Wang 2014: 278). Other medical missionaries such as John Glasgow Kerr also published medical texts in Chinese. In addition to providing medical training to students at a hospital in Canton during the 1860s and founding the Chinese Medical Missionary Association in 1886, Kerr published 34 volumes on Western medicine over a period of 30 years (Reardon-Anderson 1991).

Although missionaries' translation projects were carried out for medical training purposes, their activities did not necessarily lead to an increase in the number of Chinese practitioners of Western medicine. Medical education was viewed by Chinese as aiming at creating a pool of assistants to the missionary doctors, and it was only after the 1890s, when the Chinese government began to send young men to Japan to have them acquire 'advanced' Western medical knowledge, that the number of Chinese nationals trained in Western medicine increased (Gao 2014). Medical missionaries translated about 103 books and pamphlets on Western medicine in the second half of the 19th century, but their activities and contributions to the spread of Western medicine have received mixed evaluations (Cheng 2014).

Meanwhile, medical missionaries to Korea and their translation activities have been viewed somewhat differently by the Koreans compared to the Japanese and Chinese. From the late 19th to early 20th centuries, the two groups that led Western medical practice in Korea were medical practitioners from Japan and the Protestant medical missionaries. Japanese military doctors trained in Western medicine began practising in modern hospitals they had built in port cities such as Pusan, Incheon and Wonsan, and eventually in Seoul. The hospitals provided medical treatment for mostly Japanese nationals, especially Japanese military and government officials who lived in these cities, as well as a small number of Koreans (Kim 2013). In the latter half of the nineteenth century, missionary doctors, many of whom came from the United States and Canada, arrived in Korea. Direct proselytising was illegal at the time, so providing medical care to the traditional Korean elite groups and the general population served as an indirect means of evangelisation. As the activities of medical missionaries mostly took place at a time when Japan was the key aggressor on the Korean peninsula, the relationship between 'colonial medicine' and 'missionary medicine' was complex; these two entities competed against each other, were even confrontational at certain times, but they also enjoyed a harmonious relationship at other times. It is noteworthy that many Korean Christians who had been trained by missionaries came to play a central role in the nationalist movement against Japan (Lee 2000). Some missionaries also became advocates of Korean rights, speaking out against Japanese brutality, such as the Canadian medical missionary Frank W. Schofield who played a crucial role in the 1919 March First Movement, an anti-Japanese independence movement. Thus, Christianity became compatible with a nationalist identity in the case of Korea, whereas in China and Japan, 'nationalist rituals generated patriotic identities by attacking Christianity' (Kane and Park 2009: 365).

One example of a medical missionary translator in Korea is Oliver R. Avison (1860–1959), the fourth director of Chejungwon (Hospital of Universal Helpfulness), a Western hospital founded in 1885. After his arrival in Korea in 1893, Avison embarked on translation projects with his Korean 'helpers', and more than 30 translations of Western medical texts were produced in Chejungwon (later renamed Sebŭransŭ Ŭihakkyo, meaning 'Severance Medical School') from 1899 to 1910.[5] Avison participated in many of these projects as a translator or revisor, including Korean translations of *Yangmurhak sanggwŏn mugijil* (Materia Medica and Therapeutics Vol. 1 Inorganic Substances, 1905) and *Haebuhak* (Anatomy of the Human Body, 1906) (Kang 2017). His three Korean collaborators, Kim Pil-Soon (1878–1919), Hong Suk-Hoo (1883–1940), and Hong Jong-Eun (?–1910), all of whom were his students, worked with him in the initial stage but eventually translated independently under their own names. These Korean translators/medical students, along with four other Korean medical students, graduated from Sebŭransŭ Ŭihakkyo (formerly Chejungwon) in 1908 and became the first recipients of official medical licences in Korean history (Yeo 2009; Park and Park 2011). Chejungwon translators mostly used Korean script in their texts, using Chinese characters in combination only when necessary, although many translations and non-translations produced in Korea at the time used only Chinese characters or mixed script (a system of using both Chinese characters and Korean alphabet; see the following section on 'The translators' for more details on the connection between writing systems and translation.). This is a salient aspect of these translations, as the extensive use of the Korean script made the translations more accessible to Koreans from all walks of life.

Among the Chejungwon translators, Kim Pil-Soon's translations include *Haebuhak* (Anatomy of the Human Body, revised by Avison, 1906), *Yangmurhak sanggwŏn mugijil* (Materia Medica and Therapeutics Vol. 1 Inorganic Substances, co-translated with Avison, 1905), *Sinp'yŏn hwahakkyogwasŏ yugijil* (New Organic Chemistry Textbook, revised by Avison, 1906), and *Naegwa* (Practice of Medicine, 1906). Hong Suk-Hoo's works include *Sinp'yŏn saengnigyogwasŏ chŏn* (New Physiology Textbook, Vol. 1, revised by Avison, 1906), *Chindanhak kwŏn 1* (Physical Examination Vol. 1, revised by Avison, 1906) and *Chindanhak kwŏn 2* (Physical Examination Vol. 2, revised by Avison, 1907). Hong Jong-Eun's translations include *P'ibubyŏngjindan* (Skin Examination, 1907) and *Mussisan'gwahak* (Obstetrics by Mu, 1908). Kim Pil-Soon was hired to teach medicine at his alma mater upon graduation in 1908; however, he left academia when Korea was annexed by Japan two years afterwards. Working as a medical practitioner, Kim became an important figure in the nationalist movement and was eventually poisoned to death by an assassin believed to have been hired by the Japanese government. In fact, out of the seven graduates who became the first licensed doctors in Korea, five became active members of the anti-Japanese nationalist movement.

With the passage of time, an increasing number of Asians trained in Western medicine became translators of medical texts. Many of them had already received training in or were in the process of learning Western medicine at the time of translation. Those translators who initially collaborated with Western translators as associates later became renowned translators in their own right, as well as medical specialists, educators, government officials or activists, as shown in the examples of Kim Pil-Soon, Hong Jong-Eun and Hong Suk-Hoo. Another well-known example is Sun Yat-sen (1866–1925), the founding father of the Chinese Republic, who was a pupil of and assistant in translation for John Glasgow Kerr for a year in 1886, before he went on to study Western medicine at the newly opened Hong Kong College of Medicine for Chinese, the first teaching institution in Hong Kong to fully adopt Western medical practices (Fu 2018).

As the initial ambivalence towards Western medicine gradually waned in the late nineteenth and early twentieth centuries, East Asian countries began to send their brightest minds to the United States, Britain, Germany, and, in the case of China and Korea, to Japan, in order to acquire up-to-date medical knowledge and experience an advanced training system. The returnees were often employed as faculty members in the medical colleges or as government officials, and many of them participated in translating and authoring books on Western medicine. Those teaching and learning Western medicine in medical schools at the time were all involved in the process of translation, as the very act of making Western medical concepts comprehensible in respective languages in a learning environment implicated a process of translation (including self-translation). For Ikeda Kensai (1841–1918), one of the first nine Japanese to be awarded the Japanese government's scholarship to study abroad in 1870 and eventually the first dean of the Medical Faculty of Tokyo Imperial University, the medical school in Tokyo during the 1860s 'functioned primarily as a school for translation' (Kim 2014: 34). Students' learning involved reading out passages of medical texts and drawing out any meaning they could grasp. According to Ikeda, students 'prepared two or three lines of translations using grammar books' and if the text presented any challenges in comprehension, 'the class quickly turned into a form of discussion' (Kim 2014: 34), as they were asked by the instructor to identify gender, case, prepositions, conjunctions, and semantic meaning.

In China, numerous medical periodicals began to be published from the 1900s, which contained translations from diverse sources. The publications were dedicated to introducing Western medical concepts and treatments, pharmacological theories and policies, medical history, and general health information (Cheng 2014). In 1906, a medical student named Qian Ye organised the China Medicine Society and served as the editor for *Yiyao xuebao* (医药学报, Journal of Medicine). In 1907, Jin Ze, another medical student, established the Chinese Citizens' Health Society and published *Weisheng shijie* (卫生世界, Health World). In 1908, Wang Zixin, who had studied in Japan, established the Medical World Society and edited, compiled and distributed the journal *Yixue shijie* (医学世界, Medical World), containing articles on medical case reports, questions and answers on medical issues and short stories. Several translators who had studied in Japan worked for this journal, including the prominent translator Ding Fubao (1868–1941), who translated more than 68 Japanese medical texts (Gao 2014). His translations, which include articles in *Zhongxi yixue bao* (中西醫學報, The Journal of Sino-Western Medicine) were central in introducing Western medical knowledge to the Chinese people.

4 The translations

The subjects covered in translated texts ranged from basic sciences to medical specialities, including anatomy, pathology, pharmacology, physiology, chemistry, biology, physics, immunology, internal medicine, surgery, obstetrics, ophthalmology, dermatology and psychology. The languages of the source texts were diverse, including German, French, English, Japanese, and Chinese. One interesting aspect of the translation practice in East Asia at the time was the prevalence of indirect translation, i.e. translation based on a source which is itself a translation. From a contemporary perspective, indirect translation is a choice made reluctantly and has a lower status than direct translation due to its second-hand nature, occurring mostly when a translation from less widely spoken languages is required. In East Asia, in the second half of the nineteenth and early twentieth centuries, however, indirect translation from Japanese or Chinese translations into another East Asian language filled an important gap in the production and dissemination of Western medical knowledge. At a time when knowledge of European languages and subject expertise were scarce, indirect translation played a significant role in facilitating the spread of Western medical knowledge.

This facilitation in itself was enabled by the historical sharing of Chinese characters in East Asia. The clear distinction in speech sounds and native words among the three languages makes Chinese, Japanese and Korean mutually unintelligible, but respective users of the three languages had been able to communicate to a certain degree through the use of Chinese characters. With regard to Japan, Chinese characters, called *kanji* in Japanese, have been used to write Sino-Japanese words, which constitute a high proportion of Japanese vocabulary and are a key component of the Japanese writing system to this day. In the case of Korea, Chinese characters, presently called *hanja* in Korean, were widely used to write the Korean language before the 1446 invention of the Korean script *Hangul*, a phonetic alphabet, by King Sejong. Although Hangul is now universally used in Korea, Chinese characters were used by the ruling class up until the late 19th and early 20th centuries, i.e. even after Hangul's invention, due to their perceived prestigious status. This resulted in a high proportion of Sino-Korean words in the Korean vocabulary. When a European or American medical text translated into Chinese (using Chinese characters) or Japanese (using *kanji*) was used as source text for a subsequent translation into another East Asian language, the translation process was often facilitated by the ability of translators to retain words written in Chinese characters, and even to approximate the sound in respective languages (Wakabayashi 2016). Chinese characters are logographs that represent words or morphemes, as well as offering phonetic hints, and although they are phonetically actualised in different ways depending on the linguistic context, the historical sharing of Chinese characters often served to expedite the translation process in the three countries.

Numerous examples of indirect translations of Western medical texts and terms are found in East Asia. For example, Benjamin Hobson's Chinese translations, which were circulated during the 1850s and 1860s in the treaty ports of China and Japan, were chosen for translation by the Meiji government of Japan (Elman 2006; Tsien 1954). Japanese translation of Hobson's books on Western medicine include *Treatise on Physiology* (1851), *Natural Philosophy* (1855), *Fine Lines of the Practice of Surgery in the West* (1857), *Treatise on Midwifery and Diseases of Children* (1858) and *Practice of Medicine and Materia Medica* (1858). Meanwhile, many Korean translations of Western medical texts were based on Japanese translations. For example, translations by Kim Pil-Soon, Hong Suk-Hoo and Hong Jong-Eun were mostly based on Japanese translations of multiple source texts.

From the 1890s, the Chinese government actively adopted the Japanese model of Western medicine, translating Japanese medical texts into Chinese (Andrews 2014). This occurred in the wake of the defeat of the Qing dynasty in the Sino-Japanese War of 1894–1895, when both the Chinese court and the general public began to focus their attention on the ways in which Japan had modernised itself by adopting and adapting Western ideas, policies, and institutions. Based on similarities in political, social, and cultural conditions,

China decided that Japan would be an easy example to emulate. In 1896, the Qing government began sending students to Japan, and in 1902, when Yuan Shikai founded the Beiyang Military Medical College in Tianjin, a Japanese medical officer, Higara Seijirō, was hired to serve as its head instructor. According to Gao (2014), the hiring of Higara is significant in that it marks the beginning of the end of the era of European and American missionaries and the emergence of Japanese system-trained doctors as arbiters of Western medicine in China.[6] One such doctor who became a key figure in the adoption of Western medicine was Ding Fubao, one of the most prolific translators of Western medicine in China. Mostly based on Japanese texts, his output was so prodigious that 'with Ding's translations and publications, Japan became the main source for modern medical terminology in China' (Andrews 2015: 10).

During the Meiji era, Japan transformed into a modern, industrialised nation with unmatched military power in the region. Under the slogan 'rich country, strong army' (*fukoku kyohei*), Japan invaded neighbouring countries and acquired colonies in Taiwan, Korea and southern Manchuria by the end of the Meiji era. During the process, Japan not only adopted and institutionalised Western medicine, but also continued to dominate in other Western scientific disciplines within the region. Medicine accounted for 48 per cent of all the doctorates in science and technology between 1888 and 1920 in Japan and over a quarter of professorial chairs at imperial universities in 1905 (Bartholomew 1989).

The growing public recognition that translation and Western medicine were essential to the Japanese national interest played a crucial role in initiating translation projects and motivating translators. The translation projects were initiated by individuals and the government, and German and English medical literature continued to be important sources for translation. The University of Tokyo, the first modern institution of higher education in Japan established in 1877, and its Faculty of Medicine were central in Western medical research, practice, and education, as well as in serving national needs, shaping policy, and training government officials. The university was staffed by the young men who had returned from studying medicine in Europe, particularly in Germany. Between 1868 and 1914, as many as 1,200 Japanese medical students travelled to German cities such as Berlin, Munich, Heidelberg and Freiburg to obtain the most up-to-date medical knowledge from leading German scholars. Meanwhile, dozens of German physicians were invited to Japanese universities as instructors, to transform Japan's medical institutions and education (Kim 2014).[7]

Translators in East Asia used diverse methods to translate texts on Western medicine and often did not cite the source of their translations. In many cases, the title or the name of the author of the source text were not displayed on translation covers, although this information was sometimes provided in prefaces. In addition to the lack of bibliographic information concerning the source text, translators substantially intervened in the translation process. In the case of Japan, intervention by Meiji-era translators is mostly manifested in Japanese translators' reliance on the method of using several related works in the process of translation and drawing on their own experiential learning to further improve their translations (Meade 2015). In China and Korea, translated texts also reveal considerable additions of information from other sources and extensive omissions of content compared to the source texts. One example of such deletion is found in Japanese translations of Benjamin Hobson's works written in Chinese. In Japanese translations of *Quanti xinlun*, for instance, passages considered socially and culturally inappropriate were deleted. Hobson discusses gross anatomy from the perspective of fundamental equality among people and from the view that all human bodies share basic characteristics. As a medical missionary, Hobson had incorporated in the text Christian beliefs about God's creation of the human body, in order to convey the 'theoretical foundations of the body itself' (Bosmia *et al.* 2014: 159). Such passages were removed from Japanese translations of *Quanti xinlun* (Heinrich 2008).[8] As translation was often accompanied by a process of bringing together several sources into a single translation, the boundary between a non-translation and translation was blurred in many instances.

With regard to methods used in translating medical texts and terms, a reliance, as mentioned above, on indirect translation from Japanese or Chinese enabled translators in East Asia to translate using the same Chinese characters that were read or pronounced differently depending on the country. However, when terms that had not been previously translated required translation, which was often the case, a range of methods were used by the translators in the three countries. In the case of China, for example, common methods used in the Translation Bureau of Jiangnan Arsenal were as follows (Alleton and Alleton 1966; Wright 1997):

1) not translating the term at all (i.e. leaving the source language expressions in their original forms)
2) transliterating the source word (i.e. transcribing the sound of the source language term in Chinese characters chosen for their phonetic values)
3) using existing Chinese terms
4) creating a new term by juxtaposing two or more existing characters
5) reviving an archaic character
6) creating a new Chinese character
7) using Japanese loanwords

These methods were used in the translation of texts on science and technology in general and are not necessarily restricted to medicine; nonetheless, they offer an overall understanding of how translators in China approached translation problems at the time. The most widely used method was creating new terms by juxtaposing two or more existing characters. This was a method that Benjamin Hobson also preferred, as exemplified by his Chinese translation of 'oxygen' into *yangqi* 養氣, derived from *yang* 養 (nourish) and *qi* 氣 (vapor, gas), describing oxygen as a gas that 'nourishes' or supports combustion.[9] The use of Japanese loanwords as a translation method became prominent in China and Korea during the late 19th and early 20th centuries. In the case of China, this method was used after the 1890s when a large number of Chinese students who had gone to study medicine and other scientific fields in Japanese institutions returned to China.

5 Conclusion and future directions

This chapter has outlined the ways in which Western medical knowledge was translated during the second half of the nineteenth and early twentieth centuries in East Asia. This is a period in which Western medical knowledge was systematically introduced to the region, and China, Japan and Korea all experienced profound challenges related to imperialist encroachment, disintegrating traditional values, pressures for national development, and collapsing social and political order. The chapter has provided a comparative perspective on the transmission of Western medical knowledge in the region by focusing on the interconnections, as well as the different ways in which translations were carried out. It has described the existing discussions on Western medicine's connection to colonial/imperialist endeavours and national developments, but has also attempted to go beyond these discussions by using the lens of translation. Focusing on translation and translators, this chapter offered some insights into the specificities of the actors, processes and effects of the transnational production and circulation of Western medical knowledge in East Asia.

In the second half of the 19th and early 20th centuries, Western medicine was understood in China, Japan and Korea as a compelling tool for enabling the people to obtain health and prosperity. However, the pace of adopting this view, as well as undertaking translation activities under the goal of transmitting Western medical knowledge, differed among the three countries. Japan was the first to accommodate Western medicine in relation to national development, and the discourses circulated by its government that Western medicine enables the building of a prosperous and powerful nation led to the initiation of large governmental translation projects, creation of a pool of Japanese translators and establishment of institutions which offer Western medical training.

The situation was more complex in China, with competing views and discourses concerning Western knowledge and institutions. Medical missionaries initially played an important role as translators of Western medical knowledge. Following the defeat of the 1894–1895 Sino-Japanese War, however, Chinese nationals who had been sent to Japan to learn the Japanese system of Western medicine became crucial actors in the transmission of Western medical knowledge. Many Chinese versions of Japanese translations were produced, consequently making Japan the key source for Western medical terminology in China.

In the case of Korea, the transfer of Western medical knowledge during the late 19th and early 20th centuries was carried out by actors respectively related to Japanese colonial medicine and Protestant missionary medicine. Medical missionaries and Korean nationals affiliated with medical schools were the main actors in translation activities. Similar to the Chinese case, many Korean translation projects involved rendering Japanese translations into Korean, as Japan was deemed to possess more advanced medical institutions and training systems. At the same time, the identities of the translators and values related to translation were intertwined with articulations of a Korean national identity, revealing a tension between perceptions of Japan as a model of advancement and discourses of Korean national sovereignty.

The discussion in this chapter has shown that contrary to the lay view of translation as a one directional process from a source to target language, in which meanings contained in a source text are preserved intact in the target text, translation is a process of active renegotiation of meanings and values. In the great majority of cases, political and cultural values associated with health-seeking practices in the source text were recast and reconstituted in different ways in the process of translation. Furthermore, translation activities accompanied changes, and even conflicts, in the social identities and positions of the actors producing, mediating and circulating medical knowledge.

Although the number of historical studies of Western medicine in East Asia has been increasing in recent years, there is still much that needs to be unveiled regarding the identity of translators, the texts selected for translation, the discourses associated with translation of Western medicine, the translation processes and procedures, and the effects and consequences of translation activities. One topic that particularly requires further research is the identity of translators who participated in medical translation projects and the agency of these actors in the transnational medical knowledge production, mediation, and dissemination. Although recent research on the transmission of Western medical knowledge within the context of the modernisation processes in the region has enhanced our understanding of the identity of translators, there is still more scope for research. For example, local translators who collaborated with high-profile European translators have not been visible in many instances, despite the key role they played in the translation process. Research on translators' social status, educational background, ideological orientation, and their activities and life trajectories following their participation in translation work are some of the topics that will contribute to a more nuanced understanding of the processes and effects of the transmission of Western medicine.

Another topic that requires further research is tracing the complex textual interconnections established via translation among the three countries. The frequent use of indirect translation in the region brought the three countries into an intricate translational network of Western medical texts and terminologies. More research on the directionality of translations and the resulting connections among the terms and texts – as well as medical terminology standardisation movements and campaigns implemented from mid-20th century onwards calling for the elimination of foreign (especially Chinese or Japanese) influences on the respective countries' (Western) medical terminologies – is needed in order to better understand the relation between translation and social change, as well as the role of translation in the transmission of Western ideas and the modernisation of the region.

Another important topic that needs to be further studied is the role of traditional medicines in enabling the understanding of Western medicine and the evolving relationship between traditional medicines and Western medicine. More research is needed to understand how traditional medical concepts were incorporated into the translation processes and used to make Western medical knowledge comprehensible. Furthermore, the systematic introduction and adoption of Western medicine in East Asia led to the suppression of traditional medicines, although this happened in different ways at different times (Park *et al.* 2012). At the same time, the adoption of Western medicine in the region created opportunities to modernise traditional medicines, as efforts were made to codify and standardise them, as well as to select drugs and practices that were more in line with modern ideas. These are just a few of the many issues that require further investigation.

This contribution has emphasised that translation is far from a detached transfer of knowledge between cultural groups equal in power and resources. The act of translation is a complex process that interacts with issues of power, the discourses in circulation, and the goals and agendas of actors and institutions involved in knowledge mediation. Translations of medical texts in the second half of the 19th and early 20th centuries in East Asia recast existing perceptions of healing practices and reshaped understanding of the human body. The key point the chapter intended to make is that in China, Japan, and Korea, as in many other places in the world where Western medicine was 'introduced', the conceptualisation of Western medicine, as well as its adoption, adaptation, and use, was approached differently by the actors (e.g. the court, intellectuals, 'foreigners', and the general public) and the translation activities were deeply politicised. The approaches and reactions to translational phenomena were often a reflection of a country's or a group's self-image. It is hoped that the overview in this chapter will encourage more scholars in translation studies, medical history and East Asian studies to further engage with the complexity of the connections between translation and the production and circulation of medical knowledge.

Notes

1 The reasons behind this situation are diverse, ranging from a general lack of interest in translation in academia (Dietz 2016) to language barriers in accessing research on transnational transfer of knowledge.
2 This chapter is mostly based on English and Korean sources. It was not possible to draw on the rich discussions in Chinese or Japanese publications.
3 Although Japan's first encounter with the West began when a Portuguese ship drifted onto a Japanese island in 1543, it would be the Dutch and *rangaku* scholarship that would be the most significant in Japan's early encounter with Western science and medicine.
4 In the introduction to *Kaitai shinsho*, Sugita explains the three methods used to translate Western medical concepts. The first was the adoption of corresponding terms already existing in Japanese (e.g. the Dutch word *beendered* translated as *hone,* meaning 'bone'). The second method was the coining of new terms for concepts that had no corresponding Japanese term (e.g. *kraakbeen* was translated as *nankotsu*, meaning 'cartilage'). The third method was transliterating the source term by using Chinese characters to represent the sound (e.g. *klier* translated as *kiriru,* meaning 'gland'). Although transliteration is now widely used in Japan, this was not a preferred method in *Kaitai shinsho,* which includes relatively few instances of their use. The translation work lasted for three years, and the writing system that was chosen for translation was Literary Sinitic. The chosen writing system signals that the translation not only targeted medical experts but also a general readership of educated samurai and other learned men, with the effect of igniting an interest in Dutch learning (Clements 2015).
5 Chejungwon was established as a Western hospital in 1885 by Emperor Gojong and Horace Allen, an American surgeon and a Protestant missionary sent to Korea by the Presbyterian Church in the United States. In 1894, when the First Sino-Japanese War erupted and the Gabo Reform began, the Korean government was no longer able to finance the operation of the hospital, and Chejungwon came under the full control of the church.
6 In addition to the Japanese model-based medical schools run by the government and the missionary-operated medical schools, there were also medical schools operated by foreign governments. Examples include the German government operated Tongji German Medical College, established in Shanghai in 1908, and the German Medical School, built in Qingdao in 1911, as well as the French Catholic Zhendan Medical School, which opened in Shanghai in 1909. These schools were respectively operated under the guiding principles of the educational systems of the countries affiliated with each of the institutions.
7 Some studies have pointed out the problems concerning the adoption of Western medicine in Japan, particularly after 1880, portraying the process as 'internal colonization' (Bay 2012: 6), which is used not only to refer to the process of the medical community slowly becoming dominated by the (largely foreign-educated) medical elite of the University of Tokyo, but also to problematise the nationalisation of medicine and the regulation of citizens' bodies through legislation.
8 These passages were also removed from many Chinese reprints of *Quanti xinlun.*
9 However, Hobson's approach raised questions about the adequacy of the translation method and fuelled discussions about the need to standardise scientific jargon in the Chinese language. John Fryer, Director of the Translation Bureau of Jiangnan Arsenal, stated in his *An Account of the Department for the Translation of Foreign Books* that the terms Hobson had used in his texts were rejected by many subsequent medical practitioners and translators. This incident made standardising medical and scientific terms an important goal of Jiangnan Arsenal (Elman 2006). Nevertheless, Hobson's nomenclature is still partly used in medicine and science, e.g. the use of *qingqi* and *danqi* (diluting gas) to refer to hydrogen and nitrogen, respectively (Bosmia *et al.* 2014).

Further reading

Andrews, B. (2014) *The Making of Modern Chinese Medicine, 1850–1960*. Vancouver: University of British Columbia Press.

This text on the history of medicine in modern China provides an interesting discussion on the ways in which medicine crossed national and cultural boundaries, leading to the creation of new medical terminologies and the selective use of pre-existing terms for different purposes.

Hong, C. Y. and Wang, F. M. (2014) 'Chinese Translation of English Textbooks on Internal Medicine From the 1850s to the 1940s', *Journal of the Chinese Medical Association*, 77(6), pp. 277–282.

Offering bibliographic information on Chinese translations of books on internal medicine originally written in English, this article pieces together an account of the development of Western medicine in China from 1850 to 1949 and the identities of translators who were influential actors in the production and dissemination of Western medical knowledge in China.

Kim, H. (2014) *Doctors of Empire: Medical and Cultural Encounters Between Imperial Germany and Meiji Japan*. Toronto: University of Toronto Press.

This book provides an insightful account of the historical context surrounding Meiji Japan's translation of German medical science, concentrating on the origins, evolution and effects of its adoption of German medicine as an official model.

Yeo, I. S. (2008) 'A History of Public Health in Korea', in Lewis, M. and MacPherson K. (eds) *Public Health in Asia and the Pacific: Historical and Comparative Perspectives*. London and New York: Routledge, pp. 73–86.

This is a useful overview of the broader historical context within which translation of Western medical knowledge took place in Korea, centring on the introduction and the development of the modern public-health system.

Related topics

Dissemination of Academic Medical Research Through Translation, Medical Translations from Greek Into Arabic and Hebrew, Medical Terminology and Discourse

References

Alleton, V. and Alleton, J. C. (1966) *Terminologie de la chimie en chinois moderne*. Paris: Mouton.

Andrews, B. (2014) *The Making of Modern Chinese Medicine, 1850–1960*. Vancouver: University of British Columbia Press.

Andrews, B. (2015) 'Ding Fubao and the Morals of Medical Modernization', *East Asian Science, Technology and Medicine*, 42, pp. 7–38.

Bartholomew, J. R. (1989) *The Formation of Science in Japan: Building a Research Tradition*. New Haven, CT and London: Yale University Press.

Bay, A. (2012) *Beriberi in Modern Japan: The Making of a National Disease*. Rochester, NY: University of Rochester Press.

Bosmia, A. N., Patel, T., Watanabe, K., Shoja, M., Loukas, M. and Tubbs, R. (2014) 'Benjamin Hobson (1816–1873): His Work as a Medical Missionary and Influence on the Practice of Medicine and Knowledge of Anatomy in China and Japan', *Clinical Anatomy*, 27(2), pp. 154–161.

Bowers, J. (1980) *When the Twain Meet: The Rise of Western Medicine in Japan*. Baltimore, MD and London: Johns Hopkins University Press.

Chakrabarti, P. (2013) *Medicine and Empire: 1600–1960*. Basingstoke: Macmillan.

Cheng, H. (2014) 'The Modernization of Japanese and Chinese Medicine (1914–1931)', *Chinese Studies in History*, 47(4), pp. 78–94.

Choa, G. H. (1990) *'Heal the Sick' Was Their Motto: The Protestant Medical Missionaries in China*. Hong Kong: Chinese University Press.

Clements, R. (2015) *A Cultural History of Translation in Early Modern Japan*. Cambridge: Cambridge University Press.

Cunningham, A. (2016) *The Anatomist Anatomis'd: An Experimental Discipline in Enlightenment Europe*. London and New York: Routledge.

Dietz, B. (2016) 'Introduction: Special Issue. Translating and Translations in the History of Science', *Annals of Science*, 73(2), pp. 117–121.

Elman, B. (2006) *A Cultural History of Modern Science in China*. Cambridge, MA and London: Harvard University Press.

Fogel, J. (1996) 'Issues in the Evolution of Modern China in East Asian Comparative Perspective', *The History Teacher*, 29(4), pp. 425–448.

Fu, L. (2018) 'Medical Missionaries in China: John Glasgow Kerr (1824–1901) and Cutting for the Stone', *Journal of Medical Biography*, 26(3), pp. 194–202.

Gao, X. (2014) 'Foreign Models of Medicine in Twentieth-Century China', in Andrews, B. and Bullock, M. (eds) *Medical Transitions in Twentieth-Century China*. Bloomington: Indiana University Press, pp. 173–211.

Golvers, N. (2011) 'The Jesuits in China and the Circulation of Western Books in the Sciences (17th–18th centuries): The Medical and Pharmaceutical Sections in the SJ Libraries of Peking', *East Asian Science, Technology, and Medicine*, 34, pp. 15–85.

Hanson, M. E. (2007) '"Jesuits and Medicine in the Kangxi Court (1662–1722)". Publication of Keynote Address given 8 March 2007, for "Medicine and Culture: Chinese-Western Medical Exchange"'. Symposium at the Ricci Institute for Chinese-Western Cultural History, USF Center for the Pacific Rim, *Pacific Rim Report* 43, pp. 1–10.

Heinrich, L. (2008) *The Afterlife of Images: Translating the Pathological Body between China and the West*. Durham, NC: Duke University Press.

Hong, C. Y. and Wang, F. M. (2014) 'Chinese Translation of English Textbooks on Internal Medicine From the 1850s to the 1940s', *Journal of the Chinese Medical Association*, 77(6), pp. 277–282.

Kane, D. and Park, J. (2009) 'The Puzzle of Korean Christianity: Geopolitical Networks and Religious Conversion in Early Twentieth-Century East Asia', *American Journal of Sociology*, 115(2), pp. 365–404.

Kang, J. H. (2017) '근대계몽기 제도번역을 통한 서양의학 지식 생산 및 확산: 제중원 의학교재 번역을 중심으로 [Medical Knowledge on the Move: Institutional Translation of Medical Texts at Chejungwon During the Late Nineteenth and Early Twentieth Century]', *번역학 연구* [The Journal of Translation Studies], 18(3), pp. 7–35.

Kang, J. H. (2019) 'Institutional Translation'. In Baker, M. and Saldanha, G. (eds) *Routledge Encyclopedia of Translation Studies*, 3rd ed., London and New York: Routledge, pp. 256–261.

Kim, H. (2014) *Doctors of Empire: Medical and Cultural Encounters Between Imperial Germany and Meiji Japan*. Toronto: University of Toronto Press.

Kim, J. (2013) 'The Borderline of "Empire": Japanese Maritime Quarantine in Busan c. 1876–1910', *Medical History*, 57(2), pp. 226–248.

Kiple, K. (ed) (1993) *The Cambridge World History of Human Disease*. Cambridge: Cambridge University Press.

Kleinman, A. (1993) 'What is Specific to Western Medicine?', in Bynum, W. F. and Porter, R. (eds) *Companion Encyclopedia of the History of Medicine, Volume I*. New York: Routledge, pp. 15–23.

Kozai, T. (2009) 'C. W. Hufeland in Japan'. In Sakai, S., Sakai, T., Oberländer, C. and Ichinokawa, Y. (eds) *Transaction in Medicine and Heteronomous Modernization: Germany, Japan, Korea and Taiwan*. Tokyo: University of Tokyo Press, pp. 113–129.

Lee, T. (2000) 'A Political Factor in the Rise of Protestantism in Korea: Protestantism and the 1919 March First Movement', *Church History*, 69(1), pp. 116–142.

Lei, S. (2014) *Neither Donkey nor Horse: Medicine in the Struggle over China's Modernity*. Chicago: University of Chicago Press.

Lewis, M. and Macpherson, K. (eds) (2008) *Public Health in Asia and the Pacific: Historical and Comparative Perspectives*. London: Routledge.

Meade, R. (2015) 'Translating Technology in Japan's Meiji Enlightenment, 1870–1879', *East Asian Science, Technology and Society: An International Journal*, 9(3), pp. 253–274.

Motoo, Y., Seki, T. and Tsutani, K. (2011) 'Traditional Japanese Medicine, Kampo: Its History and Current Status', *Chinese Journal of Integrative Medicine*, 17(2), pp. 85–87.

Nakamura, E. (2013) 'The Private World of a Meiji-era Japanese Doctor: Ishii Kendō's Diary of 1874', *Social History of Medicine*, 26(2), pp. 165–181.

Park, H. L., Lee, H. S., Shin, B. C., Liu, J. P., Shang, Q. Yamashita, H. and Lim, B. (2012) 'Traditional Medicine in China, Korea, and Japan: A Brief Introduction and Comparison'. *Evidence-Based Complementary and Alternative Medicine*, 429103. DOI:10.1155/2012/429103.

Park, J. H. and Park, H. W. (2011) '제중원에서 『약물학 상권(무기질)』의 번역과 그 의미 [The Translation of Materia Medica Part. I in Jejungwon and Its Meanings]'. *의사학* [Korean Journal of Medical History], 20, pp. 327–354.

Pols, H., Thompson, C. M. and Warner, J. H. (eds) (2017) *Translating the Body: Medical Education in Southeast Asia*. Chicago: University of Chicago Press.
Reardon-Anderson, J. (1991) *The Study of Change: Chemistry in China, 1840–1949*. Cambridge: Cambridge University Press.
Shin, D. (2009) 'Korean Medical Discourses on Western Medicine, 1720–1876', *다산학* [Journal of Tasan Studies], 15, pp. 181–218.
Tsien, T. H. (1954) 'Western Impact on China Through Translation', *The Journal of Asian Studies*, 13(3), pp. 305–327.
Van Hoof, H. (1998) 'A Contribution to the History of Medical Translation in Japan', in Fischbach, H. (ed) *Translation and Medicine*. Amsterdam and Philadelphia: John Benjamins, pp. 29–36.
Wakabayashi, J. (2016) 'Script as a Factor in Translation', *Journal of World Literature*, 1(2), pp. 173–194.
Worboys, M. (1997) 'The Spread of Western Medicine', in Loudon, I. I. (ed.) *Western Medicine: An Illustrated History*. Oxford: Oxford University Press, pp. 249–263.
Wright, D. (1997) 'The Great Desideratum: Chinese Chemical Nomenclature and the Transmission of Western Chemical Concepts', *Chinese Science*, 14, pp. 45–90.
Yeo, I. S. (2008) 'A History of Public Health in Korea', in Lewis, M. and MacPherson, K. (eds) *Public Health in Asia and the Pacific: Historical and Comparative Perspectives*. London: Routledge, pp. 73–86.
Yeo, I. S. (2009) '제중원과 세브란스 의전의 기초의학 교육과 연구 [Basic Medical Science in Jejungwon and the SUMC, 1885–1945]', *연세의사학* [Yonsei Journal of Medical History], 12(1), pp. 43–57.
Yeo, I. S. (2012) '주제군징(主制群徵)에 나타난 서양의학 이론과 중국과 조선에서의 수용 양상 [Zhuzhiqunzheng (主制群徵), the Jesuit Translation of Western Medicine and Its Influence on Korean and Chinese Intellectuals]', *의사학* [Korean Journal of Medical History], 21(2), pp. 251–277.
Zhao, H. (1991) 'Chinese Versus Western Medicine. A History of Their Relations in the Twentieth Century', *Chinese Science*, 10, pp. 21–37.

3

Dissemination of academic medical research through translation throughout history and in the contemporary world

Carmen Quijada Diez

1 Introduction[1]

The definition of translation as 'the great pollinator of Science' (Fischbach 1993: 100) is a very accurate one, as it has walked hand in hand with medicine from its very beginnings. The history of medical discourse and that of translation move in parallel ways, for the transmission of knowledge (both scientific and humanistic) from civilisation to civilisation has been the common thread all throughout history, and that transmission took place through the figure of the linguistic mediator or translator (Delisle and Woodsworth 2012; Jacquart and Micheau 1996; Gutas 1998; Vickery 2000; Montgomery 2000; García Bravo 2004; Santoyo 2004 and 2009; Jacquart 2005; Burnett 2007; Daiber 2007; Saliba 2007; Pormann and Savage-Smith 2007; Valls 2007; Olohan 2009 and 2016; Gutiérrez Rodilla 1998, 2003 and 2008; Gordin 2015; Moller 2019; among many others).

This chapter aims to answer the following question: what motivates the translator's interest in medicine and its related disciplines through the ages? The answer – to transfer medical information that would otherwise remain inaccessible to other scientists around the world – will lead us through the discovery of how academic medical research was carried out, published and disseminated throughout the past all the way to the present day. This chapter will start with a historical overview, providing an examination of how medical research travelled from the ancient times until the invention of the printing press, and then describe the scientific boom that took place during the modern age and its consequences, both for medicine and for translation. The chapter then turns to the present-day dissemination of medical knowledge through a study of scientific journalism and specialised medical journals, which will inevitably lead to the current preponderance of English as the language of medicine. The chapter closes with a brief discussion on the future of medical academic research in today's interconnected world, and on the expected role of translation within these connections.

DOI: 10.4324/9781003167983-5

2 Historical perspectives

Finding a starting point from which to map when and how medical research started to spread prior to the invention of the printing press is not an easy task. However, it is clear that medicine itself is one of the oldest fields of recorded scientific activity due to the universality of the subject, since the human body and its diseases remain the same all over the world, unlike literature or religion. Medicine has also attracted more attention from translators than other scientific fields (Fischbach 1993: 92). Another issue that needs to be addressed before delving into the historical overview is to clarify the notions of 'science/scientific' and 'medicine/medical', and how these are used throughout this chapter. As Mumford correctly stated, 'at the beginning, chief, medicine man, magician, prophet, astronomer, priest were not separated functionaries' (Mumford in Vickery 2000: xvii). When mentioning the terms 'science' or 'scientific' we will always be including medicine herein, at least until we reach the specialisation and hyperspecialisation of more recent times.

Although, in line with many other Western scholars, our investigation of medical history begins with ancient Greece, we should not forget the important advancements carried out by physicians (or any other term we choose to assign to these first medical professionals) in other parts of the world. Delisle and Woodsworth (2012: 95) offer insights into some of the earliest translation activities, ranging from the Persian translator An Shigao, who is known for a translation of Sanskrit precepts into Chinese, to the Chinese Han Dynasty (206 BCE–226 CE) and later Song Dynasty (960–1280), during which some 20 Indian books on pharmacology and medicine were translated. We find an intense translation activity in India in the sixth century BCE, when the country had already established cultural ties with the Mediterranean region. The strength of this influence can be highlighted by the fact that 'the medical theories found in Plato's *Timaeus*, in works by Roman physicians and encyclopaedists, and in the writings of the Greek physicians Dioscorides and Galen are in fact of Indian origin' (Delisle and Woodsworth 1995: 108). These brief mentions highlight the obvious fact that, although it is traditional to start narratives of this kind with Greece, medicine has always been practised all over the world, particularly in the East.

Another aspect which will become relevant in the following section is that translators not only contributed to the spreading and dissemination of already existing medical research and knowledge, but that they also regarded translations as incentives for the production of their own medical texts (Jacquart and Micheau 1996: 45–54). For instance, Hunayn ibn Ishâq (ninth century, also known by his Latin name, Johannitius), the most celebrated translator of the renowned Baghdad-based House of Wisdom (see section 2.2.), wrote *Ten Treatises on the Eye* as well as the handbook *Questions on Medicine*. The latter was then translated into Latin by Constantine the African (11th century) and was referred to as the *Isagoge of Johannitius* (meaning 'Introduction' in Latin), becoming a reference book in medieval European universities (Laín Entralgo 1982: 159; Jacquart 1986; Vickery 2000: 27; Pormann and Savage-Smith 2007: 164). The Salernitan[2] commentaries written on various medical texts translated into Latin by the aforementioned monk Constantine and other translators rapidly spread to Naples and Paris and became a source of medical teaching and research for centuries to come (Vickery 2000: 38). Another well-known example is the Spanish translation of Dioscorides' *Materia Medica* by the physician Andrés Laguna published in 1555 with his own comments that doubled the size of the original work (Gutiérrez Rodilla 2009: 19–22). These are just a few examples from ancient and more recent times, but the mutual influence of translation on medicine is still strong, as will be shown below.

2.1 Greek medicine

Before referring to Greek medicine, it is important to remember that medical practice had traditionally been tied to magical and religious beliefs throughout Europe, and therefore the rational approach taken by the Greeks really was a turning point in the development of medicine. In fact, Greek was not just the language in which all kinds of medical interactions took place throughout classical antiquity, but also the etymological basis for most of our current medical terminology (both in Romance and in Germanic languages), mainly thanks to the Hippocratic Collection. This collection is composed of almost 70 books that have been traditionally ascribed to the Greek physician Hippocrates (5th and 4th centuries BCE), but which are in fact the works of different Greek schools of the 6th and 5th centuries BCE, like Knidos and Kos (López Férez 2000; Panourias *et al.* 2011). The most probable hypothesis for this attribution is that the Alexandrians who became interested in ancient medicine found numerous manuscripts written by multiple authors, and simply ascribed them all to Hippocrates (López Férez 2000; Panourias *et al.* 2011).

From the beginning of the 3rd century BCE onwards, the core of the cultural, scientific and medical world moved to Alexandria, where copyists working in its Museion[3] and Library compiled all the knowledge of the Middle East, the Mediterranean shores and even India into rolls and codices translated into Greek (García Bravo 2004: 28). By the end of that century, the Hellenisation of Rome had also affected the world of medicine, which began to be practised by Greek physicians, first as slaves and later as free citizens. This is one of the reasons why Greek has always predominated over Latin as the language of medicine and science. In fact, Latin never succeeded in becoming the language of medicine, neither in Greece nor in the other provinces of the Eastern Roman Empire (Gutiérrez Rodilla 1998: 43).

One of the most prominent figures of Greek medicine is Galen of Pergamon (2nd century CE), who remained the highest medical authority throughout the Middle Ages and whose teachings dominated medical discourse not only in Europe, but also in the Islamic world. He is often said to have a Hippocratic doctrine but an Aristotelian form (Babini 2000: 41), meaning that his work was based in the medical Hippocratic tradition, but he also relied on Platonic and Aristotelian ethical principles. Others, like Pormann and Savage-Smith, even say that 'he reshaped Hippocrates [...] in his own image' and 'succeeded in establishing himself as the "new Hippocrates"' (2007: 10). Galenism, understood as the medical theory that considers the equilibrium of four elemental humours (blood, phlegm, yellow and black bile) to be at the core of a healthy body, remained the predominant medical source until the 17th century, when the discovery of blood circulation caused its collapse. Galen's work can be considered the final synthesis of Greek medicine and its influence had a considerable impact on medical terminology due to its lasting prominence. The words used by Galen are still present in medical terminology of many languages (like *asphyxiation*/*Asphyxie*/*asfixia*/*asfissia*, *diastole*/*Diastole*/*diástole*/*diastole* [English/German/Spanish/Italian], etc. [see, for instance, López Piñero and Terrada Ferrandis 1990; Panourias *et al.* 2011; Berghammer 2006]). What is interesting however, is that Galenism became the main medical source in Europe thanks to translations of his work carried out in Baghdad, as the following section describes.

2.2 Islamic medicine

The Middle Ages experienced a rupture in science in general and in medicine in particular, roughly divided by the borders of the former Western and Eastern Roman Empire. In the West, medicine took refuge in monasteries from the 8th century onwards, where it was archived rather than practised or disseminated, causing it to fall into a lethargy from which it would take centuries to escape (Laín Entralgo 1982: 182; Moller 2019: 1–16). In contrast, the East experienced a period of rapid medical developments, both in the form of originally written works as well as through numerous translations. The Islamic world assimilated Hellenistic medical knowledge through extensive translations of medical works from Greek into Arabic (on this issue, see extensively Jacquart and Micheau 1996; Gutas 1998; Pormann and Savage-Smith 2007; Saliba 2007; and also the historiographically critical comments on this Greco-Arabic transmission of knowledge by Montgomery 2000: 89–93). These texts were usually first rendered into Semitic languages (mainly Syriac, which often served as an intermediary language, but also Pahlavi and Hebrew to a lesser extent [Taylor 2007]), and from these intermediary languages into Arabic (Laín Entralgo 1982: 158; Gutiérrez Rodilla 1998: 48; Gutas 1998: 20–24; García Bravo 2004: 30–31; Delisle and Woodsworth 2012: 106–109; Jacquart and Micheau 1996: 32–45; Montgomery 2000: 89–137; Jacquart 2005; Daiber 2007; Saliba 2007: 73; Pormann and Savage-Smith 2007: 6–79). This activity reached its peak in the 9th and 10th centuries in Baghdad with the support of the caliphs, who attracted translators and scientists of all kinds to their court (Gutas 1998). Scholars in the so-called House of Wisdom,[4] founded in the year 830, produced translations of Byzantine texts, numerous Hippocratic writings, more than a hundred works by Galen, as well as other works by Greek scientists and several Indian physicians, all under the direction of Hunayn ibn Ishâq, a 'tireless translator' (Laín Entralgo 1982: 159) and 'the master of all Islamic translators' (Delisle and Woodsworth 2012: 237). The translation of the Indian collection of Sushruta carried out during this time would later introduce Indian precepts in surgery into European medicine, and the translation of Galen's works established his practices in European and Islamic medicine for centuries to come (Jacquart and Micheau 1996: 43; Gutas 1998: 119; Pormann and Savage-Smith 2007: 43ff.; Saliba 2007: 73–129). These texts came primarily from Greek but also Sanskrit, Syriac and occasionally Egyptian, and the Arabic versions were later translated into Latin (see section 2.3.) and so travelled back to medieval Europe (Taylor 2007: 1190). This means that although Galen's scholarship dates back to the second century CE, it did not become the predominant medical practice in Europe until the 13th century, and that this Latin version of his texts was predominantly based on previous translations into Arabic.

Translation was just one of many activities that these scholars and scientists performed: they acquired Greek manuscripts (sometimes by travelling large distances), established their authenticity, compiled compendia and were also the authors of original texts (Delisle and Woodsworth 2012: 108; Jacquart and Micheau 1996: 45–54; Gutas 1998: 133–140; Gutiérrez Rodilla 1998: 52; Saliba 2007: 66–67; Pormann and Savage-Smith 2007: 13). The scholars who worked along these lines include Rhazes as well as Avicenna (Latinised name of Ibn Sina), whose *Canon of Medicine* was an important medical source until the 18th century (Sánchez Granjel 1968; Laín Entralgo 1982; Jacquart and Micheau 1996; Pormann and Savage-Smith 2007). The *Canon* was a compilation of all ancient and Arab medical knowledge that combined Greek medical experience with Aristotelian philosophy in a way that challenged the authority of their precursors, and contained critical commentaries on ancient sources (Pormann and Savage-Smith 2007: 47–50). These translators and scholars also played a didactic role through their explanations and commentaries, such as in the original works of the renowned translator Hunayn ibn Ishâq, which are frequently written in the form of questions and answers (Delisle and Woodsworth 2012: 108–109; Pormann and Savage-Smith 2007: 68). Some translators went beyond these additional commentaries and made transformations in the original texts that were supposed to 'cleanse the mistakes of the Greek tradition' (Saliba 2007: 129), which were a frequent possibility, given that dissections had not been practised in Galen's times. Many translators confronted the teachings with their own practical findings, such as al-Baghdadi's observation of just one human jawbone, where Galen had described two.

2.3 Medical research prior to the printing press: the 'forgotten ones'

Antoine Berman coined the expression 'the forgotten ones' (1989: 677), referring to the translators of the so-called School of Toledo, which played a big role in spreading (not just) medical knowledge in Europe by translating scientific achievements of the Greek and Arab world from Arabic to Latin and later to vernacular Spanish (Valls 2007). These translations were fundamental to the transmission of science in medieval Europe and those 'forgotten' translators 'radically altered the state of knowledge in the West' (Delisle and Woodsworth 2012: 110). There is some doubt regarding the existence of the School: some argue, like in the case of the House of Wisdom in Baghdad (see note 4), that it was rather a circle of translators who worked individually or in small groups under the supervision of a patron (Gutiérrez Rodilla 1998: 53; Santoyo 2004: 3 and 2009; Delisle and Woodsworth 2012:109–110). In any case, we can speak of a systematic translation movement of Arabic works and 'an organisation or "professionalism" of translation in Toledo' (Burnett 2007: 1232). Wright (2007) points out that there was little need for interlinguistic translations between Latin and the first Romance languages. Instead 'the spoken version needed merely to be "polished" rather than translated to become an acceptable text', after which 'a literate Christian originally from outside Al-Andalus would [...] elaborate a written text in the necessary formal register' (Wright 2007: 1267). This also confirms that the translation process was mainly oral.

These translations opened the door to Greek and Arabic medical knowledge in Western Europe (Laín Entralgo 1982: 197; on this School, see *in extenso* Schipperges 1961; Sangrador Gil 1985; Jacquart 1992a; Samsó 1996; Vegas González 1998). The translators of this School, such as Domingo Gundisalvo, Juan Hispano, Andrés the Jew, Pedro Gallego, Mark of Toledo and Gerard of Cremona, amongst many others, translated and in many ways co-created classical works on medicine. These included Hippocratic and Galenic treatises as well as the works of principal Arabic authors, such as Avicenna, Rhazes, Abulcasis or Al-Kindi, among many others (about the transmission of Arabic medical knowledge to medieval Latin, see the classical works by Schipperges [1964, 2003: 25–42; see also the recollection of his works related to this matter edited in 2006]; Jacquart [1992b and 2005], as well as Jacquart and Micheau [1996]). These Castilian translations ensured that texts that had previously been *auctoritate* in various medical areas continued to be so until the Renaissance (Valls 2007: 1373).

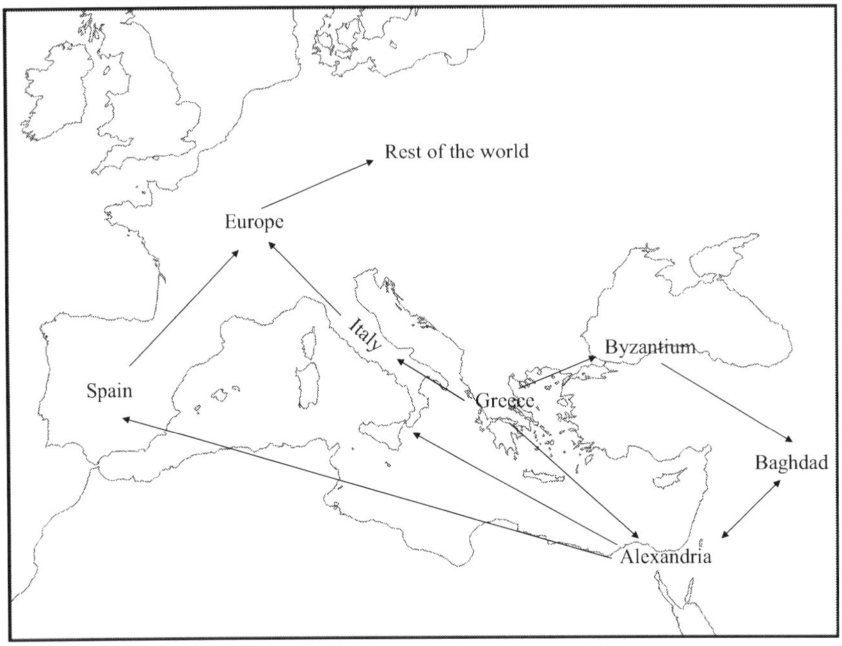

Figure 3.1 The simplified trace of scientific and medical development through time.

Figure 3.1 shows the movement of scientific (and thus medical) knowledge and its journey from Greece to Rome, then to Byzantium, Alexandria, Persia, until it arrived in Europe, and from there expanded to the rest of the world. Table 3.1 (see next page) shows the common paths that medicine and translation followed in their historical journey.

This necessarily short overview on medical research and its transmission is not only tied to translations, but also to the history of paper and the dissemination of writing, which will be the subject of the next section.

2.4 The printing press and the scientific boom during the modern age

The way in which all the medical texts mentioned so far have reached us was through copyists and booksellers, i.e. thanks to a rudimentary book trade that evolved from the Egyptian papyrus to animal skins up to the more recent parchment. In Europe, the development of cities and the world of universities in the late Middle Ages brought with it a flourishing bookstore and publishing industry which supplied the copies needed for consultation and teaching. But the invention of the printing press in the mid-15th century meant a significant change in the dissemination of knowledge in general, and of medical knowledge in particular. Indeed, the printing press had the same impact on the circulation of translation in the Renaissance as the introduction of paper had previously had in the Arabic world (Delisle and Woodsworth 2012: 96). In the case of medicine, the printing press served to exhume classical and medieval medical texts, rather than propagate works by new scholars, particularly in the last years of the 15th and throughout the 16h century.

Table 3.1 The common paths in the history of medicine and translation

Approximate date (place)	*Direction of translation (source language → target language)*
3rd century BCE onwards *(Alexandria)*	Sanskrit (all Eastern knowledge) → Greek
5th and 6th centuries CE *(Byzantium)*	Greek (original, fundamental works) → Syrian, Persian, Hindi, Syriac
8th and 9th centuries CE *(East, mainly Baghdad)*	Greek, Sanskrit, Syriac, Egyptian (original works) → Arabic
10th century *(Córdoba)*	Greek → Arabic
9th – 12th centuries *(Montecasino, Salernitan School)*	Arabic (Greek translated works and texts written originally in Arabic) → Latin
12th and 13th centuries *(Translators' School of Toledo)*	Arabic (mainly classical Greek works) → Latin → Spanish, Catalan
12th and 13th centuries *(Provence and Iberian Peninsula)*	Arabic (classical Greek works and other Arabic works) → Hebrew[a]
15th and 16th centuries *(All Europe)*	Greek → Ciceronian Latin

a It has been repeatedly claimed that translations from Arabic to Hebrew only took place in Provence, but it must be pointed out that many of these translations were carried out in the Iberian Peninsula. On this matter and on the works of medical translators into Hebrew, see Gutiérrez Rodilla (2007: 285–304), Pormann and Savage-Smith (2007: 164–165), Valls (2007: 1374) and Ferre (2012).

Out of the 3,000 books printed during the 15th century in Europe, that is, in the earliest stages of printing, 30 per cent were either medical books or texts related to medicine in some way. This fact shows the important contribution that medicine had in the scientific and book publishing activity during the Renaissance (Riera Palmero 1989: 8). In fact, medicine constituted quantitatively the most important profession and publishing activity among scientific and technical knowledge at that time (Riera Palmero 1989: 8). The majority of data indicates that physicians were always the most avid buyers of scientific publications, and that they owned almost 70 per cent of the science books of the 16th century in Europe, and up to 85 per cent in the 17th (Riera Palmero 1989: 9).

The period from the 15th to the 17th century, denoted by some as the first globalisation era (Steger 2009; Lambert 2007), was marked by European colonial expansion, the creation of the Spanish Empire, a significant reorganisation of European monarchies and religious divisions, as well as by an expansion in the circulation of medical knowledge. Although Latin continued to be the language of medical communication among the international academic elite (Gordin 2015: 167), some books were printed in vernacular languages, like Spanish, Italian, German or French. These books were aimed at the non-professional, wider readership, and included volumes such as manuals of anatomy, books about childbirth, or descriptions of new diseases. As the 17th century progressed, the works written in vernacular languages showed an important increase compared to Latin (Gutiérrez Rodilla 2005: 302; Valls 2007: 1374; Barona 2017: 15), mainly due to two facts: first, apothecaries and other laypeople practising various forms of healing had not received any higher education and could not understand treatises written in Latin in their entirety; at the same time, a number of people tried to cure themselves as they lacked access to any medical care, especially in rural areas. Vernacular languages were also the tool used to spread information on infectious diseases or epidemics, such as the bubonic plague (see, for instance, the case of Luis Mercado, whose *Opera omnia* was written in Latin, but who wrote his *Libro*

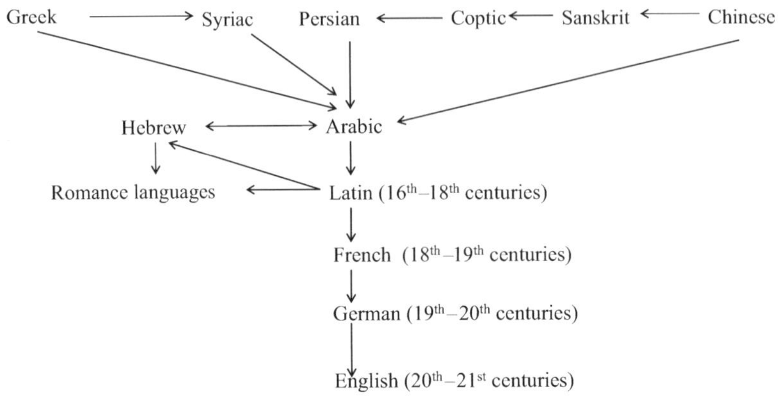

Figure 3.2 Interlinguistic movements in the history of medicine, translated and adapted from Gutiérrez Rodilla (1998: 55) and Aréchaga (2014: 23).

de la Peste [1599] in Spanish [Mariscal 1921]). These publications targeted an educated audience without a medical background who had the resources to spread information about these preventive measures amongst the general public both in cities and rural areas (Gutiérrez Rodilla 2005: 303).

For a long time, vernacular languages had little reason to compete against one another in medical publications, as they were more focused on fighting the overwhelming presence of Latin (Valls 2007: 1374). This changed in the 18th century as Latin gradually declined in its influence and a new confrontation started to emerge between the main languages of culture and wisdom, especially between French and German and, to a lesser extent and somewhat later, English. This particular fight was linked to the social, political and economic powers of the nations where those languages were spoken, rather than to the scientific advances achieved in each of them. As the Spanish humanist Antonio de Nebrija stated in his 1492 *Grammar of the Castilian Language*, language 'was always the companion of empire, and followed it such that together they began, grew, and flourished – and, later, together they fell'.[5]

Figure 3.2, illustrating the historically intense translating activities outlined in this section, shows that there has always been a dominating lingua franca in the history of medical transmission of knowledge. However, every lingua franca has co-lived with other languages, whether these belonged to other areas or were part of the emerging vulgar languages (see the aforementioned cases of Syriac, Arabic, Greek, Latin and the European vernacular languages). This echoes the current position of English as the language of leading medical research while sharing a (rather small) portion of it with other languages; a situation which, as some point out, will continue in the next years (Montgomery 2004, 2009 and 2013; Ammon 2012). One of the critical issues that will be addressed in the next section is precisely linked to this preponderance of one language over others in medical communication and the impact of this struggle on translation, especially in contemporary times.

3 Current critical issues

The origin and subsequent development of the scientific journal as the main means of communication between medical researchers is an aspect that must be studied in depth in order to know where transmission of medical research is heading, hand in hand with the interlinguistic translation that it inevitably entails. As described in the previous section, advances in medical research were spread first through manuscripts, then books, and later through encyclopaedias and dictionaries. Today, that role has been taken over by specialised journals. These publications have experienced an exponential rise since they first appeared around the middle of the 17th century: from 300 journals published in the period between 1665–1730 (Vickery 2000: 94) to millions of publications in the present day. As far back as 1981, Berry described the evolution of scientific and medical journals with the following ironic statement:

> In the beginning was the General Scientific Journal. And the General Scientific Journal begat the Specialty Journal, and the Specialty Journal begat the Subspecialty Journal. And the Subspecialty Journal begat the Single-Subject Journal, whether according to class of compound, specific disease, or methodology.
>
> *Berry 1981: 400*

He then tries to answer the question on why there is such a proliferation of new journals and gives the following reasons, most of which are as valid today as they were 40 years ago: delay in publication in the established journals frequently causing the creation of new minor ones; the growth of new specialities not easily accommodated in the already existing journals; the growth of science in general; and, last but not least, academic pressures. These elements have led to 'an epidemic of fragmentation of data' (Berry 1981: 402) that can be partly associated with Garfield's impact factor. Developed as early as 1955 (see Garfield 2006), the impact factor was originally established so that not just large journals were cited and read, but also smaller, less prominent ones; at the same time, however, the impact factor and the subsequent need of scholars to be read and cited worldwide has brought with it an unintended consequence – the requirement to publish almost exclusively in the current lingua franca. As a result, Garfield's impact factor has had, ironically, an immeasurable influence on scientific and medical research, especially in its writing and transmission (Ammon 2012), and his well-known formula 'publish or perish' has now shifted to 'publish in English or perish'.

Many scholars have already brought this issue to attention; a paper entitled 'Is Impact Factor killing the German Language?' speaks for itself (Haller, Hepp and Reinold 1999). Others have proposed local measures in order to solve the problem, such as the suggestion by the Association of the Scientific Medical Societies in Germany in 1999 to multiply the impact factor of research contributions published in German by two (Frömter *et al.* 1999: 912; Wiese 2006). Ammon (2012: 351) even proposed that Anglophones could 'be persuaded to take on an extra share of costs, perhaps for publishing or for conferences'. While these measures might seem extreme, the suggestions are perhaps understandable if we take into account studies like the one carried out by a group of Scandinavian scientists (Nylenna, Riis and Karlsson 1994). In this study, two fictional but genuine-looking short manuscripts were sent to 180 Scandinavian referees, one in English and the other in the national language; unsurprisingly, the English version was accepted more easily than the national-language version of the very same manuscript. This trend has a direct impact on medical translation, as will be seen in the next section.

3.1 Specialised journals and medical monolingualism

In 2007, Beecroft described the explosion of medical journals on the Internet as a radical change not only in the whole scientific publishing process, but also in the globalised access to medical journals. The Internet has made possible the publication and dissemination of medical research theoretically from everywhere and for any audience. However, with English being the current lingua franca of science, this also has had an impact on the evolution of national medical languages. Researchers can either choose to publish in English or as good as cease to exist for the scientific community: 'Only English-language journals achieve high impact factors, because journals in other languages are unlikely to be read and cited internationally' (Baethge 2008: 39). Beecroft (2007: 204) poses the following question: 'Is there any point in publishing in any other language than English?' He proposes that the question has a twofold answer, depending on the target audience of the paper or journal: international journals should aim at every possible reader, and therefore publish in English; national journals, on the other hand, should continue to publish in their local languages. Beecroft's ideas still obtain, more than 10 years after being proposed, as we shall see on the example of Spanish-written medical journals. Spanish is the third most spoken language in the world (around 7.8 per cent of the world's population speaks Spanish; see Instituto Cervantes 2017), after English and Chinese. However, between 2005 and 2015, an overwhelming 99.44 per cent of total publications in the field of biomedicine collected in the Web of Science database were written in English. This was followed by French with 0.13 per cent, and Chinese with 0.11 per cent, with Spanish ranking fourth and representing a meagre 0.08 per cent (Plaza and García-Carpintero 2017).

Spanish provides an interesting comparison with German, which has a much smaller number of speakers but remains important given the social, economic and political weight of Germany.[6] German-language journals make up almost one-fifth of all periodicals subscribed to by the German National Library of Medicine (Baethge 2008: 38). There is clearly a high demand for medical journals written in German, as 7 out of 10 German physicians consider it important or very important that the specialised articles they read are in German (Baethge 2008: 38; Wiese 2006). Gordin describes the dilemma of German researchers, who 'have to make the difficult choice between identity and communication, between supporting journals and educational institutions in their native language or disseminating cutting-edge research to the broadest-possible readership' (Gordin 2015: 312).

3.2 Translating medicine today

The aforementioned dilemma is directly related to translation and linked to the idea suggested by Beecroft (2007): medical journals should be written in the local languages in order to boost local research and to display geographical, socio-economic and/or national interests. In fact, taking again Spanish as an example, nearly all scientific journals aimed at Spanish-speaking researchers and physicians are related to scientific areas linked to local and geographical interests (García Delgado, Alonso and Jiménez 2013: 348). Others point out that medical research carried out in countries where English is not the official or vehicular language should not stay inside their borders or remain unknown to the international scientific community, as denounced in the paper 'Lost Science in the Third World' (Gibbs 1995; see also Horton 2000 or Ammon 2012). This brings us to the next issue. The fact that so many medical journals from non-Anglophone countries[7] are published in English brought new phenomena to the medical publishing sector, such as the so-called 'medical writers' (Daskalopoulou and Mikhailidis 2005) or 'ghost-writers' (Matías-Guiu and García Ramos 2011). These are understood as professional writers who are hired by scientists or pharmaceutical and medical companies to write medical articles on their behalf, and in which they do not appear as authors, thus questioning the notion of intellectual authorship. Another recent phenomenon linked to publishing in English is the appearance of bilingual editions of journals, which is of particular interest for translators. This is the case of the Spanish journals *Neurología* or *Revista Española de Cardiología*, both of which publish all of their articles simultaneously in Spanish and in English, and where translations from Spanish to English are carried out by a group of specialised translators (Matías-Guiu, García Ramos and Porta-Etessam 2014). There are other examples across the globe: *Deutsches Ärzteblatt* is published both in German and English since 2008; the *Revista Brasileira de Reumatologia* has published bilingual articles in Portuguese and English since 2009; *Arquivos Brasileiros de Cardiologia* provides an English translation of any article submitted in another language with no cost to the author; Turkey's *Acta Orthopaedica et Traumatologica Turcica* publishes in English but makes both English and Turkish versions of every paper available on its website (Olohan 2016: 143). Numerous journals published in Germany, Austria and Switzerland have gone a step further and changed their language of publication and in many cases even their names from German to English (Ammon 2012: 344). The role played by translators in this process has so far not been subject to any extensive studies (Olohan 2014; Olohan and Salama-Carr 2011) and further research is needed on how language-specialists are influencing not just the form, but also the content of the medical texts they are working on. Some argue that medical writers, translators and any other language or communication professionals in the medical field who are not subject experts could give advice to researchers to improve readability in their writing, but that they also 'may miss deficiencies in the logic and argumentation because they do not grasp the scientific content' (Shashok 2008). Others point to the contradictory position of some medical editors, who, on the one hand, condemn medical writers (understood as language professionals, see Laine and Mulrow [2005] or *The Lancet*'s Editorial in 1993) but, on the other, insist on having manuscripts from non-native English writers edited and proofread by an Anglophone native speaker prior to submitting it for the peer-review process (Matías-Guiu and García Ramos 2011: 258). This so-called scientific monolingualism (Vandenbroucke 1989; Gibbs 1995; Timo-Iaria 1998; Horton 2000; Ammon 2001, 2010 and 2012; Montgomery 2004, 2009 and 2013; Navarro 1998, 2001 and 2002; Gordin 2015) has as its direct consequence that most of the medical translations today have English either as their source or target language.

Apart from the translation of academic journal articles, medical translation is today a growing market segment that covers a wide range of interlinguistic communicative needs – those of publishing houses, pharmaceutical laboratories, international organisations, government or state institutions, university research groups, medical equipment companies, hospitals and other health-related centres and organisations. Some of the typical medicine and health-related products that enjoy a greater volume of translation are summaries of product characteristics, patient information leaflets, press releases or medical products advertisements, as well as original research articles and patents (Montalt and González Davies 2007; Montalt and Shuttleworth 2012).

The hyperspecialisation that Berry criticised in his 1981 paper had a direct impact on translation, the field of translation studies and on current translators' training programmes. As pointed out by Faya and Quijada (2019), Spanish universities have experienced not only growth in programmes on translation training, but specifically in courses focusing on scientific and medical subjects, both at undergraduate and postgraduate level. This increase is not accidental, but rather reflects the market's needs for specialised medical translation, and this is also demonstrated by the studies regarding this type of translation and research published in recent years (Wright and Wright 1993; Navarro 1997; Fischbach

1998; Montalt and González Davies 2007; Montalt and Shuttleworth 2012; Byrne 2012; Varela Salinas and Meyer 2015; Olohan 2016, to name a few).

4 Future directions

The previous sections have briefly described the pathways of medical translations through history as well as medical academic research in today's interconnected world. The aforementioned preponderance of the English language both in medical research and publishing has a very powerful effect on the role we expect translation to play these days. Most of the medical texts that undergo a translation process unsurprisingly have English either as their source or their target language (Montgomery 2009; Faya and Quijada 2019). These developments open questions about what our societies are losing with this linguistic reductionism from and to English. One of the consequences of this issue has already been addressed – the fact that English is a non-native language for most of its users within medical research means we can speak of an 'asymmetric global language, whose advantages are unequally distributed' (Ammon 2012: 342). Another effect of this anglicisation is that many of the leading scientists who work, research and live in languages other than English rarely or never write in their own mother tongues, which is a clear consequence of this language predominance (Montgomery 2013: 158) and in turn means that other languages lose their significance. It must also be considered that not all physicians in the world, not even in Western countries, are capable of reading and understanding medical literature in English (what Baethge [2008: 39] named 'frictional loses'), and therefore new medical knowledge is spreading far more slowly than would be desirable (Graddol 2006).

An example of the issues caused by this imbalance is the disease *brucellosis,* which affects hundreds of thousands of people and animals worldwide and has been endemic in some European areas, but which occurs very rarely in the United States. A translation of a handbook on internal medicine originally written in the United States will be unlikely to include any reference to this illness and as such be of limited use in the training of European physicians, who would instead learn about diseases that are uncommon in Europe. Similarly, scientists might be working on issues which have already been researched by scientists in other countries, as was the case of the plant hormone *gibberellin*, which the Japanese had been working on for years, just not in English (Gordin 2015: 313). Again, this is all linked to the way research is disseminated and, most importantly, cited, as measured by the aforementioned impact factor. It all seems to constitute a vicious circle from which it is very difficult to escape.

Looking back at our history, we know now that the world tends to strive for some kind of common language to communicate innovation and research. Section 2 has shown that every era in which a massive translation activity was carried out required a lingua franca to translate from or into. We are witnessing the same phenomenon today as English expands and is simultaneously challenged by languages such as Spanish or Mandarin (Montgomery 2009 and 2013; Graddol 2006: 113). Similarly to a number of examples from specialised journals which also publish in English, we can look at the cases of *Nature*, which publishes Chinese, Korean and Japanese editions, or *Science*, *Science Signaling* and *Science: Transnational Medicine*, with English and Japanese versions (Olohan 2016: 143).

As mentioned, a number of voices from the scholarly community advocate the use of national languages together with English as a lingua franca, which eases communication but does not prevent native speakers of other languages from doing research, writing and translating from and into their mother tongues (Montgomery 2000, 2004, 2009; Ammon 2001, 2010, 2012; Beecroft 2007; Gutiérrez Rodilla 2014). Medical research should be maintained in the mother tongue in order to enrich the language and, an utmost relevant factor too often forgotten, to keep research and medical knowledge available to native speakers in those countries where the research has been developed and financed. The disappearance of native languages from domestic research is a 'true diminishment' (Montgomery 2013: 116). English must be learnt, spoken and written in order to have better opportunities on the international scene and to participate in the international medical knowledge exchange, but by doing so, one is not obliged to abandon their mother tongue. Scientists and physicians must bear in mind they belong to an international community but also to a national one that they ought to defend and promote on the international stage. And for these purposes, translators will continue to play the role that historically rendered them the 'pollinators of science' and spread medical knowledge throughout the world.

Notes

1 The author wishes to acknowledge her participation in the Research Project PID2019-109565 RB-I00/AEI/10.13039/501100011033, funded by the Spanish National Research Programme.

2 The town of Salerno (near Naples, Italy) was home to one of the most renowned schools of medicine in Europe since Roman times. From the tenth century onwards, its doctors were known for their practical skills. Both the monastery of Monte Cassino and the town of Salerno played an important role in the transmission of Arab and Greek science, mainly thanks to the monk Constantine, whose work consisted not just of translating, but also of paraphrasing and adding comments on the original Arab and Greek texts and who 'formed one of the bases of medical teaching for several hundred years' (Vickery 2000: 38).

3 In 280 BCE Ptolemy founded the Museion of Alexandria, an interdisciplinary institution for teaching and research purposes where scholars would have the best working conditions to develop and widen their knowledge (free meals, housing, no taxes, high salaries, etc.; see Nesselrath 2013: 73). This centre's orientation remained Aristotelian. However, it was intended to counteract the influence of the Athenian schools of anti-monarchist ideology. Later the Library was founded, which came to have thousands of volumes and a large number of copyists, together with facilities for the dissection of corpses and for the study of plants and animals, thus becoming the most prestigious and important centre of its time. Its great rival was the Pergamon Library, founded in the 2nd century BCE (García Bravo 2004: 28).

4 Similarly to what has been written about Toledo's School of Translators, it has been argued whether this so-called House of Wisdom ever existed as such:

> Reliable evidence for this legend, however, is virtually non-existent. Dimitri Gutas, who has recently reviewed the available sources, concludes that if such a House of Wisdom ever existed, it is best explained as a library where translations from Persian into Arabic were stored. In any case, it was completely unrelated to the Graeco-Arabic translation movement of the ninth century.
>
> *Pormann and Savage-Smith 2007: 29*

In fact, Gutas in his 1998 book *Greek Thought, Arabic Culture* does not mention the House of Wisdom as such (just the Imperial Library), but instead sets out an erudite and thoroughly well-documented list of the available sources of scientific knowledge for the historical study of that period, ranging from Greek manuscripts (both in the Islamic realm and in Byzantium) to their copies and their Arabic translations (Gutas 1998: see especially Chapter 7: 151–186 and the table on pages 182–183). He concedes that there was indeed a climate that facilitated the Greco-Arabic translation movement (1998: 54–59).

5 Translation from Spanish by Armillas-Tiseyra (2016: 197).

6 With around 130 million native speakers or near-native speakers, German is the most spoken native language in the European Union, and the official language of seven countries. Data from *Tatsachen über Deutschland*, available at www.tatsachen-ueber-deutschland.de/de/rubriken/kultur-medien/attraktive-sprache (accessed 20 July 2019) and the article 'Man spricht Deutsch', from the German Foreign Office (Auswärtiges Amt), available at www.deutschland.de/de/topic/kultur/deutsche-sprache-ueberraschende-zahlen-und-fakten (Accessed: 20 July 2019).

7 'Anglophone countries' understood here in Ammon's definition (2012: 334), i.e. the 'inner-circle English-speaking countries', which include the United States, the United Kingdom, the Republic of Ireland, Canada, Australia and New Zealand.

Further reading

Delisle, J. and Woodsworth, J. (eds) (2012) *Translators Through History*. Amsterdam and Philadelphia: John Benjamins.

This monograph introduces both students and researchers to the role of translation throughout human history, from the invention of the alphabets to the emergence of national languages together with the transmission of cultural and religious values, as well as the dissemination of knowledge addressed in Chapter 4 (pages 95–124).

Montgomery, S. L. (2000) *Science in Translation: Movements of Knowledge through Cultures and Time*. Chicago: University of Chicago Press.

Like the previous monograph, this seminal work gives an insight into what translation has meant to the dissemination of knowledge in ancient and medieval times. Although a third of the book focuses on astronomy, the translation movements that took place in the past, including works on medicine, are explained in great detail.

Vickery, B. C. (2000) *Scientific Communication in History*. London: The Scarecrow Press.

This book focuses on how science made its way through history. Although not specially focused on health nor translation, both aspects play an important role throughout the work. Particularly interesting is the overview of science spreading from beyond the West and of the development and organisation of science in past and present times.

Gutiérrez Rodilla, B. M. (1998) *La ciencia empieza en la palabra. Análisis e historia del lenguaje científico.* Barcelona: Península.

Written in Spanish, it has not been translated into any other language. Although it was published more than 20 years ago, it still offers an outstanding overview of the development of medical language through history, in which translation plays a major role. This work could be a first reference point for these issues for undergraduate and postgraduate students who are new to the field.

Related topics

Medical Translations from Greek Into Arabic and Hebrew, Translations of Western Medical Texts in East Asia, Medical Humanities and Translation

References

Ammon, U. (ed.) (2001) *The Dominance of English as a Language of Science. Effects on Other Languages and Language Communities*. Berlin: De Gruyter.

Ammon, U. (2010) 'English and Other International Languages Under the Impact of Globalization', *Neuphilologische Mitteilungen*, 111(1), pp. 9–28.

Ammon, U. (2012) 'Linguistic Inequality and Its Effects on Participation in Scientific Discourse and on Global Knowledge Accumulation – With a Closer Look at the Problems of the Second-Rank Language Communities', *Applied Linguistics Review*, 3(2), pp. 333–355.

Aréchaga, J. (2014) 'Lenguaje y comunicación en la investigación biomédica básica', in Gutiérrez Rodilla, B. M. and Navarro, F. E. (eds) *La importancia del lenguaje en el entorno biosanitario*. Barcelona: Fundación Dr. Antonio Esteve, pp. 21–32.
Armillas-Tiseyra, M. (2016) 'On Language and Empire: The Prologue to Grammar of the Castilian *Language* (1492)', *PMLA*, 131(1), pp. 197–208.
Babini, J. (2000) *Historia de la medicina*. Barcelona: Gedisa.
Baethge, C. (2008) 'The Languages of Medicine', *Deutsches Ärzteblatt International*, 105(3), pp. 37–40.
Barona, J. L. (2017) 'Lo que pudo ser y no fue: el español en los albores de la ciencia moderna', *Educación Médica*, 18(2), pp. 12–16.
Beecroft, I. R. (2007) 'Globalización de las revistas médicas en línea: ¿cuál es el futuro de las revistas nacionales, continentales, internacionales?', *CirCardiov*, 14(3), pp. 203–206.
Berghammer, G. (2006) 'Translation and the Language(s) of Medicine: Keys to Producing a Successful German-English Translation', *The Write Stuff*, 15(2), pp. 40–44.
Berman, A. (1989) 'La traduction et ses discurs', *Meta*, 24(4), pp. 672–679.
Berry, E. M. (1981) 'The Evolution of Scientific and Medical Journals', *The New England Journal of Medicine*, 305(7), pp. 400–402.
Burnett, C. (2007) 'Translation from Arabic into Latin in the Middle Ages (Übersetzungen aus dem Arabischen ins Latainische im Mittelalter)', in Kittel, H., House, J. and Schultze, B. (eds) *Übersetzung – Translation – Traduction: Ein internationales Handbuch zur Übersetzungsforschung / An international Encyclopaedia of Translation Studies / Encyclopédie internationale de la recherche sur la traduction*, vol. 2. Berlin: De Gruyter, pp. 1231–1237.
Byrne, J. (2012) *Scientific and Technical Translation Explained: A Nuts and Bolts Guide for Beginners*. London and New York: Routledge.
Daiber, H. (2007) 'Die griechisch-arabische Wissenschaftsüberlieferung in der arabisch-islamischen Kultur in Übersetzungen des 8.–10. Jahrhunderts', in Kittel, H., House, J. and Schultze, B. (eds) *Übersetzung – Translation – Traduction: Ein internationales Handbuch zur Übersetzungsforschung / An International Encyclopaedia of Translation Studies / Encyclopédie internationale de la recherche sur la traduction*, vol. 2. Berlin: De Gruyter, pp. 1206–1217.
Daskalopoulou, S. S. and Mikhailidis, D. P. (2005) 'The Involvement of Professional Medical Writers in Medical Publications', *Current Medical Research and Opinion*, 21(2), pp. 307–310.
Delisle, J. and Woodsworth, J. (eds) (2012) *Translators Through History*. Amsterdam and Philadelphia: John Benjamins.
Faya, G. and Quijada, C. (2019) 'Scientific and Medical Translation', in Valdeón, R. A. and Vidal, Á. (eds) *The Routledge Handbook of Spanish Translation Studies*. London and New York: Routledge, pp. 288–310.
Ferre, L. (2012) 'The Jewish Contribution to the Transmission of the Classical Legacy', *European Review*, 20(4), pp. 552–562. DOI:10.1017/S106279871200012.
Fischbach, H. (1993) 'Translation, the Great Pollinator of Science: A Brief Flashback on Medical Translation', in Wright, S. E. and Wright, L. D. (eds) *Scientific and Technical Translation*. Amsterdam and Philadelphia: John Benjamins, pp. 89–100.
Fischbach, H. (1998) *Translation and Medicine*. Amsterdam and Philadelphia: John Benjamins.
Frömter, E., Brähler, E., Langenbeck, U., Meenen, N. M. and Usadel, K-H. (1999) 'Das AWMF-Modell zur Evaluierung publizierter Forschungsbeiträge in der Medizin', *Deutsche Medizinische Wochenschrift*, 124(30), pp. 910–915.
García Bravo, P. (2004) 'Las traducciones en la transmisión del legado médico clásico al mundo occidental', *Hieronymus*, 11, pp. 25–42.
García Delgado, J. L., Alonso, J. A. and Jiménez, J. C. (eds) (2013) *El español, lengua de comunicación científica*. Madrid: Ariel/Fundación Telefónica.
Garfield, E. (2006) 'The History and Meaning of the Journal Impact Factor', *JAMA*, 295(1), pp. 90–93.
Gibbs, W. W. (1995) 'Lost Science in the Third World', *Scientific American*, 273, pp. 92–99.
Gordin, M. D. (2015) *Scientific Babel. How Science Was Done Before and After Global English*. Chicago: University of Chicago Press.
Graddol, D. (2006) *English Next*. London: British Council.
Gutas, D. (1998) *Greek Thought, Arabic Culture. The Greco-Arabic Translation Movement in Baghdad and Early 'Abbāsid Society (2nd–4th/8th–10th centuries)*. London and New York: Routledge.

Gutiérrez Rodilla, B. M. (1998) *La ciencia empieza en la palabra. Análisis e historia del lenguaje científico.* Barcelona: Península.
Gutiérrez Rodilla, B. M. (2003) 'La historia del lenguaje científico como parte de la historia de la ciencia', *Asclepio*, 55(2), pp. 7–25.
Gutiérrez Rodilla, B. M. (2005) 'La medicina, sus textos y sus lenguas en la España de Cervantes', *Panace@*, 6(21–22), pp. 299–306.
Gutiérrez Rodilla, B. M. (2007) *La esforzada reelaboración del saber. Repertorios médicos de interés lexicográfico anteriores a la imprenta*. San Millán de la Cogolla: Cilengua.
Gutiérrez Rodilla, B. M. (2008) 'La impronta de la traducción sobre el discurso científico: toda una historia', *Puntoycoma*, 106, pp. 17–30.
Gutiérrez Rodilla, B. M. (2009) *Medicina y terapéutica en el Renacimiento: Andrés Laguna y la* Materia Médica *de Dioscórides*. Salamanca: Caja Duero.
Gutiérrez Rodilla B. M. (2014) 'El lenguaje de la medicina en español: cómo hemos llegado hasta aquí y qué futuro nos espera', *Panace@*, 15(39), pp. 86–94.
Haller, M., Hepp, H. and Reinold, E. (1999) 'Tötet der "Impact Factor" die deutsche Sprache?' *Der Chirurg*, 38(2), pp. 39–41.
Horton, R. (2000) 'North and South: Bridging the Information Gap', *Lancet* 355, pp. 2231–2236.
Instituto Cervantes (2017) *El español: una lengua viva.* Informe 2017. Available at: https://cvc.cervantes.es/lengua/anuario/anuario_17/default.htm (Accessed 16 July 2019).
Jacquart, D. (1986) 'A l'aube de la renaissance médicale des XIe–XIIe siècles: l'Isagoge Johannitii et son Traducteur', *Bibliothèque de l'École des Chartres*, 144, pp. 209–240.
Jacquart, D. (1992a) 'La escuela de traductores', in Cardillac, L. and Arántegui, J. L. (eds) *Toledo, siglos XII–XIII: musulmanes, cristianos y judíos: la sabiduría y la tolerancia*. Madrid: Alianza, pp. 183–198.
Jacquart, D. (1992b) 'La medicina árabe y Occidente', in Cardillac, L. and Arántegui, J. L. (eds) *Toledo, siglos XII–XIII: musulmanes, cristianos y judíos: la sabiduría y la tolerancia*. Madrid: Alianza, pp. 199–207.
Jacquart, D. (2005) *L'Épopée de la science árabe*. Paris: Gallimard.
Jacquart, D. and Micheau, F. (1996) *La médicine arabe et l'Occident médiéval*. Paris: Maisonnneuve et Larose.
Laín Entralgo, P. (1982) *Historia de la medicina*. Barcelona: Salvat.
Laine, C. and Mulrow, C. D. (2005) 'Exorcising Ghosts and Unwelcome Guests', *Annals of Internal Medicine,* 143(8), pp. 611–612.
Lambert, J. (2007) 'Translation and the Globalization of the Modern World', In Kittel, H., House, J. and Schultze, B. (eds) *Übersetzung – Translation – Traduction: Ein internationales Handbuch zur Übersetzungsforschung / An International Encyclopaedia of Translation Studies / Encyclopédie internationale de la recherche sur la traduction*, vol. 2. Berlin: De Gruyter, pp. 1680–1700.
Lancet, The (1993) 'Ghost With a Chance in Publishing Undergrowth', *Editorial*, 342(8886–8887), pp. 1498–1499.
López Férez, J. A. (ed.) (2000) *La lengua científica griega: orígenes, desarrollo e influencia en las lenguas modernas europeas*, vol. 1. Madrid: Ediciones Clásicas.
López Piñero, J. M. and Terrada Ferrandis, M. L. (1990) *Introducción a la terminología médica*. Barcelona: Salvat.
Mariscal, N. (1921) 'El doctor Luis Mercado y sus obras', Introduction to *Libro de la peste* by Luis Mercado. Madrid: Biblioteca Clásica de la Medicina Española, pp. 9–149.
Matías-Guiu, J. and García Ramos, R. (2011) 'Autores-fantasma, mejora de la comunicación de artículos y publicaciones', *Neurología*, 26(5), pp. 257–261.
Matías-Guiu, J., García Ramos, R. and Porta-Etessam, J. (2014) 'El idioma y la difusión de la investigación', in Gutiérrez Rodilla, B. M. and Navarro, F. E. (eds) *La importancia del lenguaje en el entorno biosanitario*. Barcelona: Fundación Dr. Antonio Esteve, pp. 33–37.
Moller, V. (2019) *The Map of Knowledge. A Thousand-Year History of How Classical Ideas Were Lost and Found.* New York: Doubleday.
Montalt, V. and González Davies, M. (2007) *Medical Translation Step by Step. Learning by Drafting*. Manchester: St. Jerome Publishing.
Montalt, V. and Shuttleworth, M. (eds) (2012) *Translation and Knowledge Mediation in Medical and Health Settings*. Antwerp: Linguistica Antverpiensia New Series – Themes in Translation Studies 11.

Montgomery, S. L. (2000) *Science in Translation: Movements of Knowledge through Cultures and Time*. Chicago: University of Chicago Press.
Montgomery, S. L. (2004) 'Of Towers, Wall, and Fields: Perspectives on Language in Science', *Science*, 303(5662), pp. 1333–1335.
Montgomery, S. L. (2009) 'English and Science: Realities and Issues for Translation in the Age of an Expanding Lingua Franca', *JoSTrans. The Journal of Specialised Translation*, 11, pp. 5–16.
Montgomery, S. L. (2013) *Does Science Need a Global Language? English and the Future of Research*. Chicago: University of Chicago Press.
Navarro, F. A. (1997) *Traducción y lenguaje en medicina*. Barcelona: Fundación Dr. Antonio Esteve.
Navarro, F. A. (1998) 'En pos de la verdadera causa de los anglicismos médicos', in Fernández, L. F. and Arjonilla, E. O. (eds) *Traducción e interpretación en el ámbito biosanitario*. Granada: Comares, pp. 451–461.
Navarro, F. A. (2001) 'El inglés, idioma internacional de la medicina. Causas y consecuencias de un fenómeno actual', *Panace@*, 2, pp. 35–51.
Navarro, F. A. (2002) 'En pos de la verdadera causa de los anglicismos médicos', *Ars Medica. Revista de Humanidades*, 1(1), pp. 53–64.
Nesselrath, H-G. (2013) 'Das Museion und die Große Bibliothek von Alexandria', in Georges, T., Albrecht, F. and Feldmeier, R. (eds) *Alexandria*. Tübingen: Mohr Siebeck, pp. 65–89.
Nylenna, M., Riis, P. and Karlsson, Y. (1994) 'Multiple Blinded Reviews of the Same Two Manuscripts. Effects of Referee Characteristics and Publication Language', *JAMA*, 272(2), pp. 149–151.
Olohan, M. (2009) 'Scientific and Technical Translation', in Baker, M. and Saldanha, G. (eds) *The Routledge Encyclopedia of Translation Studies*, 2nd ed. London and New York: Routledge, pp. 246–249.
Olohan, M. (2014) 'History of Science and History of Translation: Disciplinary Commensurability?', *The Translator*, 20(1), pp. 9–25. DOI:10.1080/13556509.2014.899091.
Olohan, M. (2016) *Scientific and Technical Translation*. London and New York: Routledge.
Olohan, M. and Salama-Carr, M. (2011) 'Translating Science', *The Translator*, 17(2), pp. 179–188. DOI:10.1080/13556509.2011.10799485.
Panourias, I. G., Stranjalis, G., Stavrinou, L. C. and Sakas, D. E. (2011) 'The Hellenic and Hippocratic Origins of the Spinal Terminology', *Journal of the History of the Neurosciences*, 20(3), pp. 177–187.
Plaza, L. M. and García-Carpintero, E. (2017) 'La producción científica biomédica en español: situación y perspectivas', *Educación Médica*, 18(2), pp. 17–22.
Pormann, P. E. and Savage-Smith, E. 2007. *Medieval Islamic Medicine*. Edinburgh: Edinburgh University Press.
Riera Palmero, J. (1989) 'La literatura científica en el Renacimiento', in *Ciencia, medicina y sociedad en el Renacimiento castellano*, Valladolid: ICE, Universidad de Valladolid, pp. 5–17.
Saliba, G. (2007) *Islamic Science and the Making of the European Renaissance*. Cambridge, MA: MIT Press.
Samsó, J. (1996) 'Las traducciones toledanas en los siglos XII–XIII', in Samsó, J. (ed.) *La escuela de traductores de Toledo*, pp. 17–22. Toledo: Diputación Provincial de Toledo.
Sánchez Granjel, L. (1968) *Historia de la medicina*. Salamanca: Gráficas Cervantes.
Sangrador Gil, J. (1985) *La escuela de traductores de Toledo y los colaboradores judíos*. Toledo: Instituto Provincial de Investigaciones Toledanas.
Santoyo, J. C. (2004) 'Sobre la historia de la traducción en España: algunos errores recientes', *Hermenēus. Revista de Traducción e Interpretación* 6, pp. 1–10.
Santoyo, J. C. (2009) *La traducción medieval en la Península Ibérica (siglos III–XV)*. León: Universidad de León.
Schipperges, H. (1961) 'Las escuelas de Toledo y su significación para la ciencia occidental', *Archivo Iberoamericano de Historia de la Medicina y Antropología Médica*, 13, pp. 41–64.
Schipperges, H. (1964) *Die Assimilation der arabischen Medizin durch das lateinische Mittelalter*. Sudhoffs Archiv für Geschichte der Medizin und Naturwissenschaften, 3, Wiesbaden: F. Steiner.
Schipperges, H. (ed.) (2003) *Gesundheit und Gesellschaft. Ein historisch-kritisches Panorama*. Berlin: Springer.
Schipperges, H. (2006) *Heinrich Schipperges Selected Writings on the Reception and Assimilation of Islamic Medicine in the Occident*. Collected and reprinted by Fuat Sezgin in collaboration with

Carl Ehrig-Eggert and Eckhard Newbauer. Frankfurt am Main: Institute for the History of Arabic-Islamic Science.

Shashok, K. (2008) 'Content and Communication: How Can Peer Review Provide Helpful Feedback About the Writing?', *BMC Medical Research Methodology*, 8(3).

Steger, M. B. (2009) *Globalization: A Very Short Introduction*. Oxford: Oxford University Press.

Taylor, D. G. K. (2007) 'Early Translations in the Ancient Orient: From Greek Into Syriac', in Kittel, H., House, J. and Schultze, B. (eds) *Übersetzung – Translation – Traduction: Ein internationales Handbuch zur Übersetzungsforschung / An International Encyclopaedia of Translation Studies / Encyclopédie internationale de la recherche sur la traduction*, vol. 2. Berlin: De Gruyter, pp. 1190–1193.

Timo-Iaria, C. (1998) 'La catástrofe del monolingüismo anglófono', *Actas Dermo-Sifiliográficas*, 89, pp. 566–570.

Valls, H. (2007) 'Medical and Scientific Texts in Translation in Medieval Europe', in Kittel, H., House, J. and Schultze, B. (eds) *Übersetzung – Translation – Traduction: Ein internationales Handbuch zur Übersetzungsforschung / An International Encyclopaedia of Translation Studies / Encyclopédie internationale de la recherche sur la traduction*, vol. 2. Berlin: De Gruyter, pp. 1371–1374.

Vandenbroucke, J. P. (1989) 'On Not Being Born a Native Speaker of English', *British Medical Journal*, 298, pp. 1461–1462.

Varela Salinas, M. J. and Meyer, B. (eds) (2015) *Translating and Interpreting Healthcare Discourses*. Berlin: Frank & Timme.

Vegas González, S. (1998) *La escuela de traductores de Toledo en la historia del pensamiento*. Toledo: Concejalía de Cultura.

Vickery, B. C. (2000) *Scientific Communication in History*. London: The Scarecrow Press.

Wiese, I. (2006) 'Zur Situation des Deutschens als Wissenschaftssprache', in Ehlich, K. and Heller, D. (eds) *Die Wissenschaft und ihre Sprachen*. Bern: Peter Lang, pp. 275–295.

Wright, R. (2007) 'Translation and the Role of Latin in Medieval Europe', in Kittel, H., House, J. and Schultze, B. (eds) *Übersetzung – Translation – Traduction: Ein internationales Handbuch zur Übersetzungsforschung / An international Encyclopaedia of Translation Studies / Encyclopédie internationale de la recherche sur la traduction*, vol. 2. Berlin: De Gruyter, pp. 1263–1270.

Wright, S. E. and Wright, L. D. (eds) (1993) *Scientific and Technical Translation*. Amsterdam and Philadelphia: John Benjamins.

Part II

Translation in medicine and medical sciences

4

Medical terminology and discourse

Joost Buysschaert

1 Introduction

The translation of medical texts poses several challenges. An obvious difficulty for medical translators is the understanding of the original text, as not all translators have had extensive medical training and the topic may be very technical. Yet, as Vandaele (2001a) has pointed out, it is often sufficient for the translators to familiarise themselves with a number of core concepts of the subject at hand. A second difficulty related to the more technical documents, such as research papers, is constituted by the syntactic complexity that is typical of 'special languages' (also called 'specialised languages', 'languages for special/specific purposes', 'LSPs' - cf. Cabré, Sager and DeCesaris 1999: 228). However, by far the most challenging aspect of medical source texts is their abundance of medical terminology. In many cases, the brunt of the translation work consists of establishing appropriate target equivalents for the technical terms.

The present chapter explores several aspects of this terminological challenge and starts with an analysis and illustration of the remarkably rich terminological variation in the medical domain. Next, the possible solutions of term normalisation or standardisation are discussed, with an overview of the main competing efforts in this respect. Term variation can, however, be functional and this is illustrated in a section on discourse issues, which illustrates how medical communication functions in a variety of discourse settings, necessitating different terminological choices. The chapter goes on to discuss the role that language technology can play in the management of medical terminology and closes with some general hints on the types of sources that may be useful in researching the meaning, usage and translation of medical terms.

2 Terminological variation as a major challenge

Not only is terminology abundant in medical texts; it is also characterised by sometimes confusing variation, with different terms referring to the same concept or the same term referring to different concepts. The present section illustrates this, starting with examples of synonymy in medical terminology. Next, the importance of usage differences is discussed,

DOI: 10.4324/9781003167983-7

followed by an illustration of polysemy, homonymy, the frequent use of abbreviations, variation in spelling, and the occasional confusion between hyponyms and hypernyms. The search for translation equivalents can also be hampered by false friends, outdated variants and lexical gaps. Each of these obstacles will be illustrated and its impact on medical translation discussed.

2.1 Synonymy

Medical dictionaries often mention one or several synonyms for the same medical term. An extreme but by no means exceptional example may be *refractory epilepsy*, which is also known as *drug refractory epilepsy, drug resistant epilepsy, medication resistant epilepsy, pharmacoresistant epilepsy* and *intractable epilepsy.* There are various reasons why synonymy is common in medical terminology. The first one is the existence of a term with a Latin or Greek root alongside a term in the vernacular, both of which are in use: e.g. *os sacrum - sacred bone; coryza – common cold; epistaxis – nosebleed; pertussis – whooping cough*. The second reason is the competition between eponymous terms and descriptive terms, particularly in the case of names for diseases and syndromes. Eponymous terms are named after the person(s) who first discovered or described the condition (e.g. *Caffey-Silverman syndrome*) or after the place where the condition was (first) encountered (e.g. *Lassa fever*; an eponym of this kind is also called a geonym). In many cases, eponymous terms also have a descriptive synonym; in the case of *Caffey-Silverman syndrome*, the corresponding descriptive label is *infantile cortical hyperostosis*. Some medical terminologists favour the descriptive terms because of their self-explanatory nature; others point out that the eponymous terms are easier to remember and, in the case of reference to persons, give credit to those who brought the condition to the fore. The issue has been heavily debated but the synonymy persists (see Whitworth 2007 versus Woywodt and Matteson 2007; see also Cappuzzo 2008). Synonymy may also arise when there are different schools of medicine with their own preferences, as also described by Bowker and Hawkins (2006), who name conceptual, linguistic and social factors as causes of medical term variation.

In choosing a preferred synonym, usage differences come into consideration (as discussed below), as does frequency of use in (recent) authoritative sources. Major languages will have respected medical journals that can be queried for clarification, or authoritative medical dictionaries and normative term collections (of the types discussed below under the heading of normalisation and standardisation).

2.2 Usage differences

The existence of synonyms does not guarantee that the variants are mutually interchangeable in all discursive contexts. Some synonyms are appropriate as informal lay terms in doctor-patient exchanges but would be replaced by more technical names in research articles. An example is the term *belly* versus *abdomen*. Languages differ in the number of lay terms they offer. In French, for example, many medical terms that are used in formal discourse are also used as lay terms; whereas English has *collarbone* alongside *clavicle*, French only has *clavicule*. Dutch, on the contrary, has many lay terms. When translating a patient-oriented text from French into Dutch, the translator will have to avoid the systematic use of Dutch cognates of the French terms in contexts where lay alternatives may be more appropriate.

Apart from differences in register (technical versus lay language), translators also encounter regional usage differences. For example, British English uses *noradrenaline*, whereas American English calls the same hormone *norepinephrine*. Similarly, differences exist between European French and Canadian French and between Netherlandic Dutch and Belgian (Flemish) Dutch, and translators have to be aware of these differences so that they can adapt the text for their target readership. The task becomes especially difficult when the readership is mixed, as with the Dutch translations commissioned by the European Medicines Agency, which are meant to be used in the Netherlands as well as Belgium. In some cases, it may be advisable to resort to alternative solutions such as the use of slashes or parentheses in order to include variants in the text.

2.3 Polysemy and homonymy

Polysemy occurs when a given term has more than one meaning and the meanings are related. Polysemy is fairly common in non-technical language but should be avoided in special languages when possible. However, several examples of polysemy are found in medical terminology. A well-known case is the term *drug*, which may refer to a therapeutic agent but also to a stimulating or depressing substance that is potentially addictive. In the case of a polysemic expression in the source text, it is important to ascertain if the target language also uses one term for both meanings, or whether it uses distinct names.

Homonymy refers to those cases where terms share pronunciation and spelling but have different meanings that are not related in an obvious way. A medical example is the term *callus*, which may refer to the formation of extra tissue at the site of a bone fracture but may also mean 'hardened skin'. There is likely to be a common etymological origin for the two meanings but the link between them is more distant than in the case of polysemy. Ideally, specialised languages should again avoid this kind of ambiguity but it may be argued that the language of medicine has evolved into a combination of various special languages (in the case of *callus,* the competing special languages are those of orthopaedics and dermatology). It is again the role of the translator to ascertain if the ambiguity persists in the target language, or whether a choice must be made between distinct equivalents.

2.4 Abbreviations

The use of abbreviations is very common in medical texts. Abbreviations may be regarded as synonyms of the full forms that they stand for. In a number of cases, the abbreviations have become more common than the full forms, like *AIDS* for *acquired immune deficiency syndrome*. However, as the domain of medicine is a combination of many subdisciplines, some abbreviations have several different meanings. The online mediLexicon[1] gives 16 possible meanings for the abbreviation *OCM*, ranging from *obstructive cardiomyopathy* to *ovine choriomammotrophin*.

Finding an equivalent abbreviation in a target language often requires a detour via the full form. In cardiology, *CPR* stands for *cardiopulmonary resuscitation*. The full term is translated into French as *réanimation cardio-pulmonaire*, and a further search for the French term reveals that the abbreviation *RCP* is in use. The German equivalent is *Herz-Lungen-Wiederbelebung*, which is abbreviated to *HLW*.

It is not uncommon for English abbreviations to be used in other languages even though the full forms of the terms are different. The English abbreviation *ACTH* for *adrenocorticotropic hormone* frequently appears in French texts, despite the fact that the full French term is *hormone corticotrope*. English acronyms, i.e. abbreviations that are pronounced as a word, are often used unchanged in other languages when they are (relatively) recent coinages (though pronunciation and spelling may be adapted to the target language). *AIDS* is an example that has already been mentioned; the acronym is also used in many other languages, including German (*AIDS*), Dutch (*aids*) and Swedish (*aids*); French and Spanish use *sida* (short for *syndrome d'immunodéficience acquise* resp. *síndrome de inmunodeficiencia adquirida*). A similar example is *SARS* for *severe acute respiratory syndrome*.

2.5 Variation in spelling

There are a number of differences between British and American spelling in English medical terms which the translators have to take into account if their target language is English. Common cases include (with UK spelling followed by US spelling):

- ae versus e: anaemia – anemia
- oe versus e: oesophagus – esophagus
- -re versus -er: titre – titer
- -our versus -or: tumour – tumor

In other languages, too, there may be variation in the degree to which originally Latin spellings have been adapted to spelling rules in the vernacular versions. The difficult Late Latin spelling *diarrhoea* (a term of Greek origin) survives in British English, loses an *-o-* in American spelling, becomes *diarrhée* in French, loses its *h* and is shortened to *diarré* in Danish; and is spelt *diarree* in Dutch. Sometimes vernacular spellings are used alongside original spellings in the same text, for example when the Latin name of a condition is added in parentheses. A Dutch source may refer to *artrose (arthrosis)*, where the vernacular form uses *-t-* and Latin *-th-*.

Some languages have also introduced spelling reforms in recent decades (amongst them German and Dutch). Older sources that are still available will use older spellings and even newer sources may not have fully adapted. A particularly thorny issue are the spelling rules for compounds and eponyms introduced in the 1995 Dutch spelling reform. The official rules prescribe *downsyndroom* but the alternative *Down-syndroom* has also remained in use. In 2011, a team of medical terminologists around the editor of the well-known medical dictionary *Pinkhof* opined that the older spellings should remain a valid alternative in medical texts (Van Everdingen and Van den Eerenbeemt 2012). The authoritative journal *Nederlands Tijdschrift voor Geneeskunde*, on the contrary, chose to adhere to the new official rules.

2.6 Hyponyms and hypernyms

Another common issue when translating medical terminology is that common subtypes of illnesses (hyponyms) are sometimes confused with main types of the condition (hypernym). Many sources list *variola major* as a synonym of *smallpox*, whereas the term only refers to the more common form of smallpox. The translator has the difficult task to decide whether it is acceptable to go along with this blurring of fine distinctions or to distinguish more rigorously between hyponyms and hypernyms in the translation.

2.7 False friends

Some terms may appear similar but have different meanings in other languages. The word *surface* is used in English as well as in French, but the *anterior surface* of an intraocular lens is not **la surface antérieure* but *la face antérieure.* Similarly, a *median section* is not **une section médiane* but *une coupe médiane*. A better-known example of false friends between French and English are the words *preservatives* (substances used to prevent decay) versus *préservatifs* (condoms).

2.8 Diachronic variation

Translators should be aware that terms they find in (especially printed) dictionaries may have been superseded by new terms. This diachronic variation may have different reasons: new normalisation efforts, changes in classification reflecting new research, or the avoidance of misnomers after research has proved that the old name gives an inaccurate description. The term *Lyme arthritis*, for example, is no longer in use for *Lyme disease*, because it is an inaccurate, or at best only a partial, description of the condition. An example of successive changes in classification together with an attempt at normalisation can be found in the types of epileptic seizures.[2] Although the term *grand mal* was replaced a long time ago by the newer classification *tonic-clonic seizure*, the old term of French origin is still common.

2.9 Lexical gaps

Rogers (2015) aptly describes the phenomenon of lexical gaps (or terminological gaps in terminology) as a common phenomenon in specialised translation. A lexical/terminological gap occurs when there is no equivalent of the source term in the target language. In the case of medicine, this gap typically occurs when a newly emerged concept receives its name in only one language, now most commonly English (*stent* or *regenerative medicine* are examples). When such a new term occurs only once in a translation, a provisional solution can be a paraphrase or a circumlocution. However, once the concept becomes established, it becomes necessary to find a fixed equivalent in the target language. Authors writing on the topic in their native languages, or translators, will then feel the need to come up with suggestions of their own, a process which is known as *secondary term formation* (Sager 1990: 80). There are three common methods of secondary term formation. The first is to simply accept the source term as a loan term, typically with minor adjustments to reflect the requirements of the target language (*stent*, originally an eponym, has been copied to many languages; German uses a capital letter [*Stent*], Spanish adjusts the term slightly to *estent*). The second method is called loan translation, where component parts of the source term are translated separately and then joined together (which is the obvious choice for *regenerative medicine*). The third method of secondary term formation, which is rarely applied, is the creation of an entirely new term not based on the source; a notable example is *taaislijmziekte*, a neologism coined as the Dutch equivalent of *cystic fibrosis*.

Resorting to loan translation can be risky in the case of multiword units. For a term like *total laryngectomy* a French translator may be tempted to opt for *largyngectomie complète*, whereas the phrase *laryngectomie totale* is the more common translation.

3 Normalisation and standardisation

3.1 The rationale behind standardisation

The proliferation of terms that denote the same medical concepts has led to various attempts at establishing standards or norms for use within a particular context. The efforts have resulted in coded term collections presented in various formats, with tree diagrams, thesauri, controlled vocabularies and ontologies amongst the most popular ones. In what follows, the neutral label 'term collections' will be used for all of them, as there can be confusion as to the exact meaning of the denominations that have been used to refer to the various term repositories (Vanopstal *et al.* 2011). What they have in common is that they try to establish preferred terms for each concept and that they assign a code (for example a number, or a combination of letters and digits) to each concept. The code serves as a unique identifier for the concept and binds all the intralingual variants that refer to the same concept and even the translations (if supplied). The overview that follows introduces some of the best-known medical term collections that aim at standardisation, and indicates how these collections can be used by a medical translator in finding a preferred term among synonyms, in finding definitions and sometimes in finding translations.[3]

3.2 Selected examples of term collections

One of the most popular early initiatives of standardisation was the *Nomina Anatomica,* which listed standard names in Latin for human anatomical parts. It started off in 1895 with a version now known as the *Nomina Anatomica Basiliensia*; subsequent versions include the *Jena Nomina Anatomica* of 1933 and the *Paris Nomina Anatomica* of 1955. It was widely used between 1956 and 1989, when it was replaced by the *Terminologia Anatomica* (TA). The TA covers more than 8,000 concepts and is available in Latin and (American) English; it was supplemented with the *Terminologia Histologica* in 2005. The collection can be consulted online.[4]

Another classification with historical roots is the *International Classification of Diseases* (ICD). Its precursor, the *International List of Causes of Death*, was adopted by the International Statistical Institute in 1893. As the title suggests, the list was intended for use in death certificates. The World Health Organisation took over the management of the list in 1948, and renamed it as *International Classification of Diseases* (ICD, World Health Organisation 2016). The ICD became the international standard for reporting diseases and health conditions. The 10th version, known as ICD-10, was released in 1990 and has been in use in over 100 countries. It is available in 42 languages, and the English and French versions can be consulted online.[5] Meanwhile, ICD-11 has also become available[6] and is expected to be implemented by WHO member states by January 2022.

A valuable medical vocabulary resource of much more recent origin, provided by the United States National Library of Medicine, is the *Medical Subject Headings*, abbreviated as MeSH.[7] It is structured as a hierarchically organised term collection, intended for indexing and cataloguing biomedical information. MeSH was started in the 1960s as an indexing tool for the bibliography *Index Medicus* and is now used in particular to index and search publications in the extensive *MEDLINE/PUBmed* database.[8] Its terms are called 'headings' or 'descriptors' and their unique IDs have been used for other purposes as well, including the structuring of medical libraries. The MeSH is constantly updated and is freely available via the MeSH Browser.[9] Translators can use the MeSH to find reliable (American) English medical terms. Apart from the 'descriptors' (i.e. the preferred terms), the Browser also supplies 'scope notes', which are in most cases definitions, as well as 'entry terms', which are synonyms or closely related terms.

The MeSH has been translated into several languages but the translations do not always cover the complete collection or do not keep track of the annual updates. Some of the translations have been criticised for having an English bias (Vandaele 2001b: 113) but they nevertheless offer a useful starting point. The translations can be found via the *Unified Medical Language System* (UMLS)[10] or via Babelmesh,[11] which offers a dozen languages. The French version is updated annually by Inserm, the *Institut national de la santé et de la recherche médicale*, and is also available via *Le MeSH bilingue.*[12]

Another collection that has established itself as an important player since 1999 is *SNOMED CT* (with CT meaning Clinical Terms), not in the least because it has been the nomenclature of choice in some of the eHealth initiatives (Cangioli *et al.* 2016). *SNOMED CT* also has the advantage of being the largest collection of its kind, covering more than 300,000 unique concepts and many medical specialties, and of being computer processable. *SNOMED CT* aims to provide the core general terminology for electronic health records. The collection, originally in English only, can be accessed via the SNOMED CT International Browser.[13] A search for a medical term yields a concept code, a description, hypernyms, hyponyms and other relationships; in the case of synonyms some will be labelled as 'preferred', others as 'acceptable'. Several translation projects are in progress to make the collection available in other languages; the SNOMED CT International Browser gives access to some of them.

SNOMED CT can also be consulted via the SNOMED CT browser[14] of UTS.[15] UTS stands for *UMLS Terminology Services*, where UMLS is short for *Unified Medical Language System*; it is one of the many useful resources provided by the United States National Library of Medicine. The UTS also contains the *Metathesaurus Browser.*[16] A search for an English medical term in the Browser offers a concept code, definitions and in some cases also translations (from the MeSH translations).

3.3 Interoperability of standards

As explained, there are many competing standards in the field of medicine, each with their own proponents. The account above is limited to the historically best-known collections and to those that cover medicine in general, leaving out other nomenclatures that focus on specific medical areas. HeTOP[17] is an interesting portal that lists many more sources and allows simultaneous searches in several of them.

Some other attempts have been made to link systems. One example is *I-MAGIC,*[18] which searches for a matching ICD-10 code starting from a SNOMED CT term. For example, typing in the term *acute necrotizing pancreatitis* first yields the SNOMED CT code for this concept (which is 7881005); clicking on 'Get ICD codes' shows the code of the same concept in ICD 10 (K85.91) and reveals that ICD 10 calls the condition *acute pancreatitis with uninfected necrosis, unspecified.* Technical committees of the ISO and the European Union are also developing standards that aim to promote compatibility and interoperability between healthcare systems (ISO/TC 215[19] and CEN/TC 251[20] in particular).

3.4 Standardisation in drug licensing documents

Another type of terminological standardisation is the one imposed on texts required for drug licensing purposes. A typical example are the templates used by the European Medicines Agency[21] for the documents needed to submit a licensing application. The templates are available in all of EU's official languages and standardise the way in which documents like Summaries of Product Characteristics or Package Leaflets have to be formulated and translated. Translation of the licensing documents is mandatory for the medicinal products in order to obtain marketing authorisation in all EU member states. This not only means that, for example, all the headings in a Summary of Product Characteristics have standard translations; it stands to reason that terms used in these headings should also be translated in the same way in the rest of the text. If a term such as *excipients* was translated in one way in the heading and in another way in the body of the text, this might cause confusion.

4 Discourse issues

When choosing appropriate medical terminology, it is important to know the target readership (or audience) of the text. Medical communication can function in a variety of discourse settings, each with its own requirements. This section will examine the following settings: communication between health professionals; communication between specialists in a subfield; communication between health professionals and patients or the general public; mixed scenarios; and interpreting doctor-patient exchanges.

4.1 Communication between health professionals

Much of the medical translation work is intended for domain specialists, i.e. readers who are themselves doctors or medical professionals. Examples include documents needed to obtain marketing authorisation for medicines, as already hinted above; research papers and their abstracts, which are also occasionally submitted for translation; and medical reports, including discharge summaries, operative reports or medical imaging reports, some of which need translation when submitted for insurance claims. The density of technical terms in these texts is striking.

Communication between doctors or other health professionals will naturally favour the more technical terms over the lay alternatives. However, given the challenges of term variation discussed above, translators should be aware of their clients' preferences even among the technical terms. It is not unusual for clients to criticise translations simply because their own preferred terms have not been used. In such cases, it may be helpful to compile a list of terms as found in the source texts, supply them with suggested equivalents in the target language and have the client vet the equivalents either prior to translation or prior to revision. Term extraction software (like Multiterm Extract,[22] SynchroTerm[23] or SketchEngine,[24] among several others) can be helpful in identifying technical terms in the source texts.

Clinical guidelines are another, now increasingly common example of medical communication aimed at health professionals. The guidelines offer evidence-based advice on a wide range of topics. Among the best-known are the Cochrane Systematic Reviews.[25]

Further guidelines of various origins can be consulted via Guidelines International Network.[26] There is a demand for the translation of these authoritative guidelines and the correct rendering of technical terms can again become an issue. An interesting account of the challenges encountered during the translation of the Cochrane reviews (or their abstracts) is found in von Elm *et al.* (2013).

4.2 Communication between specialists in a subfield

As explained above, medicine combines many subdisciplines and each may well have specific terms that are not in wider use. The subdiscipline of medical imaging may be quoted as an example, as this field uses many specific abbreviations. Translators may be called upon to translate imaging reports in the context of insurance claims, when they are likely to struggle with these abbreviations. The first point of enquiry is the meaning of the abbreviations in their source language; for English, the Royal College of Radiologists has a patient-oriented site which explains a number of common abbreviations,[27] but the actual number of abbreviations in use is much larger. Translation of medical reports is best regarded as a specialist area and translators who want to work in this area will need to develop their own termbases with abbreviations, their explanations and equivalents in the target language.

4.3 Communication between health professionals and patients or the general public

The Internet has an abundance of patient-oriented sites; even before it came into being, patients were addressed directly through medication leaflets, variously called patient package inserts, patient information leaflets or package leaflets. The question of how to make these leaflets patient-friendly has been a long-standing issue (cf. Kenny *et al.* 1998 or Gal and Prigat 2005, among many other publications; see also the European Commission's *Guideline on the readability of the labelling and package leaflet of medicinal products for human use* (2009). Problems that have been identified range from print size to the risk of misinterpretation, but the issue of clear medical terminology has inevitably been also part of the debate.

More recently, online patient-oriented medical guidelines have begun to appear,[28] and they face the same problems of readability as medical leaflets. Åhlfeldt *et al.* (2006) offer a literature review on patient-friendly documentation in general, not just leaflets, illustrating many of the challenges. Specific difficulties of translating lay-friendly medical information are discussed in Askehave and Zethsen (2011), amongst other publications. Wermuth and Verplaetse (2019: 99–104) describe the transition from technical medical documentation to lay documentation as a form of intralingual translation.

The website *Multilingual Glossary of Technical and Popular Medical Terms*[29] offers suggestions for lay equivalents to medical terms in nine European Languages. However, it is important to keep in mind that when patients are diagnosed with a particular disease or condition, they are likely to remember the term, even if it is technical, and there will be no need to replace it with a vague lay alternative in the patient leaflet or patient guideline. For example, the Glossary offers *serious skin disease* as a lay alternative for *pemphigus*; this could be used as an explanatory description in some contexts, but *pemphigus* can be retained in leaflets aimed at patients who suffer from the condition.

4.4 Mixed scenarios

The term eHealth (sometimes spelt e-Health) has been a buzzword for some time now and refers to electronic support in healthcare practice. One important aim has been to make patients' records available via online networks, for the benefit of other caregivers as well as for the patient. The electronic health record (EHR) or electronic medical record (EMR) can then serve a double purpose: fast communication between health staff as well as 'patient empowerment', as the patients also have access to their medical information. However, this double purpose presents its own set of challenges including the aforementioned term variation. Grön and Bertels (2018: 42) have noted that EHRs mix specialist terms with lay terms and even informal terms. Specialist terms might be unsuitable for the patients and limit their agency in making medical decisions; informal terms may be unsuitable for health professionals who might not be familiar with the expressions used. Avoiding these problems would need large termbases listing all the variants and making terms clickable in the records so that synonyms can be provided instantly. Similarly, if EHRs are meant to be available across language borders (so that a Spanish doctor can consult a Danish holiday maker's record), it would be useful if translations could likewise be supplied via clicking on problem terms. To make this happen, substantial work must be carried out by medical terminologists worldwide. Similar efforts have already been undertaken to support multilingual searching (Diekema 2012); an example of a cross-lingual search facility developed for PubPsych, a search engine in psychology, is discussed in España-Bonet *et al.* (2019). The facility also uses MeSH terminology.

4.5 Interpreting doctor-patient exchanges

A discourse setting that has not been discussed above is where an interpreter mediates between a doctor and a patient during a medical interview. This can be a particularly challenging experience, especially if the doctor uses technical jargon and when the cultural context of the doctor and the patient are very different. Research by Hadlow and Pitts (1991) shows that even in monolingual settings, medical staff and patients have a different understanding of common health terms. In a bilingual setting, the interpreter may try to translate technical terms using approximate lay alternatives in the target language, and risk blurring the message. Cultural considerations also play a role (cf. Kersey-Matusiak 2018). A particularly difficult problem arises when some of the topics or terms are considered taboo in the target culture, and have to be avoided through the use of paraphrases and euphemisms (Munane 2014). The International Association for Communication in Healthcare[30] is expected to publish a position paper on healthcare communication across language barriers in 2020 (Van den Muijsenbergh, Krystallidou, and Langewitz, forthcoming).

5 Medical terminology and translation technology

There is no doubt that present-day translation technology can be very helpful to medical translators, particularly for the translation of medical terminology. Most Computer-Aided Translation (CAT) programmes offer the option to store terminology in termbases which can be automatically searched during the translation process. The technology also allows the labelling of medical terms in the termbase so as to indicate their usage such as 'technical', 'lay', or 'informal', as well as to indicate regional use or clients' preferences.

Automatic term extraction has been alluded to before; given the density of terms in a typical medical source text, it is advisable to first run a term extraction, check for potentially problematic terms and add them to the termbase before embarking on the translation. In the case of English, the Medical Subject Headings site offers a 'MeSH on Demand' facility, which identifies MeSH terms in submitted texts.[31] Term extraction in medical corpora on a broader scale and involving machine learning techniques is sometimes called 'biomedical named entity recognition' (Krauthammer and Nenadic 2004; Campos, Matos and Oliveira 2012).

Translators increasingly make use of machine translation (MT), either for partial input during the translation process or for wholesale pre-translation followed by post-editing. MT output quality tends to vary considerably and will depend on language combinations and topic. Major MT providers like Google Translate and DeepL tend to perform reasonably well for medical translations between widely used languages and on a variety of medical topics, provided that the engines were trained on a substantial corpus of relevant bilingual material. However, medical terminology can again present a stumbling block. Typical problems that translators and post-editors have to be aware of are, a) inconsistent translations of the same term within the same text (i.e. one term used in a paragraph, a synonym used in the next paragraph or even the next sentence); b) wrong rendering of some multiword terms as the engine may translate the words separately and combine them into an expression that looks acceptable but is incorrect in the target language; and c) translation by means of a hypernym. All three types of mistake tend to be difficult to spot without relevant training. It is again advisable for translators and post-editors to use MT within a CAT programme that also allows for the use of their own termbases, as these can help to correct some of these terminological errors.

Alternatively, translators can build their own translation engines and train them on their own material, which in principle should also mean that their own terminological preferences will be picked up. However, it is difficult for such custom engines to match the overall quality of the major MT providers. Another issue is the integration of existing termbases into MT engines. In the case of phrase-based statistical MT engines, terms can be entered in the bilingual 'phrase tables', but it is not possible to add synonyms with the necessary usage information. If the engine is to be used for a variety of translation tasks (technical as well as patient-oriented), the method will give insufficient support. Neural MT offers even fewer opportunities for integrating terminology as it primarily focuses on fluency and in many cases prioritises natural-sounding target sentences. Although terminology could be entered in phrase tables, or a termbase could be added to the training material, Neural MT is known for regularly ignoring information supplied in this way. Recent research now aims to circumvent this obstacle (Dinu *et al.* 2019) but is unlikely to solve the problem of term variation if the engine is to perform translation tasks aimed at different readerships.

6 Sources of medical terminology

There is no dearth of monolingual medical dictionaries for the major languages and bilingual dictionaries are also available for a number of language combinations, as a search via the Internet or a library catalogue will show. Traditional paper dictionaries have the advantage of being reviewed by editors and overseen by well-established publishers, but may not list recent terminology in rapidly evolving medical subdisciplines. On the other hand, online medical glossaries and dictionaries can be of varying quality, but some can be highly relevant through their focus on very specific topics. An Internet search for a topic, adding search terms like *glossary* (for example: *neurology lexicon OR glossary OR dictionary*) often provides a wealth of resources, at least for the well-documented (especially Western) languages. Definitions can also be found via the Internet (*define + search term* often yields pertinent results in Google, and not just for English). Authoritative definitions for English medical terms can be found via sources like MeSH and UMLS, mentioned above. Translation suggestions can sometimes be found via Wikipedia (when there is a parallel article for the target term) or through one of the many online sites searching translation memory collections (Linguee,[32] Glosbe,[33] TAUS Data[34]); sites like ProZ.com[35] can also provide relevant information. It is always recommended to check the validity of these translation suggestions in reliable primary sources. Sites like Google Scholar[36] or Google Books[37] are valuable resources for confirming the use of technical terms in the target language, so is MEDLINE/PubMed.[38] For English, BioMedSearch[39] covers PubMed as well as medical dissertations and a variety of publications. Respected medical journals in the target language, also often available online, are likewise relevant resources for confirming a term and its use. Many of the sources mentioned can also be used to compare frequency of use of competing synonyms.

7 Conclusion

Supplying correct equivalents for the many technical terms in medical texts is a major challenge for medical translators (and interpreters). The problem is compounded by terminological variation: many medical concepts have more than one name within the same language. Although normalisation efforts exist, the different attempts tend to compete with each other. Moreover, terminological variation can be functional, for example when a lay synonym is more appropriate than the technical term in a text aimed at patients.

Future research will therefore have to concentrate on the best design of tools that reflect variation as well as functionality. The ideal tool will link all the terms referring to the same concept, in one language as well as across languages, and will in addition label variants to make clear in what discourse settings they are appropriate or preferred. This can for example lead to enriched termbases for use in a CAT tool; or to thesauri that boost search engine performance. Combining the enriched term collections with machine translation is a further challenge that will need to be addressed. For a number of well-documented languages, much essential information is already available, though it may be dispersed among various sources and will need to be aggregated. For other languages, the groundwork does not yet exist, or it needs further expansion.

Notes

1 www.medilexicon.com (Accessed: 21 November 2019).
2 www.ilae.org/guidelines/definition-and-classification (Accessed: 21 November 2019).
3 On the topic of medical nomenclatures, clinical terminologies and coding systems, see also Wermuth and Verplaetse (2019: 90–97).
4 http://terminologia-anatomica.org/en/ (Accessed: 21 November 2019).
5 https://icd.who.int/browse10/2016/en#/ (Accessed: 21 November 2019).
6 https://icd.who.int/browse11/l-m/en (Accessed: 21 November 2019).
7 www.nlm.nih.gov/mesh/meshhome.html (Accessed: 21 November 2019).
8 www.ncbi.nlm.nih.gov/pubmed (Accessed: 21 November 2019).

9 https://meshb.nlm.nih.gov/search (Accessed: 21 November 2019).
10 https://uts.nlm.nih.gov/metathesaurus.html (Accessed: 21 November 2019).
11 https://babelmesh.nlm.nih.gov/lookup.php (Accessed: 21 November 2019).
12 http://mesh.inserm.fr/FrenchMesh/search/index.jsp (Accessed: 21 November 2019).
13 https://browser.ihtsdotools.org (Accessed: 21 November 2019).
14 https://uts.nlm.nih.gov/snomedctBrowser.html (Accessed: 21 November 2019).
15 https://uts.nlm.nih.gov (Accessed: 21 November 2019).
16 https://uts.nlm.nih.gov/metathesaurus.htm (Accessed: 21 November 2019).
17 www.hetop.eu (Accessed: 21 November 2019).
18 https://imagic.nlm.nih.gov/imagic/code/map (Accessed: 21 November 2019).
19 www.iso.org/committee/54960.html (Accessed: 21 November 2019).
20 https://standards.cen.eu/dyn/www/f?p=204:7:0::::FSP_ORG_ID:6232&cs=18CA078392807EDD402B798AAEF1644E1 (Accessed: 21 November 2019).
21 www.ema.europa.eu (Accessed: 21 November 2019).
22 www.sdltrados.com/products/multiterm-extract (Accessed: 21 November 2019).
23 https://terminotix.com/index.asp?content=item&item=7&lang=en (Accessed: 21 November 2019).
24 www.sketchengine.eu (Accessed: 21 November 2019).
25 www.cochranelibrary.com/cdsr/reviews/topics (Accessed: 21 November 2019).
26 www.g-i-n.net/library/international-guidelines-library (Accessed: 21 November 2019).
27 www.rcr.ac.uk/public-and-media/common-medical-terms/abbreviations (Accessed: 21 November 2019).
28 E.g. www.gezondheidenwetenschap.be/richtlijnen (Accessed: 21 November 2019).
29 https://users.ugent.be/~rvdstich/eugloss/welcome.html (Accessed: 21 November 2019).
30 www.each.eu (Accessed: 21 November 2019).
31 https://meshb.nlm.nih.gov/MeSHonDemand (Accessed: 21 November 2019).
32 www.linguee.com (Accessed: 21 November 2019).
33 https://glosbe.com (Accessed: 21 November 2019).
34 https://data-app.taus.net (Accessed: 21 November 2019).
35 www.proz.com/search (Accessed: 21 November 2019).
36 https://scholar.google.com (Accessed: 21 November 2019).
37 https://books.google.com (Accessed: 21 November 2019).
38 www.ncbi.nlm.nih.gov/pubmed (Accessed: 21 November 2019).
39 www.biomedsearch.com (Accessed: 21 November 2019).

Further reading

Montalt, V., Zethsen K. and Karwacka, W. (2018) 'Medical Translation in the 21st Century – Challenges and Trends', in Montalt, V., Zethsen K. and Karwacka, W. (eds) *Retos Actuals y Tendencias Emergentes en Traducción Médica / Current Challenges and Emerging Trends in Medical Translation. MonTI*, 10, pp. 27–42.

The second section of this article deals with terminological issues as discussed in the present chapter; section 4 expands on the issue of retaining lay-friendliness in patient-oriented translations.

Wermuth, C. and Verplaetse, H. (2019) 'Medical Terminology in The Western World. Current Situation', in Alsulaiman, A. and Ahmed Allaithy, A. (eds) *Handbook of Terminology, Volume 2 [HoT2]: Terminology in the Arab world.* Amsterdam and Philadelphia: John Benjamins, pp. 84–108.

Section 4 of this chapter gives another account of medical nomenclatures, clinical terminologies and coding systems. Section 6 offers further illustration of the challenges involved in converting technical medical documentation to lay documentation.

ITI Medical and Pharmaceutical Network (no date) Available at: www.itimedical.co.uk

Medical translators can gain substantial support by joining dedicated networks, like the one of ITI (Institute of Translation and Interpreting). Most of the discussions on their e-group deal with terminological issues.

Signs and Symptoms of Translation. https://signsandsymptomsoftranslation.com.

This is an interesting blog by the Spanish to English medical translator Emma Goldsmith. Several of its regular posts deal with terminology (type in 'terminology' in the search box to find previous posts).

Biomettico. http://vandaele.biomettico.org/publications.

The research group Biomettico of the University of Montreal has produced several worthwhile publications on medical terminology; references can be retrieved via the 'Publications' section of their site, using the keyword 'terminology'.

Related topics

Inter- and Intralingual Translation of Medical Information, Machine Translation in Healthcare, Quality, Accessibility and Readability in Medical Translation

References

Åhlfeldt H., *et al.* (2006) *Literature Review on Patient-Friendly Documentation Systems.* Milton Keynes: Centre for Research in Computing, The Open University.

Askehave, I. and Zethsen, K. K. (2011) 'Lost in Translation: When Patient Information Crosses Borders', *European Industrial Pharmacy,* 11, pp. 14–16.

Bowker, L. and Hawkins, S. (2006) 'Variation in the Organization of Medical Terms: Exploring Some Motivations for Term Choice', *Terminology,* 12(1), pp. 79–110.

Biomettico (n.d.) Available at: http://vandaele.biomettico.org (Accessed: 9 August 2019).

Cabré, M. T., Sager, J. C. and DeCesaris, J. A. (1999) *Terminology: Theory, Methods and Applications*. Amsterdam and Philadelphia: John Benjamins.

Campos, D., Matos, S. and Oliveira, J. L. (2012) 'Biomedical Named Entity Recognition: A Survey of Machine-Learning Tools, Theory and Applications for Advanced Text Mining', *IntechOpen,* DOI:10.5772/51066.

Cangioli, G., *et al.* (2016) 'How Fit is SNOMED CT for eHealth Interoperability in Europe?', *MIE – Medical Informatics Europe Conference*, August 2016. www.researchgate.net/publication/308384359_How_fit_is_SNOMED_CT_for_eHealth_interoperability_in_Europe

Cappuzzo, B. (2008) 'Eponyms or Descriptive Equivalent Terms? The Question of Scientific Accuracy In Medical Discourse', in Auteri, L. (ed.) *Esercizi, Miscellanea del Dipartimento di Scienze Filologiche e Linguistiche*, vol. 2. Palermo: Luxograph, pp. 25–35.

Diekema, A. R. (2012) 'Multilinguality in the Digital Library: A Review', *The Electronic Library,* 30(2), pp. 165–181.

Dinu, G., Mathur, P., Federico, M. and Al-Onaizan, Y. (2019) *Training Neural Machine Translation to Apply Terminology Constraints*. Proceedings of the 57th Annual Meeting of the Association for Computational Linguistics. Available at: https://arxiv.org/abs/1906.01105 (Accessed: 9 August 2019).

España-Bonet C., Stiller J., Ramthun R., Van Genabith J., Petras V. (2019) 'Query Translation for Cross-Lingual Search in the Academic Search Engine PubPsych', in Garoufallou E., Sartori F., Siatri R. and Zervas M. (eds.) *Metadata and Semantic Research. MTSR 2018. Communications in Computer and Information Science,* vol 846. Berlin and Heidelberg: Springer. DOI:10.1007/978-3-030-14401-2_4.

European Commission (2009) *Guideline on the Readability of the Labelling and Package Leaflet of Medicinal Products for Human Use*. Brussels. Available at: https://ec.europa.eu/health/sites/health/files/files/eudralex/vol-2/c/2009_01_12_readability_guideline_final_en.pdf (Accessed: 9 August 2019).

Gal, I. and Prigat, A. (2005) 'Why Organizations Continue to Create Patient Information Leaflets with Readability and Usability Problems: An Exploratory Study', *Health Education Research,* 20(4), pp. 485–493. DOI:10.1093/her/cyh009.

Goldsmith, E. (n.d.). *Signs and Symptoms of Translation: A Blog by a Spanish to English Medical Translator*. Available at: https://signsandsymptomsoftranslation.com (Accessed: 9 August 2019).

Grön L. and Bertels, A. (2018) 'Clinical Sublanguages: Vocabulary Structure and Its Impact on Term Weighting', *Terminology,* 24(1), pp. 41–65. DOI:10.1075/term.00013.gro.
Hadlow, J. and Pitts, M. (1991) 'The Understanding of Common Health Terms by Doctors, Nurses and Patients', *Social Science and Medicine*, 32(2), pp. 193–196.
ITI Medical and Pharmaceutical Network (n.d.) Available at: www.itimedical.co.uk (Accessed: 9 August 2019).
Kenny, T. *et al.* (1999) 'A PIL for Every Ill? Patient Information Leaflets (PILs): A Review of Past, Present and Future Use', *Family Practice,* 15(5), pp. 471–479.
Kersey-Matusiak, G. (2018) 'Cultural Considerations When the Patient Speaks a Different Language', in Kersey-Matusiak, G., (ed.) *Delivering Culturally Competent Nursing Care.* New York: Springer, pp. 101–114.
Krauthammer, M. and Nenadic, G. (2004) 'Term Identification in the Biomedical Literature', *Journal of Biomedical Informatics,* 37(6), pp. 512–526. DOI:10.1016/j.jbi.2004.08.004.
Montalt, V., Zethsen K. and Karwacka, W. (2018) 'Medical Translation in the 21st Century – Challenges and Trends', in Montalt, V., Zethsen K. and Karwacka, W. (eds) *Retos actuales y tendencias emergentes en traducción médica / Current Challenges and Emerging Trends in Medical Translation. Mon*TI, 10, pp. 27–42.
Munane, F. A. (2014) *Cultural Taboos as a Factor in Interpretation in the Medical Field. The Case Study of the Meridian Hospital.* Master's Thesis. University of Nairobi.
Rogers, M. (2015) 'Terminology and Text: Closing the Gaps', in Rogers, M. *Specialised Translation. Palgrave Studies in Translating and Interpreting.* Basingstoke and New York: Palgrave Macmillan, pp. 110–135. DOI:10.1057/9781137478412_5
Sager, J. (1990) *Practical course in terminology processing.* Amsterdam and Philadelphia: John Benjamins.
Vandaele, S. (2001a) 'Noyaux conceptuels et traduction médicale', *Meta: Journal des Traducteurs*', 46(1), pp.16–21. DOI:10.7202/004533ar.
Vandaele, S. (2001b) 'Utilisation des bases de données bibliographiques spécialisées en traduction médicale', *Meta: Journal des Traducteurs*, 46(1), pp. 103–116. DOI:10.7202/004534ar.
Van den Muijsenbergh, M., Krystallidou, D. and Langewitz, W. (forthcoming) Healthcare Communication across Language Barriers (Position Paper). *EACH*, International Association for Communication in Healthcare.
Van Everdingen, J. J. E. and Van den Eerenbeemt, A. M. M. (2012) *Pinkhof Geneeskundig Woordenboek*. Houten: Bohn Stafleu Van Loghum.
Vanopstal, K., Vander Stichele, R., Laureys, G. and Buysschaert, J. (2011) 'Vocabularies and Retrieval Tools in Biomedicine: Disentangling the Terminological Knot', *Journal of Medical Systems*, 35(4), pp.527–543. DOI:10.1007/s10916-009-9389-z.
Von Elm, E., *et al.* (2013) 'Translating Cochrane Reviews to Ensure That Healthcare Decision-Making is Informed by High-Quality Research Evidence', *PLoS Med,* 10(9), e1001516. DOI:10.1371/journal.pmed.1001516.
Wermuth, C. and Verplaetse, H. (2019) 'Medical Terminology in The Western World. Current Situation', in Alsulaiman, A. and Ahmed Allaithy, A. (eds) *Handbook of Terminology, Volume 2 [HoT2]: Terminology in the Arab world.* Amsterdam and Philadelphia: John Benjamins, pp. 84–108.
Whitworth J. A. (2007) 'Should Eponyms be Abandoned? No', *BMJ*, 335(7617), p. 425. Available at: www.bmj.com/cgi/content/full/335/7617/425 (Accessed: 9 August 2019)
WHO (2016) *International Classification of Diseases*, 10th ed. Geneva: World Health Organisation. Available at: https://icd.who.int/browse10/2016/en#/ (Accessed: 9 August 2019).
Woywodt A. and Matteson, E. (2007) 'Should Eponyms be Abandoned? Yes', *BMJ*, 335(7617), p. 424. Available at: www.bmj.com/cgi/content/full/335/7617/424 (Accessed: 9 August 2019).

5
Quality, accessibility and readability in medical translation

Wioleta Karwacka

1 Introduction

Quality, readability and accessibility are three aspects of the patient-related dimension of medical translation. The quality of medical texts translated for lay recipients is associated with three key concepts: patient-centred care (PCC), personalised medicine (PM) and translational medicine (TM), as these involve stressing the critical impact of information transfer, including recontextualisation and communication (Montalt 2017; Montalt, Zethsen and Karwacka 2018: 28). Patient-centredness, which is the acknowledgement of the role of the patient as the focus of interest in healthcare context, is closely associated with quality, readability and accessibility; accessibility ensures that a patient is able to and knows how to access healthcare services, while readability enables a patient to comprehend their condition, understand their treatment and use medicines or medical devices in a safe way. Quality medical translation for patients needs to be readable and is a prerequisite for accessible healthcare which overcomes language barriers.

This trend is reflected in guidelines concerning language use in texts addressed to patients and can be traced in various normative acts. The European Commission Directive 2004/27/EC, for instance, includes a requirement for patient information to be 'legible, clear and easy to use' and to be also presented in Braille or another format accessible to visually-impaired patients. This directive ensures that the information on how to use a drug in an adequate and safe way is conveyed in a manner and form that enables the users to comprehend the content and comply with the recommendations for use (cf. Andriesen 2008). It also shows how readability, accessibility and quality are interrelated and interdependent concepts; high-quality documents addressed to patients are readable and accessible to various groups of patients, including visually-impaired ones or those with limited health literacy, thus securing access to health-related information.

This chapter is divided into three sections, each in turn addressing the concepts of quality, accessibility and readability in medical translations. The first section provides an overview of the problems and definitions associated with medical translation quality, followed by approaches related to factors such as compliance with legal requirements

DOI: 10.4324/9781003167983-8

or medical translator competence. The following section focuses on accessibility in healthcare, which is here primarily understood as the overcoming of language barriers in health services. The aim of this section is to explain how access is conceptualised, how it is connected to language, and what strategies can be adopted to secure healthcare accessibility. Lastly, the final section focusing on readability discusses the relevant definitions and regulations, together with an overview of studies into the readability of medical texts.

2 Medical translation quality

The quality of translated medical texts has historically received significantly less attention in the medical community than medical and pharmaceutical research or the practising of medicine (cf. Abootorabi and Moeinzadeh 2017). However, given that a mistake in medical translation may jeopardise the chances of a research paper being published or of being of clinical consequence (see for example, Wolz 2015: 248–250), the quality of translated medical texts has in recent years received increasingly more attention from researchers and translation professionals alike (see for example, Garcia-Castillo and Fetters 2007; Fernández Piera and Ardura Ortega 2012; Nisbeth Jensen 2012; Abootorabi and Moeinzadeh 2017).

Although the quality of medical translation is frequently conceptualised by researchers and specialists in the field as a requirement for literal accuracy and precision, it is conceptual accuracy (i.e. retaining the same meaning) that is actually desirable, as opposed to word-for-word rendition (Garcia-Castillo and Fetters 2007: 77). 'Cultural equivalence', which is understood as ensuring that the cultural concepts in the target text can be adequately perceived by recipients, is a frequently stressed notion in the context of medical translation quality (Garcia-Castillo and Fetters 2007: 77), alongside sensitivity to factors such as race, ethnicity, language variations, gender, age and religion. In terms of practical aspects of medical translation quality, researchers frequently mention handling intralingual variations such as dialects, or the necessity to check target texts for errors or mistranslations by means of pilot testing or the use of various quality assessment models (Garcia-Castillo and Fetters 2007: 77). What needs to be emphasised is that quality assurance starts (or should ideally start) before a translation assignment is commissioned, i.e. when the source text is drafted. This stage includes predicting potential culture-specific problems and assuring compliance with the conventions and requirements of specific text genres or functions, such as readability and clarity in expert-lay communication.

One of the factors which are critical for the quality of medical translation is the design of the project. The International Standard ISO 17100:2015 was developed to help in the implementing of quality assurance procedures at various stages of translation projects and it is followed by a number of translation agencies. The standard ensures adequate human resources (competent translators, revisers and reviewers), properly designed pre-production (e.g. managing client enquiries, assessing feasibility, drafting agreements with the client), translation (including checks, revisions, reviews and proofreading) and the post-production process. In general, the standard offers guidelines on checking the translation for the presence of omissions and semantic, grammatical or spelling mistakes. Its overall aim is to ensure 'compliance with relevant translation project specifications' (ISO 17100: 2015) rather than providing measurable parameters for assessing translation quality (Montalt, Zethsen and Karwacka 2018). The International Medical Interpreters

Association (IMIA) guide also addresses the translation project design and recommends a set of standard good practices:

1. Have a central source document repository at the institution in question
2. Establish a central translation management point
3. Prioritise translation needs
4. Recruit, qualify, select and manage vendors
5. Know how to request a quote
6. Negotiate realistic deadlines
7. Know which sources should be created and maintained to aid the translation and quality control processes (Txabarriaga 2008: 8–12).

Institutions which handle translated texts develop their own medical translation verification procedures. The IMIA applies a two-step verification process involving two editing rounds (Txabarriaga 2008: 17). Another commonly used tool for medical translation quality assurance is the back-translation procedure (cf. Fernández Piera and Ardura Ortega 2012), particularly in the sector of medical research and clinical trials, as it is required by Ethics Committees and regulatory authorities in a number of countries (Grunwald and Goldfarb 2006: 2). The procedure involves translating the target text 'back' to the source language by another translator and comparing the two source language texts to see if the message is accurately transferred (for further discussion see e.g. O'Neil 1998, Garcia-Castillo and Fetters 2007; Bundgaard and Nisbeth Brøgger 2018). Studies show that the procedure 'can improve the accuracy of translated text by highlighting different possibilities and challenging the translator's choices' (Garcia-Castillo and Fetters 2007: 79), however it also needs to be noted that its usefulness is debatable. Translators are sometimes confused about the procedure or its role in the project (Bundgaard and Nisbeth Brøgger 2018: 219–220). Back translations are also costly and time-consuming, and they do not, for instance, help reveal 'the target language contextual and usage nuances' (Txabarriaga 2008: 2) or awkward word-for-word transfer. The International Society for Pharmacoeconomics and Outcomes Research (ISPOR) uses a review method with two parallel forward translations; this means that two translators prepare their own translations independently. These are then reconciled, then two back translations are produced, compared and reconciled, and finally, after a review and a harmonisation, the target text is developed (Andriesen 2008: 15–16). Parallel translation can also be a standalone quality assurance method, where two parallel translations are produced, then compared, reconciled and accordingly adjusted (Andriesen 2008: 16). Several other instruments can be used to verify the comprehensibility of the translated material in medical translation projects, including the following: pilot testing or readability tests on focus groups of lay recipients (cf. Andriesen 2008: 15–16; Garcia-Castillo and Fetters 2007: 77–78); statistical reviews, which assess readability based on the length of sentences and words used in a document; independent evaluations e.g. by patient organisations; or an additional edit round, i.e. commissioning yet another proofreader of the source text (cf. Andriesen 2008: 15–16). Finally, cognitive debriefing can be used in the verification process of translated questionnaires or scales. This debriefing involves collecting feedback from a sample group of lay respondents on how they understand the wording of a question or statement in order to check if it is adequately readable and lay-friendly while still conveying the original concept (cf. Engel and Koester 2014).

However, despite these various guidelines and regulations, medical translation quality level still varies from project to project (cf. Andriesen 2008). Garcia-Castillo and Fetters (2007: 75) reviewed factors affecting the quality of medical translation, covering both practical aspects of medical translation and external factors which influence the process. The former include translation qualifications, checking target texts for various errors (linguistic, content-related, etc.) including mistranslations, but also the costs of these checks and the question of who is or should be financially responsible for ensuring the quality of medical translation in healthcare institutions (Garcia-Castillo and Fetters 2007: 79; Wolz 2015: 248–250). The external factors include socio-economic considerations such as discrimination or health disparities, and problems related to the patient, such as confidentiality (Garcia-Castillo and Fetters 2007: 78). Although Garcia-Castillo and Fetters (2007) mention the cost of translations amongst the practical aspects of medical translation, budget limitations may be considered an extrinsic factor as they affect the choice of the translator, the selection of quality assurance measures, and may even result in the elimination of the review stage. Extrinsic factors affecting medical translation quality also include legal issues (Garcia-Castillo and Fetters 2007: 79–100), especially the extent to which medical translation and interpreting are mandatory in particular settings or contexts. The failure to provide quality translation or interpreting may mean acting against human rights (when language barriers do not allow access to medical care), or against the Helsinki Declaration which stipulates the ethical principles for medical research involving human subjects (such as when a participant in a clinical trial is not informed about the experiment due to language barriers).

A critical factor determining the quality of medical translation is the competence of the medical translator (O'Neil 1998; Txabarriaga 2008; Garcia-Castillo and Fetters 2007). One reason why this factor is so important is that translators may be – and quite often are – the sole persons responsible for the quality of the translated material in those cases when their work is not proofread or edited (O'Neil 1998). What is more, a target text produced by a more competent translator is more likely to become a high-quality end product after editing than a poorly translated text with editing and other quality assurance procedures in place (cf. Andriesen 2008). Despite the general agreement that medical translator competence is significant in translation quality, specifying a method of testing a medical translator's language skills and other translation competences is yet to be determined in translation research (Garcia-Castillo and Fetters 2007: 77). Moreover, *ad hoc* interpreters or translators, such as family members or hospital staff, who are not properly trained are sometimes employed to facilitate communication in healthcare settings (Garcia-Castillo and Fetters 2007: 77), which potentially increases the risk of mistranslations and, consequently, the possibility of clinically relevant errors.

IMIA lists the following parameters as 'The Profile of a Competent Translator' (Txabarriaga 2008: 3):

- A native or near-native level of language proficiency in the source and target languages
- Deep cultural knowledge of the source and target languages
- Formal education in the source and target languages at least at college level (ideally including courses in translation theory and practice)
- Analytical capabilities
- Writing skills
- Expert knowledge of the subject matter terminology

- Full understanding of the source text
- Competent use of specialised dictionaries
- Preparedness to conduct terminology research to validate equivalents in the target language

Furthermore, Txabarriaga (2005, qtd in Txabarriaga 2008: 3) emphasises the following indicators of medical translation proficiency:

> knowledge of the subject matter, knowledge of relevant terminology, the ability to discern meaning in context and transfer it within the target language constraints, i.e., accurately (all meaning has been transferred), precisely (all nuances of the language, tone, intent, style have been preserved in the target language), correctly (grammar, syntax, orthography rules have been observed), completely (no part of the original was omitted and nothing has been added to the target text), and consistently (specific terms, stylistic elements and language-specific norms have been consistently used throughout).

An even wider range of competences deemed conducive to producing high-quality translation can be found in the model developed by PACTE (Procés d'Adquisició de la Competència Traductora i Avaluació, PACTE 2003, 2005, 2008), which proposes a range of various sub-competencies. Table 5.1 presents the definitions and examples of

Table 5.1 Medical translator sub-competences based on the PACTE model of translator sub-competences (Karwacka 2018; cf. PACTE 2003, 2005, 2008)[1]

Sub-competence (PACTE model)	*Description (PACTE model)*	*Medical translation sub-competence*
Bilingual sub-competence	Procedural knowledge required for communication in two languages	Specialised medical language in source and target languages, including terminology and acronyms; lay and professional terms; registers; controlled terminologies and classification
Extra-linguistic sub-competence	Declarative knowledge; general knowledge, domain-specific knowledge, bicultural competence, etc.	Background medical knowledge, bicultural competence: culture-specific concepts
Knowledge about translation	Declarative knowledge of translation function and aspects of the profession	Standards, conventions and procedures relevant to medical translation
Instrumental sub-competence	Procedural sub-competence; use of resources, information and communication technologies	Use of medical databases, repositories of texts, dictionaries, CAT tools, etc.
Strategic sub-competence	Procedural sub-competence; ability to identify translation problems and apply procedures to solve them	Ability to apply medical translation procedures appropriately
Psychophysiological components	Memory, perception, attention, intellectual curiosity, perseverance, rigour, creativity, logical reasoning, analysis and synthesis, etc.	Decision-making, thoroughness, honesty, punctuality, etc.

each of those sub-competences alongside examples pertaining specifically to medical translation.

These skills address the critical factors affecting the quality of medical translation and allowing for the production of conceptually equivalent texts in which information and culture-specific elements are handled in compliance with target conventions. The competence model also includes sub-competences which are necessary in larger translation projects. For example, CAT tools can positively impact the end product quality, as the use of a termbase ensures a consistent use of terminology throughout a project. Some of the psychophysiological components are not specific only to medical translation, but they remain a crucial aspect of medical translator competence.

Nisbeth Jensen (2012) maps medical translation sub-competences on the PACTE model and compares the competence of translators who are also medical professionals with the set of sub-competences ideally possessed by professional translators. Her study indicates that although medical professionals are more likely to have sufficient background knowledge to perform medical translation tasks, they might not have the other sub-competences crucial in medical translation, such as knowledge about translation or some of the instrumental or strategic sub-competences. Consequently, neither medical nor linguistic certification seems to reliably ensure medical translation competence, which is why interviews, questionnaires and sample translation tests provide more adequate information on the competence profile of a translator.

Various analyses of source and target texts show that certain areas pose particular problems in medical translations. They include the incorrect use of specialised medical language and terminology, problems in managing polysemy, inadequate use of evidence-based medicine (EBM) language, inadequately managed implied information in medical texts (Karwacka 2013, 2016), insufficient readability (Karwacka 2016, Kościałkowska-Okońska 2018), and discourse-related problems (Walkiewicz 2018). For these reasons, it is important to ensure that translation quality assurance begins at the pre-translation stage, based on contribution from clients, translators, proofreaders, project managers and other invested parties, but that it also includes a well-planned translation and editing stage, and that this continues until feedback from clients is collected, translators informed and translation memories updated.

3 Medical translation and accessibility

Accessibility in healthcare can be understood as an unobstructed possibility of using a service or to reach a provider or an institution when necessary, in a manner which is adequate to the needs of an individual patient or the whole community (Levesque, Harris and Russell 2013: 1). Accessibility involves approachability ('people facing health needs can actually identify that some form of services exists, can be reached, and have an impact on the health of the individual', Levesque, Harris and Russell 2013: 5), acceptability ('cultural and social factors determining the possibility for people to accept the aspects of the service', Levesque, Harris and Russell 2013: 5), availability, accommodation, affordability, and appropriateness ('the fit between services and clients' need, its timeliness, the amount of care spent in assessing health problems and determining the correct treatment and the technical and interpersonal quality of the services provided', Levesque, Harris, Russell 2013: 6). These correspond with specific ability dimensions: ability to perceive, ability to seek, ability to reach, ability to pay, and ability to engage (Levesque, Harris and Russell 2013: 5).

The World Health Organisation specifies accessibility as follows:

> Health facilities, goods and services have to be accessible to everyone without discrimination, within the jurisdiction of the State party. Accessibility has four overlapping dimensions:
>
> - Non-discrimination
> - Physical accessibility
> - Economic accessibility (affordability)
> - Information accessibility.
>
> *WHO 2002: 12*

Information accessibility 'includes the right to seek, receive and impart information and ideas concerning health issues' (WHO 2002: 13). This access to information, however, 'should not impair the right to have personal health data treated with confidentiality' (WHO 2002: 13), which may be jeopardised e.g. when health information is transferred via *ad hoc* interpreters, such as other patients or hospital staff. Consequently, medical translation (including interpreting) is the *sine qua non* condition for overcoming language barriers and securing accessibility for ethnic minorities, migrants or other persons with limited language proficiency. Sign language interpreting and intralingual transcription into Braille ensure information accessibility for severely hearing-impaired or visually-impaired patients. Intralingual translation secures information accessibility for those with limited health literacy through lay-friendly, easy to read materials. Meaningful access does not only involve the availability of translation services, but also ensures that the target texts satisfy the needs of the recipients. If the postulate of affordability is to be met, translation and interpreting services in healthcare settings should be free of charge for the patients who require them, and the most efficient way of ensuring this is by introducing a reimbursement system for language services within healthcare settings (Chen, Youdelman and Brooks 2007: 366).

The right to full access to medical services results from a number of regulatory acts, including the Universal Declaration of Human Rights, the International Convention on the Elimination of All Forms of Racial Discrimination, the Convention on the Rights of the Child, the Framework Convention for the Protection of National Minorities and the International Covenant on Economic, Social and Cultural Rights, as well as from the European Constitution, the European Convention on Human Rights, and from other country-specific constitutions and laws (Baráth *et al.* 2007: 21–38). According to these regulatory acts, everyone should have access to relevant documents and interlingual communication with medical staff, however studies show that patients are not always sufficiently assisted. For instance, a study which investigated the availability of interpreters at 240 healthcare services in 16 European countries in 2012 revealed that 42 per cent of them provided no links to interpreting services (Kluge *et al.* 2012: 258–259). A number of researchers report insufficient linguistic accessibility or inadequate linguistic services as a barrier directly affecting the quality of medical services (see for example, Chen, Youdelman and Brooks 2007: 362–366; Brisset *et al.* 2013: 1238–1246; Wolz 2015: 248–250). That means that language barriers prevent patients from obtaining quality healthcare or even from seeking medical help and make them vulnerable, therefore proving that interpreting is an important factor in the provision of health-related services (Al-Sharifi *et al.* 2019). Such barriers also adversely affect provider effectiveness and satisfaction, as they prevent providers from meeting professional standards of care (Bowen 2001). Consequently, they also increase exposure to liability risks. What is more, language barriers may also affect healthcare costs through their effects on service utilisation and health outcomes. However, the potential economic advantages of employing skilled interpreters have not been assessed in detail yet, and such an evaluation would need to be country-specific as the results of estimates for one country might not be transferable to other countries (Bowen 2001). Language barriers may indirectly affect the process of healthcare provision in other ways. For example, they may lead to socio-demographic exclusion and consequently insufficient research participation of language minorities in medical studies, which in turn may cause a bias in study results which do not accurately represent the entire population, or lead to conclusions which erroneously ignore risk factors, disease prevalence or treatment response in certain ethnocultural groups (Bowen 2001). It is especially important in those cases when a minority is particularly likely to be affected by a disease but is underrepresented in a study, and raises serious doubts about the generalisability of research results.

The problems of accessibility are complex, which is why recommended approaches include a number of strategies to address their various aspects. The first step to counteract the consequences of insufficient accessibility is the identification of the issue itself (Wolz 2015: 249), which can be done for instance by means of surveys addressed to healthcare providers and patients. The strategies that are proposed as potential solutions include adequate financing mechanisms, increasing the number of properly qualified medical interpreters (Chen, Youdelman and Brooks 2007: 365–366), ensuring cultural competence training (Wolz 2015: 249), increasing medical interpreting quality by coordinating and standardising applicable practices followed by medical interpreters (Chen, Youdelman and Brooks 2007: 364–366), and raising awareness on the effects of language barriers including their medical, social and legal dimensions, both for institutional service providers and for patients.

4 Readability

Securing access to healthcare involves ensuring readability of texts addressed to patients or other lay recipients such as patients' parents, guardians or caregivers, and thus making them user- and patient-friendly. The US Food and Drug Administration (FDA) defines readability as 'the ease of understanding or comprehension achieved by the style of writing' (2001: 23); they further specify that 'reading involves both decoding and comprehension. The reader must be able to recognize (decode) the words in the medical device patient labelling as well as comprehend the meaning of the text' (US Food and Drug Administration 2001: 23). Readability of medical information is regulated by law in a number of countries, and this section discusses regulations in the EU and the US.

In the EU, readability requirements and the related issue of accessibility are particularly delineated in the case of package leaflets and labels:

> Pack design and labelling ensure that the critical information necessary for the safe use of a medicine is legible, easily accessible and that users of medicines can easily assimilate this information so that any risk of confusion and error is minimised. For non-prescription medicines the clear identification and selection of the appropriate medicine is very important, especially in cases where there is no pharmacist

> intervention, therefore, pack design and labelling are considered key elements to ensure the safe use of this type of medicines.
>
> *European Medicines Agency 2011: 3*

The European Medicines Agency's (EMA) Working Group on the Quality Review of Documents (QRD group) has developed specific guidelines and templates in order to harmonise content presentation in summaries of product characteristics, package leaflets, pack design and labels (cf. Wolf, Fuchs and Schweim 2014: 1; European Medicines Agency n.d.; European Medicines Agency 2016). QRD's guidelines outline the critical readability and accessibility-related aspects of the written materials for patients. These guidelines are relevant to medical translation as the labels are often translated into various (not only European) languages, and the target text needs to be clear and easily understood in order to ensure that patients understand all the important information and can use a medicine in a safe way:

> A good combination of clear/comprehensive information and pack design ensures that the information considered critical for the safe and effective use of a medicine is easily accessible by the consumer or healthcare professional selecting the product, and helps differentiate medicines within the same range (e.g. umbrella brands) to minimise the risk of confusion.
>
> *European Medicines Agency 2011: 3*

QRD recommendations include clear and cohesive presentation of key information such as the name of the active substance, route of administration, indications, dosage and contraindications, including graphically presented information (pictograms), etc. The regulatory basis for this document is Directive 2001/83/EC, which regulates the requirements relevant to package labelling and packaging information, including detailed mandatory information, logos and pictograms. Moreover, layout, font type, and other graphic considerations are regulated by the 'Guideline on the readability of the labelling and package leaflet of medicinal products for human use' (Revision 1, 12 January 2009), also called the 'Readability Guideline' and 'Guideline on the packaging information of medicinal products for human use authorised by the Union' (Revision 14.3, July 2015).

The 'Readability Guideline' (European Commission 2009) provides extensive recommendations on those aspects of drug leaflets and labels which affect readability and user-friendliness. These include design, layout, style and syntax, recommendations for preparing the materials for visually-impaired and blind patients, outline for pilot tests of leaflets, etc. The guideline is also a source of templates for labels and leaflets. Medicinal product package labels and patient leaflets in all language versions should conform to the guideline, which makes it a prominent quality-related medical translation norm for EU countries.

The linguistic requirements introduced in the guideline of the European Commission (2009), such as the use of simple vocabulary and the avoidance of long sentences and paragraphs, should be met by both the source and target texts. The guideline does not specify how long a sentence or a paragraph should be, but recommends the use of lists rather than long paragraphs, and these should consist of a maximum of 5–6 bullet points. Side effects should be listed in order of frequency, not by system or class. Sentences should be written in active rather than passive voice and reasoning should be provided for specific recommendations in the leaflet. Instead of repeating the name of the drug, the guidelines recommend the use of 'this medicine' or 'your medicine', and all abbreviations, acronyms and medical terms should be followed by an explanation. The document also provides specific guidance on adapting the materials to the needs of blind patients: the Marburg Braille system is recommended, and the packaging should include name of the medicinal product and its strength in Braille. Pharmaceutical companies can also make other information available for the blind and visually impaired, such as leaflets which are provided to patient organisations upon request.

The guideline recommends patient consultations to 'identify whether or not the information as presented, conveys the correct messages to those who read it. Testing itself does not improve the quality of the information but it will indicate where there are problem areas which should be rectified' (European Commission 2009: 20). The main purpose of the test is to make sure that the materials are legible, clear and easy to use, and, consequently, ensure compliance with Directive 2001/83/EC as amended and Directive 2004/27/EC.

The guideline also specifically addresses the issue of translation which is subject to quality verification and testing:

> The package leaflet should be legible, clear and easy to read in all EEA languages. As a matter of principle it is normally sufficient to undertake patient consultation in one EEA language. [...] In the centralised, decentralised and mutual recognition procedure, only the English language version of the package leaflet will be agreed during the scientific assessment. The quality of translation should be the focus of a thorough review by the applicant/marketing authorisation holder once the original package leaflet has been properly tested and modified. During the drafting of the original package leaflet every effort should be made to ensure that the package leaflet can be translated from the original to the various national languages in a clear and understandable way. It is important that the outcome of the user consultation is then correctly translated into other languages.
>
> *European Commission 2009: 21–22*

It is worth emphasising that only one target language version has to be verified and consulted, but the expectation remains that all target texts will be equally readable. However, as various analyses of patient leaflets show (see for example Kościałkowska-Okońska 2018), not all target texts meet this criterion.

The translated versions are expected to be accurate renditions of the original message and use natural language, but they do not specify which particular features are expected to be present in a translation, nor how to achieve this accuracy:

> Strict literal translations from the original language may lead to package leaflets which contain unnatural phrases resulting in a package leaflet which is difficult for patients to understand. Therefore, different language versions of the same package leaflet should be 'faithful' translations allowing for regional translation flexibility, whilst maintaining the same core meaning.
>
> *European Commission 2009: 22*

The linguistic features of other medical documents, such as patient brochures or discharge summaries, are not subject to specific readability regulations, although QRD decisions (European Medicines Agency 2019) also concern the wording of the Summary of Product

Characteristics (SmPC). This includes the use of abbreviations and acronyms, subscript and superscript, foreign terms, grammatical gender, measures, health information or the translation of international non-proprietary names (i.e. official standard names for drugs which are not registered brand names). The overall purpose of the QRD decisions seems to be to avoid recurring linguistic (especially stylistic) issues and to ensure consistency, but some attention is given to readability, such as that '[i]nformation on the disease should normally be limited to a patient-friendly description of the sections "indications" and "pharmacotherapeutic group" of the SmPC, under their respective headings' (European Medicines Agency 2019: 5).

In the United States, readability is regulated in FDA documents such as MG (Medication Guide), PPI (Patient Package Insert) and PIFU (Patient Instructions for Use), which concern 'outpatient Rx products with serious and significant public health concerns and based on (not in conflict with) Professional Information (PI)' (US Food and Drug Administration). It is emphasised that adequate patient labelling contributes to preventing serious adverse events, improves patient adherence to drug application instructions, and affects the patient's decision to use a given product (US Food and Drug Administration 2001). Prescription medication labels should be typed in at least 12-point font size, written in non-technical language and organised in question-and-answer format (US Food and Drug Administration 2001). Readability level of patient labelling should be close to the proficiency level at 6th to 8th grade of US education. The guidelines also indicate the importance of appropriate spacing or bullet points (US Food and Drug Administration n.d.).

FDA also regulates the labelling of the more complex medical devices that are aimed at direct patient use, such as insulin pumps or test kits. The regulations emphasise comprehensibility in their safe use and disposal which include explanations for any terminology or jargon and a writing style that takes the patients' expectations into account. Recommended strategies to facilitate comprehension include repeating and summarising the most important information, organising complex information in tables, concise writing, and the use of lay words with professional terminology in parentheses, italics or otherwise highlighted to signal the appearance of specialised terms (US Food and Drug Administration 2001).

Readability and comprehensibility can be tested in pilot studies which are recommended both by EU and US authorities. The readability of EU package leaflets is verified in legibility and usability tests to ensure that information is presented in a clear, simple and comprehensible manner from the perspective of medicine users and with special focus on the main topics, i.e. indications and contraindications (Pires, Vigário and Cavaco 2015: 3). The Readability Guideline (European Commission 2009: 24) discusses the profile of test participants consisting of at least 20 subjects who are not professionally involved in healthcare and who represent the population sample that is most likely to use the medication in question (thus avoiding socio-demographic exclusion). The group should also include geriatric patients and those with limited health or language proficiency. If the test results suggest that the recipients find it difficult to identify or understand the information in the leaflet, the text needs to be amended and tested again. The threshold value for the readability test result is 90 per cent, i.e. it is assumed that the text is comprehensible if 90 per cent of answers are correct (Pires, Vigário and Cavaco 2015: 3). As mentioned above, readability tests are required for one European language version only (European Commission 2009), which means that readability of different language versions of the same text may vary.

FDA offers guidance for comprehension studies concerning non-prescription drug labelling focusing especially on 'the major communication message with the greatest clinical consequence to the consumer' (US Food and Drug Administration 2010: 4). The target level of comprehension is determined at the stage of study planning and it may vary depending on the 'clinical significance of the primary communication objective' (US Food and Drug Administration 2010: 4), which may include the understanding of indications and contraindications, dosage, warnings, drug interactions, etc. (US Food and Drug Administration 2010: 4.). Secondary communication objectives, which are not obligatory, concern less critical information such as general health information (e.g. when using this product, continue a healthy diet and exercise). The questions designed to check comprehension can be closed or open-ended, but should be 'direct, specific, and unambiguous' (US Food and Drug Administration 2010: 8). Multiple-choice questions should not be overused, and the questions should not be biasing or leading. The purpose of these questions is to check understanding, not to test behaviour. If an incorrect answer is provided, there should be follow up questions to identify the source of the comprehension problem (US Food and Drug Administration 2010: 8).

Despite these regulations being in place, package leaflets of medicinal products, and especially sections concerning dosage or adverse drug reactions, can still be difficult to understand, particularly for low-literacy patients (Pires, Vigário and Cavaco 2015: 1–3). Furthermore, although it is commonly agreed that the readability of patient information is important, user tests or readability checks are not always performed on translated texts. Wolf, Fuchs and Schweim (2014) tested QRD template versions 8 and 7.3.1 together with a shorter model template, and concluded that QRD templates can be improved and condensed. They also suggest readability testing of the templates (not only the documents based on them) before they are used. Readability can be checked in pilot studies with comprehension questions, or with the use of readability formulas, for example, the Flesch-Kincaid formula or Simple Measure of Gobbledygook (SMOG), which are based on the length of words and sentences used in a particular text (Wang *et al.* 2013: 503–514).

Although there are no specific guidelines concerning the quality of texts translated for the purposes of conducting clinical trials (Andriesen 2008), there are European recommendations related to the readability of patient information and the informed consent form (ICF). This information must be presented in writing and should be 'comprehensive, concise, clear, relevant, and understandable to a layperson' (European Patients' Forum 2016: 4–5). The quality and quantity of the information provided to patients are still subject to debate, and the process of obtaining informed consent is sometimes treated as a formality involving rushed box-ticking rather than a meaningful and informative presentation of risks and benefits (European Patients' Forum 2016: 3). The US regulations state that the 'information must be in language that is understandable to the research subject' (US Food and Drug Administration 2018). If information is not provided in the language a participant understands, language barriers adversely affect or even hinder the informed consent process, which illustrates the interdependence of readability and accessibility.

5 Conclusions

Medical translation quality, readability and accessibility are important factors in patient safety, influence a patient's decision to use a medicine or a service, have an impact on the quality of healthcare services, and can determine the representation of various groups in clinical trials. For these reasons, all three issues deserve interest and concern of various stakeholders, including translation scholars, health scientists, patient organisations, ombudspersons, etc. As discussed in this chapter, research into quality, readability and accessibility is ontological, descriptive and prescriptive – authors attempt to conceptualise what those phenomena essentially are, describe the various aspects of those problems, and formulate recommendations or strategies for increased patient-centredness, which frequently indicate the need to improve quality, readability and accessibility and raise awareness about those aspects of medical translation. The problematic areas include, in particular, the gap between the needs or expectations and the reality, the friction between literal and semantically accurate translations, as well as verification procedures and pilot tests. Future research will hopefully shed light on those gaps and contribute to more patient-centred medical translation.

Note

1 The description of sub-competences was developed by PACTE (Procés d'Adquisició de la Competència Traductora i Avaluació, PACTE 2003, 2005, 2008) and the division of medical subcompetences discussed in this chapter is based on the PACTE model. The medical subcompetence division presented in Table 1 was also described and published in Polish (Karwacka 2018).

Further reading

Garcia-Castillo D, and Fetters, M. D. (2007) 'Quality in Medical Translations: A Review', *Journal of Health Care for the Poor and Underserved,* 18, pp. 74–84.

An overview of research into medical translation quality and of approaches to the problem.

Levesque, J-F, Harris, M. F. and Russell, G. (2013) 'Patient-Centred Access to Health Care: Conceptualising Access at the Interface of Health Systems and Populations', *International Journal for Equity in Health,* 12(18).

An analysis of the issue of access to healthcare from the perspective of patient-centredness.

Montalt, V. (2017) 'Patient-Centred Translation and Emerging Trends in Medicine and Healthcare', *The EST Newsletter*, European Society for Translation. Available at: www.est-translationstudies.org/commit-tees/news_editors.html (Accessed: 4 May 2019).

Patient-centredness in medical translation.

Wolf A., Fuchs, J and Schweim, H. G. (2014) 'Readability of the European QRD Template. The European QRD Template Version 8 in Comparison to Its Predecessor and a Shorter Model Template', *Pharmazeutische Industrie*, 76(8), pp. 1312–1322.

Readability testing of package leaflet templates.

Wolz, M. (2015) 'Language Barriers: Challenges to Quality Healthcare', *International Journal of Dermatology,* 54, pp. 248–250.

The influence of linguistic communication shortcomings on healthcare.

Related topics

Medical Terminology and Discourse, Machine Translation in Healthcare, Inter- and Intralingual Translation of Medical Information

References

Abootorabi, E. and Moeinzadeh, S. N. (2017) 'Quality Assessment of Medical Translations Performed by the Two Groups of Medical Translators and Physicians', *Journal of Paramedical Sciences (JPS)*, 8(4), pp. 26–35.

Al-Sharifi, F., Winther Frederiksen, H., Knold Rossau, H., Norredam, M. and Zwisler, A. D. (2019) 'Access to Cardiac Rehabilitation and the Role of Language Barriers in the Provision of Cardiac Rehabilitation to Migrants', *BMC Health Services Research*, 19(1), p. 223. DOI:10.1186/s12913-019-4041-1.

Andriesen, S. (2008) 'Quality Control in Medical Translations', *Innovation in Pharmaceutical Technology*, 25, pp. 12–16.

Baráth, Á., Gajewska, A., Jones, A., Macáková, S., Moisă, F., Ondrušová, M. and Szilárd, I. (2007) *Budowanie zdrowych społeczności romskich. Podręcznik szkoleniowy.* Brussels: International Organization for Migration (IOM).

Bowen, S. (2001) *Language Barriers in Access to Health Care.* Health Canada. Available at: www.canada.ca/en/health-canada/services/health-care-system/reports-publications/health-care-accessibility/language-barriers.html (Accessed: 4 May 2019).

Brisset, C., *et al.* (2013) 'Language Barriers in Mental Health Care: A Survey of Primary Care Practitioners', *Journal of Immigrant Minority Health.* 16, pp. 1238–1246. DOI:10.1007/s10903-013-9971-9.

Bundgaard, K. and Brøgger, M. N. (2018) '"Don't Fix Bad Translations": A Netnographic Study of Translators' Understandings of Back Translation in the Medical Domain', *MonTI*, 10, pp. 205–224.

Chen, A. H., Youdelman, M. K. and Brooks, J. (2007) 'The Legal Framework for Language Access in Healthcare Settings: Title VI and Beyond', *Journal of General Internal Medicine*, 22(2), pp. 362–367.

Engel, U. and Koester, B. (2014) 'Response Effects and the Cognitive Involvement in Answering Survey Questions', in Engel, U., Jann, B., Lynn, P., Scherpenzeel, A. and Sturgis, P. (eds.) *Improving Survey Methods Lessons from Recent Research.* London and New York: Routledge.

European Commission (2009) *Guideline on the Readability of the Labelling and Package Leaflet of Medicinal Products for Human Use.* Revision 1, 12 January 2009. https://ec.europa.eu/health/sites/health/files/files/eudralex/vol-2/c/2009_01_12_readability_guideline_final_en.pdf (Accessed: 4 May 2019).

European Commission (2015) *Guideline on the Packaging Information of Medicinal Products for Human Use Authorised by the Union.* Revision 14.3, July 2015. https://ec.europa.eu/health//sites/health/files/files/eudralex/vol-2/2015-07_14_3_packaging.pdf (Accessed: 4 May 2019).

European Medicines Agency (n.d.) *Product Information Templates.* www.ema.europa.eu/en/human-regulatory/marketing-authorisation/product-information/product-information-templates (Accessed: 4 May 2019).

European Medicines Agency (2011) 'QRD Recommendations on Pack Design and Labelling for Centrally Authorised Non-Prescription Human Medicinal Products', *Quality Review of Documents (QRD).* www.ema.europa.eu/en/documents/regulatory-procedural-guideline/draft-quality-review-documents-recommendations-pack-design-labelling-centrally-authorised-non_en.pdf (Accessed: 4 May 2019).

European Medicines Agency (2016) 'QRD Product-Information Annotated Template (English) Version 10', *Centralised Procedures – Quality Review of Documents (QRD) Templates.* www.ema.europa.eu/en/documents/template-form/qrd-product-information-annotated-template-english-version-10_en.pdf (Accessed: 4 May 2019).

European Medicines Agency (2019) *Compilation of QRD Decisions on Stylistic Matters in Product Information.* www.ema.europa.eu/en/documents/regulatory-procedural-guideline/compilation-quality-review-documents-decisions-stylistic-matters-product-information_en.pdf (Accessed: 4 May 2019).

European Patients' Forum (2016) *Clinical Trials Regulation: Informed Consent and Information to Patients.* www.eu-patient.eu/globalassets/policy/clinicaltrials/epf_informed_consent_position_statement_may16.pdf (Accessed: 4 May 2019).

European Parliament and Council (2001) *Directive 2001/83/EC of 6 November 2001 on the Community Code Relating to Medicinal Products for Human Use.* Luxembourg: Office for

Official Publications of the European Communities. Available at: https://ec.europa.eu/health/sites/health/files/files/eudralex/vol-1/dir_2001_83_consol_2012/dir_2001_83_cons_2012_en.pdf (Accessed: 4 May 2019).

European Parliament and Council (2004) *Directive 2004/27/EC of 31 March 2004 amending Directive 2001/83/EC on the Community Code Relating to Medicinal Products for Human Use.* Luxembourg: Office for Official Publications of the European Communities. https://ec.europa.eu/health/sites/health/files/files/eudralex/vol-1/dir_2004_27/dir_2004_27_en.pdf (Accessed: 4 May 2019).

Fernández Piera, M. and Ardura Ortega, M. (2012) 'Adaptación del consentimiento informado a la legislación española en los ensayos clínicos internacionales', *Panace*, 36(13), pp. 291–293.

Garcia-Castillo D, and Fetters, M. D. (2007) 'Quality in Medical Translations: A Review', *Journal of Health Care for the Poor and Underserved,* 18, pp. 74–84.

Grunwald, D. and Goldfarb, N. (2006) 'Back Translation for Quality Control of Informed Consent Forms', *Journal of Clinical Research Best Practices*, 2(2).

International Organization for Standardization (2015) *Translation Services-Requirements for Translation Services*. Technical Committee, ISO 17100:2015.

Karwacka, W. (2013) 'Constructing Translation Research with the Use of Keystroke Logging: A Case Study', *Forum Filologiczne Ateneum*, 1(1), pp. 93–111.

Karwacka, W. (2016) *Przekład tekstów medycznych. Normy, standardy i problemy*. Gdańsk: Gdańsk University Press.

Karwacka, W. (2018) 'Medical Translation Training: From a Translation Student to a Medical Translation Professional', in Karwacka, W. (ed.) *Towards Understanding Medical Translation and Interpreting.* Gdańsk: Gdańsk University Press, pp. 177–190.

Kościałkowska-Okońska, E. (2018) 'Translating Patient Information Leaflets: Expectations of Users and the Reality', in Karwacka, W. (ed.) *Towards Understanding Medical Translation and Interpreting.* Gdańsk: Gdańsk University Press, pp 137–159.

Kluge, U., *et al.* (2012) 'Health Services and the Treatment of Immigrants: Data on Service Use, Interpreting Services and Immigrant Staff Members in Services Across Europe', *European Psychiatry*, special issue 'Migration and Mental Health', 27(2), pp. S56–S62. DOI:10.1016/S0924-9338(12)75709-7.

Levesque, J.-F., Harris, M. F. and Russell, G. (2013) 'Patient-Centred Access to Health Care: Conceptualising Access at the Interface of Health Systems and Populations', *International Journal for Equity in Health*, 12(18) https://equityhealthj.biomedcentral.com/articles/10.1186/1475-9276-12-18.

Montalt, V. (2017) 'Patient-Centred Translation and Emerging Trends in Medicine and Healthcare', *The EST Newsletter*, European Society for Translation. Available at: www.est-translationstudies.org/commit-tees/news_editors.html (Accessed: 4 May 2019).

Montalt, V., Zethsen, K. K. and Karwacka, W. (2018) 'Medical Translation in the 21st Century-Challenges and Trends', *MonTI. Monografías de Traducción e Interpretación*, 10, pp. 27–42.

Nisbeth Jensen, M. (2012) 'Patient Information Leaflet Translators in the EU: Mapping the Hypothetical Competences of Professional Translators and Pharmacists-Cum-Translators', in Fischer, B. and Nisbeth Jensen, M. (eds) *Translation and the Reconfiguration of Power Relations: Revisiting Role and Context of Translation and Interpreting.* Zurich: LIT Verlag, pp. 237–257.

O'Neil, M. (1998) 'Who Makes a Better Medical Translator: The Medically Knowledgeable Linguist or the Linguistically Knowledgeable Medical Professional? A Physician's Perspective', in Fischbach, H. (ed.) *Translation and Medicine*. Amsterdam and Philadelphia: John Benjamins.

PACTE (2003) 'Building a Translation Competence Model', in Alves, F. (ed.) *Triangulating Translation: Perspectives in Process Oriented Research*. Amsterdam and Philadelphia: John Benjamins, pp. 43–66.

PACTE (2005) 'Investigating Translation Competence: Conceptual and Methodological Issues', *Meta*, 50(2), pp. 609–619.

PACTE (2008) 'First Results of a Translation Competence Experiment: "Knowledge of Translation" and "Efficacy of the Translation Process"', in Kearns, J. (ed.) *Translator and Interpreter Training: Issues, Methods and Debates*. New York: Continuum, pp. 104–126.

Pires, C., Vigário, M. and Cavaco, A. (2015) 'Readability of Medicinal Package Leaflets: A Systematic Review', *Revista de Saúde pública*, 49(4). DOI:10.1590/s0034-8910.2015049005559.

Txabarriaga, R. (2008) *IMIA Guide on Medical Translation.* International Medical Interpreters Association. Available at: www.imiaweb.org/uploads/pages/823..pdf (Accessed: 4 May 2019).
US Food and Drug Administration. (2001) *Guidance on Medical Device Patient Labeling; Final Guidance for Industry and FDA Reviewers.* Center for Devices and Radiological Health. www.fda.gov/media/71030/download (Accessed: 4 May 2019).
US Food and Drug Administration. (2010) *Guidance for Industry Label Comprehension Studies for Nonprescription Drug Products.* Center for Drug Evaluation and Research. www.fda.gov/media/75626/download (Accessed: 4 May 2019).
US Food and Drug Administration (2018) *Informed Consent for Clinical Trials.* www.fda.gov/patients/clinical-trials-what-patients-need-know/informed-consent-clinical-trials#What_is_Informed_Consent_(Accessed: 4 May 2019).
US Food and Drug Administration. (no date) *Patient Labeling 101.* Center for Drug Evaluation and Research. www.fda.gov/media/88986/download (Accessed: 4 May 2019).
Wang, L. W., Miller, M. J., Schmitt, M. R. and Wen, F. K. (2013) 'Assessing Readability Formula Differences with Written Health Information Materials: Application, Results, and Recommendations'. *Research in Social and Administrative Pharmacy*, 9(5), pp. 503–516. DOI:10.1016/j.sapharm.2012.05.009
Walkiewicz B. (2018) 'Translation of Medical Texts from Discourse Perspective', in Karwacka, W. (ed.) *Towards Understanding Medical Translation and Interpreting.* Gdańsk: Gdańsk University Press, pp. 85–108.
Wolf A., Fuchs, J and Schweim, H. G. (2014) 'Readability of the European QRD Template. The European QRD Template Version 8 in Comparison to Its Predecessor and a Shorter Model Template', *Pharmazeutische Industrie*, 76(8), pp. 1312–1322.
Wolz, M. (2015) 'Language Barriers: Challenges to Quality Healthcare', *International Journal of Dermatology,* 54, pp. 248–250.
World Health Organisation (2002) 'Questions and Answers on Health and Human Rights', *Health & Human Rights Publication Series,* 1(July).

6

Inter- and intralingual translation of medical information

The importance of comprehensibility

Matilde Nisbeth Brøgger and Karen Korning Zethsen

1 Introduction

The past decades have seen an increasing focus on the importance of health communication, especially the communication of health matters to lay people and the general public. Patients today increasingly demand sufficient information to make informed choices on whether to go ahead with a medical procedure, take a specific medication, etc., and they want the communication of this information to be tailored for them, i.e. written in an understandable manner. This demand for understandable patient information and communication comes not only from patients, but is part of a larger societal push to involve the wider public in their own health. Consequently, in recent years, the concepts of patient empowerment and patient-centred communication have become increasingly popular, as will be described below. This means that healthcare professionals and authorities need to tailor their communication to laypeople, and also that medical knowledge and texts must be translated intralingually *within* the same national language, from expert language to plain language. Many of these medical texts are translated interlingually as well (i.e. between languages, for example from English into Danish), and often, a combination of inter- and intralingual translation takes place, putting additional demands on the time and effort of the translators.

In this chapter, we will first explain the paradigmatic shift towards patient-centredness and patient empowerment within written health communication, and the ensuing increased focus on lay-friendly and comprehensible information. We will further explain the concepts of intralingual and interlingual translation, and discuss the various complexities of translating medical texts for lay people. Lastly, we will illustrate some of the many challenges and pitfalls surrounding intralingual/interlingual medical translation with the help of authentic examples.

2 From the biomedical paradigm to patient-centredness

The idea that medicine should be patient-centred is not new; it was proposed by Balint already in 1969 as an alternative to the biomedical paradigm which focused solely on the

 DOI: 10.4324/9781003167983-9

discovery of illness and its subsequent treatment. As an alternative to this illness-oriented approach, the main notion of patient-centred medicine was to consider the 'whole' person, i.e. both the physical and the mental wellbeing of the patient, and to see the patient as a unique human being (Balint 1969: 269). Similarly, Engel (1977) highlighted the limitations of the biomedical model, characterising it as dualistic and reductionist (1977: 320), and argued for replacing it with a biopsychosocial model, in which the doctor attends not only to the biomedical needs of the patient but also to their psychological and social needs (Engel 1977: 324). This shift from doctor-centred care to patient-centred care naturally leads to a shift from monologic to dialogic consultations, and thus communication is increasingly seen as 'the royal pathway to patient-centred medicine' (Bensing *et al.* 2000: 1). Today, patient-centredness is an established way of considering the practice of communication in healthcare. Closely linked to the concept of patient-centred communication is the concept of patient empowerment (e.g. Funnell *et al.* 1991). Patient empowerment is defined by WHO as 'a process in which patients understand their role, are given the knowledge and skills by their healthcare provider to perform a task in an environment that recognises community and cultural differences and encourages patient participation' (WHO 2009). This shows a link between empowerment and communication; patients need some degree of empowerment in order to be able to participate in decisions about their own health as well as to challenge healthcare providers when needed, and communication can lead to this greater empowerment.

3 The importance of comprehensibility

It is a natural consequence of the paradigmatic shift to patient-centredness and patient empowerment that the patient needs to understand relevant communication. In the context of this chapter on translation, we focus on written communication directly aimed at the general population and patients, i.e. lay people. Although some illnesses have a socio-economic bias, i.e. are much more common among certain socio-economic groups, it is generally fair to say that most written health communication is a form of mass communication, as any member of the society could potentially be at the receiving end. This is why the concept of health literacy is crucial not only for patients, but also for those producing health communication, including translators. Health literacy, as established by Nutbeam in 1998 in his definition for the WHO (1998: 10), is defined as the ability to access, understand and act on information about one's own health. Nutbeam (2000: 265) established three levels of health literacy, namely functional, interactive and critical health literacy, and the three levels represent a continuum which moves from basic to more advanced. Basic health literacy, i.e. functional health literacy, is described as a situation where a patient can read, understand and act on health-related information. At the other end of the continuum is critical health literacy where patients are able to critically evaluate health information and use this information to take control of their own health, illness and living conditions. Thus, even the basic level of functional health literacy requires that the patient understands relevant information. Sometimes this information is provided orally, but today much information is given in written form (often electronically) as one-way communication where the patient does not have the possibility to ask questions while reading. This is for instance the case with brochures, emails, websites, electronic patient records (in countries where these can be accessed by patients) and so on.

It seems reasonable that medical information aimed at lay people should be written in a language actually intelligible to lay people, but such a seemingly obvious understanding is in fact fairly recent, and coincides with the shift from the biomedical paradigm to patient-centredness. The Plain Language Movement, which advocates for a clear writing style, only started to gain momentum within the English-speaking world in the 1970s. According to Stewart (2010), people increasingly needed to deal with complex documents concerning their finances, health or legal matters, and these documents needed to be written in a style intelligible to the target group. The Movement demanded that plain language should be used by the authorities when writing documents either directly addressing or in other ways relevant to the public, and that professionals such as lawyers or doctors should adopt a clear writing style in their interactions with their clients and patients. In 1998, the EU launched its own plain language campaign 'Fight the Fog', and the relatively recent 2010 EU Clear Writing campaign bears witness to the fact that there is still some way to go before this goal is achieved. This brings us to the reason why intralingual translation is of such importance.

4 Intra- and interlingual translation

The practice of 'intralingual translation' has presumably existed since time immemorial, but the term itself was introduced by Roman Jakobson; he categorised translation as interlingual, intralingual and intersemiotic (Jakobson [1959] 2012: 114). Interlingual translation, or the translation between national languages, is considered 'translation proper' and thus the prototypical form of translation. Intralingual translation has, in spite of its many similarities with 'translation proper', lived a life on the periphery of translation studies for many years. However, Zethsen (2007, 2009, 2018), Zethsen and Hill-Madsen (2016) and others during the past decade (e.g. Berk Albachten 2019; Whyatt, Kajzer-Wietrzny and Stachowiak 2016) argue that intralingual translation is fundamentally a translational activity which belongs to the field of translation studies. There are many similarities between intralingual and interlingual translation and the same micro-strategies are applied in both to a large extent (Zethsen 2009; Ersland 2014). For instance, the strategies available when translating terminology between two languages are no different from rewriting an expert text for lay people or intralingually translating a work of classic literature into a simplified version. The main differences seem to be a question of degree rather than type (Zethsen 2009: 809), to the effect that some micro-strategies, especially those related to simplification and explicitation (Zethsen 2009: 809; Ersland 2014: 84–85), are used much more in intralingual than in interlingual translation. Intralingual translation has a strong tendency to involve a form of simplification where it becomes the main purpose of the translation, and because of this tendency the micro-strategies applied (additions, omissions, restructuring, etc.) seem to be much more radical than what is seen in the majority of interlingual translations where simplification is only one of many available micro-strategies.

5 Translating medical texts for lay people

When training to become an expert within a field, mastering the relevant terminology and style is an important tool for precise and efficient communication; this mastery furthermore signals that the communicator is an accepted member of the discourse community in question. It is difficult for experts to put aside their knowledge and remember how much they would have understood before they became experts. Bromme, Jucks and Wagner (2005: 571) state that:

> [T]here is a good deal of evidence that experts have difficulty in adapting their advice to the information needs of laypersons. One can assume that experts' extensive and highly integrated knowledge of their own domain makes it very difficult for them to comprehend the completely different perspective of a layperson.

This viewpoint is supported by researchers such as Hinds (1999), Nickerson (1999), Hayes and Bajzek (2008), and Lentz and de Jong (2009), who argue that experts are often unaware of what poses problems for lay people, and might overestimate the knowledge of their receivers. All this can be summed up as a phenomenon which Hinds (1999: 205) labels as *the curse of expertise*, and this is exactly why a mediator – an intralingual translator – is often needed.

Expert medical language is in Western European languages characterised by the use of terminology, often of Latin or Greek origins, and, as is the case with many other languages for specialised purposes, by the passive voice, heavy premodification, nominalisation, long and compact sentences containing large amounts of information, etc. (Askehave and Zethsen 2000a, 2010; Montalt and González-Davies 2007; Nisbeth Jensen 2013, 2015). To the medical expert, this language is precise and often economical with words, and as such, it serves its specialised function. For the lay person, however, medical language can be challenging in varying degrees. Some lay people may be familiar with Latin and may therefore be able to deduct the meaning of some medical terminology; others suffer from a chronic disease and may have gradually become acquainted with the terminology of that particular disease, but may know little about medical language in general; and still others may not be able to read any medical texts at all. Some languages (e.g. Spanish or English) are more Latin-based than others (such as German and the Nordic languages), and speakers of the more Latin-based languages may be able to figure out what a Latin word means or the Latin word may already be part of everyday language. In Nordic languages, for instance, everyday language does not make use of Latin medical terminology; instead, lay terms with Nordic roots and with no connection to Latin are widely used. This means that in many cases, most people will literally not have a clue about what a medical term with Latin roots means, and it is crucial that everyday words are used instead (Zethsen 2004). In Danish, for instance, an ulcer is called 'mavesår', literally 'stomach wound', and hardly anyone knows the Latinate term. Appendicitis is called 'blindtarmsbetændelse', i.e. not remotely Latinate. In addition to the above-mentioned (and many more) lexical and syntactic features, which characterise expert language, the phenomenon of presupposition also plays an important role. In other words, what is absent from the text is in fact just as important as what is present, as is seen in those cases where an author presupposes that patients understand certain words or expressions where they would, in fact, need an explanation. Again, it may be difficult for experts to gauge exactly what lay people know and do not know. Presupposition is very common and may well be one of the main reasons why medical texts are often so inaccessible to lay people. In such instances, the intralingual translator will typically use the strategy of explicitation to help the readers.

Common to all lay target groups is the fact that they are either not able to understand a medical text in full or the potential for misunderstandings is high. Additionally, some lay people have very low health literacy (often young people, old people, non-native speakers, people with little schooling and people with varying levels of learning or reading difficulties) and their extralinguistic situation may also be a stressful one, especially due to an illness, sleep deprivation or old age. These target groups need a translation, sometimes within their own language (intralingual translation), and sometimes intralingual translation coupled with a translation between languages (interlingual translation). Within translation studies, functionalism (e.g. Reiss and Vermeer 1984; Vermeer 1989) has become the most common approach when translating specialised texts. It is the skopos (purpose) of a text in the target culture which determines the nature of the translation. Once the translator knows the purpose of the translation (ideally through the commissioner), i.e. how the text is to function in the target culture, the translator can determine the style of the translation, including the level of formality, the correct use of terminology, etc. This means that if a medical text is translated for a target group consisting of semi-experts within that particular field, a certain amount of medical terminology and syntactical complexity may be in order. However, if the target group potentially consists of the entire population of a country, the translator has to aim for the lowest common denominator to ensure that as many members as possible of this very broad target group will understand the information. In Denmark, for instance, the health authorities recommend writing so that the text would be understandable to an 11 to 12-year-old in cases of mass communication (Sundhedsstyrelsen 2009). It should be emphasised that when the target language is not English, many of these texts are translated interlingually as well, and so we often see a combination of inter- and intralingual translation – a situation which does of course place additional demands on the translator. In the following section, we shall illustrate and discuss intra- and interlingual medical translation using examples from patient information leaflets.

6 Patient information leaflets as a case study

As a result of the increased focus on health communication as well as because of various legislative measures, new patient communication genres have come into existence during the past 30 years. One of these genres is the Patient Information Leaflet (PIL), which came into existence as a legal requirement in 1992 and was fully adopted by the EU in 1999 (Council of the European Communities 1992). EU PILs are therefore so-called mandatory genres and as such are heavily regulated by law (Askehave and Zethsen, 2003). A PIL must accompany all medication; it contains information about dosage, contraindications, side effects, etc. aimed at patients. The PIL has been described as the most important source of information about medication for the patient (Bjerrum and Foged 2003: 58). Despite the legal requirement that PILs are 'written and designed to be clear, understandable and enable the users to act appropriately' (Article 63(2) of EU Directive 2001/83/EC, European Parliament and of the Council, 2001), a growing body of research suggests that many PILs are linguistically complex and difficult to understand for lay people (Askehave and Zethsen 2000a, 2000b, 2002, 2003, 2010, 2014; Clerehan and Buchbinder 2006; Consumers' Association 2000; Dickinson, Raynor and Duman 2001; Harwood and Harrison 2004; Horwitz, Reuther and Andersen 2009; Nisbeth Jensen 2013; Pander Maat and Lentz 2010; Raynor 2007; Zethsen and Askehave 2010). This is of course in direct contrast to the function and purpose of the genre.

Within the EU framework, a PIL is the result of an intralingual translation process as it must be drawn up in accordance with the Summary of Product Characteristics (SPC).

The SPC document includes pharmaceutical information about the medicinal product in question, the chemical composition of the drug, dosage instructions, etc. It is written by and for medical experts, in a very specialised medical register. The PIL is produced based on the SPC, and it is a much shorter document with a new audience and a new communicative purpose. When a pharmaceutical company applies for marketing authorisation through the so-called Centralised Procedure in the EU, it must submit a dossier which includes the draft SPC, labelling, and a PIL in English. The European Medicines Agency (EMA) then has 210 days to decide whether marketing authorisation should be granted; this is called 'CHMP (The Committee for Medicinal Products for Human Use) opinion'. Five days later, translations from English into all other languages must be submitted, which means *after* the EMA has granted the marketing authorisation. This means that the source text for the SPC and the PIL is always in English, irrespective of home country, and it also means that the English version is the approved version.

Another intralingual translation process can be identified for PILs in instances where there is not a shift in audience, but where the original PIL is too linguistically complex, i.e. has not been successfully targeted at the intended audience (as is often the case, cf. the growing body of research mentioned at the beginning of this section), and must be rewritten. In such cases, the English-language PIL is the source text and a more intelligible English-language PIL is the target text. Furthermore, as mentioned above, an interlingual translation process also takes place, as EU PILs must be available in all EU languages. Here, the English-language PIL is the source text and the Spanish/Latvian/Danish/etc. PIL is the target text. In the following, we will give examples from authentic SPCs and English (EN) and Danish (DK) PILs found online, with English back translations in square brackets. This means that these examples come from authorised documents. It is not possible to find information on who the translators are, but we know that PILs are most often translated by pharmacists and only occasionally by professional translators (Nisbeth Jensen 2013). We will show how intralingual translation, and, when relevant, interlingual translation (here, into Danish), take place and discuss the appropriateness of the strategies applied.

Example 1

- SPC: severe hypotension
- EN PIL: if you have severe low blood pressure (hypotension)
- DK PIL: hvis du har meget lavt blodtryk (hypotension) [if you have very low blood pressure (hypotension)]

In Example 1, we see an intralingual translation from SPC to PIL of 'severe hypotension' by the addition of the more lay-friendly term 'severe low blood pressure'. The expert term is maintained but placed in parentheses. This might seem like a good choice in the name of patient education and empowerment; however, as we know that many patients do not even have health literacy at the functional level, some receivers might be confused by the expert term. If one does not know what hypotension means, it is not clear from the sentence whether the term in parentheses is a synonym or extra information. If we look at the Danish PIL, the choice to include 'hypotension' is even more problematic as Danes are less exposed to Latin-based terminology. Example 1 thus shows how PILs are translated intralingually from SPC to PIL, and how this translation sometimes needs even further intralingual translation. We also see that in the interlingual translation into Danish (EN

PIL to DK PIL), the translator needs to be aware of intralingual translation, i.e. the need for lay-friendly PILs, as a direct translation is likely to be problematic.

Example 2

- SPC: toxic epidermal necrolysis and Stevens-Johnson syndrome
- EN PIL: inflammation of the mucous membranes (Stevens-Johnson syndrome, toxic epidermal necrolysis)

In Example 2, the same intralingual translation strategy is used, i.e. maintaining the expert terms, but placing them in parentheses ('toxic epidermal necrolysis' and 'Stevens-Johnson syndrome') in the PIL. In this case, there could be good reasons for maintaining at least 'Stevens-Johnson syndrome' as it might be a condition that the patient has, and thus knows. In addition to the maintained expert terms, the intralingual translation used an explicitation by adding the explanation 'inflammation of the mucous membranes'. However, this explicitation includes two other medical terms 'inflammation' and 'mucous membranes'. In addition to being a medical term, 'inflammation' is also a nominalisation – a syntactic choice which is known to be complex (Coleman 1964: 186; Charrow 1988: 98; Halliday 1994: 353). Again, the intralingual translation might need further intralingual translation in order to be intelligible for the target group.

Example 3

- SPC: Subcutaneous use. Apidra should be given by subcutaneous injection [...]
- EN PIL: Apidra is injected under the skin (subcutaneously)
- DK PIL: Apidra injiceres under huden (subkutant) [Apidra is injected under the skin (subcutaneously)]

In Example 3 we again see that the medical term 'subcutaneously' is placed in parentheses in the intralingual translation; however, in this case, we are not dealing with an illness that the receiver might have. If one does not understand the term 'subcutaneously', one does not know what (or how much of the preceding sentence) it refers to. Syntactically, the intralingual translation is also problematic as the passive construction 'is injected' makes it difficult to judge who the performing agent is. The interlingual translation into Danish actually increases the complexity as the term 'injiceres' is translated directly. In Danish, the Latin-based term 'injicere' would only be used by experts whereas the lay term 'indsprøjte' (a word with Nordic roots which could be literally translated into 'squirt into') would be the one used by lay people. Thus, in Example 3, we see both problematic intra- and interlingual translations, on lexical and syntactic levels.

Example 4

- EN SPC: Repaglinide is indicated in adults with type 2 diabetes mellitus [...]
- EN PIL: Repaglinide Accord is an oral antidiabetic medicine containing repaglinide [...]

In the intralingual translation from SPC to PIL in Example 4, the translator has introduced a premodification 'oral antidiabetic medicine'. While the modifiers might not consist of highly complicated terms, there are no good arguments for such wording, as it may be difficult to deconstruct and thus to understand. Instead, the translator could simply have written 'Repaglinide Accord is a medicine used for diabetes. It is taken orally'.

Example 5

- EN SPC: When a patient stabilised on any oral hypoglycaemic medicinal product is exposed to stress such as fever, trauma, infection or surgery, a loss of glycaemic control may occur
- EN PIL: [...] If you are about to have major surgery or you have recently suffered a severe illness or infection. At such times diabetic control may be lost

In Example 5, we see the words 'surgery' and 'infection' being modified in the target text using 'major' and 'severe', respectively. The use of these strategies presupposes that the reader knows what 'major surgery' and 'severe infection' entail as opposed to 'minor surgery' or just 'surgery'. We also see the expert medical term has been intralingually translated, i.e. 'glycaemic control' into 'diabetic control', which is more lay-friendly; however, again, it presupposes knowledge of what 'diabetic control' means.

In these examples, we see several instances of medical terms being directly translated or moved into parentheses. The use of specialised terminology is often quoted as one of the main reasons why medical texts are difficult for lay people to understand (Bromme, Jucks and Wagner 2005; Bromme, Rambow and Nückles 2001; MHRA 2005). Some might argue that patients today are more knowledgeable about medical terms than before; however, specialised expert medical terminology is still a source of confusion (Dahm 2011: 24). This means that even though patients are more involved in their own health and in health-related topics today, the use of medical terms may still constitute a comprehension barrier. Just as certain micro-strategies may be recommended for certain types of interlingual medical translation (Montalt and González-Davies 2007), it is possible to make recommendations concerning medical intralingual translation. For instance, several strategies can be applied in order to 'de-terminologise' the text (Montalt and González-Davies 2007: 251–253). Here is an example of strategies for intralingual translation of the expert term in the sentence 'If you experience tachycardia':

1. Expert term + (lay term): If you experience **tachycardia (fast heartbeat)**
2. Replace with a lay term: If you experience **fast heartbeat**
3. Lay term + (expert term): If you experience **fast heartbeat (tachycardia)**
4. Keep expert term + explanation: If you experience **tachycardia, which means that your heart is beating fast (over 100 beats per minute)**
5. Explanation + (expert term): If you experience **that your heart is beating fast (tachycardia)**
6. Explanation: If you experience **that your heart is beating fast**

This shows that the intralingual translator has several strategies available when translating medical terms. For mass communicated texts, we recommend that strategy 1 is avoided and that 3, 4 and 5 are only used when the expert term is really necessary. This could be in situations where a chronic illness makes it relevant for the patient to be gradually educated about their illness and/or where the resourceful patient may want to look up more information and may thus need to know the expert term. In many cases, strategy 2 (lay term) or 6 (just explaining the expert term) are perfectly suitable. Of course, these are merely guidelines, not prescriptive rules. Our point is that all translation situations are *ad hoc* and contextual, which means that the translators must use their competence to tailor the text for the target group.

The examples above demonstrate that it is not only medical terminology that is problematic in intra- and interlingual medical translations; syntactical choices such as passive voice, nominalisation and premodification can also unnecessarily complicate target texts. The same is true for presupposition and information-dense sentences. As medical texts are often produced by experts (for PILs, often by pharmacists) who may be influenced by the writing style of their expert discourse community as discussed above, and may not have the linguistic skills or knowledge required to produce optimally comprehensible texts, the need for translators possessing intra- and interlingual competence becomes even more imperative.

7 Conclusion and future directions

Research on intralingual translation has up until now not been very prolific, though the past decade has seen increased interest in this topic. As far as practical intralingual medical translation is concerned, there is still much work to be done as regards specific micro-strategies for some of the numerous pitfalls such as medical terminology, syntactical choices (e.g. passive voice, nominalisation and premodification), as well as presuppositions and information-dense sentences. On a more general level, digital access to e.g. electronic patients' records or other expert texts is increasing day by day and it seems that lay people are uncritically given access to large amounts of information which they may not understand, or worse, misunderstand. Research looking at comprehensibility and reception in connection with such electronic access would be extremely relevant. Finally, the lack of appropriate intralingual translation is interesting from a more socio-political perspective; certain medical genres, such as the patient information leaflet, are legally regulated, clearly meant for lay people, but at the same time used by medical companies as a means of avoiding legal responsibility, for instance by including long and complex lists of side effects, which remain fairly incomprehensible to patients. This means that even though the apparent skopos of the text is patient information, there may be a strongly competing different skopos, which results in the creation of long and complex texts that are incomprehensible to many laypeople.

It is important for researchers to help create awareness about the need for comprehensible information and it is the right of patients to be able to understand communication relevant to their health. Either experts have to write in a more accessible way when writing for lay people or intralingual translation must be carried out professionally. Expert-lay intralingual translation is crucial at a time where there is easy electronic access to large amounts of texts often written by experts, and it is time to bring intralingual translation out of the shadows so to speak, and name it as a skill interlingual translators of health information should possess.

Further reading

Montalt, V. and González-Davies, M. (2007) *Medical Translation Step by Step: Learning by Drafting*. Manchester: St. Jerome.

This textbook explains the basics of medical translation and the different ways of teaching how to translate medical texts.

Muñoz-Miquel, A., Ezpeleta-Piorno, P. and Saiz-Hontangas, P. (2018) 'Intralingual Translation in Healthcare Settings: Strategies and Proposals for Medical Translator Training', in Montalt, V., Zethsen, K. and Karwacka, W. (eds) *Retos actuales y tendencias emergentes en traducción médica / Current Challenges and Emerging Trends in Medical Translation. MonTI*, 10, pp. 177–204.

This article shows the importance of intralingual translation skills. It presents an empirical study in which a series of intralingual strategies were used to make real fact sheets for cancer patients more comprehensible and effective. It concludes with a proposal for training medical translators to deal with this type of intralingual translation.

Nisbeth Jensen, M. (2015) 'Optimising Comprehensibility in Interlingual Translation: The Need for Intralingual Translation', in Maksymski, K., Gutermuth, S. and Hansen-Schirra, S. (eds) *Translation and Comprehensibility*. Berlin: Frank and Timme.

This paper uses Plain Language research to operationalise the skopos of comprehensibility in Patient Information Leaflets. It is argued that Plain Language, which has mainly been used for intralingual translation, can be broadened to also be applied in the field of interlingual translation.

Zethsen, K. K. (2007) 'Beyond Translation Proper – Extending the Field of Translation Studies', *TTR: Traduction, Terminologie, Redaction*, 20(1), pp. 281–308.

This article discusses how intralingual translation or 'rewording' is de facto peripheral to translation studies and argues that the relationship between inter- and intralingual translation is a neglected area of research, as is a thorough description of intralingual translation. An attempt to formally define translation, including intralingual translation is made (further elaborated in Zethsen and Hill-Madsen 2016).

Zethsen, K. K. (2018) 'Access Is Not the Same as Understanding. Why Intralingual Translation Is Crucial in a World of Information Overload', *Across Languages and Cultures*, 19(1), pp. 79–98.

This article discusses the role of intralingual translation within health communication by means of two specific cases: patient information leaflets and electronic medical patient records. It argues that providing access to information is not necessarily the same as providing the patient with information, and that providing access, but not accessible information, is at best due to ignorance, at worst due to negligence.

Related topics

Knowledge Translation, Quality, Accessibility and Readability in Medical Translation, Medical Terminology and Discourse

References

Askehave, I. and Zethsen, K. K. (2000a) *The Patient Package Insert of the Future. Report for the Danish Ministry of Health*. Aarhus: The Aarhus School of Business.

Askehave, I. and Zethsen, K. K. (2000b) 'Medical Texts Made Simple – Dream or Reality?', *Hermes, Journal of Linguistics*, 25, pp. 63–74.

Askehave, I. and Zethsen, K. K. (2002) 'Translating for Laymen', *Perspectives: Studies in Translatology*, 10(1), pp. 15–29.

Askehave, I. and Zethsen, K. K. (2003) 'Communication Barriers in Public Discourse', *Document Design*, 4(1), pp. 23–42.

Askehave, I. and Zethsen, K. K. (2014) 'A Comparative Analysis of the Lay-Friendliness of Danish EU Patient Information Leaflets From 2000 to 2012', *Communication and Medicine*, 11(3), pp. 209–222.

Balint, E. (1969) 'The Possibilities of Patient-Centered Medicine', *Journal of the Royal College of General Practitioners*, 17(82), pp. 269–276.

Bensing, J., Verhaak, P. F. M., Van Dulmen, A. M. and Visser, A. P. (2000) 'Communication: The Royal Pathway to Patient-Centered Medicine', *Patient Education and Counseling*, 39(1), pp. 1–3. DOI:10.1016/S0738-3991(99)00107-X.

Berk Albachten, Ö. (2019) 'Challenging the Boundaries of Translation and Filling the Gaps in Translation History: Two Cases of Intralingual Translation From the 19th Century Ottoman Literary Scene', in Dam, H. V., Nisbeth Brøgger, M. and Zethsen, K. K. (eds) *Moving Boundaries in Translation Studies*. London and New York: Routledge, pp. 168–180.
Bjerrum, L. and Foged, A. (2003) 'Patient Information Leaflets: Helpful Guidance or a Source of Confusion?' *Pharmacoepidemiology and Drug Safety,* 12(1), pp. 55–59.
Bromme, R., Jucks, R. and Wagner, T. (2005) 'How to Refer to "Diabetes"? Language in Online Health Advice', *Applied Cognitive Psychology,* 19, pp. 569–586.
Bromme, R., Rambow, R. and Nückles, M. (2001) 'Expertise and Estimating What Other People Know: The Influence of Professional Experience and Type of Knowledge', *Journal of Experimental Psychology: Applied,* 7(4), pp. 317–330.
Charrow, V. (1988) 'Readability vs. Comprehensibility: A Case Study in Improving a Real Document', in Davidson, A. and Green, G. M. (eds) *Linguistic Complexity and Text Comprehension*. Hillsdale, NJ: Lawrence Erlbaum, pp. 85–114.
Clerehan, R. and Buchbinder, R. (2006) 'Toward a More Valid Account of Functional Text Quality: The Case of the Patient Information Leaflet', *Text and Talk,* 26(1), pp. 39–68.
Coleman, E. B. (1964) 'The Comprehensibility of Several Grammatical Transformations', *Journal of Applied Psychology,* 48(3), pp. 186–190.
Consumers' Association (2000) *Patient Information Leaflets: Sick Notes?* London: Consumers' Association.
Council of the European Communities (1992) *Council Directive 92/27/EEC of 31 March 1992.*
Dahm, M. R. (2011) *Exploring Perception, Use and Understanding of Medical Terminology Among Native and Non-Native English Patients and Physicians in Australia. A Mixed Methods Investigation.* PhD Thesis. Macquarie University, Sydney.
Dickinson, D., Raynor, D. T. and Duman, M. (2001) 'Patient Information Leaflets for Medicines: Using Consumer Testing to Determine the Most Effective Design', *Patient Education and Counseling,* 43(2), pp. 147–159.
Engel, G. (1977) 'The Need for a New Medical Model: A Challenge for Biomedicine', *Science*, 196, pp. 129–135.
Ersland, A. (2014) *Is Change Necessary? A Study of Norms and Translation Universals in Intralingual Translation.* Master's Thesis. University of Bergen.
European Parliament and Council (2001) *Directive 2001/83/EC of the European Parliament and of the Council of 6 November 2001.*
Funnell, M. M. *et al.* (1991) 'Empowerment: An Idea Whose Time Has Come in Diabetes Patient Education', *Diabetes Education*, 17, pp. 37–41.
Halliday, M. A. K. (1994) *An Introduction to Functional Grammar*. London: Arnold.
Harwood, A. and Harrison, J. E. (2004) 'How Readable Are Orthodontic Patient Information Leaflets?', *Journal of Orthodontics,* 31(3), pp. 210–219.
Hayes, J. R. and Bajzek, D. (2008) 'Understanding and Reducing the Knowledge Effect: Implications for Writers', *Written Communication,* 25, pp. 104–118.
Hinds, P. J. (1999) 'The Curse of Expertise: The Effects of Expertise and Debiasing Methods on Predictions of Novice Performance', *Journal of Experimental Psychology: Applied*, 5(2), pp. 205–221.
Horwitz, A., Reuther, L. and Andersen, S. E. (2009) 'Patienters Vurdering af Medicinpakningernes Indlægssedler', *Ugeskrift for Læger,* 171(8), pp. 599–602.
Jakobson, R. (2012) 'On Linguistic Aspects of Translation', in Venuti, L (ed.) *The Translation Studies Reader*. London: Routledge, pp. 126–131.
Lentz, L. and de Jong, M. (2009) 'How Do Experts Assess Usability Problems? An Empirical Analysis of Cognitive Shortcuts', *Technical Communication,* 56(2), pp. 111–121.
MHRA. (2005) *Always Read the Leaflet: Getting the Best Information With Every Medicine.* London: The Stationery Office.
Montalt, V. and González-Davies, M. (2007) *Medical Translation Step by Step: Learning by Drafting*. Manchester: St. Jerome Publishing.
Nisbeth Jensen, M. (2013) *Translators of Patient Information Leaflets: Translation Experts or Expert Translators? A Mixed Methods Study of Lay-Friendliness*. PhD thesis. Aarhus University, Aarhus School of Business and Social Sciences.

Nisbeth Jensen, M. (2015) 'Optimising Comprehensibility in Interlingual Translation: The Need for Intralingual Translation', in Maksymski, K., Gutermuth, S. and Hansen-Schirra, S. (eds) *Translation and Comprehensibility.* Berlin: Frank and Timme.
Nickerson, R. S. (1999) 'How We Know – and Sometimes Misjudge – What Others Know: Imputing One's Own Knowledge to Others', *Psychological Bulletin,* 125(6), pp. 737–759.
Nutbeam, D. (2000) 'Health Literacy as a Public Health Goal: A Challenge for Contemporary Health Education and Communication Strategies into the 21st Century', *Health Promotion International,* 15(3), pp. 259–267. DOI:10.1093/heapro/15.3.259.
Pander Maat, H. and Lentz, L. (2010) 'Improving the Usability of Patient Information Leaflets', *Patient Education and Counseling,* 80(1), pp. 113–119.
Raynor, D. T. (2007) 'The Importance of Medicines Information for Patients', *Prescriber,* 18(2), pp. 60–62.
Reiss, K. and Vermeer, H. J. (1984) Grundlegung einer allgemeinen Translationstheorie. *Linguistische Arbeiten,* 147. Tübingen: Max Niemeyer Verlag.
Stewart, J. (2010) 'Plain Language. From "Movement" to "Profession",' *Australian Journal of Communication,* 37(2), pp. 51–72.
Sundhedsstyrelsen (2009) *Health Literacy – Begrebet, Konsekvenser Og Mulige Interventioner.* København: Sundhedsstyrelsen. Available at: www.sst.dk/publ/publ2009/cff/dokumentation/healthliteracy_notat.pdf.
Vermeer, H. (1989) 'Skopos And Commission in Translational Action', in Chesterman, A. (ed.) *Readings in Translation Theory.* Helsinki: Oy Finn Lectura Ab, pp. 173–187.
Whyatt, B., Kajzer-Wietrzny, M. and Stachowiak, K. (2016) 'Similar and Different: Cognitive Rhythm and Effort in Translation and Paraphrasing', *Poznań Studies in Contemporary Linguistics,* special issue 'Language Processing in Translation', 52(2), pp. 175–208.
WHO (1998) *Health Promotion Glossary.* Geneva: World Health Organization.
WHO (2009) *Patient Empowerment and Health Care.* Geneva: World Health Organization.
Zethsen, K. K. (2004) Latin-Based Terms: True or False Friends? *Target,* 16(1), pp. 125–142. DOI:10.1075/target.16.1.07zet.
Zethsen, K. K. (2007) 'Beyond Translation Proper – Extending the Field of Translation Studies', *TTR: Traduction, Terminologie, Redaction,* 20(1), pp. 281–308.
Zethsen, K. K. (2009) 'Intralingual Translation: An Attempt at Description', *Meta,* 54(4), pp. 795–812.
Zethsen, K. K. (2018) 'Access Is Not the Same as Understanding. Why Intralingual Translation Is Crucial in a World of Information Overload', *Across Languages and Cultures,* 19(1), pp. 79–98.
Zethsen, K. K. and Askehave, I. (2010) 'PIL of the Month: A Study of Best Practice in EU Patient Information Leaflets', *Journal of Applied Linguistics and Professional Practice,* 7(1), pp. 97–120.
Zethsen, K. K. and Hill-Madsen, A. (2016) 'Intralingual Translation and its Place Within Translation Studies – a Theoretical Discussion', *Meta,* 61(3), pp. 692–708.

7

Machine translation in healthcare

Barry Haddow, Alexandra Birch and Kenneth Heafield

1 Introduction

In the healthcare domain, there is often a need to have information translated into one or more different languages, for example healthcare websites and reports, or where healthcare professionals do not speak the same language as their patients. In many cases, whilst human translation would be the ideal solution, it is not always available. Human translation is expensive, and resources enabling translation into all potential languages may not be always available. Also, healthcare information changes, and so texts need to be updated, requiring further costly translation. In a setting where translation is needed immediately, an interpreter may not be available when required, or the patient may prefer to discuss the matter directly with a clinician, rather than involving a third party.

For these reasons, we consider whether machine translation (MT) can have a role in translation for healthcare. The idea of MT is that we have a computer program which can read in text (or speech) in one language (known as the 'source' language) and translate it to an equivalent text (or speech) in another language (known as the 'target' language). In this chapter we mostly describe text-to-text translation, although such a system can translate speech-to-text or even speech-to-speech by adding appropriate automatic speech recognition (ASR) and text-to-speech (TTS) components. An MT system does not necessarily replace a human translator, but may operate as an assistant to a human translator, with the aim of reducing the cost of translation and increasing its availability.

In this chapter, we will provide a brief overview of machine translation, its different paradigms and an evaluation of the current state-of-the-art. We will discuss the different usage models of MT, and how it can fit into the translation workflow. Finally, we will show how MT has been used in healthcare settings through a selection of projects, with an extended discussion of two projects that we have been involved in.

DOI: 10.4324/9781003167983-10

2 Overview of machine translation

2.1 Development

Machine translation has a long history, dating back to the early days of computing science when researchers first pondered on whether machines would be able to translate human languages. Given that one of the first uses of computers was for code-breaking, the natural question was whether a foreign language (e.g. Russian) could simply be seen as an 'encoded' version of English. It quickly became quickly apparent that 'decoding' human language was considerably more difficult than cracking codes, however the statistical models developed in code-breaking and signal processing eventually provided the inspiration for the statistical MT models developed in the 1990s and early 2000s.

The earliest commercially successful MT systems were not statistical, however, but *rule-based* (otherwise known as RBMT). RBMT is based on the idea that the knowledge of translators is expressed as a collection of rules such as *'le chat' in French translates to 'the cat' in English*, or *French adjectives come after their nouns, whereas in English they come before the nouns.*[1] The MT system has many thousands of such rules, and is able to apply them efficiently in order to produce a translation. In the 1970s, RBMT systems were developed that were useful enough to be exploited commercially by companies such as Systran, one of the oldest and best known machine translation companies in the world.

The advantages of RBMT systems over later statistical models are that it is much simpler to explain and debug their reasoning, and they can be easily tweaked and updated to suit the users' needs. In situations where the input to the translation system can be tightly restricted and controlled, RBMT can potentially produce good results. However the development of RBMT systems for new languages requires considerable effort, and it is unfeasible to provide systems that can deal with idiomatic language and have a broad coverage of a large range of relevant vocabulary and grammar.

In common with other applications in natural language processing, RBMT was eclipsed by statistical approaches in the early 2000s, and only survives in niche areas. These statistical approaches are developed (or 'trained') using large corpora, so are often referred to as 'data-driven' or 'corpus-based' approaches.

Following the development of statistical models for speech recognition in the 1980s and 1990s, researchers at IBM developed a statistical approach to MT based on word-to-word translation (Brown *et al.* 1994). These word-based systems modelled the translations of individual words and their position in the target sentence. The development of statistical models was helped by the increases in computing power, and by the availability of machine-readable 'parallel' corpora, i.e. corpora with corresponding sentences in two different languages. Much of this early research on statistical MT used the Canadian Hansards, an English-French parallel corpus. Given large numbers of translated sentences, the translation of a word can be identified by looking at the frequency of terms appearing in those sentences. If the term 'chat' appears in many French sentences, with corresponding English translations containing the word 'cat', then the co-occurrence of these two words results in a high probability of them being translations of one another.

The word-based statistical models developed at IBM were mathematically elegant, but the resulting translations were not of good quality. Indeed the output was often referred to as 'word salad'. In order to improve the quality of MT, researchers sought to increase the size of the chunks translated by the models from words to small continuous segments known as 'phrases'.[2] These phrase-based models (Koehn, Och and Marcu 2003) still relied on parallel corpora, and used the word-based models as part of their training process, but using the larger chunks enabled them to produce more natural output.

The introduction of PBMT (phrase-based machine translation), coupled with the availability of still more powerful computers and larger corpora, led to rapid gains in the quality of MT, and the launch of the now ubiquitous Google Translate in 2006. MT systems could now be created with relative ease for any language pair with a parallel corpus, and multilingual organisations such as the European Parliament and the United Nations were mined for parallel corpora. Open-source implementations of PBMT such as Moses (Koehn *et al.* 2007), which is a software toolkit for translation model training and experimentation, drastically lowered the barrier to entry and stimulated further research.

PBMT had its limitations though. The output, whilst often fairly readable, frequently lapsed into what was referred to as 'phrase salad'. Language pairs with a large degree of reordering (such as English-German, with the movement of verbs causing particular problems) produced poor results since PBMT's search did not allow long-range movement. Researchers repeatedly attempted to add linguistic knowledge to PBMT (creating syntax-based MT), eventually providing some improvements (Williams *et al.* 2016), but such systems offered a relatively small increase in quality in exchange for a large increase in complexity and running time.

2.2 Current state-of-the-art: neural machine translation

In 2014/2015 a new paradigm in MT, known as neural machine translation (NMT) (Sutskever, Vinyals, and Le 2014; Bahdanau, Cho and Bengio 2015; Lu-ong, Pham and Manning 2015) was developed, and very quickly showed better performance than all the earlier statistical models. NMT represents translation as a neural network and it benefits from new developments in deep learning and neural network modelling and training that are sweeping across many fields of AI, including natural language processing. Within the next few years NMT systems replaced PBMT in major commercial systems such as Google (Wu *et al.* 2016), Facebook, Microsoft etc. and almost the entire MT research community switched to using NMT. For an extended description of NMT, aimed at translators, readers can refer to Forcada (2017).

Neural MT is, like PBMT, a data-driven approach, and depends on statistics of the training corpora. However, for many writers, the term 'statistical MT' includes approaches like PBMT and syntax-based MT, but does not include neural MT.

A neural network is essentially a complicated non-linear mathematical function, constructed from simpler units and parameterised by vectors and matrices (i.e. large tables of numbers). In NMT, translation is modelled by a specific type of neural network. This neural network enables us to assign a 'score' (or probability) to any source-target sentence pair, so that translation can be achieved by finding the highest scoring target sentence for a given source sentence. The parameters of a neural network are set during the training phase, where we use an iterative procedure to find the set of parameters which assigns the highest possible score to the training data (a large parallel corpus). The idea is that, if the neural network assigns a high score to the training sentence pairs produced by professional translators, then it will assign a high score to any good source-target sentence pair, and a low score to a bad sentence pair.

NMT models are trained in an end-to-end fashion, as opposed to the collection of heuristics used to estimate a PBMT model. In other words, they model words, phrases, word ordering and alignments all in one model, making them conceptually simpler and easier to extend than phrase-based models where all these things were modelled separately and then combined. The models themselves are more powerful than those used in PBMT, enabling them to represent phenomena like long-distance dependencies and word ordering differences that PBMT frequently failed to capture. The increase in modelling power allows the models to balance the needs of fluency (producing a good sentence in the target language) and adequacy (staying 'faithful' to the source language) in a way that PBMT could not, since it imposed a rigid trade-off between the two. Also, many NMT models are built using standard components from toolkits which are developed by the greater AI community. Because they use these common building blocks, they are simpler and more reliable to implement.

Whilst NMT has largely displaced earlier statistical and rule-based approaches as the most commonly used MT paradigm, it is not without its problems. The output of NMT can sound very natural and fluent at times, but the system will sometimes achieve this at the cost of ignoring the source. In other words, the output sounds great, but the translation is wrong. NMT is also data hungry, in the sense that it thrives when it is provided with large quantities of high-quality training data. For many language pairs that we wish to translate, however, there is very little parallel text available, and the available text is either of poor quality, or it is very different from the text we wish our system to translate.

Furthermore, NMT systems are naturally opaque, in the sense that we cannot provide a useful explanation of how the system came up with a particular output.

The increasing quality of MT has led some to suggest that we are approaching human quality of translation. For example, recent paper titles directly included claims of 'bridging the gap between human and machine translation' (Wu *et al.* 2016) and 'achieving human parity' (Hassan *et al.* 2018). However, follow-up studies (Läubli, Sennrich and Volk 2018; Toral *et al.* 2018; Bojar, Federmann *et al.* 2018) cast doubt on these claims, showing that such 'human parity' could only be obtained with very narrowly defined evaluation criteria, and is highly unlikely to be true in general. Nevertheless, there is no doubt that MT has reached the stage where it is a very usable technology in many contexts.

3 Usage models for machine translation

We can identify two main usage models[3] for MT: *dissemination* and *assimilation*, also known as *outbound* and *inbound* translation. We could also consider the usage of MT in dialogue, which combines both inbound and outbound translation in the same application. In this section we discuss these usage models, and in Section 5 we will see examples of them from healthcare settings.

The dissemination model pertains to the situation where we have created content in one language, and wish to translate it into one or more other languages in order to reach a wider audience. This is known as MT for dissemination. For example, we may have written a news article or press release in English, and would like it to be available for speakers of other languages, or we may be posting a product advert (in English) on a site like eBay or Amazon, and would like to reach other, non-English speaking markets.

Very often, when MT is used for dissemination, it is not published in 'raw' form, but is 'post-edited' by a translator to produce a high-quality text in the target language. The idea is that by using MT in this way, translation time, and therefore cost, can be reduced. There may be other benefits in addition to cost-saving; for instance using MT may provide more consistent translations, with better control over domain-specific terminology.

Whether post-editing actually makes the whole translation process more efficient is dependent on many factors, obviously including the quality of the translation itself, but also the user interface employed and the receptiveness of the translator to post-editing. If translators are presented with poor translations and asked to edit them to produce good content, they are likely to waste time trying to make sense of this poor translation, before deleting it and starting from scratch. This can give them a bad impression of MT and discourage them from using it in the future. Some ways in which researchers have tried to improve post-editing is through interactive MT (where the MT predictions change as the translator types) and quality estimation (where the system estimates a confidence score in its output, and only translations reaching a threshold are shown to the user). See Specia, Scarton and Paetzold (2018) for further details on quality estimation.

Related to post-editing is the idea of *monolingual post-editing* (MPE). In this case, the content is passed through an MT system, producing target language output, which is edited for fluency by a speaker of the target language who does not understand the source text. This process is quite different from post-editing since no translator is involved, and the process is fully dependent on the MT system for ensuring that the meaning of the source sentence is preserved. MPE could be risky for NMT systems, where in some cases the system produces fluent output which is very different in meaning from the source sentence. MPE has had some success in academic studies (e.g. Schwartz 2012) but it is not clear if it is usable in practice.

The other main usage model for MT is for assimilation, also known as inbound translation or *gisting*. In this case, the user of the MT system has a text in a language that they do not understand, and they wish to translate it to a language they do understand, in order to read the text. For example, an English speaker wishes to learn about current affairs in Germany but does not speak German, so they can use MT to translate German news. For the general public, this is likely to be the usage of MT that they are most familiar with. It is also possibly the largest usage of MT, by words translated.[4]

The requirements of MT for assimilation are likely to be different from those of MT for dissemination. For the latter use-case, if we assume that the translation is going to be post-edited by a translator, small and easily corrected mistakes that affect meaning are acceptable, since the translator will fix these. However in the assimilation use-case, it may be that the user does not understand the source language at all, so errors in the MT that affect the meaning can be crucial. On the other hand, bad MT output may be understandable (if it contains translations of all the elements of the source text) but may require drastic editing (e.g. if the usual word-order is very different in the target language).

4 Evaluation

In MT studies, evaluation plays a crucial role. How good is the output really? How useful is it? The common assumption in MT research is that human translation is perfect (often referred to as the *gold standard*) and so the aim of MT evaluation is to measure to what extent it compares to human translations. There are many different evaluation protocols and measures that are used in the MT literature, often making comparison difficult.

Evaluation in MT serves several different purposes. During system development, MT developers and researchers need rapid methods of evaluation to determine which system variants perform best, and whether the innovation that they have just added to the system has improved translation. They would also like to have a diagnostic evaluation, to determine where the system is failing so that they can address specific errors. When piloting the use of MT for a real-world situation, developers would like to know whether MT is achieving its intended purpose, for example if it is really improving communication. Or, if the MT system is being used for post-editing, if it is really making translation faster, whilst preserving or increasing quality. For this type of evaluation, it would also be useful to have some diagnostics – if MT does not help communication, what are the problems with it?

The difficulties in evaluating MT are similar to the difficulties in evaluating translation by humans. How do you measure the 'quality' of a translation, when there are multiple ways of saying the same thing, and therefore multiple 'correct' translations? And how is the evaluation of MT influenced by its intended purpose? As we noted at the end of the previous section, small errors in MT output that radically change its meaning may be easily caught by an editor, but problematic if the MT is to be consumed in its unedited state. So the evaluation of MT should really consider how it is to be used. Evaluation should also consider what type of text the MT system will be used for. This is important in specific domains like healthcare, where the MT system may have been developed and optimised for a generic text, but never tested in healthcare context.

MT evaluation methods are typically divided into automatic and manual evaluation. The idea of automatic evaluation is that it can be performed with minimal human intervention, and with the evaluator having little or no knowledge of the languages being translated. This is usually accomplished through the use of *reference* translations. A representative set of sentences in the source language are translated into the target language by professional human translators, and this is known as the reference set. To evaluate the MT system, we apply the system to the same set of source sentences and compare the resulting output to the reference translations, using an automated procedure. There are many ways of comparing MT output to the reference translation – these are typically known as *metrics* – and amongst the commonly used ones are bleu, ter, chrf3 and meteor. The metrics are implemented as computer software, and calibrated by comparing them to human assessment of sets of translations. Automatic evaluation in this way is inevitably imperfect, since it is hard to assess whether two natural language sentences are saying the same thing, and to what extent, but using a large enough set of source–reference pairs can help smooth out some of the uncertainties. Using several different references produced by different translators also helps, but such sets are expensive to produce.

Manual evaluation of MT means that the system output is given to a human to ask them to rate its quality. Since MT is generally destined for human consumption, manual evaluation is preferred as the definitive measure of the usefulness of the MT output. However manual evaluation is expensive (since it is time consuming, and ideally performed by linguists) so it cannot be applied at every stage in a system's development. Manual evaluation also presents its own difficulties. For instance, it is difficult to make it completely objective, and so differences between evaluators must be taken into account. Also, it is hard to design evaluation protocols which completely reflect the intended usage of the MT, which means that we often use somewhat artificial scenarios, and so have to verify that they correlate with our intended usage.

Typical protocols to evaluate MT are either to ask the evaluator to rate the MT on a linear scale, say for adequacy and fluency, or to make comparative judgements between different MT system variants. In both cases we are arguably measuring the users' perception of the quality of the MT, rather than the actual quality of the MT. In other words, the evaluators are being asked to make a judgement about how useful the translations would be to achieve their intended goal (e.g. communication, post-editing), and that judgement is subjective.

To develop a more ecologically valid evaluation of MT, we could ask translators to post-edit MT output and measure the time and effort required to produce a high-quality translation, if we are interested in post-editing. Alternatively, if we are more interested in gisting performance, we could ask evaluators to use the MT output to perform a task, such as a reading comprehension. One attempt to make reading comprehension based MT evaluation easier to apply was based on the idea of cloze tests (Forcada *et al.* 2018).

Given the abundance of evaluation measures, protocols and data sets used to evaluate MT, readers should be careful when drawing comparisons between different works. The annual shared tasks organised in the research field (Barrault *et al.* 2019; Niehues *et al.* 2019) help to bring researchers together to test their systems on common data sets, and to drive the development of evaluation protocols. There are still many open problems in MT evaluation. For instance almost all MT evaluation is based on sentences, and does not pay any attention to how those sentences fit together in context. The recent debate in the MT community on 'human-level' performance has raised questions as to how well discerning our evaluation is with really strong systems, and how we design our test sets to properly stretch these systems. At the same time, extending MT research to new languages, new text types and trying to address new types of phenomena also shows up limitations of the automatic metrics used.

5 Machine translation in healthcare

5.1 Overview

We now turn our attention to the usage of MT in healthcare settings. For the reasons outlined in the introduction (i.e. the non-availability or prohibitive cost of human translation/interpreting), there have been many attempts to apply MT in healthcare settings. In this section, we will survey several research projects on MT in healthcare, concentrating in particular on two recent projects where we have first-hand knowledge.

Applications of MT for healthcare mostly fall into three categories, which intersect with the usage models proposed in Section 3. These will be discussed in more detail in the rest of this section, but at a high-level, the application types are:

1. Usage of MT to assist in translation of healthcare-related information for the general public. This could be the publishers of the information using MT to help reduce translation costs, or users of the information translating it themselves, typically with online translation services.
2. Applying MT to translate more specialist healthcare-related publications such as scientific papers, patents and disease reports. This is often inbound translation (because healthcare professionals would like to read the works not written in their own language) but could be outbound translation (the publisher may use MT to assist translation).
3. Using MT for doctor-patient communication. Often this means that the MT is intended for live interaction between doctor and patient, implying that the MT needs

to operate in both language directions. Furthermore, it may be necessary to combine it with automatic speech recognition (ASR) and text-to-speech (TTS) if spoken dialogue is to be supported.

Reviewing the history of MT usage in healthcare, we found no healthcare-specific projects before the 2000s. It is likely that this reflects the fact that, before this time, researchers were mainly engaged in trying to improve the basic technology rather than thinking about specific applications. In the 2000s, MT quality improved fairly rapidly, with rule-based systems developing to higher quality, and with corpus-based approaches appearing and later becoming dominant. This led to several different groups experimenting with MT in healthcare, using a variety of different approaches to MT.

5.2 Selected projects in MT for healthcare

One early system for applying MT to healthcare was proposed by Somers and Lovel (2003). This system, proposed in a collaboration between a computational linguist and a healthcare researcher, was never fully built, but shows many features of later systems. It was envisaged as a means to improve doctor-patient communication with immigrant populations in the UK, focusing in particular on the Somali and Urdu languages (and translating to/from English). The system as described is primarily text-based, but leaves open the possibility for a speech-based extension.

The idea was that the doctor would be able to use their desktop computer to access a translation system which would supply MT in both directions using a mixture of rule-based MT, example-based MT (an early type of data-driven MT) and translation memories. A corpus of translated doctor-patient interviews would be used to help train the system, recognising the need for domain-specific training data. The text-entry interface for the doctors was proposed to be partially free text, and partially menu-based, representing the need to control the input text in order to assist the MT. The interface for patients was not fully developed in this work, but the authors recognised that some patients would not be computer-literate, and that one of their target groups (i.e. Urdu speakers) may not be comfortable with the Latin alphabet.

In a later work (Somers 2006), the first author of the above paper sets out the difficulties of creating a translation system for doctor-patient dialogues, and reports on lessons learnt (partly whilst developing the above system, partly from other similar efforts which are referenced). He argues that the user interface is vitally important, and that this should be designed with both doctor and patient in mind. He also emphasises the importance of evaluation, and not just an intrinsic evaluation of the MT system, but evaluation of the usefulness of the system in improving doctor-patient communication. Finally, Somers argues that there is much more to healthcare communication than the doctor-patient dialogue, and translation needs arise in many other parts of the healthcare journey.

Another system from the 2000s aimed at doctor-patient communication was MedSLT,[5] which was developed by Bouillon, Rayner and colleagues at the University of Geneva (Bouillon *et al.* 2005; Rayner *et al.* 2008). This was a speech-speech system that supported several language pairs. Since MedSLT used rule-based MT and rule-based components in the speech recognition, it had the advantage of high accuracy, but at the cost of low coverage: it was limited to certain healthcare topics, had a small vocabulary (up to 1,000 words per domain and language), and the patients could only provide yes/no answers.

A different kind of healthcare application of MT was explored in the translation part of the GPHIN (Global Public Health Intelligence Network) project (Blench 2008). The idea of this application is to automatically monitor news around the world for notifications of disease outbreaks. For instance, GPHIN helped to provide early warning of the SARS outbreak in 2002 – although this was before MT was added to GPHIN. GPHIN monitors many news feeds, and when it detects a relevant article (according to a language-specific topic classifier) it sends it for automatic translation and then to a human analyst. The GPHIN description notes that the translation provided by the machine is usually only suitable to obtain the 'gist' of the original article, and that the human analyst edits the translation to improve its comprehensibility before passing it to the report. The description of multilingual GPHIN (*ibid.*) does not provide any explicit data on the value of MT, but implies that it enables analysts to process articles more rapidly, and in a wider range of languages.

One healthcare scenario where MT can be very useful is in a crisis. Here, there is the need to scale up translation and interpreting very rapidly, possibly in languages that are not frequently supported by human translators. Developing an MT system to support aid workers on the ground can be part of the solution since such systems can be expanded rapidly to support many users once developed. With modern data-driven MT, systems can be developed quickly, assuming that appropriate data (i.e. parallel corpora) is available.

An important case study of crisis translation was the Microsoft translator system[6] developed in response to the 2010 Haitian earthquake. Text messages were being used to coordinate relief efforts, but there were insufficient Haitian Creole translators to handle the volume of translation, even after enlisting volunteer help. To assist with the translation, the Microsoft MT team developed a system for translating English to/from Haitian Creole, producing a first version within five days. Rapid system development was made possible by data-driven approaches to MT, since the system can be learnt directly from parallel text, as opposed to earlier knowledge-based approaches where the system developers needed to encode the translation lexicon and syntax directly into the system. The problem for languages such as Haitian Creole, however, is that there is very little parallel text, that is to say, the language is 'under-resourced' or 'low-resourced', with respect to MT. The Microsoft researchers had to address this lack of data by chasing down whatever resources they could obtain, for instance from government agencies and volunteers, and persuading organisations to make data and dictionaries available with as few restrictions as possible. The primary resource for data-driven MT is parallel text (Section 2.1), but there are techniques for making use of other resources, such as dictionaries and terminology lists.

A more recent effort on MT for crisis scenarios is within the Interact[7] project. The aim of this project was to learn how translation could improve the flow of information in the aftermath of a crisis, such as an earthquake or a nuclear accident. The project was not limited to machine translation, but included it as part of its overall strategy for distributing information. The Interact project also considered text simplification (both manual and automatic) as a useful method for improving machine translation.

An even more recent crisis-related MT initiative has seen researchers at Dublin City University develop and deploy MT systems specifically tuned for documents related to COVID-19 (Way *et al.* 2020). These MT systems are supplied for several European languages to/from English.

The growth of online healthcare information provided by government funded providers has led to an accompanying need for translation, and an investigation of MT as a means to reduce costs and increase coverage. The principal need is to reach out to immigrant populations, since the diverse and changing linguistic makeup of these groups make it difficult for health services to cover all possible languages. The dilemma for health services is that they want to provide timely, accurate, clearly written information, preserving the respect for their 'brand', yet MT is always imperfect.

In England and Wales, online healthcare information was first provided by NHS Direct (starting in 1998), later rebranded as NHS Choices, and now by the NHS website (www.nhs.uk). NHS Choices had a 'translate this page' button at the top of the page, powered by Google Translate, and a warning about the potential unreliability of MT (in English). At the time of writing, the NHS website has a page[8] which suggests that readers can use an online translator (without recommending a specific service), with a warning:

> Although online translators can accurately translate individual words and phrases, they may not always be able to interpret the meaning of larger or more complex pieces of information.

This warning is clearly instructing readers to take care in relying on automatic translation, although the warning about specific types of errors is not entirely accurate – it is true that the quality of MT will be on average worse in complex sentences, but it can also mistranslate important terms, especially if their meaning is domain-dependent.

In the United States, researchers at the University of Washington examined how MT could be used to increase the availability of public health information, first for the Spanish-speaking and later for the Chinese-speaking community (Kirchhoff *et al.* 2011; Laurenzi *et al.* 2013; Turner, Desai, *et al.* 2015; Turner, Brownstein *et al.* 2015). Their conclusion was that post-editing of MT could speed up production of Spanish language resources, but was less helpful for Chinese translation, since the then state-of-the-art English to Chinese MT (based on phrase-based MT) was not of good enough quality. An error analysis of the English to Spanish translations indicated that the most important issues were word-sense errors.

Also published by the University of Washington was a useful systematic review of the usage of MT in healthcare settings (Dew *et al.* 2018). This review conveniently covers almost exactly the period (2006–2016) when (non-neural) statistical MT was the dominant paradigm; before this period, rule-based systems were more common, and after this period, neural MT systems dominated. Of the 27 papers covered in the review, there was an even split between using MT for health education (i.e. translation of public health information, or health-related research) and MT for communication, generally between doctors and patients. The general conclusion was that MT needed to be combined with post-editing, or pre-editing (i.e. simplifying the source to make it easier for the MT to handle) in order to be useful.

A series of shared tasks in MT for biomedical research papers (Bojar, Buck *et al.* 2014; Bojar, Chatterjee, Federmann, Haddow *et al.* 2015; Bojar, Chatterjee, Federmann, Graham *et al.* 2016; Jimeno Yepes *et al.* 2017; Neves *et al.* 2018; Bawden *et al.* 2019), provide an insight into the development of MT for this particular task between the years 2014 and 2019. The idea of a shared task is that researchers in a particular area test their systems on a common data set, and then gather at a conference or a workshop to compare results and experiences. In this particular shared task, the data set has consisted of biomedical and health-related research paper abstracts. In each year of the task, human assessment of the translations produced by the systems has been performed. In the most recent edition (Bawden *et al.* 2019), the human evaluation reported that in several cases the MT systems were performing as well as, or better than, the human-created references. The claims of human-like performance of the MT system should be treated with caution though – the quality of the references was questionable in some cases.

We now turn our attention to recent healthcare-related MT projects which involved the authors. The first (Health in my language – HimL) applied MT to the dissemination of health information, whereas the second (Medical MT – MeMaT) addressed doctor-patient communication. Both projects took place at a time when NMT was just eclipsing earlier methods; in fact HimL started out as a PBMT project.

5.3 The health in my language project

5.3.1 Overview

Health in my Language (HimL) was an EU-funded Horizon 2020 project, which ran from 2015 to 2018, and aimed to trial the usage of MT in the healthcare domain. It brought together three research groups (Charles University in Prague, Ludwig Maximilian University of Munich and the University of Edinburgh), two healthcare organisations with translation needs (NHS 24 and Cochrane) and an integration partner (Lingea – a language service provider based in the Czech Republic).

We describe the healthcare user partners in more detail below, but both are organisations that create content mainly in English, but for different reasons would like to disseminate it in a variety of other languages. In HimL we wanted to enable the wider dissemination of content through the use of machine translation. In particular, the project focused on translation from English to languages of Central and Eastern Europe – specifically Czech, German, Polish and Romanian. At the start of the project, the state-of-the-art paradigm in MT was phrase-based MT (PBMT), and the plan was to advance this technology in aspects that were important to the domain (i.e. healthcare) and the target language pairs:

- Morphology: the MT systems needed to be able to translate from a morphologically impoverished language (English) into morphologically rich languages
- Accuracy: it would be important that the MT systems stay faithful to the source, i.e. we prioritised *adequacy* (possibly at the expense of *fluency*, if necessary)
- Domain Adaptation: the MT systems had to perform well in a specific domain (healthcare) yet taking advantage of training data gathered opportunistically from many domains

The project was structured so that the research partners would work on all of these topics, feeding the results into annual system releases. These were then to be integrated by Lingea, and made available for translating the content produced by the two user partners. These partners would evaluate the usefulness of the MT in their particular context.

When the project was launched, it was envisaged that the MT systems would mainly be PBMT, with the possibility of using syntax-based MT if the extra computational cost could be justified by quality gains. However, in the first year of HimL, NMT started to gain in popularity, and by the second year it was clear that NMT could offer significant gains in performance. HimL had to move to NMT or risk providing a substandard experience for the user partners, and losing relevance. This entailed a significant amount of project re-planning as many details of the plan assumed that we would be working with PBMT. The third and final set of MT systems created in HimL were NMT, and showed a significant quality improvement over the first two years' releases.

5.3.2 Background to the user partners

COCHRANE

Cochrane is a global non-profit organisation which aims to improve healthcare by publishing high-quality, independent reviews of the best available evidence. These are known as *systematic reviews* and Cochrane has published more than 7,000 of them since its establishment more than 20 years ago. The reviews are published in the Cochrane Library,[9] with abstracts and plain language summaries also made available on the Cochrane website.[10] The target audience includes healthcare professionals, policy makers and healthcare consumers.

Cochrane reviews are normally written in English, which is a major barrier for much of the potential audience. Readers may have no knowledge of English. It might be insufficient to be able to trust their reading of a crucial topic, or they may not wish to take on the extra burden of foreign language reading. With this difficulty in mind, Cochrane established a translation strategy in 2014 with the aim of making their content available to as wide an audience as possible. Translation efforts have mainly concentrated on the plain language summaries.

Since Cochrane have limited resources available for translation, especially as they can require specialist medical knowledge, most of the translation has been performed by volunteers. A wide range of languages are available in the Cochrane Library, with the largest amount of translated content available in French and Spanish. However, there is still a large amount of content untranslated, and many languages have quite poor coverage. An additional problem is that Cochrane reviews are regularly revised as new research becomes available, so, in order for the translated summaries to reflect the current best practice, they must be regularly updated.

In order to address this scaling problem, Cochrane wanted to experiment with automated translation. The idea was that an MT system, specialised to the particular domain of Cochrane reviews, could either produce content which could be published immediately, or could be post-edited by a human translator into a publishable format. The MT system would need to be integrated into Cochrane's content management workflow so that Cochrane could select which content should be translated, and then route the text through the MT, the editing and acceptance process, and finally to publication. Because of the European focus of HimL, and Cochrane's desire to expand into Central and Eastern Europe, we selected German and Czech as the most important languages for the project to focus on, from Cochrane's perspective.

NHS 24

NHS 24 is responsible for providing a range of telehealth services to the residents of Scotland, on behalf of NHS Scotland (National Health Services for Scotland). It provides health support via phone, email, webchat, social media and SMS, on a 24 × 7 basis. All public sector organisations in Scotland have a mandate to ensure equality of access, and for NHS 24 this means providing support for people whose first language is not English.

NHS 24 manages the NHSInform[11] website to provide people in Scotland with accurate and up-to-date healthcare information. It comprises about 3,500 pages of information covering clinically validated health advice, as well as information about health and care rights and about the services provided by hospitals, pharmacies, health centres, general practitioners, etc. Much of the information on NHSInform is specific to Scotland, and not available anywhere else. The content on NHSInform is written in plain English, targeting a reading age of 9, in order to have the maximum possible reach.

Many users and potential users of NHS 24 services are immigrants and do not necessarily have a good knowledge of English. NHS 24 do produce translations of some leaflets, but the production of translated content is limited by cost, and such content may not be updated as frequently as the English content. In theory, any resident can ask for a translation of a particular piece of NHSInform content, but in practice this requires the person to be aware that the content exists, and there will inevitably be a significant delay while the content is translated.

In HimL, we explored whether MT would be a viable way to extend the availability of healthcare information in Scotland, particularly by translation of the NHSInform website. As with Cochrane, we wanted to insert MT into the content management workflow of NHS 24, so that when webpages were created or updated, the content officer would be able to mark them for translation by the automated system, then merge the resulting translated content back into the site. Given the backgrounds of European immigrant population of Scotland, we decided to focus on translation into Polish and Romanian for NHS 24.

5.3.3 Building, deploying and evaluating MT for healthcare

In the three years of the project, there were three different system releases; PBMT systems in the first two years, and then NMT in the final year. The change from PBMT was not straightforward, partly because NMT was quite a different technology for the researchers, and also because it was not initially clear whether NMT would offer better performance.

To enable the NMT systems to out-perform PBMT, two key innovations had to be refined and applied to the HimL MT systems. The first innovation was to use 'subwords' in translation, as opposed to full words, as the basic unit (Sennrich, Haddow and Birch 2016). Neural networks require a fixed vocabulary size, but because of proper names, morphological variants and language-specific problems like compounding and transliteration, translation requires a very large, even unlimited, vocabulary. Allowing the neural network to operate on subwords means that it can cope with these productive linguistic phenomena using a small, finite vocabulary, by splitting unknown and rare words to smaller units, even to characters where necessary. The second innovation was a method for using monolingual text to create extra synthetic training data. The way this works is that we train a first version of the system with just the parallel data, then we use this system to translate monolingual data (in the target language) in order to create synthetic parallel data. A second version of the system is trained using a combination of the true parallel data and the synthetic parallel data. Normally the second version performs better than the first. Part of the improvement comes because the synthetic data can be chosen to be 'in-domain', i.e. healthcare-specific texts in this case. Applying these two innovations gave NMT a clear edge over PBMT in lab-based comparisons.

The deployment of the MT systems differed between the two user partners, but in both cases reflected the caution from the organisations about using MT. For Cochrane, the translation was integrated into their in-house CMS Archive. This provided the Cochrane website administrators with a 'translate this' button next to each article, which would send the article off for translation, and reload the results into the article database when it was ready. Care had to be taken to separate the machine-translated articles from the human-translated articles since they were handled by a similar process, but it was important that they should be distinguished when presented on Cochrane's website.

A less-automated process was used for NHS 24's integration. The content officers were provided with a web form for requesting translations. This caused the content to be sent to the HimL server, with the translation returned by email. The content officer then had to paste the translated text back into the database using another web form. This manual solution was sufficient for the project, but a more automated solution would be required for real-life usage.

Several types of evaluation were employed during HimL. The system developers applied automatic evaluation during development, since this provided quick results, and new evaluation measures were developed to measure the specific aspects of MT that were being targeted. HimL also applied human evaluation in order to assess how useful the MT was for users, and to gauge their attitude towards translated content.

At Cochrane, human evaluation in the early part of the project showed that the translation could not be published unedited, especially given Cochrane's high editorial standard. In the latter part of the project, Cochrane evaluated the use of HimL MT for post-editing. In other words, Cochrane translators were provided with the HimL MT output (as well as the source sentence) and asked to edit it into a high-quality translation of the original source sentence. In a comparison of post-editing using HimL MT, with the standard Cochrane workflow, which includes access to Google Translate, as well as Cochrane's translation memories and glossaries, we showed that productivity improvements were possible with HimL MT. In the translation of plain language summaries from English to all project languages apart from Polish, speedups of between 30 per cent and 60 per cent were observed. For Polish, post-editing did not help so much, most likely because the MT systems were of poorer quality in Polish. Feedback from translators reflected these speedups – about 70 per cent of translators preferred using the HimL MT for post-editing; the rest preferred to translate from scratch.

5.3.4 User reaction

We will discuss two different user studies undertaken by NHS 24 to gauge attitudes to machine translation. The first was a user survey where participants were recruited through several different user groups to complete an online questionnaire focused on Polish and Romanian HimL translations. The second was a needs impact study, where we recruited Polish and Romanian speakers for in-depth interviews to discuss their information needs, and if and how machine translation should be incorporated into NHS 24.

The user survey consisted of two parts; the first asking about access to health information and NHS services, and the second asking about a test website translated with the HimL Y3 (Year 3) system. We advertised the survey in several NHS community partnerships, including some targeted at Polish or Romanian speakers. We obtained 46 responses from Polish speakers, but only two incomplete responses from Romanian speakers, not enough to draw any conclusions.

In questions about the access to services, we found that nearly half had used the Internet for health information, and all of these had used NHS websites. However, about 40 per cent of those responding to the question reported it as 'difficult' or 'very difficult' to access health information in their own language. This indicates that there is a need for translation, at least amongst the Polish community.

As regards the HimL test translations shown to respondents, we found that whilst over 60 per cent stated that they would recommend the translations to others in their community, a similar proportion reported that the translations were not accurate. Respondents reported that the language in the translations was 'awkward and difficult to follow' and that, whilst simple sentences are often 'translated in an acceptable way and could be understood', translation got worse for longer sentences. One respondent reported that 'Some translations are so bad that they're confusing and misleading' and yet '... this could be some sort of help'.

The needs impact study consisted of in-depth interviews (using an interpreter) with 22 Polish and 17 Romanian speakers, in addition to six interviews with community group workers. Interviewees were asked about their strategies for accessing health information, as well as their opinions on the HimL translations on a test website. The translations were generated using the Y2 (PBMT) systems, although we had follow-up interviews with the community group workers on the Y3 (NMT) systems.

On the users' information needs, all literate respondents liked the idea of online health information in their own language. Currently some used Google Translate, and some used Polish or Romanian sites, since they did not have sufficient English to understand the NHS 24 sites. To make a translated website suitable for these language communities, respondents were concerned that the translations should be accurate, that the website be endorsed by NHS, and that it be sufficiently promoted within the community and available in leaflet form. Some of the Romanian respondents were illiterate, so clearly would need information provided in other formats, such as audio or video.

The general perception of the MT on the Y2 test site was that it was clearly machine translated, and interviewees often had trouble working out what was meant. Common errors include wrong verb tenses, missing words, and a meaning which is the opposite of the one intended. The Y3 was seen as an improvement over Y2, with better grammar and fluency, easier to understand, and with no instances of the translation meaning the opposite of the original. However there was still concern about using the machine-translated site as a sole source of information. Respondents would prefer to have access to the English version as well.

The overall message from the user survey was that, whilst the translations could be useful in parts, the overall level of quality was not high enough for an NHS 24 branded website. Improvements had been made between Y2 and Y3, but errors still remained. Most respondents felt that NHS 24 should only publish translations if they could be guaranteed to be equivalent quality to human translation. This means that post-editing is the only reasonable way to use MT in this context.

COCHRANE

Similar to the NHS 24 user studies, we surveyed Cochrane users about the impression they have of the raw MT, and its perceived usefulness. This was the original aim of HimL: to deploy, improve and evaluate the use of raw MT for these demanding use-cases.

The survey centred on machine-translated plain language summaries (PLS), which were displayed on the Cochrane website. We translated a number of PLSs using HimL translation systems, and uploaded the translated output onto the Cochrane website. The machine-translated summaries contained a notice explaining the origin of the translation, as well as a link to the survey, but in other respects the content was treated the same as other Cochrane translations. This means that these summaries still appeared in searches of the Cochrane article database along with human-created content and translations, and were indexed by search engines.

We ran three different surveys with different versions of the HimL system, and with extra questions added in later surveys. The three versions of the system were the Y2 system (phrase-based MT), an early version of our neural MT system and the Y3 (neural MT) system. The questions in the survey concerned the understandability of the text (on a five-point scale), the usefulness of having the MT (yes/no) and an open-ended question to explain the usefulness. We also applied the survey to PLSs translated by volunteers (i.e. human translations) to give an idea of the upper bound of quality and usefulness. The surveys were promoted through Cochrane communication channels, such as newsletters and social media.

For the phrase-based systems, quality ratings were relatively low (around 2). For the later evaluations, with the neural MT systems, quality ratings improved to 3–3.5 for all language pairs apart from English→Polish.

This should be contrasted with the ratings of volunteer human translations, which, using the same scale, achieved mean ranks of 4.5/4.8 for en-de/en-pl. This clearly indicates that the quality of machine-translated text is still lower than the quality of text translated by humans, but it is catching up. Of course, the fact that MT is of lower quality than human translation is not really a surprise, but the more important question is, even at this quality level, is the MT useful?

To answer this question, we added an extra question about the usefulness of the MT to the later user surveys on the NMT systems. Specifically, we asked whether it was more useful to see the MT in addition to the English source, compared to just seeing the English source. We also asked the same question about the human-translated articles, to gauge an upper bound for MT usefulness. When we limited the survey to respondents with a low knowledge of English, we found that at least 85 per cent of respondents found the human translation in their own language useful, but the results for MT were more mixed. The en-pl translation was found useful by only 8 per cent of respondents, reflecting its low quality, but for other pairs, proportions were higher: en-ro (49 per cent), en-cs (57 per cent) and en-de (81 per cent).

In the final version of the survey, we introduced an additional open question which asked why respondents did not consider the provided translation to be useful. Common reasons were that it was of low quality, difficult to understand, unnatural, not fluent, or contained incomprehensible terms or sentences. Others reported that they found the English easier to understand, showing that these respondents had sufficient knowledge of English. For the human translations, the most common reason given for the translation not helping was that the respondents were used to reading documents in English. Some reported that the original was more fluent, or that they just preferred it.

5.4 Medical machine translation

The Medical Machine Translation (MeMaT) project was a UK Research Council funded project, run under the umbrella of the Global Research Challenges fund. It was a short pilot project that ran from September 2017 to March 2018. It was a collaboration between the University of Edinburgh, the University of Cape Town and the Gugulethu Community Health (GCH) centre in Cape Town, South Africa.

With 11 official languages, doctors in South Africa rarely share a language with their patients. Despite the official status of the other languages, services are delivered in English or Afrikaans with little budget for translators into widely-spoken local languages, such as isiXhosa. Nurses, cleaners, and patients are often pressed to serve as interpreters, even for private matters like HIV. A consultation lasts 10 minutes, so care is impacted when *ad hoc* interpreters cannot be reached in time or are unfamiliar with medical terms: 'Lots of people have already died because they cannot understand or say what is the matter with them' (Schlemmer and Mash 2006).

GCH serves a large, low socio-economic status community which is predominantly isiXhosa speaking, which means doctor-patient communication can be severely affected by the language barrier. To address this, one of the doctors at GCH (Saadiq Moolla) created the *Mobile Translate MD* app which provides canned translations of common sentences. The app has been downloaded over 2,000 times from the Google Play Store, and used by many more.

The MeMaT project aimed to further improve doctor-patient interaction by empowering doctors to translate arbitrary sentences, as opposed to just canned sentences. The project engaged with medical practitioners to test the usefulness of the machine-translation (MT) system with expert language speakers.

Building a quality machine translation system in this context posed two main research challenges: the small size of available training data and linguistic differences from English. Since all modern approaches to MT require training data in the form of parallel sentences, and whilst this enables systems to be built quickly, the results are strongly influenced by the size and quality of the data. An aim of this research project was to improve performance on low-resource data sets.

5.4.1 Building and evaluating MT systems

Our first challenge was to collect appropriate monolingual and parallel training data. The situation for isiXhosa is typical of many low-resource languages – parallel data is available only from Bible translations, and from the localisation of open-source software such as the Ubuntu Linux distribution. A significant amount of effort in the project was directed at scraping and cleaning data from a number of websites with parallel data (the University of Cape Town, Wikipedia, Western Cape Government websites and the South African Constitution). We also had a very small amount of data (a few hundred words and phrases) from the Mobile Xhosa project, and also anonymised conversations from health webchat sites. The data we gathered for the project was released as a corpus to aid future research in this language.

Using the isiXhosa–English parallel corpus we built for the project, we created some initial MT systems. Using automatic evaluation though, we could see that the results were quite poor, and we applied two main techniques to improve the translation. The first technique was the same as in HimL, i.e. the use of synthetic parallel data created by back-translating using the first version of the system. The second technique we applied was to exploit the similarity between the isiXhosa and Zulu languages, and the fact that there is a lot more parallel data for English–Zulu than for English–isiXhosa. Using this related language data alongside the isiXhosa data, we were able to show further significant improvements in automatic measures of translation quality. The resulting translation systems were not tested with users, partly because this was only a short pilot project and user-testing was not foreseen, and partly because the quality of the systems was not high enough. Nevertheless, the project was an early indicator that the technique of 'transfer learning', where MT for a low-resource language is improved by using data from a higher resource language pair, was an effective way of improving quality.

6 Outlook

In this chapter we have described the development, current status, and typical usage of machine translation (MT). We have also presented several research projects in which MT has been applied to the healthcare domain. We have observed that MT has greatly improved in quality as the development of the technology proceeded through distinct phases: first rule-based MT, then statistical MT (with phrase-based MT being the most common version of this) and finally neural MT which is dominant today. Despite these improvements, MT is still imperfect in many situations, and will perform particularly poorly when there is insufficient training data (i.e. parallel sentences) in the domain and language that we require.

In the healthcare domain, we expect that the two main uses for MT will be the same as in other domains; for dissemination and for assimilation (gisting). For the former use-case, publishing raw (i.e. unedited) MT is unlikely to be feasible in the near future. Any publishing in this domain is already subjected to intensive editing, in other words, content written by humans is highly unlikely to be published without oversight, and so machine created content will definitely not be published without prior editing. However, MT has the potential to speed up the translation process, enabling a reduction in costs and/or an increase in the availability of content, as well as streamlining the updating process.

In light of the NHS 24 survey results, we expect that MT will be an important way for healthcare consumers to obtain service and health information, when it is not written in their main language. They will typically do this by using online translation services such as Google Translate to translate web pages. Whilst organisations like NHS 24 are unwilling to put their 'seal of approval' on raw MT of their content, they need to allow for the fact that consumers will apply MT to their content themselves. Making sure that the content is written in plain, simple English is one way to help MT systems, as well as making it easier for non-English speakers to read the content themselves. Medical professionals also need to be aware that their patients may be accessing machine-translated information, and be prepared for misunderstandings.

The case study in South Africa presents quite a different context for MT. In that situation, we are trying to translate into and out of a language (isiXhosa) which has very few written resources, and even fewer parallel texts, and is radically different from English. The MT problem is much harder than even for the English–Polish task considered in HimL, and more research will be needed to enable high-quality translation in such under-resourced languages. The South African use-case also raises another question: that of spoken language translation (SLT). In principle, this is just a pipeline of services – automatic speech recognition, machine translation and text-to-speech – however assembling the pipeline raises many more difficulties, for example the compounding of errors as they are passed through the pipeline, the often radically different nature of the spoken language compared to written, and the unavailability of the technologies in many world languages.

The state of MT today is that it can produce often fluent and readable translations of (say) French newspapers in English, but for many domains and languages, translation can still be poor. Current techniques rely on large quantities of training data, which is generally parallel texts in the languages being translated, preferably of a similar topic and genre to the text to be translated. Rule-based MT systems can be produced without parallel data, but require significant effort to encode human language knowledge into the system, and typically can only cover a very limited range of expressions. We do not have straightforward routes to incorporate linguistic and domain knowledge into NMT systems, nor to improve them with user feedback. These topics are all part of current research, and we are optimistic that progress will be made. However, we do not expect MT to replace human translators and interpreters at any time in the foreseeable future; rather, we expect that translation and interpreting will increasingly be performed with machine assistance, making the process more efficient and reliable.

List of abbreviations

ASR	Automatic Speech Recognition
CMS	Content Management System
GCH	Gugulethu Community Health
HimL	Health in my Language
LM	Language Model
MeMaT	Medical Machine Translation
MPE	Monolingual Post-editing
MT	Machine Translation
NHS	National Health Service
NLP	Natural Language Processing
NMT	Neural Machine Translation
PBMT	Phrase-based Machine Translation
PLS	Plain Language Summary
RBMT	Rule-based Machine Translation
TTS	Text to Speech

Notes

1 Yes, this rule has exceptions, because sometimes French adjectives come *before* their nouns. This is one of the dificulties facing RBMT – whenever you write a rule, you have to write new rules to cover its exceptions.
2 Perhaps confusingly, these are not phrases in the linguistic sense, but can be any continuous sequence of words.
3 It is possible to identify a third usage model, where MT output is not consumed by humans, but by a different piece of software, for example a document index for an information retrieval system. An example of this from the medical domain is the KConnect (www.kconnect. eu/) project.
4 In 2016, Google Translate claimed to be translating 100 billion words per day (www. blog. google/products/translate/ten-years-of-google-translate/), and it is just one provider of translation. It is unlikely that such a quantity of words is being post-edited, even if we include amateur translators.
5 www.issco.unige.ch/en/research/projects/medslt/about.html
6 www.microsoft.com/en-us/research/blog/translator-fast-tracks-haitian-creole/
7 https://sites.google.com/view/crisistranslation/home
8 www.nhs.uk/accessibility/health-information-in-other-languages/
9 www.cochranelibrary.com
10 www.cochrane.org
11 www.nhsinform.scot/

Further reading

Forcada, M. (2017) 'Making Sense of Neural Machine Translation'. *Translation Spaces*, 6(2), pp. 291–309.

In this article, the author offers an explanation of neural machine translation (NMT) aimed at translators and students of translation studies.

Dew, K. *et al.* (2018) 'Development of Machine Translation Technology for Assisting health communication: A systematic review'. *Journal of Biomedical Informatics*, 85, pp. 56–67

This is a systematic review of research on MT in healthcare settings between the years 2006–2016, describing 27 different studies.

Läubli, S. *et al.* (2020). 'A Set of Recommendations for Assessing Human–Machine Parity in Language Translation'. *Journal of Artificial Intelligence Research*, 67, pp. 653–672

This article discusses the problem of MT evaluation, and the recent claims of 'human parity' in the MT literature.

Lewis, W. (2010) 'Haitian Creole: How to Build and Ship an MT Engine from Scratch in 4 days, 17 hours, and 30 minutes'. *Proceedings of European Association for Machine Translation*. Available at: www.mt-archive.info/EAMT-2010-Lewis.pdf (Accessed: 6 January 2021).

This gives an account of the building of the rapid development of a Haitian Creole system to assist aid workers in the aftermath of the 2010 earthquake.

Somers, H. (2006) 'Language Engineering and the Pathway to Healthcare: A User-Oriented View'. *Proceedings of the First International Workshop on Medical Speech Translation*. Available at: http://citeseerx.ist.psu.edu/viewdoc/download?doi=10.1.1.503.2586&rep=rep1&type=pdf (Accessed: 6 January 2021).

This position paper presents a view on how MT-based assistants for clinical settings should be developed.

Related topics

Post-editing of Machine Translation, Evaluation of Machine Translation, Computer Assisted Translation, Risks of Machine Translation Usage, Automatic Translation of Spoken Language

References

Bahdanau, D., K. Cho and Y. Bengio (2015) 'Neural Machine Translation by Jointly Learning to Align and Translate'. *Proceedings of International Conference on Learning Representations*. Available at: https://arxiv.org/pdf/1409.0473.pdf (Accessed: 6 January 2021)

Barrault, L. *et al.* (2019) 'Findings of the 2019 Conference on Machine Translation (WMT19)'. *Proceedings of the Fourth Conference on Machine Translation (Volume 2: Shared Task Papers, Day 1)*, Florence.

Bawden, R. *et al.* (2019) 'Findings of the WMT 2019 Biomedical Translation Shared Task: Evaluation for MEDLINE Abstracts and Biomedical Termi-nologies'. *Proceedings of the Fourth Conference on Machine Translation (Volume 3: Shared Task Papers, Day 2)*, Florence.

Blench, M. (2008) 'Global Public Health Intelligence Network (GPHIN)'. *Proceedings of the Association for Machine Translation of the Americas*.

Bojar, O. and Buck, C. *et al.* (2014) 'Findings of the 2014 Workshop on Statistical Machine Translation'. *Proceedings of the Ninth Workshop on Statistical Machine Translation*, Baltimore.

Bojar, O., Chatterjee, R. Federmann, C., Graham, Y. *et al.* (2016). 'Findings of the 2016 Conference on Machine Translation'. *Proceedings of the First Conference on Machine Translation*, Berlin.

Bojar, O., Chatterjee, R. Federmann, C. and Haddow *et al.* (2015) 'Findings of the 2015 Workshop on Statistical Machine Translation'. *Proceedings of the Tenth Workshop on Statistical Machine Translation*, Lisbon.

Bojar, O., Federmann, C. *et al.* (2018) 'Findings of the 2018 Conference on Machine Translation (WMT18)'. *Proceedings of the Third Conference on Machine Translation: Shared Task Papers* Brussels.
Bouillon, P. *et al.* (2005) 'A Generic Multi-Lingual Open Source Platform for Limited-Domain Medical Speech Translation'. *Proceedings of European Association for Machine Translation.*
Brown, P. F. *et al.* (1994) 'The Mathematic of Statistical Machine Translation: Parameter Estimation'. *Computational Linguistics,* 19(2), pp. 263–311.
Dew, K. *et al.* (2018) 'Development of Machine Translation Technology for Assisting Health Communication: A Systematic Review'. *Journal of Biomedical Informatics*, 85, pp. 56–67.
Forcada, M. (2017) 'Making Sense of Neural Machine Translation'. *Translation Spaces*, 6(2), pp. 291–309.
Forcada, M. *et al.* (2018) 'Exploring Gap Filling as a Cheaper Alternative to Reading Comprehension Questionnaires When Evaluating Machine Translation for Gisting. *Proceedings of the Third Conference on Machine Translation, Volume 1: Research Papers.*
Hassan, H. *et al.* (2018) 'Achieving Human Parity on Automatic Chinese to English News Translation'. In: *ArXiv e-prints*. Available at: https://arxiv.org/pdf/1802.05368.pdf (Accessed: 6 January 2021).
Jimeno Yepes, A. *et al.* (2017) 'Findings of the WMT 2017 Biomedical Translation Shared Task'. *Proceedings of the Second Conference on Machine Translation, Volume 2: Shared Task Papers*, Copenhagen.
Kirchhoff, K. *et al.* (2011) 'Application of Statistical Machine Translation to Public Health Information: A Feasibility Study'. *Journal of the American Medical Informatics Association,* 18(4), pp. 473–478.
Koehn, P. *et al.* (2007) 'Moses: Open Source Toolkit for Statistical Machine Translation'. *Proceedings of the 45th Annual Meeting of the Association for Computational Linguistics Companion Volume Proceedings of the Demo and Poster Sessions*, Prague.
Koehn, P., Och, F.J. and Marcu, D. (May 2003) 'Statistical Phrase-Based Translation'. *Proceedings of the 2003 Human Language Technology Conference of the North American Chapter of the Association for Computational Linguistics*, Edmonton.
Läubli, S. *et al.* (2020) 'A Set of Recommendations for Assessing Human–Machine Parity in Language Translation', *Journal of Artificial Intelligence Research,* 67, pp. 653–672.
Läubli, S., Sennrich, R. and Volk, M. (Oct. 2018) 'Has Machine Translation Achieved Human Parity? A Case for Document-level Evaluation'. *Proceedings of the 2018 Conference on Empirical Methods in Natural Language Processing*, Brussels.
Laurenzi, A. *et al.* (2013) 'A Web-based Collaborative Translation Management System for Public Health Workers'. *ACM SIGCHI Conference on Human Factors in Computing Systems*, Paris.
Lewis, W. (2010) 'Haitian Creole: How to Build and Ship an MT Engine from Scratch in 4 days, 17 hours, and 30 minutes'. *Proceedings of European Association for Machine Translation*, 24.
Luong, T., Pham, H. and Manning, C. D. (2015) 'Effective Approaches to Attention-based Neural Machine Translation'. *Proceedings of the 2015 Conference on Empirical Methods in Natural Language Processing*, Lisbon.
Neves, M. *et al.* (2018) 'Findings of the WMT 2018 Biomedical Translation Shared Task: Evaluation on Medline Test Sets". *Proceedings of the Third Conference on Machine Translation, Volume 2: Shared Task Papers*, Brussels.
Niehues, J. *et al.* (2019) 'The IWSLT 2019 Evaluation Campaign'. *Proceedings of International Workshop on Spoken Language Translation.*
Rayner, M. *et al.* (2008) 'The 2008 MedSLT System'. *Coling 2008: Proceedings of the workshop on Speech Processing for Safety Critical Translation and Pervasive Applications.*
Schlemmer, A. and Mash, B (2006) 'The Effects of a Language Barrier in a South African District Hospital', *South African Medical Journal*, 96(10), pp. 1084–1087.
Schwartz, L. (2012) 'Monolingual Post-Editing by a Domain Expert is Highly Effective for Translation Triage'. *Proceedings of the Association for Machine Translation of the Americas.*
Sennrich, R., Haddow, B. and Birch, A. (2016) 'Neural Machine Translation of Rare Words with Subword Units'. *Proceedings of the 54th Annual Meeting of the Association for Computational Linguistics (Volume 1: Long Papers)*, Berlin.
Somers, H. (2006) 'Language Engineering and the Pathway to Healthcare: A User-Oriented View'. *Proceedings of the First International Workshop on Medical Speech Translation*, New York.

Somers, H. and Lovel, H. (2003) 'Computer-based Support for Patients with Limited English'. *Proceedings of the 7th International EAMT Workshop on MT and Other Language Technology Tools, Improving MT Through Other Language Technology Tools, Resource and Tools for Building MT at EACL 2003*.

Specia, L., Scarton, C. and Paetzold, G. H. (2018) *Quality Estimation for Machine Translation*. Williston, VT: Morgan and Claypool.

Sutskever, I., Vinyals, O. and Le, Q. V. (2014) 'Sequence to Sequence Learning with Neural Networks'. *ArXiv e-prints*.

Toral, A. *et al.* (2018) 'Attaining the Unattainable? Reassessing Claims of Human Parity in Neural Machine Translation'. *Proceedings of the Third Conference on Machine Translation: Research Papers*, Brussels.

Turner, A. M., Brownstein, M. *et al.* (2015) 'Modeling Workflow to Design Machine Translation Applications for Public Health Practice'. Journal of Biomedical Informatics, 53, pp. 136–146.

Turner, A. M., Desai, L. *et al.* (2015) 'Machine Assisted Translation of Health Materials to Chinese: An Initial Evaluation'. *MEDINFO 2015: eHealth-enabled Health –Proceedings of the 15th World Congress on Health and Biomedical Informatics*, São Paulo.

Way, A. *et al.* (2020) 'Facilitating Access to Multilingual COVID-19 Information via Neural Machine Translation'. *ArXiv e-prints*, 25.

Williams, P. *et al.* (2016) *Syntax-based Statistical Machine Translation*. Morgan and Claypole.

Wu, Y. *et al.* (2016) 'Google's Neural Machine Translation System: Bridging the Gap between Human and Machine Translation'. *ArXiv e-prints*.

8

Medical humanities and translation

Vicent Montalt

In loving memory of my father,
who, while living with Parkinson's disease,
remained an enthusiastic storyteller in his native Catalan.

1 Introduction[1]

In this chapter I will explore some of the intersections and entanglements between medical translation, as part of the established academic discipline of translation studies, and the interdisciplinary and intercultural field of medical humanities. I will do so both from historical and contemporary perspectives. Professional medical translators have traditionally focused on biomedical science, a top-down, standardised and autonomous body of knowledge that has dominated medicine and healthcare for a long time. However, biomedical science is the result of often complex historical processes and exists in socially, culturally and linguistically rich and varied contexts. Beyond its professional dimension, translation can also be understood in broader terms, both as an educational tool for health professionals and as a critical frame of analysis, as this chapter will demonstrate. In an era of growing automation and machine translation, my aim is to broaden the topic of health and medicine within the field of translation studies, foreground the human factor, and expand the frame of critical thinking. With this aim in mind, I will first outline the historical perspectives which have preceded biomedical science, with an emphasis on language and translation. Then, I will turn to more recent times, during which the evolution towards a more holistic and humanised view of medicine and health has been accompanied by the emergence of personalised and translational medicine. Medical humanities and some of its entanglements with translation will be the next step in my overview. In the last few years, medical humanities has widened its scope to include critical and reflective factors, which offer an expanded framework for a more proactive presence of the humanities – and consequently, of translation – in the forging of medical and healthcare knowledge. Finally, I will argue that narrative medicine, one of the main contributions of medical humanities, is opening up a rich seam to be mined for translation practice and research.

DOI: 10.4324/9781003167983-11

2 Historical intersections

A paper published recently in *Le journal des médecines cunéiformes* (Arbøll 2019) reports on a 2,700-year-old cuneiform tablet from ancient Iraq written in Akkadian, describing medical treatments, and containing a drawing of a demon which Assyrians and Babylonians called Bennu, and which was thought to cause epilepsy. It is the earliest illustration of devilish associations with this condition. The term *bennu* might also have been used to describe 'convulsions' (Arbøll 2019: 5). At the time, healers were responsible for expelling what they understood as supernatural forces and treating the medical symptoms they caused with drugs, rituals or incantations. The Assyrians and Babylonians believed that there was a connection between the moon, epilepsy and insanity (Arbøll 2019). They also believed that the one who knew the true name of things, and of the demons that modified them, possessed magical powers; by pronouncing the true name of a thing one would become the master of it and could rule over it (Laín Entralgo 1958: 47). The power of naming things and the art of the word – *ars dicendi* – are crucial aspects of both these ancient forms of medicine and the contemporary ones, although in different ways.

Before science reached the point when it became able to demonstrate the mechanisms of disease, supernatural forces often provided causal explanations. It was perfectly acceptable and believable to state that convulsions due to epilepsy – a neologism originating in classical Greece with which we now name the disease – were in fact caused by the gods, or indeed, in some cases, by the devil himself.

The oldest detailed account of epilepsy is on a Babylonian tablet dating as far back as at least 2000 BCE. According to the Cuneiform Digital Library Initiative,[2] the earliest known medical text dates from the third dynasty of Ur (also *c.*2000 BCE) and is written in Sumerian. Other early (14th century BCE) Sumerian texts have been found at Hattusa (Boğazkale, Turkey), but it is not known whether they were originally composed in Sumerian or copied and translated from Babylonian originals – an open question that seems to suggest a very remote origin of medical translation.

From the viewpoint of medical humanities and translation, what is most relevant about this archaeological discovery is the critical importance of interpreting the meaning of the cuneiform tablet and its magical-medical content through a hermeneutically complex process of translation and exegesis. The whole of the first section of the paper mentioned above (Arbøll 2019) consists of a semantic analysis of the Akkadian words referring to illness, diagnosis and symptoms, and the various translations into English provided by different scholars. One of the most frequently recurring expressions is '[Akkadian word] can be translated as [English word]'. Finding the meaning and making sense of the cuneiform writing require not only translation as a mere lexical tool to establish direct equivalences – in this case between Akkadian and English – but also a translational frame of inquiry in which remote concepts and explanations are critically scrutinised, re-contextualised, reformulated and brought to the here-and-now of new target readers.

In Western medical traditions, supernatural views of medicine can be traced back to ancient times through *The Iliad* and *The Odyssey* of Homer (8th century BCE), who composed his epic poems some four or five centuries before Hippocrates. In his seminal book *La curación por la palabra en la antiguedad clásica* (*The Therapy of the Word in Classical Antiquity*, 1958), Pedro Laín Entralgo, a Spanish psychiatrist and classical Greek scholar, outlined the presence and role of therapeutic speech in Greek culture. Together with surgical, pharmaceutical and dietetic methods, disease was also cured with charms, spells and incantations. Spells were linked to imperative or coercive intentions when trying to modify phenomena, such as averting the action of a demon or staunching the flow of blood. Charms were used when the dominant intention was to plead for help from divine powers. In these pre-Homeric traditions, words used therapeutically could sometimes be accompanied by music. According to Laín Entralgo (1958), the use of such words in Homer's epic poems was not always of a magical nature. Sometimes words were used to evoke in the patient a state of mind that would help them to cope with the effects of the illness. Both in magical and non-magical uses of the word the purpose of the healer was to achieve a psychosomatic change in the patient. In current linguistic terminology, these are examples of the performative power of language in action, language as a force capable of transforming minds and bodies. Current uses of language in healing include, for instance, cognitive behaviour therapy (CBT) and mindfulness in psychiatric medicine.

Plato recognised the therapeutic power of the word and its emotion-stirring qualities, and allowed it a place in his Republic (*c.*375 BCE). However, he excluded poets and playwrights from his ideal Republic, because he believed no good could come from words that excited passions and obscured reason. Aristotle, on the other hand, thought that emotional catharsis had therapeutic value. According to Laín Entralgo (1958), Aristotle's *Rhetoric* (4th century BCE), a treatise devoted to the power of the word, may be considered as a therapeutic oratory. For Aristotle, any doctor whose words were capable of producing psychological reactions in certain patients similar to those of tragic poems, would be more effective than one who only considered therapeutic practice as a silent art: *muta ars*. In Aristotelian verbal catharsis, the action of the word can be of such intensity that it can work as if discourse itself were a drug (Laín Entralgo 1958: 338–343).

Just a few centuries after the inscription on the Akkadian clay tablet mentioned above, Hippocrates wrote *On the Sacred Disease* (*c.*400 BCE), where he dismissed the religious origin of epilepsy and other diseases in favour of natural causes accessible to rational thought and understanding:

> It is thus with regard to the disease called Sacred: it appears to me to be nowise more divine nor more sacred than other diseases, but as natural cause from the originates [*sic*] like other affections. Men regard its nature and cause as divine from ignorance and wonder, because it is not like to other diseases. And this notion of its divinity is kept up by their inability to comprehend it [...].[3]

According to *Diccimed*,[4] the medical term prior to Hippocrates was *hiròs nósos*, the sacred disease; and, one of the first tasks Hippocratic doctors undertook was to rename it avoiding any religious connotations. They adopted the medical term 'epilepsy' from Greek epi- (over, upon) and -lepsi (take). Even this intentionally more descriptive, biomedical word retains traces of its magical origins, as if sufferers were 'taken over' by some supernatural power. Interestingly, Hippocrates' view of epilepsy as a brain disorder, and not as a divine punishment, did not begin to take root until the 18th and 19th centuries, the intervening 2,000 years being dominated by the earlier supernatural views.

The Hippocratic tradition thus departs from the magical and religious, focuses on the physical in its understanding and explanation of disease, and, despite Plato and Aristotle, abandons the possibility of curing by the word. *Physis*, the knowledge of nature in classical Greece, takes centre stage and medicine gradually becomes a *muta ars* – or, as Petrarch puts it, *herba, non verba* [herbs, not words]. Nowadays, the muteness of the corpses on which medical students get to know human anatomy shape their purely physical concepts about the human body during their university training. For centuries, this orientation away from words and discourse has greatly influenced healthcare, and in particular, doctor-patient communication.

The emergence of Hippocratic medicine as *muta ars* in classical Greece and its subsequent historical development driven by *physis* – and apparently excluding *ars dicendi* – eventually gave rise to current biomedical science. However, when examined from the perspective of the history of translation, medicine can hardly be defined as *muta ars* but its opposite, *ars dicendi*. Translation has been a historical driving force of scientific advancement. Over the centuries, the development of medical knowledge has depended on the transmission of discoveries and ideas through texts across languages and cultures, starting in Ancient Mesopotamia, which, at the moment, is as far back as we can go for material evidence. Modern science and medicine are indivisible from translation; in fact, they began as translation (Montgomery 2000). At every milestone, 'translation was the key to scientific progress as it unlocked for each successive inventor and discoverer the minds of predecessors who expressed their innovative thoughts in another language' (Fischbach 1993: 90). In historical terms, translation has been defined as the borrowing or appropriating of the findings of others (Delisle and Woodsworth 1995), a process that often involved innovation and further development, as is the case of Islamic medicine drawing on Hellenic medical tradition to form its own (Savage-Smith 1997). Likewise, medieval and early modern scholars in Europe drew upon Islamic traditions and translations as the foundation of their medical undertaking. It was through Arabic translations that the West learned of the Hellenic medicine (Savage-Smith 1997).

Historically, translation has always been entangled in the process of knowledge production, albeit in rather covert ways. In contrast with the so-called 'diffusionist' models of knowledge production and distribution, Delisle and Woodsworth (1995: 101) point out that 'The translators of history should not be regarded as passive conduits of specialised information, but rather as agents fully implicated in the works they reformulated in another language.' The very process of circulation produces new knowledge. Wisnovsky (2017) argues that even when translators declare themselves to be faithful interpreters, individual acts of recreation and transformation inevitably occur during the process of translating a philosophical work from one language to another. Drawing on Aristotle's categories of textual kinesis or motion, he shows that in Greek-Arabic translation of philosophical works in the Middle Ages, the interplay between translating, commentating/glossing and transcribing/copying has caused expansions, contractions and mutations in concepts and arguments that can explain some substantive developments of philosophy in general, and natural philosophy and medicine in particular.[5] Focusing attention on the creative aspects of the reception of medical texts in other languages and cultures throughout history helps us to think more critically about the dominant diffusionist, instrumentalist and subservient view that reduces translation to no more than a conduit of previous knowledge.

3 Biomedical science and beyond

The biomedical model has been around since the mid-19th century and still dominates our scientific understanding of health and disease. It focuses on the physical aspects of disease (anatomy, biochemistry, physiology, pathology, genetics, etc.) and adopts a positivist stance in its search for objective biomedical truth, mostly ignoring non-clinical factors. It assumes disease to be fully accounted for by deviations from the norm of measurable biological (somatic) variables (Engel 1977). Biomedical research provides data which health professionals can use when making decisions of all sorts, giving rise to Evidence-Based Medicine (EBM), which prevails in current approaches to diagnosis and treatment. In the biomedical model, a patient is seen as an object under treatment, a body that is sick and can be managed independently from its mind, family and social circumstances. Biomedicine is presented as a hierarchical, top-down, research-initiated model; it is deemed to be objective, standardised and eschewing cultural and experiential factors. Biomedicine has its own ontological and epistemological norms, and excludes other medicines and forms of knowing and understanding health and disease, such as those with traditional and local roots. In biomedicine, diseases are pigeonholed into categories in which a particular narrative, often predicated on a reductive or mechanistic account, dominates the discourse (Bowman 2014). This can lead to what Carel and Kidd (2014) describe as 'epistemic injustice' in healthcare: patients are vulnerable to the privileging of particular ways of describing illness or disease. This occurs, for example, when society as a whole, or health professionals in particular, lack the interpretative framework to understand particular experiences. For instance, this was the case in the 1960s, and later, with sexual harassment. Society did not acknowledge it and the behaviour of the perpetrators was typically tolerated and even excused. As a result, women were victimised, because the wider social context did not label such behaviour as sexual harassment (Carel and Györffy 2014: 1256).

In the past, translators mainly operated within the framework of biomedicine, owing to its economic and political power and prestige. They focused mainly on expert-to-expert communication, that is, on highly specialised text genres, in which the abstract language of biomedical research excludes the human, lived experience of patients and obscures the fact that where illnesses are unique, disease labels are classificatory terms only (Haggerty *et al.* 2003). That is why for decades, at least in countries such as Spain, trained doctors with some knowledge of foreign languages were at an advantage in the field of medical translation and led the biomedical translation market, whereas trained linguists and translators tended to be marginalised on the grounds that they did not have the disciplinary knowledge nor the terminological command required to understand and translate biomedical texts in an accurate and reliable way. The development of translation studies as a discipline and the provision of specialised training programmes have meant that more linguists are now involved in biomedical translation. Although these recent developments are encouraging, factual accuracy, conceptual precision, terminological equivalence and adherence to strict textual norms of the biomedical genres continue to be the core concerns of translators working in biomedicine, whether they are health professionals or linguists.

Between 1960 and 1980, George Engel, an American internist and psychiatrist, published a set of papers in which he outlined the limitations of the biomedical model and called for a new, more holistic approach, which he called the 'biopsychosocial model'. Through this model, he introduced psychosocial factors which would be taken into account without sacrificing the advantages of the biomedical approach, so that patients would continue to be cared for from a disease standpoint, but, additionally, psychological and social information would be given equal standing in the care process (Farre and Rapley 2017). Subsequently, today's patient-centred care (PCC) took these principles on board. Patient-centred doctors aim at eliciting and understanding their patients' psychosocial context and perspectives, taking into account their ideas, concerns and expectations

(Epstein *et al.* 2005). They aim at reaching a shared understanding of the problem with their patients and involve them in decision making and management of their illnesses. Patient-centred care has galvanised some new thinking and prompted responses in translation studies, which I will come back to in the next section.

Two distinct, and sometimes opposing, perspectives constantly interact in clinical communication: that of health professionals, doctors in particular, and that of patients. Or, in Jürgen Habermas' theory of communicative action (2015), that of expert systems and that of lifeworld (*Lebenswelt*), respectively. Both have their own particular motivations, expectations, resources, values, conceptual systems, discourses, stories, strategies for public presentation and social roles; and, this dichotomy of socio-professional cultures causes problematic asymmetries that can be understood and bridged in intra- and interlingual translation terms. Intralingual translation, or genre shift (Montalt and González-Davies 2007), is particularly relevant in some intergeneric relationships, such as between a Summary of Product Characteristics (SPC, a technical genre describing the properties and officially approved conditions of use of a medicine that forms the basis of information for healthcare professionals) and a patient information leaflet (a genre derived from the SPC typically aimed at patients taking medicines) (Montalt and González-Davies 2007; Ezpeleta-Piorno 2012). It is also relevant in translational medicine precisely because it can help to bridge the gap between experts who write the information they want to convey and their lay readers, who may require a register more suited to their needs.

In recent years, biomedical science has diversified into Personalised Medicine (PM) and Translational Medicine (TM). PM springs from the notion that, in biomedical and pharmacological terms, one size no longer fits all. PM can then be defined as targeted medicine. What at first sight might seem a radical move towards patient-centred care is, in fact, a biomedical model that uses characterisation of individuals' phenotypes and genotypes (e.g. molecular profiling, medical imaging, etc.) for tailoring the right therapeutic strategy for the right person at the right time, and/or to determine predisposition to disease, and/or to deliver timely and targeted prevention. Personalising therapeutic strategies, and pharmacological treatment in particular, does not necessarily mean reinforcing patient-centred care or including the psychosocial factors mentioned above. No matter how much PM individualises diagnosis and treatment, it is still very much within the biomedical paradigm of *muta ars*. Patients are still the individual recipients and beneficiaries of biomedical innovation, the silent bodies that passively receive the targeted cure based on the best possible biomedical evidence. Biomedical translators are there to facilitate this impersonal, detached, and 'neutral' flow of information and knowledge. Their main objectives are to target specific groups of patients, or even to convey individualised diagnoses, prognoses and treatments.

Translational Medicine (TM) goes a step further than either Evidence-Based Medicine (EBM) or PM. It aims to transform scientific discoveries arising from laboratory, clinical or population studies into new clinical tools and applications that will hopefully bridge laboratory and clinical practice, and improve human health by reducing the incidence of disease, morbidity and death. It is focused on ensuring that proven strategies for disease treatment and prevention are eventually implemented within a patient population. Ensuring this translatability of knowledge involves encouraging the flow of information from the laboratory to the clinic ('bench to bedside'), and from the clinic back to the laboratory ('bedside-to-bench'). TM is based on the notion of knowledge translation (KT), whose aim is to bring pure scientific knowledge from 'bench to bedside', by testing its validity in clinical practice, while at the same time keeping the scientific knowledge 'intact' throughout the process of translation across various social fields and sectors of the healthcare system (Engebretsen, Sandset and Ødemark 2017). KT reflects a subordinate and mechanistic view of translation as no more than a conduit for knowledge dissemination, in which true scientific knowledge remains 'uncorrupted' after crossing multiple social, cultural and linguistic barriers. In translational terms, the 'target culture' (that of clinical practice and the sphere of the patient) is subordinated to the 'source culture' (that of biomedical research). The aim of the translation is to be a hermetically sealed container and a safe carrier of the original message from the source to the target culture. Engebretsen, Sandset and Ødemark (2017) critique TM in the following terms:

> We maintain that KT relates to the 'original scientific content' as a double supplement. On the one hand, KT offers new approaches to the communication of scientific knowledge to different groups in the healthcare system with the aim of supplementing a lack of knowledge among clinicians (and patients). On the other, it demonstrates that a textual and cultural supplement, namely a concern with target audiences (clinicians and patients), is inevitable in the creation of an 'autonomous' science. This creates an inherent paradox in existing KT models – while these models presuppose that the principal duty of adequate KT is to implement the original scientific message in new social contexts and textual forms without altering its content, the same models, paradoxically, also state that it is through translational modifications and adaption to new audiences, i.e. through synthesis and development of guideline recommendations, that the message becomes scientifically trustworthy. Hence, translation both threatens and fulfils the original scientific message.

This paradox reflects the current entanglements between biomedicine and translation, and the need to think about them in critical terms. Further research is needed to expand the critique to the 'bedside-to-bench' dimension of TM. Translation-oriented research and critical thinking are also needed to address the issue of patients reporting outcomes in clinical trials through genres such as PRO (Patient Reported Outcomes). The patient is not only the recipient of a treatment in a clinical trial, but also plays an active role by contributing feedback in the form of personal experience on issues of interest to the pharmaceutical company. This subjective data, called health outcomes, is of vital importance in determining the benefits and risks of a drug, providing better understanding of diseases, improving adherence to a course of treatment and, most importantly for pharmaceutical companies, obtaining approval for a drug.

4 Medical humanities and its entanglements with translation

The increasing specialisation of the different branches of biomedicine, together with their growing social prestige and economic and institutional power, have caused a fragmentation of knowledge, a narrowing of perspectives on health and wellbeing, and a hegemonic relationship with other medicines and other ways of knowing about sickness and health. This reductionism has been identified as a driver of change in the direction of rebalancing between biomedicine and humanities: '[…] there has been a paradigm shift away from what might be called medical reductionism to medical holism, where patients are not reduced to diseases and bodies but rather are seen as whole persons in contexts and in relations' (Cole, Carlin and Carson 2015: 8). In the 'Introduction' to *Medicine, Health and Being Human*, Lesa Scholl presents her project as 'a conversation between medical practitioners and researchers, alongside humanities and social science scholars, from across the globe, who are concerned about the narrowing of medicine to medical science that has been occurring since the early modern period' (2018: 2). This monological (and largely monolingual, i.e. mainly in English) limitation of medicine to medical science has affected, in a somewhat negative way, how we currently understand, teach and research medical translation.

The move towards a more holistic, comprehensive and inclusive model of medicine and healthcare, together with a burgeoning interest in ethics and values, is the main driving force behind the emergence and consolidation of the field of medical humanities, more recently also called 'health humanities', in academia. In 'The Almost Right Word: The Move from Medical to Health Humanities', Jones *et al.* (2017) offer a detailed discussion on the name the field should adopt. They argue that medicine is but one component of health and wellbeing, and that health humanities is a more encompassing label than medical humanities, because it accurately captures theoretical and pedagogical developments in the education of health professionals. The publication of several peer-reviewed journals such as the *Journal of Medicine and Philosophy* (since 1976), *Journal of Medical Humanities* (since 1980), *Literature and Medicine* (since 1982) and *Medical Humanities* (since 2000) shows the vigour of the field and the successful expansion it has undergone in the last few decades.

The field of medical humanities provides an interdisciplinary approach to understanding and investigating the effects of illness and disease on patients, health professionals and the societies in which they live and work. Medical humanities includes areas as diverse as medical ethics and law, pedagogy in physician training, medical anthropology, narrative medicine, history of medicine, cultural studies, science and technology studies, sociology, economics, philosophy, literature, theatre, film and visual art. In the introductory chapter of *Medical Humanities. An Introduction*, Cole, Carlin and Carson (2015: 12) define medical humanities as follows: '[...] an inter- and multidisciplinary field that explores contexts, experiences, and critical and conceptual issues in medicine and health care, while supporting professional identity formation'. In *The Edinburgh Companion to the Critical Medical Humanities*, Whitehead and Woods (2016) synthesise these elements in what they call 'the three Es' of medical humanities: Ethics, Education and Experience. Translation and multilingual communication intersect with these main components of medical humanities in a variety of ways, as I shall explain below.

Perhaps the most long-lasting of these intersections is the translation of the works of doctor-writers who have written about the great dramas of human existence and the practice of medicine, such as John Keats, Anton Chekhov, Arthur Conan Doyle, William Carlos Williams, Oliver Sacks, and Nawal el Saadawi. The study, translation, adaptation and staging of the works of playwrights such as Shakespeare (Montalt 2015, 2016), who used the medical knowledge of their time to reflect upon the connections between body, mind and emotions in their characters, is another fruitful area which crosses disciplinary boundaries.

Medical humanities strives to better understand contexts and bring to the fore critical and conceptual issues in medicine and health. In this endeavour, translators are well placed, since they are aware of the usefulness of text genre, a notion that helps them to critically understand language in action and the connection between text and context.

Beyond the naive, uncritical idea that medical language is uniform, univocal and non-rhetorical, translators tend to be very discerning, both within a given language and between different languages, of its great textual and terminological variability and intentionality. They understand the influence that the situations and contexts in which texts are embedded exert on both 'original' writing and translating. Formal and critical analysis of the myriad genres used in medical and health communication in multilingual and multicultural settings is paramount for translators; first, to become aware of the variations between genres, not only in different languages and cultures, but even within the same language and culture; second, to accommodate their target texts to the implicit and explicit norms of what is considered adequate and acceptable in a given context. In addition to the down-to-earth uses of genres in translation practice, such as the use of parallel texts for different purposes, medical humanities can nurture other critical perspectives on genres, in particular their historical and ethical dimensions. Text genres are dynamic rhetorical constructs. The genres we are familiar with today are the result of social and textual developments throughout time. Take, for instance, a biomedical research article. Scientists in the 18th and 19th centuries did not report their findings in the same form as they currently do. What we understand by a research article at present is the result of many diachronic changes that have shaped it structurally and rhetorically into a highly useful tool for creating and spreading knowledge, and also for establishing given conventions that affect writer-reader interactions and hierarchies. In addition to this historical dimension, different text genres have different ethical priorities. Ensuring that experiments can be repeated through the provision of detailed and accurate explanations is a central issue in an original article (OA), but in a patient information leaflet (PIL), comprehensibility and reliability of information take centre stage as ethical priorities, which affect the notion of quality as well as the methods and resources to achieve it.

Communication with the patient is the origin of mainstream medical humanities, which is rooted in ethical principles and is closely linked to patient-centredness. Ethical considerations are important in areas such as access to healthcare through adequate provision of information and means of communication, decision making and informed consent in clinical practice, participation in clinical trials and end-of-life care. In all these areas, communication plays a central role; and, the medical consultation, with its doctor-patient interactions, is the central genre of healthcare in which many of these ethical issues unfold. Expert-lay translation (Askehave and Zethsen 2002), intralingual translation (Zethsen 2009, 2018) and patient-centred translation (PCT) (Montalt, 2017a) are developments which are linked with the more holistic and ethically-oriented approach to medicine and healthcare promoted by medical humanities. In PCT, for example, the target patient's perspective takes centre stage. It aims at empowering patients by making texts comprehensible and empathetic through grammatical, terminological, stylistic, textual and pragmatic choices as well as by the use of non-verbal resources, such as diagrams and drawings. It takes into account educational backgrounds, clinical situation, specific needs, and preferences in the presentation of information of both individual and well-defined subgroups of patients. Intralingual translation (Zethsen 2009) is a fundamental component of PCT, which relies on constant testing and feedback from real target patients (Montalt 2017a; García-Izquierdo and Montalt 2017).

Another area that intersects with medical humanities' ethical dimension is translation and multilingual communication in crisis situations – from climate-change-induced disasters to wars and pandemics – in which there is a growing awareness of the moral need to respond in a spirit of international solidarity and collaboration. Translation in crisis scenarios is becoming a global priority. Federico Federici, a leading researcher in this emerging area of translation studies, sees an 'urgent need to establish a concerted and multidisciplinary debate on the role of intercultural communication in international multilingual missions that respond to emergencies across the world' (2016: 3). In *Intercultural Crisis Communication. Translation, Interpreting and Languages in Local Crises* (2019), editors Christophe Declercq and Federico Federici address diverse issues of multilingual, multicultural and multimodal infrastructure in all stages of the crises. This collection includes a contribution in the field of medical translation where three main components are established to plan for the complexity of medical and health communication and translation in such critical situations: *logos*, *ethos* and *pathos* (Montalt 2019). *Logos* (Greek word for 'reason', 'discourse') refers both to content and communication logistics. The focus is on accuracy, reliability and clarity of the medical content and the terminology of the messages. Paramount here are logistics and accessibility, and more particularly, the rational organisation and distribution of relevant information, the creation of effective messages and coordinated communication, using the most appropriate resources. *Ethos* (Greek word for 'attitude', 'character') refers to the set of values and attitudes of a particular individual or group, and the ethical codes that regulate multiple professions (translators, interpreters, doctors, nurses, etc.) and communication in crisis scenarios. *Pathos* (Greek word for 'suffering') brings to the fore personal and collective suffering and empathy. Feelings and emotions should not be overlooked nor removed from the logos and ethos dimensions in multilingual and multicultural communication in crisis scenarios. Medical humanities can contribute to the much-needed multidisciplinary debate on how to respond to crises and enhance the human factor.

Education is another principal interest of mainstream medical humanities. It focuses on new curricula and educational materials, which aim to draw on the perspectives and methods of inquiry of the humanities and social sciences, and bring them into medical and health education (Whitehead and Woods 2016). The link between medical translation and the training of doctors in communication skills can be illustrated in a recent study (Bittner *et al.* 2016), in which 57 medical students from German universities participated in the following experiment: 25 of them translated medical documents for real patients on a platform[6] using plain and understandable language, while the other 30 did not translate such documents. All the students then engaged in communicative interactions in a virtual consultation with six simulated patients, who connected via Skype and evaluated the students' communication skills. Based on the transcripts of the conversations, an expert conducted a blind assessment of the communication skills of all 57 students. In addition, all participants answered a self-assessment questionnaire focusing on their own communication skills. According to the authors of the study, students in the first group (i.e. those who had translated patient documents) obtained a significantly higher assessment result than students in the second group, which shows that written translation of medical documents for patients is associated with significantly more frequent use of plain, comprehensible language in doctor-patient interactions.

That 'all the world's a stage' is well known in the sociological tradition of Kenneth Burke and his theory of dramatism (1969), and Erving Goffman and his dramaturgical perspective in the study of social interactions (1978), as well as in the sociological understanding of health provision and health communication. In clinical interactions, patients play different roles from those performed by health professionals. Simulated interactions between patients and medical students aimed to enhance the latter's communication skills have been developed by linguists such as John Skelton (2008). Role-plays have been used in professional development programmes in multilingual and multicultural settings, such as the Building Bridges Programme of the Refugee Council (UK).[7] The programme provides a useful model conceived for refugee doctors and nurses wanting to work for the National Health System in the UK that is transferable to other countries (Butt *et al.* 2019). Role-plays can also be used as a research tool to investigate mediated and unmediated interactions in consultation processes and informed consent. The GENTT (Text Genres for Translation Purposes) research team (Universitat Jaume I, Spain)[8] has used this methodological tool in a number of funded research projects involving doctors, nurses, actors, interpreters, translators and linguists, in order to investigate the multiple dimensions of clinical interactions (non-verbal and verbal language, comprehensibility, ethics, empathy, implicit and explicit norms of the health system, cultural factors and medical content) in multidisciplinary teams.

Efforts to bridge the gulf between biomedical science and experience in the medical humanities can be seen in the distinction between pain and suffering (bodies feel pain but people suffer), as has been argued by Cassell in *The Nature of Suffering and the Goals of Medicine* (1998), and between disease and illness. Disease happens to bodies and is described and understood through biomedical science, whereas illness refers to what people feel and experience, and is understood through eliciting their stories. It is through language that both patients and professionals are able to shape and express what they experience in their own narratives. This will be explored in the next section in more depth, but first let me conclude this section by focusing on some more recent responses to medical humanities.

In the last few years, mainstream medical humanities has been criticised by some scholars (Viney, Callard and Woods 2015; Whitehead and Woods 2016; Kristeva *et al.* 2018) on the grounds that it has been limited to a subsidiary role of ‘repairing’, as a soft, ‘subjective’ and cultural supplement to a stable body of ‘objective’, biomedical and scientific knowledge (Kristeva *et al.* 2018), and that it should be proactive in embracing more fundamental issues of knowledge production. In ‘Critical Medical Humanities: Embracing Entanglement, Taking Risks’, Viney, Callard and Woods (2015) challenge the utilitarian model on which medical humanities is based, i.e. providing a service to biomedical sciences. They argue that it should intervene more explicitly in ontological questions, in particular, aetiology, pathogenesis, intervention and cure, rather than, as has commonly been the case, leaving such questions largely to the domains of life sciences and biomedicine (*ibid.* 3).

According to these critical scholars, this more radical programme should acknowledge the pathological and healing powers of culture, and consider the body as a complex biocultural fact. Issues of race and ethnicity, sexuality and gender, disability, mental health, technology and media, economics, and social and environmental inequalities are central to the production of medical knowledge as well as to the experience of health and illness (Viney, Callard and Woods 2015). Other key aspects in such a programme are non-medical notions of health, illness and wellbeing; rethinking of the concept of ‘evidence’ in healthcare; and, the acknowledgement that humanities and social sciences may play a more proactive, constitutive role in shaping such knowledge.

5 Narrative, medicine and translation

Interlingual translation in medicine deals with communication problems between and among patients and healthcare professionals interacting in different languages and with different cultural backgrounds. However, difficulties can also occur when the language and culture is the same; intralingual translation helps – often unacknowledged – to bring participants together by adapting texts and contents for the lay reader. Narratives of patients and health professionals also make a contribution by bridging divides between them and by promoting mutual understanding. Patients and health professionals removed from their original societies, cultures and languages living in foreign countries often feel the need to make sense of – and perhaps modify their own systems of values and beliefs to accommodate to – the target healthcare system. Some of them may recount their experiences in oral, written or multimodal narratives, thus making their voices heard in the society. These in turn may prompt questions that not only mobilise conventional biomedical research but also contribute to a better understanding of illness and health. Biomedical research and healthcare can be seen as intertwined chains of translations and narratives. The entanglements between translation, narrative and medicine are the main themes of this section.

In his essay 'The Storyteller', Walter Benjamin (1986) states that the art of storytelling is reaching its end because the epic side of truth – wisdom – is dying out. This profound distinction invites us to think about the difference between biomedical truth and the wisdom in the embodied and culturally embedded experiences individual patients and health professionals have of that abstract truth – a wisdom that can be revealed through personal narratives.

The relationship between medicine and narrative is as old as ancient myth. Homer's epic narratives in *The Iliad* and *The Odyssey* – the root and seed of Western civilisation and medicine of the last 25 centuries (Laín Entralgo 1958: 11) – contain some of the earliest ideas about health and illness that we have inherited from the past. In current scientific medicine, narrative, as opposed to argumentation or instruction, is a rhetorical strategy used to organise events chronologically – such as the course of a disease or the steps carried out in an experiment – in a number of genres, including the clinical case. In it, the author, typically a physician, gathers relevant clinical information about a patient, who is turned into a 'case', and translates them into a narrative with a conventionalised structure and form for their peers to read. Other medical genres also have a strong narrative element, such as original articles reporting on current biomedical research.

In recent times, some authors have expanded the links between medicine and narrative beyond the conventions of biomedical genres. Because of his humanistic approach to neurology and his ability to combine scientific accuracy with narrative excellence, Oliver Sacks is a good example to mention here. In the preface to *The Mind's Eye* (2010), he states:

> I grew up in a household full of doctors and medical talk – my father and older brothers were general practitioners, and my mother was a surgeon. A lot of the dinner table conversation was inevitably about medicine, but the talk was never just about 'cases'. A patient might present as a case of this or that, but in my parents' conversation, cases became biographies, stories of people's lives as they responded to illness or injury, stress or misfortune. Perhaps it was inevitable that I myself became both a physician and a storyteller.
>
> *Sacks 2010: ix*

His 'case histories', as he calls them, are based on real patients and told in non-academic narrative prose taking advantage of literary techniques to make them truly understandable and appealing to the lay reader. Thanks to their literary quality and readability,

Oliver Sacks' narratives have been bestsellers for decades and have contributed to the public understanding of rare neurological disorders and how they impact on the lives of sufferers and their families. His patients are not presented simply as people displaying symptoms that require treatment. He is interested in their social, cultural and psychological dimensions and gives us authentic characters who come to life in the text.

More recently, the exploration of the links between medicine and the patient seen as a person has led to the development of narrative medicine in consultations. Rita Charon (2004) tells the story of one of her patients and summarises the essence of narrative medicine:

> A 36-year old Dominican man with a chief symptom of back pain comes to see me for the first time. As his new internist, I tell him, I have to learn as much as I can about his health. Could he tell me whatever he thinks I should know about his situation? And then I do my best not to say a word, not to write in his chart, but to absorb all he emits about his life and his health. I listen not only for the content of his narrative, but for its form – its temporal course, its images, its associated subplots, its silences, where he chooses to begin in telling of himself, how he sequences symptoms with other life events. I pay attention to the narrative's performance – the patient's gestures, expressions, body positions, tones of voice. After a few minutes, he stops talking and begins to weep. I ask him why he cries. He says, 'No one has ever let me do this before'.

Her patient's narrative revealed to Charon 'the connections among his symptoms, his illiteracy, his failures as a breadwinner, his familial losses, and his life in an alien culture' (2004: 863). In other words, through active listening and viewing she was able to understand not only her patient's musculoskeletal symptoms from the angle of disease but also the complexities of his illness. Through observing the way in which the patient performed his narrative, she was better able to understand his most pressing concerns. Such performances – with voice, gestures and silences – provide relevant information about the patients' feelings and emotions, attitudes and values, and their ability to make sense of (or misunderstand) what goes on in the interaction. Health narratives like this can help narrow the gap between disease (as a concept referred to by professionals) and illness (as the 'same' thing experienced by individual patients), between biomedical and lay discourses and terminologies. Narrative medicine focuses on active listening to patients' accounts of their suffering rather than merely considering abstract pain as a symptom. According to Charon (2004), without the narration not only treatment but suffering, too, might be fragmented.

Narrative medicine has led to a resurgence of interest in writings both by patients and physicians (Shapiro 2012: 309). Beyond the oral interaction between patient and doctor in a consultation, patients have increasingly chosen to reclaim their voices from the healthcare system by telling their own stories on different platforms. This has also stimulated many physicians to cross the disciplinary and professional boundaries and to tell stories about their patients and about themselves both as doctors and, in some cases, as patients or relatives. In books such as Henry Marsh's *Do No Harm* (2014), Atul Gawande's *Being Mortal* (2014) and Paul Kalanithi's bestseller *When Breath Becomes Air* (2016), doctors and surgeons share with lay readers and colleagues their anxieties and fears, insights and reservations, insecurities and ethical dilemmas. All these narratives have a clear educational value to help the medical professionals and trainees '[…] develop critical thinking, challenge facile assumptions, think more deeply about patients and themselves in relation to their patients, become more aware of their and patient's emotions, and ward off cynicism and disillusionment' (Shapiro 2012: 309). They also offer non-specialists rare glimpses of the difficulties experienced by those practising the art of medicine. Narrative medicine can contribute to humanising healthcare, because it can provide a deep and therapeutic understanding of the people who display symptoms, as well as of the people who 'treat' them.

In addition to narrative medicine, the term 'life narrative' is used in the field of autobiographical studies. In *Reading Autobiography. A Guide for Interpreting Life Narratives,* Smith and Watson (2010) enlist more than 60 genres of life narrative, some of which are especially relevant to medical humanities and translation: addiction narrative (254–255), autobiography (256), case study (264–265), digital life stories (268), gastrography[9] (271), or scriptotherapy (279). Patients' autobiographies are becoming a very dynamic field of study. Emotional and spiritual healing may sometimes be as effective as physical curing. Holistic healing can be particularly useful in some cases of trauma. For example, pianist and public intellectual James Rhodes recounted his traumatic childhood experiences in the form of a memoir and shared it with the general public (2015). Rhodes launched into circulation a series of motifs, themes, styles, discourses, narrative structures, presentations of the 'I', and rhetorical strategies of all kinds, which can be used and adapted later by others to advance the process of discovering repressed causes of suffering when recovering from trauma (Montalt 2017b). Above all, his memoir suggests that it is possible to construct a personal and sincere voice that empowers others who decide to make their own audible, however scattered and incoherent this voice may seem on the surface. The coherence (and also the difficulty) lies precisely in the continuity between personal experience and the way the author uses language in the telling of his own story (*ibid.*).

Many teenage cancer patients relate their experiences in online blogs. Inspired by Susan Sontag's ideas about health, illness and metaphor (2009), a recent study (Sapiña, Domínguez and Montalt 2017) analysed the types of metaphors patients use in English and Spanish in two comparable corpora. In another recent study, Moreno (2019) looked at a similar set of examples in German and Spanish. One of the most relevant findings in both studies is that patients use a wide range of metaphors to talk about their experiences and that their choice of metaphors varies between languages and cultures. Patients who communicate on the Internet discover how others coping with the same disease express themselves in other languages. New narrative and experiential models can thus be combined with the ones they are already familiar with. Exploring how patients construct their narratives in different languages, cultures and healthcare systems can shed light on the variability and richness of such stories.

In this context, beginning and end-of-life narratives are particularly interesting, because in many Western societies both occurrences have become medicalised and bureaucratised over the centuries, and in that process their human dimension has been eroded. Neither birth nor death are *per se* health problems, but both have largely been removed from the family and society, and, to a considerable extent, have lost their experiential meaning. Gynaecology, obstetrics, gerontology and geriatrics are fertile grounds for research in the medical humanities from a multilingual and multicultural angle. Recent lines of research in this field include the study and translation of birth narratives (Susam-Saraeva 2020), translating the experience of dying into a performative phenomenology (Robinson 2017) and the exploration of aging in theatre and its intersections with translation, adaptation and dramaturgy (Montalt 2020). Mental health is another area of potential interest. Its historical, cultural and social dimensions are more complex and intertwined than in other, more 'physical' diseases, and biomedical and pharmacological approaches can provide only partial indications of the best treatment to adopt.

6 Final remarks

Muta ars was a fundamental principle in Western medical knowledge and for centuries shaped the relationship between body, health, language, culture and being human. Today, the biomedical paradigm is still largely influenced by muteness in its approach to understanding disease and restoring health. However, science in general, and biomedical science in particular, have always used words to generate and circulate knowledge, especially in a multilingual and multicultural world. The entanglements between translation and medical humanities reviewed in this chapter point in the direction of re-introducing the human element which has been eroded both in healthcare and in translation. This will entail developing a holistic view in which the biomedical coexists with the historical, ethical, emotional, cultural and social dimensions of language and communication. It also means putting the patient centre stage and ensuring that medical technology and machine translation are always used in their best interest.

Medical humanities has shown doctors how they can approach patients in a more sensitive and humane manner, and restore the human face of the physician without detracting from their clinical expertise. It is now expanding its scope in a more critical and reflexive way to play a proactive role in the generation and shaping of medical knowledge and the provision of healthcare. Likewise, using translation as a tool for communication in the professional arena is fully compatible with developing it as an educational tool for health professionals, and as a frame of critical enquiry about how medical knowledge is generated, circulated, received and put to good use. Translation studies can benefit from medical humanities in its move to a more critical and plural approach to medicine and healthcare. Similarly, medical humanities can benefit from translation studies' focus on the semiotic (verbal and non-verbal), hybrid, dynamic and transformative nature of knowledge, by learning from the work of writers such as Walter Benjamin (1992), Roman Jakobson (1959) and George Steiner (1992). What seems to be the 'original' is in fact linked to a long tradition of words, texts and ideas; and, what seems to be the 'target' is no more than a step further in the transformation of that particular text, concept or argument, beyond which more transformations will occur.

As I finish this chapter, the COVID-19 outbreak is spreading rapidly around the world. Pandemics show us in a clear and poignant way how our individual bodies (which may be carriers of the virus) are entangled with our collective body, the rest of society. Biological and societal ecologies coexist. In the COVID-19 pandemic, the epidemiological and medical debate has suddenly gone well beyond the expert circles and is uppermost in the thoughts and actions of every member and facet of the society: family, health organisations, government, education, transport, business and commerce, and the press. We are witnessing the extent to which many aspects of the outbreak lie beyond the scope of biomedicine. Understanding the causes and effects of pandemics and responding to them globally require people from all academic fields to pull together. This crisis is bringing about a growing awareness on at least three fronts: the limits of science and the need for multidisciplinary research; the importance of strong healthcare systems; and the crucial role of both national and international communication. There will be opportunities for people with imagination and flair to embrace change, increase knowledge, and find new and more effective ways of communicating within and beyond the medical profession.

In these uncertain times, the rapid technological innovations in areas such as e-Health and machine translation may submerge the advances made in humanising healthcare and alter the translator's role and ethos in unexpected ways. Once we get through the initial stages of this crisis, however, there will be patients whose illnesses will be exacerbated by their changed personal, familial and economic circumstances. Some elements of patient-centred care may have to be set aside for a time, but what will continue to be needed is the holistic treatment of patients. What will be cherished, most of all, is the memory of nurses and doctors who, in frightening and exhausting conditions, were still moved to offer those dying in isolation many small acts of kindness.

Notes

1 I would like to acknowledge support from two funded research projects I participated in: Generalitat Valenciana (AICO/2019/182) and Ministerio de Ciencia, Innovación y Universidades (PGC2018-098726-B-I00).
2 https://cdli.ucla.edu.
3 http://classics.mit.edu/Hippocrates/sacred.html, translated by Francis Adams (1796–1861), a Scottish doctor and translator of Greek medical works.
4 *Diccionario médico-biológico, histórico y etimológico* [Medico-biological, historical and etymological dictionary), University of Salamanca, https://dicciomed.usal.es.
5 For evidence of these transformations, see the articles in Wallis and Wisnovsky (2016).
6 https://washabich.de.
7 www.refugeecouncil.org.uk/get-support/services/refugee-health-professionals-building-bridges-programme/.
8 www.gentt.uji.es.
9 In this context, the term means '[...] life writing in which the story of the self is closely linked to the production, preparation, and/or consumption of food' (Smith and Watson 2010: 271).

Further reading

Cole, T. R., Carlin, N. S. and Carson, R. A. (2015) *Medical Humanities: An Introduction*. Cambridge: Cambridge University Press.

In this textbook Cole *et al.* use concepts and methods from the humanities to explore ethical and existential issues related to the experience of disease, care of the dying, health policy, religion and health, and medical technology. Case studies, images, questions for discussion, and role-playing exercises help readers to engage in the practical, interpretive and analytical aspects of the material, developing skills for critical thinking as well as compassionate care.

Montalt, V. and González-Davies, M. (2014) *Medical Translation Step by Step: Learning by Drafting*. London and New York: Routledge.

Medical Translation Step by Step provides a pedagogical approach to medical translation based on learner and learning-centred teaching tasks. Starting from a broad communication framework, the book follows a top-down approach to medical translation: communication → genres → texts → terms and other units of specialised knowledge. It is positively focused in that it does not insist on error analysis, but rather on ways of writing good translations and empowering both students and teachers.

Robinson, D. (2017) *Translationality. Essays in the Translational-Medical Humanities*. London and New York: Routledge.

Robinson offers four essays exploring four complementary dimensions of the links between translation and medical humanities: 'The Medical Humanities', 'The Translational Humanities of Medicine', 'The Medical Humanities of Translation', and 'The Humanities of Translational Medicine'. The history of medical literature understood humanistically through both the act and the pretence of translation, or, as Robinson (2017: 47–128) terms it, 'the translational humanities of medicine (literary history as performed translationality)' is another line of inquiry entangling translation and medical humanities.

Whitehead, A. and Woods, A. (eds) (2016) *Edinburgh Companion to the Critical Medical Humanities*. Edinburgh: Edinburgh University Press.

Whitehead *et al.* comprehensively introduce the ways in which interdisciplinary thinking across the humanities and social sciences might contribute to, critique and develop medical understanding of the human individually and collectively. The 36 chapters in this book range widely within and across disciplinary fields to explore the intersections between medicine, as broadly defined, and critical thinking.

Related topics

Knowledge Translation, Disability in Translation, Dissemination of Academic Medical Research Through Translation

References

Arbøll, T. P. (2019) 'A Newly Discovered Drawing of a Neo-Assyrian Demon in BAM 202 Connected to Psychological and Neurological Disorders'. *Le journal des médecines cunéiformes*, 33, pp. 1–31.

Askehave, I. and Zethsen, K. K. (2002) 'Translating for Laymen', *Perspectives: Studies in Translatology*, 10(1), pp. 15–29.

Benjamin, W. (1986) 'The Storyteller. Reflections on the Works of Nikolai Leskov', Translated by H. Zorn, in Arendt, H. (ed.) *Illuminations*, New York: Harvard University Press and Harcourt, pp. 83–107.

Benjamin, W. (1992) 'The Task of the Translator. An Introduction to the Translation of Baudelaire's *Tableaux parisiens*', in Arendt, H. (ed.) *Illuminations*. London: Fontana Press, pp. 70–82

Bittner, A., Bittner, J., Jonietz, A., Dybowski, C. and Harendza, S. (2016) 'Translating Medical Documents Improves Students' Communication Skills in Simulated Physician-Patient Encounters', *BMC Medical Education*, 16(1), pp. 72.

Bowman, D. (2014) 'On Identity in (the) Medical Humanities', *Medical Humanities*, 40, pp. 1–2. DOI:10.1136/medhum-2014–010540.

Burke, K. (1969) *A Grammar of Motives*. Berkeley: University of California Press.

Butt, M. F., Salmon, L., Mulamehic, F., Hixon, A., Moodambail, A. R. and Gupta, S. (2019) 'Integrating Refugee Healthcare Professionals in The UK National Health Service: Experience From A Multi-Agency Collaboration', *Advances in Medical Education and Practice*, 10, pp. 891–896.

Carel, H. and Györffy, G. (2014) 'Seen but not Heard: Children and Epistemic Injustice', *The Lancet*, 384(9950), pp. 1256–1257.

Carel, H. and Kidd, I. J. (2014) 'Epistemic Injustice in Healthcare: A Philosophical Analysis', *Medicine, Health Care and Philosophy*, 17(4), pp. 529–540.

Cassell, E. J. (1998) 'The Nature of Suffering and the Goals of Medicine', *Loss, Grief and Care*, 8(1–2), pp. 129–142.

Charon, R. (2004) 'Narrative and Medicine', *The New England Journal of Medicine*, 350, pp. 862–864. DOI:10.1056/NEJMp038249.

Cole, T. R., Carlin, N. S. and Carson, R. A. (2015) *Medical Humanities: An Introduction*. Cambridge: Cambridge University Press.

Declercq, C. and Federici, F. M. (eds) (2019) *Intercultural Crisis Communication: Translation, Interpreting and Languages in Local Crises*. London: Bloomsbury Publishing.

Delisle, J. and Woodsworth, J. (eds) (1995) *Translators Through History*, vol. 13. Amsterdam and Philadelphia: John Benjamins.

Engebretsen, E., Sandset, T. J. and Ødemark, J. (2017) 'Expanding the Knowledge Translation Metaphor', *Health Research Policy and Systems*, 15(19). https://health-policy-systems.biomedcentral.com/track/pdf/10.1186/s12961-017-0184-x.pdf.

Engel, G. L. (1977) 'The Need for a New Medical Model: A Challenge for Biomedicine', *Science*, 196(4286), pp. 129–136.

Epstein, R. M., Franks, P., Fiscella, K., Shields, C. G., Meldrum, S. C., Kravitz, R. L. and Duberstein, P. R. (2005) 'Measuring Patient-Centered Communication in Patient-Physician Consultations: Theoretical and Practical Issues', *Social Science and Medicine*, 61(7), pp. 1516–1528.

Ezpeleta-Piorno, P. (2012) 'An Example of Genre Shift in the Medicinal Product Information Genre System', *Linguistica Antverpiensia, New Series-Themes in Translation Studies*, 11, pp. 167–187.

Farre, A. and Rapley, T. (2017) 'The New Old (And Old New) Medical Model: Four Decades Navigating the Biomedical and Psychosocial Understandings of Health and Illness', *Healthcare*, 5(4), pp. 88.

Federici, F. M. (ed.) (2016) *Mediating Emergencies and Conflicts*. Basingstoke: Palgrave Macmillan.

Fischbach, H. (1993) 'Translation, the Great Pollinator of Science: A Brief Flashback on Medical Translation', *Scientific and Technical Translation*, 6, p. 89.

García-Izquierdo, I. and Montalt, V. (2017) 'Understanding and Enhancing Comprehensibility in Texts for Patients in an Institutional Health Care Context in Spain', *Revista Española de Lingüística Aplicada (RESLA)*, 30(2), pp. 592–610.

Gawande, A. (2014) *Being Mortal: Medicine and What Matters in the End*. New York: Metropolitan Books.

Goffman, E. (1978) *The Presentation of Self in Everyday Life*. London: Harmondsworth.

Habermas, J. (2015) *The Theory of Communicative Action: Lifeworld and Systems, a Critique of Functionalist Reason*,vol. 2. Hoboken, NJ: John Wiley and Sons.

Haggerty, J. L., Reid, R. J., Freeman, G. K., Starfield, B. H., Adair, C. E. and McKendry, R. (2003) 'Continuity of Care: A Multidisciplinary Review', *BMJ*, 327(7425), pp. 1219–1221.

Jakobson, R. (1959) 'On Linguistic Aspects of Translation', *On Translation*, 3, pp. 30–39.

Jones, T., Blackie, M., Garden, R. and Wear, D. (2017) 'The Almost Right Word: The Move from Medical to Health Humanities', *Academic Medicine*, 92(7), pp. 932–935.

Kalanithi, P. (2016) *When Breath Becomes Air*. New York: Random House.

Kristeva, J., Moro, M. R., Ødemark, J. and Engebretsen, E. (2018) 'Cultural Crossings of Care: An Appeal to the Medical Humanities', *Medical Humanities*, 44(1), pp. 55–58.

Laín Entralgo, P. (1958) *La curación por la palabra en la antigüedad clásica*. Madrid: Revista de Occidente.

Marsh, H. (2014) *Do No Harm: Stories of Life, Death and Brain Surgery*. London: Hachette.

Montalt, V. (2015) 'Shakespeare y la medicina: dramaturgias del cuerpo y la mente (I): "Let's Purge This Choler Without Letting Blood"', *Panace@*, 16(41), pp. 73–77.

Montalt, V. (2016) 'Shakespeare y la medicina: dramaturgias del cuerpo y la mente (II): "The Senators of Rome Are This Good Belly"', Panace@, 17(43): pp. 46–50.

Montalt, V. (2017a) 'Patient-Centred Translation and Emerging Trends in Medicine and Healthcare', *The EST Newsletter*, European Society for Translation Studies.

Montalt, V. (2017b) 'Traducir el trauma y el estigma a escritura autobiográfica: una lectura de James Rhodes', *eHumanista/IVITRA*, 11, pp. 319–336

Montalt, V. (2019) 'Medical Translation in Crisis Scenarios', in Declercq, C. and Federici, F. M. (eds) *Intercultural Crisis Communication: Translation, Interpreting and Languages in Local Crises*. London: Bloomsbury.

Montalt, V. (2020) 'Aging Minds and Bodies in Shakespeare', in Salvador, V. and Sanpietro, A. (eds) *Understanding the Discourse of Aging. A Multifaceted Perspective*. Newcastle-upon-Tyne: Cambridge Scholars Publishing.

Montalt, V. and González-Davies, M. (2007) *Medical Translation Step by Step: Learning by Drafting*. St Jerome: Manchester.

Montalt, V. and González-Davies, M. (2014) *Medical Translation Step by Step: Learning by Drafting*. London and New York: Routledge.

Montgomery, S. L. (2000) *Science in Translation: Movements of Knowledge Through Cultures and Time*. Chicago: University of Chicago Press.

Moreno, J. (2019) *La metáfora en las narrativas de pacientes: estudio de corpus desde una doble perspectiva lingüística y cultural*. Master's thesis. Universitat Jaume I.

Rhodes, J. (2015) *Instrumental*. London: Canongate.

Robinson, D. (2017) *Translationality: Essays in the Translational-Medical Humanities*. London and New York: Routledge.
Sacks, O. (2010) *The Mind's Eye*. London: Picador
Sapiña, L., Domínguez, M. and Montalt, V. (2017) 'More Than a Battle: Intercultural and Interlingual Issues in the Use of Metaphors in the Narratives of Young Cancer Survivors'. *Genealogies of Knowledge I: Translating Political and Scientific Thought across Time and Space Conference*, University of Manchester, 7–9 December 2017. Abstract available at: http://genealogiesofknowledge.net/events/gok2017conference/abstracts/ (Accessed: 15 December 2020).
Savage-Smith, E. (1997) 'Medicine in Medieval Islam', in Lindberg, D. C. and Shank, M. H. (eds) *The Cambridge History of Science*, vol. 2. Cambridge: Cambridge University Press, pp. 139–67.
Scholl, L. (ed.) (2018) *Medicine, Health and Being Human*. London and New York: Routledge.
Shapiro, J. (2012) 'Narrative Medicine and Narrative Writing', *Family Medicine*, 44(5), pp. 309–311.
Skelton, J. (2008) *Role Play and Clinical Communication: Learning the Game*. Abingdon: Radcliffe Publishing.
Smith, S. and Watson, J. (2010) *Reading Autobiography: A Guide for Interpreting Life Narratives*. Minneapolis: University of Minnesota Press.
Sontag, S. (2009) *Illness as Metaphor and AIDS and its Metaphors*. London: Penguin.
Steiner, G. (1992) *After Babel. Aspects of Language and Translation*. Oxford: Oxford University Press.
Susam-Saraeva, Ş. (2020) 'Translating Birth Stories as Counter-Narratives', *Mutatis Mutandis. Revista Latinoamericana de Traducción,* 13(1), pp. 45–63. doi: 10.27533/udea.mut.v13n1a03.
Viney, W., Callard, F. and Woods, A. (2015) 'Critical Medical Humanities: Embracing Entanglement, Taking Risks', *Medical Humanities*, 41(1), pp. 2–7.
Wallis, F., and Wisnovsky, R. (eds) (2016) *Medieval Textual Cultures: Agents of Transmission, Translation and Transformation*, vol. 6. Berlin: Walter de Gruyter.
Whitehead, A. and Woods, A. (eds) (2016) *Edinburgh Companion to the Critical Medical Humanities*. Edinburgh: Edinburgh University Press.
Wisnovsky, R. (2017) 'Commentaries, Translation and Philosophical Change: The Case of Greek-into-Arabic', *Genealogies of Knowledge I: Translating Political and Scientific Thought across Time and Space Conference*, University of Manchester, 7–9 December 2017. Available at: https://genealogiesofknowledge.net/events/gok2017conference/video-recordings (Accessed: 15 December 2020).
Zethsen, K. K. (2009) 'Intralingual Translation: An Attempt at Description', *Meta: journal des traducteurs/Meta: Translators' Journal*, 54(4), pp. 795–812.
Zethsen, K. K. (2018). 'Access Is Not the Same as Understanding. Why Intralingual Translation Is Crucial in a World of Information Overload', *Across Languages and Cultures*, 19(1), pp. 79–98.

9

Knowledge translation[1]

John Ødemark, Gina Fraas Henrichsen and Eivind Engebretsen

1 Introduction: medical knowledge translation

'Translation' has emerged as a key word in disciplines such as cultural studies, anthropology and science and technology studies (STS). Moreover, from around the year 2000 it has become institutionalised in medicine, leading to the development of the field of 'knowledge translation'. The turn to translation in the humanities can be seen as an index of the requirement to cross cultural and disciplinary boundaries in a purportedly global age. As the concept of 'translation' has become increasingly important in the human sciences, we could perhaps also regard knowledge translation as forming part of a new translational paradigm. The turn to translation in medicine is, however, of a different kind, aimed at preserving the identity of the scientific message, not at celebrating epistemic or cultural difference.

This chapter is about knowledge translation (hereinafter KT) in medicine and healthcare. KT refers to a variety of scientific practices and research activities bound together by the common goal of 'bridging the gap' between science in laboratories and clinical application, and, more generally, putting research-based knowledge into policy and practical care (Straus, Tetroe and Graham 2009; Woolf 2008). The all-important task for KT is to reduce the gap between theory and practice, by making medical practice knowledge-based. We see this clearly in WHO's definition of KT:

> Knowledge translation (KT) has emerged as a paradigm to address many of the challenges and start closing [*sic*] the 'know-do' gap. KT is defined as 'the synthesis, exchange, and application of knowledge by relevant stakeholders to accelerate the benefits of global and local innovation in strengthening health systems and improving people's health'.
>
> *World Health Organisation 2019*

While interlingual translation crosses boundaries between languages, KT aims to cross the space between biomedical science and practical healthcare. Ideally, there should be an 'equivalence' of some sort between the message produced by science and its application in practice in hospitals and clinics. In other words, the aim of KT as a form of translation is to close or bridge the gap between *knowing* and *doing*.

DOI: 10.4324/9781003167983-12

In this chapter, we will describe different theories and practices associated with KT in medical contexts. Moreover, we will also discuss how views on translation from translation studies and human sciences more broadly can supplement current models of translation in medicine and health. We will first give a description of KT and its emergence as a theory *and* practice in medicine. Next, we will discuss KT more critically by contrasting it with models of translation developed in translation studies and human sciences. Our aim is thus both to give an introductory description of KT and to suggest some new ways of conceiving translation in medicine. While we argue that KT is based on a simplistic view of translation and knowledge dissemination, we also maintain that KT, as a practical form of knowledge production and knowledge transmission, might benefit from incorporating more theoretical notions of translation as a complex material, textual and cultural process, which inevitably impacts upon the 'original scientific message'. We need such an expanded version of KT in order to cope with contemporary epistemic and cultural differences, as well as with the inevitable entanglement of the socio-cultural and biomedical aspects (cf. Engebretsen, Sandset and Ødemark 2017; Kristeva *et al.* 2019; Ødemark and Engebretsen 2018).

2 The history of KT

To understand KT as a theory of knowledge dissemination and a medical practice, we need to turn to the history of medicine. More precisely, we must identify the problem KT was – and still is – supposed to solve. So-called translational research first emerged in the biomedical field in the 1990s. This research was, from the very beginning, explicitly presented as a solution to the slow and insufficient uptake of research discoveries in everyday clinical practice. Translational research emerged as a possible solution to both a temporal and a quantitative problem; the flow from science to practice was too slow, and the amount of knowledge transported too small. Accordingly, translational research set out to solve these two problems relating to the social efficiency of biomedical research (e.g. Mankoff *et al.* 2004).

Around the year 2000, several prominent researchers drew further attention to the fact that many innovative research results never left the laboratory setting (e.g. Bero *et al.* 1998; Zerhouni 2005; Woolf 2008). There was now an increased concern about the 'disconnection between the promise of basic science and the delivery of better health' (Sung *et al.* 2003: 1279). It was the recognition of this 'disconnection' that inspired a new range of knowledge production in medicine, which became increasingly referred to as 'translation' (*ibid.*). In addition, there was also a growing concern that treatments offered to patients were too often inadequate because physicians did not base their decisions on recent research results. Patients were denied treatments with proven benefits, or they might even receive unnecessary or potentially harmful treatments (Graham *et al.* 2006).

2.1 KT and evidence-based medicine

In order to understand KT, we need to see it as part of a new scientific model for knowledge production in medicine, and, most importantly, relate it to a radically new conception of *evidence* formed in 'evidence-based medicine' (hereinafter EBM). As noted, an increasing concern with evidence along with its social and clinical efficiency formed part of a new biomedical research paradigm that gradually became hegemonic in medical research after the Second World War. The growth of epidemiological methods, notably randomised controlled trials (see below), was instrumental to this development. The shift towards EBM began in Canada, and it is hardly a coincidence that this was also the place where KT was first defined,[2] with the Canadian Institute of Health Research becoming a pioneer in its conceptualisation.

The epistemological premise of EBM is that *all forms of knowledge are inherently biased*, and that bias and subjectivity need to be balanced by expert claims that are *intersubjectively valid*. As defined by David Sackett in a seminal paper from 1997,

> The practice of evidence-based medicine means integrating individual clinical expertise with the best available external clinical evidence from systematic research. By best available external clinical evidence we mean clinically relevant research, often from the basic sciences of medicine, but especially from patient centered clinical research into the accuracy and precision of diagnostic tests [...].
>
> *Sackett 1997: 3*

The term 'external' is important here. The inherent bias of individual decisions must be counterbalanced by evidence drawn from an origin *external* to the case of the individual patient, i.e. from systematic research. This necessarily implies some kind of transposition of knowledge from one domain (research) to another (clinical application). Moreover, it also 'requires new skills of the physician, including efficient literature searching and the application of formal rules of evidence evaluating the clinical literature' (Guyatt *et al.* 1992: 2420). KT, then, must be seen as the operationalisation of EBM principles, making research evidence available for clinical use *through translation* – or, as one paper has it in its title, it is about '*shortening* the journey from evidence to effect' (Davis *et al.* 2003, our emphasis). KT is the instrument used in this 'shortening'.

EBM and KT are also linked in a more fundamental and ideological manner, and with radical consequences for the role of the medical practitioner. Until the 1950s, the medical professional was the embodiment of knowledge, and they did not need any proof of their epistemological authority beyond their medical degree and their professional experience (Weisz *et al.* 2007). Characteristic of the EBM paradigm is an increasing emphasis on knowledge as something that is independent of the expert, i.e. knowledge does not dwell in the body of the 'initiated' doctor, but in texts available to the expert, but also to laypersons who, as consumers of health services, should be able to choose the best treatment available (Timmermans and Berg 2003). Hence, the EBM paradigm actively sought to undermine the personal and 'traditional' authority of medical experts, and to control bias and prejudice by constructing a new textual authority, also accessible to people outside the medical profession, the new consumers of medical services.

3 The tools of KT

The processes described above constructed new standards for the production of medical knowledge and its practical and social application. Three crucial tools of medical KT were developed:

3.1 Randomised controlled trials (RCTs)

RCTs are often referred to as the 'gold standard' of modern clinical medicine and they are currently the only proper way of testing knowledge produced by science. A well-known method is the comparison of the effects on a group of patients that are offered a specific intervention or drug with a group that is given a placebo. The first example of an RCT in medicine is the study conducted by Marshall and colleagues in 1948 on the effects of streptomycin (antibiotics) on tuberculosis. One group of patients (the treatment group) was offered antibiotics and the effects were compared with a group that was given a placebo (the control group). Results after six months showed better healing in the treatment group (Marshall *et al.* 1948).

With further institutionalisation of RCTs in the 1950s, knowledge became increasingly independent of the individual human subject. It was, we could say, dislocated from the individual professional, and relocated to collective institutions (e.g. expert panels), at the same time as new genres of texts were created to communicate state-of-the-art science (e.g. clinical guidelines). A further consequence of this was that the new type of medical evidence was considered *translatable* and so accessible to everybody, enabling patients and relatives to make their own informed decisions.

Translational research formed a supplement to two traditional fields of medical research, namely basic research and clinical research. The aim of this new type of research was to integrate methods and knowledge from basic sciences, such as genetics and molecular biology, into clinical research and interventions, which then could be further tested through RCTs. A crucial element of the new translational method was *stepwise* testing of findings which were developed through basic research in the laboratory setting, first on animals, and next on humans (e.g. a new drug). In order to gain clinical significance, it was claimed, results from laboratory research should be prepared for testing on large populations through RCTs (Solomon 2015). This use of RCTs is the dominant model for testing and implementing research in our current epistemological order.

3.2 Literature reviews

Following on from the development of RCTs, new manners of communicating the science emerged. Proponents of KT and translational research devised a new set of textual genres with the aim of summarising research for clinical use. Different forms of cognition and text production were set to work; both *content analysis* (in systematic literature reviews) and *statistical analysis* (meta-analysis) were introduced as methods for evaluating RCTs of a particular treatment or intervention. While a systematic review describes and categorises state-of-the-art research by collecting and summarising all empirical evidence that fits pre-specified eligibility criteria, meta-analyses use statistical methods to summarise the results of these studies. This textualising of medical knowledge formed the basis for 'clinical guideline recommendations'. In these texts, reviews of several trials are operationalised into normative practical guidance for clinicians. Through this new methodology, based on statistical meta-analysis of clinical trials, evidence became detached from the expert (Timmermans and Berg 2003; Solomon 2015).

3.3 Clearing houses

Another tool used by KT are the newly established institutions bringing together scientists, clinicians and bureaucrats in 'Clearing houses' or 'knowledge centres' with the aim of facilitating the production of research reviews. So-called guideline development groups were also established, either as new institutions or as departments in already established units, such as national health agencies, in order to promote and organise guidelines (Weisz *et al.* 2007). An example of one such institution is the Cochrane Collaboration in Oxford, established in 1992 as one of the first and certainly the most famous Clearing house. Another important epistemic practice were consensus meetings, taking place primarily in the 1980s and 1990s (Solomon 2015). Here specialists came together to discuss contested issues and offer clinical recommendations. These meetings were, on the one hand, a result of this new realisation of knowledge bias (thought to be compensated for by the presence of many experts), but on the other, were still based on the authority of collective expert opinions.

With the rise of evidence-based medicine and the concomitant idea of an evidence-based practice, medical knowledge became *translatable* in a new way. The ability to translate – from basic science to practical health care action – is now the key to the mobilisation and use of medical knowledge. Although very different, all these methodological, technical *and* textual practices share the common purpose of translating knowledge from 'bench to bedside', or from basic research into clinical practice. In this process, RCTs, literature reviews and Clearing houses are particularly important tools of translation.

4 Critical perspectives upon KT

KT had an enormous impact on medicine and knowledge policy. A critical examination of the conceptions of knowledge and translation that inform KT is consequently of great academic and societal significance. In the following sections, we will turn to some critical perspectives on KT. We aim to demonstrate that notions of translation developed in translation studies and in the humanities more broadly can become resources for a more critical interrogation of medical KT.

As discussed above, KT has been conceptualised as a process with distinct stages of production (basic research), testing (RCTs) and the dissemination of knowledge (guidelines). The most common model moves from the production of scientific knowledge to its practical application in three stages:

- T1: A transfer from basic science in laboratories to clinical research on populations (this is also known as translational research), and further onto
- T2: A transfer from clinical research to clinical recommendation, often in terms of the development of clinical guidelines based on systematic reviews of clinical trials, and ending in
- T3: A transfer from clinical recommendations to routine clinical practice (e.g. Woolf 2008)

In this model, medical translation of knowledge is construed as a process of testing and synthesising scientific results produced in the laboratory and preparing it for sound clinical application and scientifically warranted healthcare. Hence, the directionality of translation is from the places where science is produced to its application. We observe that this is viewed as a linear process of knowledge production and transmission. The process begins in a place emblematic of modern science, the laboratory, and with basic science ('pure science' in its most iconic form) as its foundation.

Another influential model is the *Knowledge-to-Action-Model* developed by the Canadian Institute of Health Research. This proposes a knowledge creation pyramid, divided into three stages of 'knowledge creation' (knowledge inquiry, knowledge synthesis and knowledge tools), which is set to interact with what the institute calls an 'application cycle', which is depicted as wholly external to the production of knowledge. Hence, the application of knowledge can never have an impact upon knowledge creation – KT is neither creative nor productive (e.g. Graham *et al.* 2006).

In both models, the idea is that concrete practices should be governed by science, and that application should follow from, and be what we will call a *supplement* to, biomedical knowledge creation. As Derrida observed, the word 'supplement' implies both 'adding on to the original' and 'compensating for a lack in the original'. The supplement is at the same time an addition from the outside to something natural and original, *and* a compensation for an insufficiency inscribed *within* the origin (Derrida 1997: 141–157). Derrida regarded translation as an integral part of all textual *production*. According to him, translation is not an accidental event that can happen to a text in the empirical cases where the text is turned into another (target) language. On the contrary, translation and textual productivity is an essential part of the text's mode of being in the world. The struggle to create meaning in the text, to interpret it 'correctly', is simultaneous with the birth of the text (*ibid.*).

The idea of translation as a supplement – conceived in the double sense described above – has potentially broad implications for KT. The *translation* aspect of KT does not only duplicate and disseminate the original knowledge; it also *completes* the original 'scientific text' by fulfilling it with a possible interpretation in a particular context. Indeed, this supplementary logic is implicit in existing KT models. While KT models presuppose that the principal duty of adequate KT is to implement the original scientific message in new social contexts and textual forms without altering its content, the same models, paradoxically, also state that it is *through translational modifications* and adaption to new audiences, that is, through synthesis and development of guideline recommendations, that the message becomes scientifically trustworthy. However, existing KT models fail to draw the necessary consequences from this paradox.

5 Seeing KT from translation studies

It is a truism in translation studies that the original source text can never be fully recovered by the target text, that interlingual translation always implies semantic shifts, and that the source text is inevitably rewritten in registers and styles pertaining to the target text and target culture (e.g. Venuti 2009). With this understanding of translation in mind, we could say that KT as a translational practice resembles interlingual translation practices that aim for semantic and pragmatic equivalence between an original source text and a new target text (e.g. Nida and Taber 1969). Using another analogy from interlingual translation, we could say that the current construal of knowledge production and translation in KT resembles the now highly contested literary view of translation where the translator's work is 'invisible' (Venuti 1995) and/or the where the translator is merely an 'ancillary' (Berman 1984) to the reproduction of meaning and knowledge. Indeed, in this view, the translator is doomed to be the proverbial traitor (traduttore, traditore!) also in KT – not of artistic genius but of the scientific logos – since all changes and translational shifts will change the original 'message'.

Analogous to the literary model, translation in KT should – if it is to be felicitous – be a mere transfer that does not add nor detract from the evidence and findings produced by basic research and RCTs. Rather, the purpose of translation in KT is to preserve and implement the original, scientific content in new socio-cultural contexts. The act of translation is a process of 'copying the original' where the translational act itself is a non-act, the translator a non-actor and the purpose of translation is to be a 'container' of the original message without adding, transforming or in any other ways 'betraying' the original.

This lack of attention to how the process of translation inevitably will affect the original message is perhaps due to an uncritical acceptance of models of translation, knowledge production and knowledge dissemination that combine elements from two of the most persistent paradigms in the Western history of ideas: romanticism and the Enlightenment. In the case of KT, we find a combination of:

- Notions from aesthetic and literary romanticism, which purport that translation is the art of preserving, of 'carrying across', the artistic genius behind the original masterpiece
- An unquestioned Enlightenment model of knowledge dissemination, which assumes that knowledge should trickle down from elites and theory into 'popular' practice, the bedside of everyday care

Thus, it is possible to identify a persistent cultural topology, a set of notions that privileges the original over the copy or translation, still having an impact upon KT as a scientific and (purportedly) non-cultural practice (Steiner 1975: 448–449). The new medical and scientific KT distributes value and translational directionality in ways that resemble ancient literary and philosophical ideologies of translation: the original is the source of value, and its admired qualities should be kept intact in every process of translation and/or transmission (cf. Ødemark and Engebretsen 2018). This, however, presupposes that it is possible to separate the production of knowledge from its transfer; the scientific content to be translated is construed as being outside the process of translation. Knowledge, moreover, is said to have reached its culmination in the secluded space of the laboratory or the more mobile 'seclusions' of RCTs (testing the effect, transferability, reproducibility and relevance of knowledge) – and it is the *findings* that should be transported to, and implemented in, situations of practical care. In line with this, so-called 'barriers' and 'drivers' of KT are essentially understood as social and cultural factors *external* to the production of knowledge (Davis 2003).

6 Future directions of KT – or KT with other kinds of translation

The lack of attention to the textual and socio-cultural aspect of translation in KT has led medical researchers to argue that the time has come to 'drop the knowledge translation metaphor' (Greenhalgh and Wieringa 2011). Contrary to this, it has also been claimed that an expanded notion of the 'translation metaphor' might help devise forms of KT more attuned to biological, epistemological and cultural complexities (Engebretsen, Sandset and Ødemark 2017). In this final section of the contribution, we will sketch a version of KT more able to tackle the cultural and textual complexities of the translation process.

KT is a scientific and purportedly non-cultural practice that regards the social and cultural as a 'barrier' to the transmission of knowledge already formulated in the laboratory and confirmed by randomised controlled trials. In the humanities, however, 'translation' has emerged as a key theoretical concept to deal with epistemic and cultural difference – well beyond discussions on interlingual translation. In this situation, attention to concepts and practices of translation have an unexploited potential for bridging the gap between medicine and social/human sciences. Such interdisciplinary exchange can in turn contribute to an increased understanding of the interplay between scientific and cultural factors of KT and thereby ultimately enhance the flow of knowledge within healthcare.

As we have seen, KT aims to cross the space between scientific knowledge and social practice; the know-do gap. Etymologically speaking, translation has always been about crossing spaces. The Latin derived term 'translation' simply implies that an agent carrying some (undefined) thing crosses a spatial boundary, and that the transferred object does not have to be of a linguistic nature (Cheyfitz 1997: 35; Evans 1998; Wintroub 2015). Questions concerning the transfer of knowledge in the spaces between different disciplines, sciences and paradigms have long been associated with 'translation' in the history and philosophy of science (Severi and Hanks 2015). Moreover, the concept of 'cultural translation' has been deployed in both anthropology and cultural history to study interactions in the spaces between cultures (Burke 2007: 8).

In the humanities, 'translation' has thus emerged as a key theoretical concept to deal with epistemic and cultural difference – and to thematise problems of interpretation and understanding well beyond discussions on 'mere' interlingual translation (cf. also Buden *et al.* 2009). Even in the discipline of translation studies 'proper', Lefevere maintained that problems in translation are not primarily of a linguistic nature. Lefevere describes a situation in translation studies where a concern about the pragmatic situation of a given translation has supplanted a prior, more formal approach focusing on the linguistic rules governing the target and the source text. 'In other words', he writes, 'the rules to be observed during the process of decoding and reformulation depend upon the actual situation, on the function of translation, and on who wants it made and for whom' (Lefevere 1999: 75). If the concern with the pragmatics of translation now has become part of the current state of the art, some additional factors should be brought into consideration, Lefevere maintains:

> I would like to challenge [...] the supposedly primary or fundamental role played by linguistic codes in the operation known as translating. [...]. It is my contention that people who translate texts do not, first and foremost, think on the linguistic level, the level of individual words and phrases. Rather, they think in terms of what I would like to call two grids. I do not want to speculate on the primacy of one grid over the other; rather, I would suggest that we think of them as intertwined. One is what I would like to call a 'conceptual grid', the other a 'textual grid'.
>
> *Lefevere 1999: 75 and 76–77*

The grids are the results of socialisation, and are therefore in the last instance culture specific:

> An educated member of any culture in the West, for instance [...], will know that certain texts are supposed to contain certain markers designed to elicit reactions on the reader's part, and that the success of communication depends on both the writer and reader of the text agreeing to play their assigned parts in connection with these markers. The writer is supposed to put them in, the reader is supposed to recognise them. Texts that start with 'Once upon a time', for instance, will elicit quite different expectations in the reader than texts that start with 'Leave Barcelona 8:15 a.m.; Arrive Amsterdam 11.30 a.m.'
>
> *Lefevere 1999: 76*

Lacking the concept of a 'fairy tale', it is surely difficult to translate 'once upon a time' and its connotation to a particular cultural genre. Thus, the formula assigns and elicits a particular commitment from the audience that has acquired the adequate cultural competence. It is crucial to understand that what comes after such a formulaic opening line is not actually 'coded' in the formulaic phrase itself; the knowledge and expectation that what follows is fiction and belongs to the genre of fairy tales are acquired through habitual encounters with tales that start this way and the rituals that accompany them. Such cultural and textual framings cannot be read out of the sentence as 'mere linguistic data'; i.e. 'once upon a time' would not, on its own, signify 'this is a fairy tale/fiction', if there were no cultural conventions to categorise texts beginning with this phrase as pertaining to a particular genre. Linguistic translation, then, also has to account for cultural factors and metadiscursive practices for producing and classifying genres (Briggs 1993).

New work in the history of science, like Wintroub's work on early modern colonialism, navigation and science (2017) has also been concerned with translation taken in a cultural and material sense. By following 'science in action', empirically orientated scholars have come to focus their attention on the construction of science, and they have focused upon the productive role of translation in the construction of science and knowledge. Influenced by science and technology studies (STS) and Actor Network Theory (ANT) such work has underscored that translation is never simply a discursive process, but a material and cultural practice conducted in complex contexts (Wintroub 2015). ANT and STS have actually asserted that translation is the very condition for all knowledge and scientific effects (Latour 1993). Latour even maintains that his understanding of translation has done away with the 'old beast of relativism' (Latour 1993: 113) by presenting a pragmatic solution to the problem of cultural (as well as other forms of) translatability. He simply points to the fact that cultures and natures *have always been related or translated*, and that the activity of relating/translating is undertaken with reference to criteria and yardsticks that do not belong to the 'nature' of the things compared but to the instruments of translation bringing them together:

> Worlds appear commensurable or incommensurable only to those who cling to measured measures. Yet all measures, in hard and soft science alike, are also measuring measures, and they construct a commensurability that did not exist before their own calibration. Nothing is, by itself, either reducible or irreducible to anything else. Never by itself, but always through the mediation of another. How can one claim that worlds are untranslatable, when translation is the very soul of the process of relating?
>
> *Latour 1993: 113*

In practice, the problems of commensurability/incommensurability are solved. The task is therefore defined as identifying what instruments of translation are at work *in particular, empirical acts of relating*; how the instruments are calibrated and what social and intellectual structures they produce and/or forms a part of (Latour 1993: 113).

If we use this notion of instruments of translation to examine KT, we find a particularly important instrument of translation, namely texts. Various textual genres function as instruments of translation in KT. The translation process in KT begins in literary reviews and ends in so-called clinical guidelines, which prescribe manners of intervention in concrete cases (e.g. particular diagnoses) based upon the systematic reviews of the scientific state-of-the-art as expressed in the literature. Hence, the translation process hinges upon systematic reviews and guidelines, and on the fact that such texts, in increasingly condensed and vernacular forms, are able to transmit the science necessary to implement state-of-the-art care. Generally, this text production is conceived as *supplementing* a lack of knowledge among clinical practitioners. Thus, a textual and cultural supplement, namely a concern about target audiences (practitioners and patients), is inevitable even in an 'autonomous' biomedical science restricted to the body as a biomedical phenomenon, because communicating with individual patients in particular socio-cultural contexts is the practical end of medicine (Engebretsen, Sandset and Ødemark 2017).

As we have observed above, most current versions of KT are actually closer to the now highly contested literary view of translation as a practice that aims at creating a semantic or pragmatic equivalence between an original ST and a new TT. Arguably then, KT in its current forms is based on an inadequate understanding of the various *textual and cultural supplements* that affect the construction, dissemination and application of knowledge. Moreover, we have also seen that Derrida sees translation as an integral part of all textual production. The translation or target text relates to the source text in what Derrida has referred to as a double supplement: it both adds on to the original and compensates for a lack in the original (Derrida 1997). The translation does not only duplicate the original message; it also *completes* the original message by filling in one of the source texts' possible interpretations. This also implies that the necessity of interpreting and translating texts – the fact that texts do not speak for themselves, but are constantly the objects of interpretation and scrutinised for their true meaning – 'always already' characterises the source text.

If shifts of meaning are an inevitable outcome of the transport of signs between texts, KT could become more effective if such shifts were defined as a creative potential rather than as a mere 'barrier'. There is an inherent paradox in existing KT models. While these models presuppose that the principal duty of KT is to implement the original scientific message in new social contexts and textual forms without altering its content, the same models, paradoxically, also state that it is *through translational modifications* and adaption to new audiences, i.e. through synthesis and development of guideline recommendations, that the message becomes scientifically trustworthy. Hence, *translation both threatens and fulfils the original scientific message*. However, existing KT models fail to draw the consequences from this paradox: translation is inherent in science and the division between science and its translation is both impossible and unproductive to maintain.

7 Conclusion

In this chapter, we have asserted that the practice of KT might benefit from incorporating more theoretical notions of translation as an entangled cultural process that inevitably affects the 'original scientific message'. Moreover, we have shown that the current dominant model of KT presupposes that it is possible to separate the production of knowledge from its transfer; the scientific content to be translated is construed as being outside the process of translation. Knowledge is said to have reached its culmination in the controlled trials (RCTs), and it is the results from these trials that should be transported to, and implemented in, practical care situations. To accomplish this, various textual genres are mobilised in the different stages of the translation process, culminating in so-called clinical guidelines, which prescribe means of intervention in concrete cases (e.g. particular diagnoses, prognoses or treatments) based on systematic reviews of the scientific state of the art. Hence, the translation process hinges upon textualisation in such genres as systematic reviews and guidelines, and that such texts, in increasingly condensed and vernacular forms, are able to transmit the science necessary to implement state-of-the-art care.

Understanding KT as a cultural and textual supplement, as we suggest, is to acknowledge that altering the scientific message is a necessary and integral part of KT. Modifications and changes that occur through the translational process should therefore not be viewed as 'barriers' to accurate translation; rather, such changes are prerequisites for evidence-based healthcare. Inspired by recent theories of translation in the human sciences, we claim that KT can be more adequately understood in terms of a 'double supplement'. On the one hand, KT offers new approaches to the communication of scientific knowledge to different groups in the healthcare system with the aim of supplementing a lack of knowledge among clinicians (and patients); on the other, it demonstrates that a textual and cultural supplement, namely a concern with target audiences (clinicians and patients), is inevitable in the creation of an 'autonomous' science. Hence, the division between science and its translation is unproductive and impossible to maintain.

Notes

1 The article was finished during a stay at the Centre for Advanced Study in Oslo (CAS). Thanks are due to CAS for their funding and to our colleagues in the project group THE BODY IN TRANSLATION.

2 More precisely, this took place at McMaster University with the Evidence Based Medicine Working Group in 1992 (Solomon 2015).

Further reading

Greenhalgh, T. and Wieringa, S. (2011) 'Is It Time to Drop the "Knowledge Translation Metaphor"? a Critical Literature Review', *Journal of the Royal Society of Medicine,* 104(12), pp. 501–509. DOI:10.1258/jrsm.2011.110285

A seminal and illuminating criticism of KT coming from biomedicine and the health sciences concluding that the time has come to drop the metaphor of translation in medicine.

Kristeva, J., Moro, M. R., Ødemark, J. and Engebretsen, E. (2019) 'The Cultural Crossings of Care: A Call for Translational Medical Humanities', in Bleakley, A. (ed.) *Routledge Handbook of the Medical Humanities*. London and New York: Routledge.

A position paper in the medical humanities calling for a critical use of translation and translation studies to explore the boundaries between biomedicine and the humanities.

Solomon, M. (2015) *Making Medical Knowledge*. New York: Oxford University Press.

A short introduction to the history of translational research with an illuminating discussion of the philosophical assumptions of this major paradigm in modern medicine.

Timmermans, S. and Berg, M. (2003) *The Gold Standard: The Challenge of Evidence-Based Medicine and Standardization in Health Care*. Philadelphia, PA: Temple University Press.

Provides a historical overview of the growth of evidence-based medicine, especially the development and use of clinical guidelines.

Wintroub, M. (2015) 'Translations: Words, Things, Going Native and Staying True', *The American Historical Review*, 120(4): pp. 1185–1217. DOI:10.1093/ahr/120.4.1185

A conceptual history of 'translation' as well as an application of the sociology of translation to historical material.

Related topics

Medical Humanities and Translation, Inter- and Intralingual Translation of Medical Information, Dissemination of Academic Medical Research Through Translation

References

Berman, A. (1984) *L'épreuve de l'étranger: culture et traduction dans l'Allemagne romantique*. Paris: Gallimard.

Bero, L. A., Grilli, R, Grimshaw, J. M., Harvey, E, Oxman, A. D. and Thomson, M. A. (1998) 'Closing the Gap Between Research and Practice: An Overview of Systematic Reviews of Interventions to Promote the Implementation of Research Findings', The Cochrane Effective Practice and Organization of Care Review Group, *BMJ*, 317(7156), pp. 465–468. DOI:10.1136/bmj.317.7156.465.

Briggs, C. (1993) 'Metadiscursive Practices and Scholarly Authority in Folkloristics', *The Journal of American Folklore*, 106(422), pp. 387–434. DOI:10.2307/541905.

Buden, B., Nowotny, S., Simon, S., Bery, A. and Cronin, M. (2009) 'Cultural Translation: An Introduction to the Problem, and Responses', *Translation Studies*, 2(2), pp. 196–219. DOI:10.1080/14781700902937730.

Burke, P. (2007) 'Cultures of Translation in Early Modern Europe', in Burke, P. and Po-chia Hsia, R. (eds.) *Cultural Translation in Early Modern Europe*. Cambridge: Cambridge University Press, pp. 7–38.

Cheyfitz, E. (1997) *The Poetics of Imperialism: Translation and Colonization from The Tempest to Tarzan*. Philadelphia: University of Pennsylvania Press.

Davis, D. *et al.* (2003) 'The Case for Knowledge Translation: Shortening the Journey from Evidence to Effect', *BMJ*, 327(7405), pp. 33–35. DOI:10.1136/bmj.327.7405.33.

Derrida, J. (1997) *Of Grammatology*. Baltimore, MD: Johns Hopkins University Press.

Engebretsen, E., Sandset, T. and Ødemark, J. (2017) 'Expanding the Knowledge Translation Metaphor', *Health Research Policy and Systems*, 15(1), p. 19. DOI:10.1186/s12961-017-0184-x.

Evans, R. (1998) 'Metaphor of Translation', in Baker, M. (ed.) *Routledge Encyclopedia of Translation Studies*. London and New York: Routledge, pp. 149–153.

Graham, I. D. *et al.* (2006) 'Lost in Knowledge Translation: Time for a Map?', *Journal of Continuing Education in the Health Professions*, 26(1), pp. 13–24. DOI:10.1002/chp.47.

Greenhalgh, T. and Wieringa, S. (2011) 'Is It Time to Drop the "Knowledge Translation Metaphor"? a Critical Literature Review', *Journal of the Royal Society of Medicine*, 104(12), pp. 501–509. DOI:10.1258/jrsm.2011.110285.

Guyatt, G. *et al.* (1992) 'Evidence-Based Medicine: A New Approach to Teaching the Practice of Medicine', *JAMA*, 268(17), pp. 2420–2425. DOI:10.1001/jama.1992.03490170092032.

Kristeva, J., Moro, M. R., Ødemark, J. and Engebretsen, E. (2019) 'The Cultural Crossings of Care: A Call for Translational Medical Humanities', in Bleakley, A. (ed.) *Routledge Handbook of the Medical Humanities*. London and New York: Routledge.

Latour, B. (1993) *We Have Never Been Modern*. Boston: Harvard University Press.

Lefevere, A. (1999) 'Composing the Other', in Bassnett, S. and Trivedi, H. (eds.) *Post-Colonial Translation: Theory and Practice*. London and New York: Routledge, pp. 75–94.

Mankoff, S. P., Brander, C., Ferrone, S. and Marincola, F. M. (2004) 'Lost in Translation: Obstacles to Translational Medicine', *Journal of Translational Medicine*, 2(14). DOI:10.1186/1479-5876-2-14.

Marshall, G. *et al.* (1948) 'Streptomycin Treatment of Pulmonary Tuberculosis', *British Medical Journal*, 2(4582), pp. 769–782. DOI:10.1136/bmj.2.4582.769.

Nida, E. A. and Taber, C. R. (1969) *The Theory and Practice of Translation, With Special Reference to Bible Translating*. Leiden: Brill.

Ødemark, J. and Engebretsen, E. (2018) 'Expansions', in Gambier, Y. and D'Hulst, L. (eds) *A History of Modern Translation Knowledge*. Amsterdam and Philadelphia: John Benjamins, pp. 85–90. DOI:10.1075/btl.142.09ode.

Sackett, D. (1997) 'Evidence-Based Medicine', *Seminars in Perinatology*, 21(1), pp 3–5. DOI:10.1016/S0146-0005(97)80013-4.

Severi, C. and Hanks, W. F. (2015) 'Introduction', in Severi, C. (ed.) *Translating Worlds: The Epistemological Space of Translation*. Chicago: Hau Books, pp.1–17.
Solomon, M. (2015). *Making Medical Knowledge*. Oxford: Oxford University Press.
Steiner, G. (1975) *After Babel: Aspects of Language and Translation*. Oxford: Oxford University Press.
Straus, S., Tetroe, J. and Graham, I. (2009) 'Defining Knowledge Translation', *CMAJ: Canadian Medical Association Journal*, 181(3–4), pp. 165–168. DOI:10.1503/cmaj.081229.
Sung, N. *et al.* (2003) 'Central Challenges Facing the National Clinical Research Enterprise', *JAMA*, 289(10), pp. 1278–1287. DOI:10.1001/jama.289.10.1278.
Timmermans, S. and Berg, M. (2003) *The Gold Standard: The Challenge of Evidence-Based Medicine and Standardization in Health Care*. Philadelphia, PA: Temple University Press.
Venuti, L. (1995) *The Translator's Invisibility*. London: Routledge.
Venuti, L. (2009) 'From Translation, Community, Utopia', in Damrosch, D., Melas, N. and Mbongiseni, B. (eds) *The Princeton Sourcebook in Comparative Literature*. Princeton: Princeton University Press, pp. 358–379.
Weisz, G., Cambrosio, A., Keating, P., Knaapen, L., Schlich, T. and Tournay, V. J. (2007) 'The Emergence of Clinical Practice Guidelines', *The Milbank Quarterly,* 85(4), pp. 691–727. DOI:10.1111/j.1468-0009.2007.00505.x.
Wintroub, M. (2015) 'Translations: Words, Things, Going Native and Staying True', *The American Historical Review,* 120(4), pp. 1185–1217. DOI:10.1093/ahr/120.4.1185.
Wintroub, M. (2017) *The Voyage of Thought. Navigating Knowledge across the Sixteenth-Century World.* Cambridge: Cambridge University Press.
Woolf, S. H. (2008) 'The Meaning of Translational Research and Why It Matters', *JAMA*, 299(2), pp. 211–213. DOI:10.1001/jama.2007.26.
Zerhouni, E. A. (2005) 'Translational and Clinical Science. Time for a New Vision', *The New England Journal of Medicine,* 353(15), pp. 1621–1623.
WHO (2019) *Ageing and Life Course. Knowledge Translation.* Available at: www.who.int/ageing/projects/knowledge_translation/en/(Accessed: 7 June 2019).

Part III

Translation and interpreting in healthcare settings

10

Community/liaison interpreting in healthcare settings

Bruce T. Downing

1 Introduction

Interpreting[1] is the real-time spoken or signed counterpart of written translation. It is the act of re-expressing in a second language what a speaker/signer of one language has said, for the benefit of others who have limited or no comprehension of the original language.[2] An interpreter enables speakers of different languages to communicate by attending to the words of someone speaking one language and re-expressing the speaker's message, immediately or soon after, in another language, for the benefit of one or more listeners who do not share the speaker's language.

One-way interpreting, from a single speaker to an audience (conference interpreting), is a well-established professional occupation. Conference interpreters usually interpret in the simultaneous mode, beginning to interpret soon after a speaker begins and continuing to interpret as the speaker continues. They also most often interpret from a sound-proofed booth, listening via headphones and connected electronically to their audience. Two-way interpreting of dialogue, i.e. assisting individuals who speak one language in communicating back and forth orally with other individuals speaking a different language, is likewise carried out in diplomatic, scientific, and commercial settings by both professional and non-professional interpreters. This chapter, however, is concerned with *community interpreting*, the kind of interpreting that takes place in everyday community settings where a bilingual person enables individuals speaking different languages to understand each other.

1.1 Community interpreting

Community interpreting frequently takes place informally in a wide variety of settings, as when a person who speaks the local language helps a tourist with their shopping. Yet community interpreting becomes essential, and is more likely to be prescribed, regulated and professionalised, in interactions between members of the public and providers of public services, such as medical care, or authorities such as the police and in the courts.[3]

DOI: 10.4324/9781003167983-14

The central role of the community interpreter is to assist individuals through their services by enabling them to communicate almost as if there were no language barrier. Thus, the term *liaison interpreting* is often used as a synonym of *community interpreting*, to emphasise how interpreters in the community provide a linkage between individuals. Another label, preferred in some European countries, is *public service interpreting*; this label recognises that the focus of attention in the field of community interpreting is on interactions between a person who provides a service to the public, such as a teacher or a nurse, and someone in need of their services who is not able to speak their language proficiently or to understand it without assistance. In this context, interpreters also provide a public service.

Community interpreting typically takes place in two-way interactive communications and thus is also often referred to as *dialogue interpreting*. Whereas conference interpreters normally interpret unidirectionally from their weaker language (the so-called B-language) into their stronger A-language, dialogue interpreters are challenged to interpret bidirectionally, alternately from language A to language B and then from B to A. Furthermore, while conference interpreters mainly use the *simultaneous mode*, interpreting what has just been said as the speaker continues to speak, the mode of interpreting most commonly used in dialogue interpreting is the *(short) consecutive mode*: one party speaks briefly and pauses, the interpreter relays the content of what has just been said in a second language; when an addressee responds in their own language, the interpreter again interprets what was said but in the other direction. This is thus a form of triadic communication, with the interpreter participating as an intermediary between two or more primary interlocutors, typically a service provider and a recipient of services. In contrast to the typical limited role of the interpreter in other settings, a community interpreter is frequently seen to be an active participant in the communication, helping to guide, and to varying degrees actively entering into, the interaction, as first shown through empirical research beginning in the 1990s (Wadensjö 1998; Roy 2000; Davidson 2003; Angelelli 2004). Since every language, and every variety of a language, is accompanied by its distinct culture, the interpreter is often seen as both a linguistic and a cultural bridge, with responsibilities that go beyond simply re-expressing the utterances of speakers of different languages.

The term ‘community interpreting’ is commonly used as a label for any and all ways of dealing with a language mismatch (‘non-congruent languages’) that involve a bilingual intermediary in a community setting. Empirical research has revealed that often the bilingual intermediary, instead of interpreting what one party says to another, engages in two intermingled conversations: one with the service provider in one language, and another with the seeker of services in their own language. How much information is actually passed between the two principal parties is often left to the discretion of the intermediary. It is characteristic of this sort of indirect communication that one speaker will speak to the intermediary *about* the other party or ask the bilingual to obtain information from the other. The intermediary reports to the other party (in the third person) what has been said, rather than actually interpreting (directly relaying) the message. Thus, much of what is called community interpreting (or healthcare interpreting) is not interpreting in the strict sense at all. Rather, a sort of free-flowing mixed-language communication takes place in which information and perspectives of the principal parties are shared – or not shared – in a haphazard fashion. Pöchhacker and Kadric (1999) provide a carefully analysed case study of one such encounter.

1.2 Healthcare interpreting

For the purposes of this chapter, we will now focus on community interpreting in the context of healthcare. The subfield of *healthcare interpreting* is also referred to with the narrower descriptor *medical interpreting*, perhaps because the bulk of research on interpreting in the field of healthcare as well as programmes of training for service in the health area are centred around the crucial face-to-face verbal interactions between doctors and their patients. However, the field of healthcare is clearly much broader than physician-patient encounters. It includes such diverse areas as physical therapy, dentistry, laboratory visits, hospice care, appointment scheduling over the phone, etc. Venues in which healthcare interpreters work include hospitals, private practices, home health visits, mobile clinics, and others. Currently healthcare interpreters may work remotely, connected to other parties via telephone, two-way video, or computer linkage, provided that the infrastructure is in place in any given country.

Healthcare is about caring for the patient or seeker of health services. In contrast with police work or the courts, where encounters are often adversarial, in the field of healthcare the focus must be on the welfare of the patient. The 'Do no harm' principle applies to the provider of language services as well as to the physician. The interpreter may be considered as a member of the healthcare team, with shared responsibility for health outcomes. Achieving clear communication (and cultural understanding) across different languages and cultures is not easy; that is why training and professionalism of healthcare interpreters is important, just as it is for all others who contribute to providing health services to the public. People's lives are often at stake.

It is generally acknowledged that clear and unimpeded communication between healthcare providers and those who seek their services is essential for quality care. In spite of this, when healthcare providers and their patients do not speak the same language, it is still very often the case that only partial and *ad hoc* accommodations are available, such as calling upon bilingual friends and family members of the patient to assist, as will be discussed below. Under favourable social, economic, and political circumstances, however, interpreting services are provided by dedicated professionals. This approach would seem to offer the best likelihood of successfully bridging the language gap in the interest of improved healthcare for immigrants, refugees, and other speakers of minority languages.

1.3 Professional healthcare interpreting

What is a professional healthcare interpreter? On some points there is considerable agreement. We will list some of these first and then discuss areas of ongoing controversy concerning professional roles and behaviours.

A professional healthcare interpreter:

1. Has a strong command of both languages being utilised, including a reasonable command of technical medical language and concepts as well as spoken varieties of the patient's language
2. Accurately and completely interprets what is said by a healthcare provider and a patient and any other participant in the encounter
3. Knows and follows a code of ethics/standards of practice established for the healthcare interpreting profession

4. Uses consecutive mode in most dialogue situations but is able to interpret simultaneously when appropriate (e.g. in mental health encounters)
5. Is able to sight-translate short texts such as dosage instructions
6. Maintains confidentiality and impartiality, and shows respect for all parties
7. Has formal education, at least to secondary school level, preferably two to four years at university level, and ideally a professional degree in translation/interpreting
8. Holds a licence or certification from a government or appropriate professional body, if available, based on criterion-referenced testing

A global survey of ethical codes and standards of practice for interpreters (Bancroft 2005) found substantial commonalities among standards that addressed healthcare interpreting, but also some important differences. Three principles are shared by the documents included in this review: confidentiality, accuracy/completeness, and impartiality (*ibid.*: 18). Others widely shared are maintenance of role boundaries and limited interventions to deal with misunderstandings and cultural issues. Recognising that bias may be present and that cultural misunderstandings between the parties do arise, some published practice standards for professional interpreters offer guidance regarding measured kinds of intervention by the interpreter.

Healthcare interpreters are often called upon to interpret for multiple speakers when people other than a provider and a patient are present, such as auxiliary healthcare staff and/or family and friends of the patient (including parents whose child is the patient). In the United States, professional interpreters are encouraged to observe a principle of transparency: '…during the encounter the interpreter informs all parties of any action he or she takes, including speaking for him- or herself, outside of direct interpreting' (NCIHC 2005: 12). See also Hsieh (2016: 286–288), who offers a 'multi-party model' of interpreted interactions.

A central part of the interpreter's role is obviously to re-express in a second language what a speaker has just said. For this reason, interpreters have sometimes been thought of (by themselves and others) as essentially a machine-like conduit of communication. However, it does not follow that a healthcare interpreter can or should serve *merely* as a conduit. The interpreter is a person, necessarily an active participant in the communication (Wadensjö 1998; Roy 2000; Angelelli 2004). Nor does it make sense that the healthcare interpreter is or should be invisible – an impossibility in this setting. The conference interpreter working in an isolated booth, or the courtroom interpreter restricted to 'merely interpreting' may be more or less invisible or strive to be 'just a conduit' for the words of others, but the interpreter in healthcare settings cannot reasonably avoid active involvement in the discourse, even while endeavouring to maintain accuracy and completeness in relaying what is said, as well as impartiality in serving the interests of all parties.

The terms '(mere) conduit' and 'invisible' have been used in the research literature mainly to reject the notions that these terms imply (Ozolins 2016). Interpreters may strive to limit their personal involvement in what is essentially a privileged communication between a professional and client (the patient). However, standards of practice and interpreter training commonly recognise the active involvement of the interpreter, including (at minimum) greetings, introductions that may include explanation of one's role, requests for clarification, redirection, and sometimes cultural explanations and intervention as needed. The best training for healthcare interpreters includes attention to 'ethical decision-making' as a skill to be mastered by the interpreter: how to balance neutrality/impartiality with active intervention in the interest of safety, fairness, and comprehension (CHIA 2002: 11–12). Hsieh (2016: 301), however, offers a note of caution:

> When and how interpreters can best provide their intervention ... may be dependent on various contexts (e.g., clinical, interpersonal, organisational, sociocultural, and ethical). [...] As a result, interpreter training cannot offer standardized solutions to interpreter interventions. Rather, we can only educate interpreters about the variety of issues they need to consider as they contemplate whether, when, and how they should intervene in provider-patient interactions.

Some published healthcare interpreting standards include 'advocacy' on behalf of the patient as an action that an interpreter may choose to adopt in support of 'the health, well-being or dignity of the patient' (NCIHC 2005: 10). The California Standards for Healthcare Interpreters (CHIA 2002) identifies four distinct roles for the healthcare interpreter: *message converter*, *message clarifier*, *cultural clarifier*, and *patient advocate* 'presented in order of increasing complexity and controversy'. Interpreters are advised to adopt the advocacy role, if at all, only 'after considering their advocacy skills and potential risks and benefits' (*ibid.*: 46). To move from one of these roles to another requires 'increasing skill, experience and caution on the part of the interpreter'. A similar concept of *incremental intervention* (Beltran-Avery 2001: 9–10) is incorporated into the Bridging the Gap Medical Interpreter Training offered widely across the USA by the Cross Cultural Healthcare Program (The Cross Cultural Health Care Program, no date). In this model, the interpreter is seen as 'changing hats' from *conduit* to *clarifier* to *culture broker* to *advocate* as necessary to aid communication and address cultural misunderstandings and conflicts.

The greatest disagreement among scholars and practitioners concerning the role of the professional healthcare interpreter relates to these notions of neutrality vs. advocacy and active cultural mediation. Language is a component of culture; when different languages are spoken, their speakers come from different cultures. One can argue that Western medicine is a (sub)culture in itself, with its own discourse, jargon, social expectations, etc. Therefore, cultural misunderstandings may arise just as linguistic ones do. An immigrant or refugee or member of an indigenous minority may need the services of a culture broker or advocate as much or more than any assistance in direct communication with a healthcare provider. The issue is whether one and the same intermediary can serve both as cultural adviser and advocate for a patient's viewpoint, and neutral, accurate conveyor of direct communications between parties with different worldviews and possibly different agendas.

Professional guidelines for healthcare interpreters emphasise enabling clear and direct communication between healthcare providers and patients, as well as their families. Interpreters therefore aim for accuracy and impartiality in relaying what is said. Both the provider and the patient and their family members can directly ask questions, express doubts and disagreements, and negotiate differences with the help of the interpreter.

1.4 Linguistic accommodations in healthcare a broader view

For a wide variety of reasons, the services of professional healthcare interpreters are not always available, are not always called upon even though available, or are not even preferred as a response to language barriers that could impede the provision of quality healthcare. There exists a whole range of possible responses to the situation where the language normally spoken by a healthcare provider (e.g. a doctor) does not match the primary language of an individual seeking care (e.g. a patient). Ways of addressing the language mismatch, some of which are more satisfactory than others, include:

1. The doctor knows and uses the language of the patient (bilingual provider)
2. The doctor knows a little of the patient's language and uses it along with their own primary language (semi-bilingual provider)
3. The doctor uses only their own primary language, perhaps supplemented by gestures and a loud voice
4. The patient knows a little of the provider's language and uses it along with their own primary language (semi-bilingual patient)
5. A more or less bilingual family member or friend, often a child, accompanying the patient, mediates between provider and patient (family mediator, child language brokering)
6. Other bilinguals are called upon - e.g. from a nearby ethnic restaurant or from custodial/janitorial staff (non-professional interpreter)
7. Bilingual members of the medical staff are called away from their regular duties (*ad hoc* interpreter)
8. Staff members who are assigned interpreting duties in addition to other duties are called upon (dual-role interpreter)
9. An interpreter from the on-site interpreting staff is called upon (staff interpreter, also called a dedicated interpreter)
10. An interpreter is hired from outside the institution – a freelancer or one sent by an interpreting agency or a service organisation (on-call or contract interpreter)
11. A remote interpreter is connected via telephone, video hook-up or computer (including a staff interpreter working remotely)

Only interpreters drawn from categories 8–11 can be expected to perform professional[4] interpreting to some degree. Dual-role interpreters (category 8) include staff employed as intercultural mediators, working directly with patients, who also interpret. In published research, those in categories 5–7 are often grouped together as '*ad hoc* interpreters' or 'non-professional interpreters'. However, family members, so often relied upon to interpret, are likely to behave quite differently from unaffiliated individuals and should be considered separately. Downing and Roat (2002) elaborate upon and evaluate these various alternatives.

A somewhat simpler classification developed by Hsieh (2016: 93–116) distinguishes types of interpreters as follows: professional interpreters (in-person interpreters and technology-based interpreters); bilingual medical professionals (bilingual healthcare providers and bilingual medical employees); and non-professional interpreters (chance interpreters and family members who interpret). Hsieh (*ibid.*: 109–110) urges researchers not to confound these distinct types of players while studying the medical consequences of language discordance.

The organisation and practice of cross-linguistic and cross-cultural communication in healthcare is clearly varied and complex. The quality of communication that can be expected under these various alternatives is further complicated by consideration of the motivations, language proficiency, cultural competence, social status, general education and relevant training, if any, of the particular individual who serves as intermediary in a given healthcare encounter.

2 Historical perspectives

For as long as human beings have spoken different varieties of language, those able to speak more than one have been called upon to assist others in communication. The participation of family and community members in this way existed in the past as it does now. However, the relevant history of community interpreting begins essentially in the latter half of the 20th century, with the first efforts to move toward specialisation and professionalisation of the role of language mediator and to refine ideas of what professional community interpreting is or might become.

In a major publication on court interpreting in 1991, community interpreting was described as 'any interpretation provided by non-professional interpreters' (González, Vásquez and Mikkelson 1991: 29). This was an accurate description for the most part for that early period. Immigrants and speakers of minority languages within a country, it was assumed, would learn the official language or would manage encounters with informal '*ad hoc*' language assistance. Later on, change has come about from at least three principal sources, with variations in different countries. First, members of certain linguistically and culturally distinct communities, such as the deaf and hard-of-hearing community or indigenous minorities, demanded better access to services. Second, the often unanticipated arrival in many countries of refugees from other parts of the world, such as Indochinese refugees after the war in Vietnam ended in 1975, overwhelmed hospitals and other public services, some of which began adding 'translators' or 'bilingual aides' to their staffs. Third, political movements in some countries (e.g. Australia, Sweden, Canada and the United States) pushing for minority rights, including language rights, brought about the establishment of legal rights to language accommodations (e.g. the provision of election ballots and government publications in multiple languages) and availability of interpreting services without charge to those not proficient in the language(s) spoken by public servants, educators and healthcare providers.

Efforts in the direction of professionalisation seem to have begun first in Australia and Sweden. In Australia, a national accreditation authority (NAATI) was established in 1977 to register and accredit interpreters and translators and to approve courses of training. A national professional organisation of interpreters and translators, AUSIT, was founded in 1987. The first-ever textbook on community interpreting was published by Melbourne University Press (Gentile, Ozolins and Vasilakakos 1996). In Sweden, interpreting service agencies appeared in the late 1960s and state authorisation of community interpreters began in 1976 (Niska 2004). Since 1986, public authorities have been required by law to use an interpreter 'if necessary' in dealings with non-speakers of Swedish (Niska 2007: 298).

In the USA, it was among ASL (American Sign Language) interpreters that community interpreting (beyond the courts) first began to be thought of as a profession like translation and conference interpreting. The Americans with Disabilities Act of 1999 mandated various accommodations including interpreting services for the deaf and hard-of-hearing. Meanwhile, Title VI of the Civil Rights Act of 1964, which prohibited discrimination on the basis of national origin, has been interpreted by the federal Supreme Court, and a subsequent Executive Order, as requiring all recipients of federal funding (including virtually all hospitals and clinics) to provide appropriate language assistance for anyone with 'limited English proficiency' (LEP; for details, see Chen, Youdelman and Brooks 2007). While some healthcare institutions lagged behind, others quickly organised departments of language services and hired bilingual staff to assist speakers of the locally predominant languages or began to contract with freelancers or interpreting agencies to provide interpreters as needed.

Meanwhile, community interpreters, as well as supporters, advocates and researchers from many parts of the world, came together at the first Critical Link Conference (Carr *et al.* 1997) held in Orillia, Ontario, Canada, in 1995, where it became apparent that there was little agreement on the appropriate roles for and practices of community interpreters. At that conference, Roberts (1997) proposed six essential steps for the development of community interpreting as a profession:

1. Clarification of terminology
2. Clarification of the role(s) of the community interpreter
3. Provision of training for community interpreters
4. Provision of training for trainers of community interpreters
5. Provision of training for professionals working with interpreters
6. Accreditation of community interpreters

The history of the National Council on Interpreting in Health Care (NCIHC) in the United States, organised around the time of the first Critical Link Conference, illuminates how at least some of these essential steps have been successfully pursued (Downing 2009; Downing and Ruschke 2012), specifically in the healthcare field. The NCIHC is not a professional organisation of interpreters; its membership is composed of interpreters, healthcare providers, educators, and researchers. The NCIHC began its work by compiling the first glossary of healthcare interpreting terminology (NCIHC 2001). Commissioned by the NCIHC, Beltran-Avery (2001) explored and clarified issues in the ongoing debate concerning the interpreter's role. The consensus role and standards of practice of healthcare interpreters were laid out in a published code of ethics (NCIHC 2004) and standards of practice (NCIHC 2005), both extensively vetted through convenings and surveys of working interpreters. Comparable standards had earlier been published by two regional associations, the Massachusetts Medical Interpreters Association in 1986, later revised (International Medical Interpreters Association and Education Development Center 2007) and the California Healthcare Interpreters Association (CHIA 2002).

Interpreter training in the United States has expanded slowly from a single 40-hour course developed in Seattle, Washington (The Cross Cultural Health Care Program, n.d.; now offered nationally) and a handful of short non-degree tertiary-level courses. A study of community interpreter training conducted through surveys and on-site visits in 1990–1991, limited to the United States, Canada, the UK, Denmark and Sweden (Downing and Tillery 1992), had found only a similar mix of entry-level training programmes. Today in the United States a large number of programmes are offered on-site and online by universities, colleges, and independent training organisations (Downing and Ruschke 2012), yet most practising healthcare interpreters in the United States still have received only a modicum of formal training. Beginning in 2007 the NCIHC surveyed existing interpreter preparation programmes in the United States. Based on that survey, along with a 'job task analysis' conducted among working interpreters nationwide and consultation with a panel of experts, the NCIHC published national standards for healthcare interpreter training (NCIHC 2011).

While the NCIHC training guide references essential qualifications of interpreter trainers, there are few programmes designed specifically to prepare teachers in this field (the fourth step for development of the profession in Roberts 1997, cited above). In line with Roberts' fifth step, various research reports and other publications seek to educate healthcare providers as to what to expect from professional interpreters and how to work with them. One example is a guide prepared jointly by the NCIHC and the American Translators Association (2010).

Meanwhile, accreditation/authorisation of interpreters (called in the United States 'certification') is now available after a long development process. Two separate organisations, the Certification Commission for Healthcare Interpreters (CCHI) and the National Board of Certification for Medical Interpreters (NBCMI), each offer certification testing in a small range of languages paired with English. Youdelman (2013) recounts the development process and how there came to be two competing certifying organisations.

Other nations have followed similar paths regarding legal status, utilisation, professionalisation and accreditation of community interpreters. Corsellis (2008) presents an overview and a case study of similar developments in Europe. Schuster (2014) offers a sociological model of progress in this field, tracing steps toward professionalisation in Israel, influenced by developments elsewhere.

3 Main research areas and methods

Many disciplines intersect around healthcare communication and interpreting, but two mostly distinct strands of research are evident: research in the medical field and research in translation and interpreting studies. This section will first elaborate on these two strands, introducing the major developments and key works within them. It will give brief information about various studies on interpreting in general that have emerged within the last two decades and then delve deeper into more recent studies focusing on healthcare interpreting in particular.

3.1 Research in the medical field

The first category is research, mostly but not always quantitative, largely published in standard medical journals. Medical research has focused on relationships between mediated bilingual provider-patient communication and medical outcomes, compliance, patient satisfaction and repeat visits, as well as costs, etc. In the late 20th century, some studies addressed the consequences of a 'language gap' or 'language dissonance', and of 'non-congruent' languages being spoken. If there was a bilingual intermediary present, little note was taken of how the third person's involvement affected the communication or outcomes.

As the use of interpreters expanded, the medical literature has paid increasing attention to the presence or absence of a professional interpreter and the completeness and accuracy of the interpreter's renditions of what others have said. For example, Flores *et al.* (2012), identifying and rating the seriousness of interpreting errors in recorded and transcribed clinical interviews, found significantly fewer errors of clinical significance in the performance of interpreters with over 100 hours of relevant training. Comparable results are reported by Pham *et al.* (2008), who prefer to speak of 'alterations' rather than 'errors', and by Nápoles *et al.* (2015). More recent research has begun to explore just how the participation of a professional interpreter and the nature and quality of the overall triadic interaction can influence medical outcomes. Summarising the results of a number of studies, Terui (2017: 218) reaches this conclusion:

> Using professional interpreters can lead to better care, higher satisfaction, fewer errors that lead to clinical consequences, fewer misattributions of psychiatric symptoms and diagnoses, increased patients' adherence to follow up, reduced disparities in utilisation of services, lowering medical expenses, and improved clinical outcome.

Hsieh (2016) investigates in detail the interactions among participants in interpreter-mediated healthcare services, drawing out implications for both healthcare providers and interpreting services. She advocates assessment of the quality and outcomes of *the interaction among all participants in a clinical encounter* rather than a narrower focus on errors of interpretation.

3.2 Translation and interpreting studies

The other principal strand of research on mediated bilingual encounters in healthcare has come from the growing field of interpreting studies, including approaches from applied linguistics, discourse studies, sociology and ethnography. In 2004, Pöchhacker's pioneering *Introducing Interpreting Studies* (2004) gave a broad and thorough overview of the field, not limited to community interpreting, which remains a valuable resource and a landmark in the discipline. In 2007, Hale's textbook *Community Interpreting* came out, Part III of which offers a concise summary of research topics and publications, describes principal methods (discourse analysis, ethnographic studies, survey research and experimental studies), and offers practical advice on the conduct of research.

Hale and Napier's book *Research Methods in Interpreting* (2013), designed essentially as a practical guide to graduate-level research, breaks down research methods into the following broad categories: the use of questionnaires, qualitative ethnographic methods, discourse analysis and experimentation. It also includes a section on research on education and assessment. Also valuable, as an explication of research methods broadly in the field of translation and interpreting as a whole, is the book *Researching Translation and Interpreting*, edited by Angelelli and Baer (2016). In Part I, the editors offer an overview of new and expanded theoretical approaches. They invited leading researchers to offer chapters in Part II outlining research domains such as bilingualism, cognitive processes, pedagogy, and professional identity, and in Part III the contributors describe research methods, including methods relevant to community interpreting research such as case studies, conversation analysis, interviews and focus groups, and survey-based studies, among others.

Research on interpreting today is primarily concerned with the role and behaviour of the bilingual intermediary and the nature and quality of the communication itself. In their introduction to the volume of selected papers from the sixth Critical Link conference, the editors refer to 'the sociological turn in Translation and Interpreting Studies whereby focus on settings and people in increasingly multilingual societies is deemed more important, or at least more pressing, than focus on language per se' (Schäffner, Kredens and Fowler 2014: 4). They also note that research methods have evolved, as exemplified in papers in their book, to include recorded interviews, questionnaires, recorded and transcribed clinical interactions and observations, reports and documents of participants.

3.3 Current contributions and research on healthcare interpreting

Research on healthcare interpreting has expanded in the past decade both in quantity and geographical range. A literature review of healthcare interpreting studies published between 2007 and 2017 (Liu and Zhang 2019) noted the close correlation between governmental support and enhanced interpreting services and research, mainly in the United States and Europe. That research found important variations also in specific settings, such as mental health, and found both positive and negative evaluations of *ad hoc* versus professional interpreters. For example, providers felt that patient empowerment could be achieved through the greater accuracy of communication provided by professional interpreters, while patients generally felt more empowered by the advocacy and support provided by informal interpreters (Liu and Zhang 2019: 2).

Research continues, however, to reveal inadequacies in cross-cultural healthcare communication in virtually every location studied. Problems are attributed to lack of funding, lack of appropriate training, supervision and remuneration of interpreters, and the continued use of untrained staff and family members as interpreters. It is interesting that research participants often express satisfaction with the communication even when transcription and analysis of recorded interactions reveal critical communication lapses; Lesch and Saulse (2013), in a study of interpreting in South Africa, offer an illustration of this. The authors recommend improved policies for interpreting services and better training for providers on how to work with interpreters.

Taibi (2014) has brought attention to the situation in the Arab world, where, he says, community interpreting services are generally lacking. This lack exists despite a sizeable national language minority in Tunisia, a large migrant population in the United Arab Emirates, and the large numbers of religious pilgrims in Saudi Arabia. Taibi suggests strategies for change based on the experiences of Australia, Canada, and those European countries that have developed such services.

In much of Western Europe, however, language services remain uneven and varied in nature from country to country. An extensive survey in 2014–2015 by Angelelli (2018) investigated translation and interpreting services available in five EU member states (Germany, Greece, Italy, Spain and the UK) for EU citizens when they cross borders from one member state to another. The study revealed great diversity and widespread failure to attain EU human rights goals. Thus, in these five countries the survey found that EU citizens who crossed national borders frequently did not receive the quality language services promised under Directive 2011/24/EU. Specifically, except for the UK, where translation and interpreting services are 'mandated by the country's Equality Act 2010, language services are neither mandatory nor frequent in healthcare organisations' in the countries studied (Angelelli 2018: 121). When study participants were asked to indicate to what extent translation and interpreting services were utilised, the response 'only as a last resort' was selected by 57 per cent of those working in Spain, 41 per cent in Greece, and 70 per cent in Germany, as opposed to only 22 per cent of participants in the UK (*ibid.*).

Gentile (2017) describes cutbacks in legal interpreting in the UK and in healthcare interpreting in the Netherlands, where privatisation of interpreting services has led to decreases in service quality and pay rates, leaving many qualified interpreters to quit the field. Thus, in the Netherlands, 'informal interpreters' are increasingly relied upon in healthcare settings rather than professional interpreters, previously available through government funding.

Research at the University of Amsterdam focused on patients' perspective on interactions between General Practitioners and female Turkish-speaking immigrant patients supported by informal interpreters, whose role 'besides providing linguistic translation' was to 'perform the roles of advocates and caregivers of the patients' (Zendedel *et al.* 2018: 158). The focus in a series of interviews was on patient satisfaction with respect to trust and perceived empowerment, rather than on interpreter accuracy, neutrality and confidentiality as in many previous studies. Although none of the women interviewed had ever had the services of a professional interpreter, all indicated a preference for informal interpreters, nearly all of whom were family members, mainly on the basis of trust and the feeling that they were empowered through their interpreter-advocate (*ibid.*: 165–166); some indicated that they would trust professional interpreters more with respect to confidentiality.

In a journal article, Pöchhacker (2006) succinctly outlines the development of research specific to healthcare interpreting, encompassing such diverse disciplines as nursing, linguistics, mental health, medical and social sciences, and communication studies, in addition to more traditional interpreting studies, citing prominent examples in each area. His review also distinguishes the varying *themes* of research such as interpreter performance, communication practices, and goals and outcomes with respect to the service provided. Pöchhacker concludes by emphasising the overarching focus of this research on *quality*, which must ultimately be assessed in terms of *benefits* and the associated *costs*.

To close this sampling of recent research, a US study published in the *Journal of Transcultural Nursing* (Estrada and Messias 2018) looked at goal-directed triadic communication between providers (nurse-practitioners), well-qualified interpreters (also serving as patient navigators), and Hispanic patients with limited English proficiency, through examination of recorded and transcribed sessions and post-session interviews. The study revealed productive joint efforts at problem-solving. In the authors' words, 'three modes of co-constructed, collaborative knowledge generation [took place]: constructing connections, constructing mutual understanding, and constructing effective system navigation strategies' (Estrada and Messias 2018: 500). Both the interactional model and the research design in this study appear worthy of emulation.

4 Critical issues

This section will look at some of the issues that have a bearing on the provision and effectiveness of healthcare interpreting, such as the availability, or otherwise, of language services in diverse immigrant languages; achieving balance between interpreting, cultural mediation and advocacy; and the development of training and assessment.

4.1 Adequate language services in diverse immigrant languages

The diversity of languages and dialects and their associated cultures across the world presents a unique challenge for the field of community interpreting when combined with the scope and scale of migration in today's world that is bringing so many diverse languages into proximity within a given local community. Newcomers, or their children, may learn the dominant language(s) of their new home in due course; the problem is the linguistic and cultural barriers that arise immediately upon arrival for immigrant adults with respect to the dominant local community.

This is a problem unique to community services, which need to be able to reach all individuals equally regardless of their language. National governments can conduct their core functions in one or a handful of languages. International conferences routinely make their communications accessible to attendees in a small number of languages through the services of professional conference interpreters. Such a broad organisation as the European Union has, with considerable cost and difficulty, been able to accommodate an increasing number of languages in its deliberations and communications. Any service that requires face-to-face interaction with any and all members of the general public, however, is increasingly likely to face a unique challenge: that significant, and often growing, proportions of their local population do not share a common language with those who provide public services such as healthcare. Moreover, the languages and dialects spoken may be highly diverse.

For instance, well over one hundred distinct languages are spoken at home by public school students in New York City (some estimate that as many as 800 languages may be spoken in the city by all age groups).[5] Parents of these students may not speak English or may speak it with a limited degree of proficiency. Therefore, such routine functions as parent-teacher conferences and healthcare encounters cannot be performed equitably without some linguistic accommodation. For a widely spoken minority language such as Spanish in New York City and in many parts of the United States, a hospital may be able to hire full-time Spanish-English interpreters with appropriate skills and training. For other languages not widely spoken in a given area (languages of limited diffusion, or LLDs) the same solution may be unavailable. Today, this kind of communication barrier is common in major cities, and even in villages and rural areas, in many parts of the world.

From the point of view of the potential interpreter of an LLD (for example, Tigrinya, Khmer or Nuer in the United States) there likely will be no language-specific skills training available. Moreover, the demand for interpreting in a given LLD may be so low that it would be unprofitable for a bilingual speaker of this language to seek training or accreditation, even if available, or to envision a career in interpreting. This is the obvious reason why volunteers and family members with some command of the provider's language are so often called upon and is part of the rationale for providers choosing to 'make do' without needed language assistance.

As a consequence, it may be very difficult to locate anyone able to interpret with professional competency between a provider of health services and a given patient who may show up to receive healthcare. Remote interpreting via telephone, video or a computer link offers a partial solution by linking an interpreter of an LLD, located anywhere in the world, with a patient who speaks that language and a service provider. Remote interpreting assignments may thus provide enough work for the interpreter of a less widely spoken language to support a career in interpreting.

With respect to widely spoken language pairs, the ethical mandate to offer professional interpreting services in healthcare is only countered by costs, political will, awareness of need, and sometimes the reluctance of providers to utilise services already available. The critical problem is how to provide equivalent services in the case of the many other languages, with respect to which cultural barriers may be greater. There may be fewer educated bilinguals ready to be trained and employed as interpreters, and demand for their services may be limited in a given geographical area. Until solutions can be found for this imbalance, language services will remain unequal for speakers of different languages in the same locality.

4.2 Finding the right balance between interpreting and cultural mediation/ advocacy

A second critical issue facing the field of healthcare interpreting centres around the role(s) of the professional interpreter is the possible contributions of bilingual family members, and needed support for immigrant and minority patients in addressing cultural conflicts and misunderstandings.

Studies have shown that bilingual family members accompanying a patient can contribute in many ways, such as clarifying cultural viewpoints and patient complaints and advocating for the patient (or the provider). However, research has also shown that, untrained in interpreting and not reticent to assert their own views, family members who interpret often inhibit clear, direct, and accurate communication between provider and patient. Accompanying relatives of the patient can be given the opportunity to offer their perspective without being expected to interpret as well. What reason other than cost-saving and convenience is there to call upon bilingual adult family members to take the role of interpreter? This important question becomes more urgent in face of what Gentile (2017) describes as the de-professionalisation of interpreting under nationalistic political pressures and budget constraints even in countries that have previously supported professional interpreting.

A related issue is this: to what extent can a professional interpreter be expected to provide accurate and impartial interpreting (suppressing personal opinions) and also to provide cultural brokering and guidance for the benefit of patients unfamiliar with Western healthcare? Can the interpreter do both or are these two distinct roles?

Verrept (2008) discusses the establishment and history of a government-sponsored intercultural mediation programme in Belgium in which bilinguals trained as culture brokers are employed rather than professional interpreters filling a more limited role. Culture brokers meet separately with patients to share information and learn about their concerns in addition to interpreting where needed. A major obstacle from the beginning has been the reluctance of providers to bring in the mediators rather than continuing to rely on family members for interpreting. However, evaluations found significant improvements in quality of care when the mediators' services were used. Patients were more willing and able to discuss their concerns with the mediators than directly with their physicians. To adequately fulfil their broad role, mediators needed extensive training. In this type of programme, support and advocacy for individual patients are emphasised over the usual impartial role of the interpreter (which by contrast may appear to serve the needs of the provider over those of the patient). This is a model that might work well in other settings.

Other solutions to the problem of providing both cultural support for patients and interpreting services have also been implemented. A paediatric specialty hospital in Seattle, Washington (USA), established a separate position of 'bilingual patient navigator' to serve alongside the regular interpreting staff (Crezee and Roat 2019). Bilingual navigators are assigned to assist selected families – those judged most likely to benefit from their services – by guiding, teaching, and supporting them, as well as interpreting as needed. Other patient families receive the usual professional interpreter services. An external evaluation of the programme at the end of two years (in 2011) showed 'significant improvement' in multiple areas including a lower no-show rate, shorter average length of stay, a greater number of interpreted encounters, and significant cost savings (*ibid.*: 7–8).

4.3 Development of training and assessment

A third critical need is to work toward agreement on adequate levels of general education and professional training for interpreters. While good models and practices regarding certification of skills exist, there is a need for new ideas on the best ways of training interpreters and on how to prepare interpreter trainers. These questions are most acute with respect to initial training and assessment of interpreters of LLDs where the barriers include the lack of qualified trainers who speak these languages and bilingual training materials, as well as the problems of adequate testing and certification for multiple language pairs.

5 Future directions

The field of community interpreting has come into its own over the past 30 or so years with respect to both practice and research. Yet clearly major issues remain, and development is uneven. The fundamental issue of whether professional interpreters or (trained) cultural mediators (or untrained volunteers and family members) should be preferred to assist bilingual communication in healthcare still demands attention. Legal requirements, social priorities, the extent of cultural differences between providers and seekers of their services, and the number of speakers of particular minority languages in a given area will all continue to influence the choices being made. Nevertheless, further research bearing on the issues, especially with regard to ethical questions, barriers to understanding, and health outcomes, is needed.

In addition, there is a need for better understanding of each party's active role in mediated bilingual communication. This can lead to improvements in the design of interpreter training and the creation of instructional materials (role plays, glossaries, readings, etc.) as well as making appropriate training and educational programmes for prospective community interpreters more widely available.

Notes

1 The preferred term is *interpreting* rather than *interpretation*. One reason for preferring the participle is to emphasise the interactive and transitory nature of interpreting, which unlike translation does not result in a permanent record. Another reason is to avoid confusion with other meanings of the word *interpretation*, as in the interpretation of a work of art or of a body of medical data (NCIHC 2001: 5).
2 To simplify the phrasing in the remainder of this chapter, I will refer to speakers and hearers, without direct reference to communication involving signed languages. Much of what is said here applies equally to interpreting into and out of signed languages.
3 The demands on court interpreters are in many ways unique. Court interpreting is thus sometimes included under the community interpreting label and sometimes not. Since our focus here is on the medical setting we will not enter into this discussion.
4 Categories 1, 2 and 7 would also perform 'professionally' but according to their own *medical profession*'s standards, not according to the standards of the interpreting profession.
5 www.nytimes.com/2010/04/29/nyregion/29lost.html (Accessed: 31 March 2020).

Further reading

Beltran Avery, M.-P. (2001) *The Role of the Healthcare Interpreter: An Evolving Dialogue. The National Council on Interpreting in Health Care*. Available at: www.ncihc.org (Accessed: 29 May 2019).

This article traces how, over time, open discussion among interpreters and other stakeholders led to broad agreement on healthcare interpreters' roles.

Hsieh, E. (2016) *Bilingual Health Communication: Working with Interpreters in Cross-Cultural Care*. London and New York: Routledge.

This important book investigates interpreting from the perspectives of both interpreters and medical providers and proposes a new theoretical framework for future research and practice.

Flores, G., et al. (2012) 'Errors of Medical Interpretation and Their Potential Clinical Consequences: A Comparison of Professional vs Ad Hoc vs No Interpreters', *Annals of Emergency Medicine*, 60(5), pp. 545–553.

A study of the quality of communication in bilingual medical interviews, showing the value of interpreter training in reducing transmission errors.

Hale, S. B. (2007) *Community Interpreting*. Basingstoke and New York: Palgrave Macmillan.

A thorough treatment of medical and legal interpreting, including contexts of practice, ethics, training, and research.

National Council on Interpreting in Health Care (2005) *National Standards of Practice for Interpreters in Healthcare*. NCIHC. Available at: www.ncihc.org (Accessed: 28 May 2019).

An influential document guiding current practices of professional healthcare interpreters.

Related topics

Child Language Brokering in Healthcare Settings, Healthcare Interpreting Ethics, The Impact of Interpreters and the Rise of Deaf Healthcare Professionals

References

Angelelli, C. V. (2004) *Medical Interpreting and Cross-Cultural Communication*. Cambridge: Cambridge University Press. DOI:10.1017/CBO9780511486616.

Angelelli, C. V. (2018) 'Cross-Border Healthcare for All EU Residents? Linguistic Access in the European Union', *JALPP*, 11(2), pp. 113–134. DOI:10.1558/japl.31818.

Angelelli, C. V. and Baer, B. J. (eds) (2016) *Researching Translation and Interpreting*. London and New York: Routledge.

Bancroft, M. (2005) *The Interpreter's World Tour: An Environmental Scan of Standards of Practice for Interpreters*. The National Council on Interpreting in Health Care. Available at: www.ncihc.org/assets/documents/publications/NCIHC%20Environmental%20Scan.pdf (Accessed: 31 March 2020).

Beltran Avery, M.-P. (2001) *The Role of the Healthcare Interpreter: An Evolving Dialogue*. The National Council on Interpreting in Health Care Working Paper Series. Available at: https://memberfiles.freewebs.com/17/56/66565617/documents/The%20role_of_health_care_interpreter.pdf (Accessed: 31 March 2020).

Carr, S. E., Roberts, R. P., Dufour, A. and Steyn, D. (eds) (1997) *The Critical Link: Interpreters in the Community: Papers From the 1st International Conference on Interpreting in Legal, Health and Social Service Settings, Geneva Park, Canada, 1–4 June 1995*. Amsterdam and Philadelphia: John Benjamins.

Chen, A. H., Youdelman, M. K. and Brooks, J. (2007) 'The Legal Framework for Language Access in Healthcare Settings: Title VI and Beyond', *Journal of General Internal Medicine*, 22, pp. 362–367. DOI:10.1007/s11606-007-0366-2.

CHIA (2002) *California Standards for Healthcare Interpreters*. Available at: http://www.chiaonline.org/Resources/Documents/CHIA%20Standards/standards_chia.pdf (Accessed: 2 February 2021).
Corsellis, A. (2008) 'Developing Interpreting in the Public Services: A Case Study', in Corsellis, A. (ed.) *Public Service Interpreting*. London: Palgrave Macmillan, pp. 11–23. DOI:10.1057/9780230581951_2.
Crezee, I. H. M. and Roat, C. E. (2019) 'Bilingual Patient Navigator or Healthcare Interpreter: What's the Difference and Why Does It Matter?', *Cogent Medicine*, 6(1), pp. 1–15. DOI:10.1080/2331205X.2019.1582576.
Davidson, B. (2003) 'The Interpreter as Institutional Gatekeeper: The Social-Linguistic Role of Interpreters in Spanish-English Medical Discourse', *Journal of Sociolinguistics*, 4(3), pp. 379–405. DOI:10.1111/1467–9481.00121.
Downing, B. and Roat, C. E. (2002) *Models for the Provision of Language Access in Health Care Settings*. The National Council on Interpreting in Health Care Working Paper Series. Available at: https://www.ncihc.org/assets/documents/workingpapers/NCIHC%20Working%20Paper%20-%20Models%20for%20Provision%20of%20Language%20Access.pdf (Accessed: 31 March 2020).
Downing, B. and Ruschke, K. (2012) 'Professionalizing Healthcare Interpreting Between Spoken Languages: Contributions of the National Council on Interpreting in Health Care', in *In Our Hands: Educating Healthcare Interpreters*. Washington, DC: Gallaudet University Press, pp. 209–228.
Downing, B. T. (2009) 'Community Interpreting in the USA: Contributions of a Broad-based National Organization', in Anamur, H., Bulut, A. and Uras-Yilmaz, A. (eds) *International Colloquium of Translation: Translation in all its Aspects with Focus on International Dialogue*. Istanbul: Association of Translation, pp. 373–377.
Downing, B. T. and Tillery, K. H. (1992) *Professional Training for Community Interpreters*. Minneapolis, MN: Center for Urban and Regional Affairs, University of Minnesota.
Estrada, R. D. and Messias, D. A. K. H. (2018) 'Language Co-Construction and Collaboration in Interpreter-Mediated Primary Care Encounters with Hispanic Adults', *Journal of Transcultural Nursing*, 29(6), pp. 498–505. DOI:10.1177/1043659617747523.
Flores, G., Abreu, M., Barone, C. P., Bachur, R. and Lin, H. (2012) 'Errors of Medical Interpretation and Their Potential Clinical Consequences: A Comparison of Professional Versus Ad Hoc Versus No Interpreters', *Annals of Emergency Medicine*, 60(5), pp. 545–553. DOI:10.1016/j.annemergmed.2012.01.025.
Gentile, A., Ozolins, U. and Vasilakakos, M. (1996) *Liaison Interpreting: A Handbook*. Melbourne: Melbourne University Press.
Gentile, P. (2017) 'Political Ideology and the De-Professionalisation of Public Service Interpreting: The Netherlands and the United Kingdom as Case Studies', in Valero-Garcés, C. and Tipton, R. (ed.) *Ideology, Ethics and Policy Development in Public Service Interpreting and Translation*. Clevedon: Multilingual Matters, pp. 63–83. DOI:10.21832/9781783097531-008.
González, R. D., Vásquez, V. F. and Mikkelson, H. (1991) *Fundamentals of Court Interpretation: Theory, Policy and Practice*. Durham, NC: Carolina Academic Press.
Hale, S. B. (2007) *Community Interpreting*. Basingstoke: Palgrave Macmillan.
Hale, S. and Napier, J. (2013) *Research Methods in Interpreting: A Practical Resource*. London and New York: Bloomsbury.
Hsieh, E. (2016) *Bilingual Health Communication: Working with Interpreters in Cross-Cultural Care.* London and New York: Routledge. DOI:10.4324/9781315658308.
International Medical Interpreters Association and Education Development Center (2007) *Medical Interpreting Standards of Practice*. Available at: https://www.imiaweb.org/uploads/pages/102.pdf (Accessed: 2 February 2021).
Lesch, H. M. and Saulse, B. (2013) 'Revisiting the Interpreting Service in the Healthcare Sector: A Descriptive Overview', *Perspectives: Studies in Translatology*. 22(3), pp. 332–348. DOI:10.1080/0907676X.2013.822008.
Liu, Y. and Zhang, W. (2019) 'Unity in Diversity: Mapping Healthcare Interpreting Studies (2007–2017)', *Medical Education Online*, 24(1). DOI:10.1080/10872981.2019.1579559.
Nápoles, A. M., Santoyo-Olsson, J., Karliner, L. S., Gregorich, S. E. and Pérez-Stable, E. J. (2015) 'Inaccurate Language Interpretation and Its Clinical Significance in the Medical Encounters of Spanish-Speaking Latinos', *Medical Care*, 53(11), pp. 940–947. DOI:10.1097/MLR.0000000000000422.

NCIHC (2001) *The Terminology of Health Care Interpreting A Glossary of Terms*. Available at: https://www.ncihc.org/assets/documents/NCIHC%20Terms%20Final080408.pdf (Accessed: 2 February 2021).
NCIHC (2004) *A National Code of Ethics for Interpreters in Health Care*. Available at: https://www.ncihc.org/assets/documents/publications/NCIHC%20National%20Code%20of%20Ethics.pdf (Accessed: 2 February 2021).
NCIHC (2005) *National Standards of Practice for Interpreters in Health Care*. Available at: https://www.ncihc.org/assets/documents/publications/NCIHC%20National%20Standards%20of%20Practice.pdf (Accessed: 31 March 2020).
NCIHC (2011) *National Standards for Healthcare Interpreter Training Programs*. Available at: https://www.ncihc.org/assets/documents/publications/National_Standards_5-09-11.pdf (Accessed: 30 January 2021).
NCIHC and ATA (American Translators Association) (2010) *What's in a Word? A Guide to Understanding Interpreting and Translation in Health Care*. Available at: https://www.ncihc.org/assets/documents/publications/Whats_in_a_Word_Guide.pdf (Accessed 2 February 2021).
Niska, H. (2004) *Community Interpreting in Sweden: A Short Presentation*. Stockholm: Institute for Translation and Interpreting Studies, Stockholm University.
Niska, H. (2007) 'From Helpers to Professionals', in Wadensjö, C., Englund Dimitrova, B. and Nilsson, A.-L. (eds) *The Critical Link 4: Professionalization of Interpreting in the Community. Selected Papers From the 4th International Conference on Interpreting in Legal, Health and Social Service Settings, Stockholm, Sweden, 20–23 May 2004*. Amsterdam: Benjamins Translation Library, pp. 297–310. DOI:10.1075/btl.70.32nis.
Ozolins, U. (2016) 'The Myth of the Myth of Invisibility?', *Interpreting. International Journal of Research and Practice in Interpreting*, 18(2), pp. 273–284. DOI:10.1075/intp.18.2.06ozo.
Pham, K., Thornton, J. D., Engelberg, R. A., Jackson, J. C. and Curtis, J. R. (2008) 'Alterations During Medical Interpretation of ICU Family Conferences That Interfere With or Enhance Communication', *Chest* American College of Chest Physicians, 134(1), pp. 109–116. DOI:10.1378/chest.07-2852.
Pöchhacker, F. (2004) *Introducing Interpreting Studies*. London and New York: Routledge. DOI:10.4324/9780203504802.
Pöchhacker, F. (2006) 'Research and Methodology in Healthcare Interpreting', *Linguistica Antverpiensia, New Series*, 5, pp. 135–159.
Pöchhacker, F. and Kadric, M. (1999) 'The Hospital Cleaner as Healthcare Interpreter: A Case Study', *The Translator*, 5(2), pp. 161–178. DOI:10.1080/13556509.1999.10799039.
Roberts, R. P. (1997) 'Community Interpreting Today and Tomorrow', in Carr, S. E., Roberts, R. P., Dufour, A. and Steyn, D. (eds) *The Critical Link: Interpreters in the Community: Papers From the 1st International Conference on Interpreting in Legal, Health and Social Service Settings, Geneva Park, Canada, 1–4 June 1995*, pp. 7–27. DOI:10.1075/btl.19.03rob.
Roy, C. B. (2000) *Interpreting as a Discourse Process*. Oxford: Oxford University Press.
Schäffner, C., Kredens, K. and Fowler, Y. (2014) 'Interpreting in a Changing Landscape: Challenges for Research and Practice', in Schäffner, C., Kredens, K. and Fowler, Y. (eds) *Interpreting in a Changing Landscape*. Amsterdam and Philadelphia: John Benjamins, pp. 1–11. DOI:10.1075/btl.109.02sch.
Schuster, M. (2014) 'From Chaos to Cultural Competence', in Schäffner, C., Kredens, K. and Fowler, Y. (eds.) *Interpreting in a Changing Landscape: Selected Papers From Critical Link 6*. Amsterdam and Philadelphia: John Benjamins, pp. 61–82. DOI:10.1075/btl.109.07schu.
Taibi, M. (2014) 'Community Interpreting and Translation in the Arab World', *Babel* 60(1), pp. 52–69.
Terui, S. (2017) 'Conceptualizing the Pathways and Processes Between Language Barriers and Health Disparities: Review, Synthesis, and Extension', *Journal of Immigrant and Minority Health*, 19(1), pp. 215–224. DOI:10.1007/s10903-015-0322-x.
The Cross Cultural Health Care Program (n.d.) *Bridging the Gap Training Program*. Available at: https://xculture.org/medical-interpreter-training/ (Accessed: 5 June 2019).
Verrept, H. (2008) '10. Intercultural Mediation: An Answer to Healthcare Disparities?', in Valero-Garcés, C. and Martin, A. (eds) *Crossing Borders in Community Interpreting: Definitions and Dilemmas*. Amsterdam and Philadelphia: John Benjamins, pp. 187–201. DOI:10.1075/btl.76.10ver.

Wadensjö, C. (1998) *Interpreting as Interaction*. London and New York: Longman. DOI:10.4324/9781315842318.
Youdelman, M. (2013) 'The Development of Certification for Healthcare Interpreters in the United States', *Translation and Interpreting*, 5(1), pp. 114–126. DOI:10.12807/ti.105201.2013.a06.
Zendedel, R., Schouten, B. C., van Weert, J. C.M. and van den Putte, B. (2018) 'Informal Interpreting in General Practice: The Migrant Patient's Voice', *Ethnicity and Health*, 23(2). DOI:10.1080/13557858.2016.1246939.

11

Child language brokering in healthcare settings

Rachele Antonini and Ira Torresi

This chapter focuses on non-professional interpreting and translation performed by children from migrant backgrounds, between healthcare providers who speak the host country's language(s), and their own families and/or communities who may lack the necessary proficiency in these language(s). We will first offer a definition of this type of interpreting and translation, called Child Language Brokering (henceforth, CLB) in general (Section 1). We will then review the legal frameworks (Section 2) and the literature on CLB, specifically within the healthcare sector (Section 3). Finally, before reflecting on future directions, we will present some of the findings of our own research on CLB in Italy, with special reference to healthcare (Section 4).

1 Child language brokering: a definition

CLB is an umbrella term for all non-professional interpreting and translation practices performed by children and adolescents (for the purposes of this chapter, we will set the age limit of CLB at 18). Such practices range from describing TV programmes at home to sight-translating bank documents (i.e. translating them orally from a written text). The term became widespread in the 1990s (Shannon 1990; Tse 1995, 1996). Until this point, brokering children and adults were grouped together under various terms such as 'natural translators' (Harris 1976, 1980), 'para-phrasers' (Orellana, Dorner and Pulido 2003; Orellana *et al.* 2003), 'family interpreters' (Valdés 2003) or just 'bilinguals' (Malakoff and Hakuta 1991); some of this terminology is still in use. Within interpreting studies, occurrences of CLB have traditionally been dealt with only when they emerged in larger studies of *ad hoc*, family, or non-professional interpreting (e.g. Meyer, Pawlack and Kliche 2010; Pöchhacker 2008) rather than being awarded separate attention.

Typically, child language brokers come from migrant families and have attended school in the host country; they thus participate in both the host country's and their family's languages and cultures. For this reason, their families or communities may call upon them to serve as linguistic and cultural facilitators whenever a professional interpreter or translator is not available, or not desirable because it is easier to rely on a family member

DOI: 10.4324/9781003167983-15

than seeking out professional interpreting services. Similarly, host country institutions, including healthcare providers, may accept CLB as a 'lesser evil', particularly because it is free and because it saves the time and effort of arranging for professional interpreting services (Cirillo, Torresi and Valentini 2010; Antonini 2015: 100). Additionally, in certain settings such as schools or other educational institutions, CLB may be a way to ensure migrant children's inclusion through their active participation in the community, at first as beneficiaries of other children's brokering and later, when they master their new language, as providers of CLB (Rossato 2014; Cirillo 2017: 307).

As is the case with all non-professional translation and interpreting, child language brokering is seldom covered in translation and interpreting handbooks, because it lies outside the boundaries of professional practice that translation and interpreting students are usually trained in. CLB is frequently considered inappropriate particularly in the healthcare sector, as the kind of interpreting and translation required in these settings may be too demanding for a child, both in terms of the medical vocabulary and the emotional strain involved in the process (See Section 3 for a detailed discussion and references). Above all, it is generally understood that personal involvement with the patient receiving treatment is best avoided when providing healthcare services (La Puma *et al.* 1991: 1290). Regardless of such perceptions, however, CLB does occur in real-life healthcare settings, particularly within the context of the recent rise in immigration and the refugee crisis, as will be described in the following sections.

2 Legal frameworks

The provision of interpreting and translation services in healthcare differs widely across countries. Generally speaking, in countries where there is more experience in dealing with multilingualism and superdiversity, there is also greater awareness of the risks posed by non-professionals providing language services. The general provision of language services depends on whether a government will take action by devising and implementing specific policies (Ozolins 2010). In countries with a historically higher migration rates (e.g. Australia, Sweden and the UK), a range of policies has been put into place to help immigrants and minority language speakers in overcoming their language and cultural barriers, such as the use of printed material and interpreters (Hall and Sham 2007: 18). Unfortunately, a systematic implementation of similar language policies is an exception rather than the rule in other parts of the world. In many countries grappling with the more recent influx of migrants such as Italy, Spain or France, the provision of language services in healthcare is based on *ad hoc* measures and random initiatives (Rudvin 2006). The constantly growing demand for language services is not met by an adequate provision of professional interpreting and translation services; instead, the task of interpreting is relegated to family members (including children), friends, untrained members of support staff, and even strangers found in waiting rooms or on the street (Flores 2006).

Countries that actively oppose the use of non-professional interpreters in healthcare settings, and CLB in particular, attempt to limit these practices through a number of guidelines and measures that aim to ensure accessibility with the use of professional interpreters (Rice 2014). In the United States, for instance, the use of bilingual children and family members is opposed on the grounds that their health literacy is not adequate for undertaking this task, since they are put in a position where they try 'to absorb information and transmit it while emotionally upset' (Levetown 2008: e1448). The use of hospital employees is likewise opposed, because 'their educational levels, even in their own country, may be low, and they [...] will be assaulted emotionally with confidential and difficult information' (Levetown 2008: e1448). More recently, the US Department of Health and Human Services ruled with Section 1557 of the Patient Protection and Affordable Care Act that:

> In many circumstances family members, friends, and especially children, are not competent to provide quality, accurate oral interpretation. For communications of particularly sensitive information, oral interpretation by an individual's family or friend often also implicates issues of appropriateness, confidentiality, privacy, and conflict of interest. Thus, covered entities may not rely on family members, friends, or other informal interpreters to provide language access services.
>
> *Department of Health and Human Services 2016: 31417–31418*

Despite these regulations, children continue to language broker in healthcare settings in the United States, as will be illustrated in Section 3. This can be partly ascribed to a lack of political will to take the legislative debate all the way to final implementation. For instance, the bill banning CLB from California hospitals, discussed by the California Assembly and Senate in 2003/04 (Yee, Diaz and Spitzer 2003), and mentioned by Angelelli (2010), was never lifted from appropriations suspense, meaning that the measures contained in it were never funded, and therefore the bill never came into effective force.

Across the EU, the problem does not seem to be the infringement of regulations on CLB, but the lack of any regulations that would limit this practice or in other ways ensure that patients' language rights are respected. As Yubo Liu and Wei Zhang observe, 'while the US is widely acknowledged as the country most proactive in state and federal efforts in ensuring the rights and interests of patients with limited English proficiency to access interpreting services in healthcare settings, European countries have experienced more fluctuations in the level of government support' (Liu and Zhang 2019: 1–2).

Studies have demonstrated that the lack of provision of professional interpreting and translation services and the ensuing use of minor or adult non-professionals can lead to unequal access to healthcare services and discrimination. The European Union Agency for Fundamental Rights' report (2013), based on qualitative social research and legal analysis in five EU Member States, reveals 'the operation of multiple grounds of discrimination, particularly concerning healthcare' (European Union Agency for Fundamental Rights 2013: 3). The report shows that '[l]anguage was the most relevant communication barrier mentioned by migrants in all the EU Member States surveyed' (European Union Agency for Fundamental Rights 2013: 47). The report also shows that informal interpretation and CLB are reported as one of the most common forms of mediation use in healthcare in Austria, the Czech Republic and Italy (European Union Agency for Fundamental Rights 2013: 50). As these insights into the situation in the United States and the EU show, CLB is still frequently considered to be either the only viable alternative to professional interpreting or the most convenient way to deal with language barriers in the health sector, despite the nascent legal framework and the broad acknowledgement of the possible negative effects of this practice. We will explore this issue in more depth in the following two sections devoted to research on CLB in healthcare, and to our own case study of the phenomenon in Italy.

3 Literature review

As indicated in Section 1, the existence and occurrence of CLB in healthcare settings are typically mentioned in studies that focus on other research areas, such as informal interpreting and medical practice. More recently, the discussion started appearing in works focusing on discriminatory practices within the theoretical framework of human rights, equality and quality of care, and medical ethics. Studies from these areas usually describe CLB as a practice which should be discouraged and prevented (e.g. European Union Agency for Fundamental Rights 2013; Juckett and Unger 2014).

The few studies that have investigated CLB in healthcare as their main focus have highlighted the cognitive, psychological, relational and sociological impact of CLB on children and their families through qualitative methodologies, primarily interviews. The existing research has developed along two main lines: (1) the views of healthcare professionals and, more recently, (2) the views of children (and parents/guardians in a more limited manner). A qualitative study that assessed the reasons for the limited use of professional interpreters by US physicians (Diamond *et al.* 2008: 258) identified four recurrent themes: (1) a general acknowledgement of the underuse of professional interpreting services, which the physicians described as a need to 'get by'; (2) the perceived value of the benefits of using a professional interpreter against their own time constraints and workload; (3) the convenience of relying on family members, including children, or on the physician's second language skills; (4) the normalisation of the underuse of professional interpreting services, despite acknowledging that this situation prevents patients with limited English proficiency from receiving equal care. Another study, which involved 77 bilingual young people in the UK (Free *et al.* 2003), identified the main healthcare settings in which children are likely to interpret/translate. These include: 'translating instructions on medicines, helping complete surgery registration forms, and interpreting in hospital, dental and general practice settings' (Free *et al.* 2003: 531). Their research also shows that:

> While some young people reported that they were sometimes used for interpreting because of deficiencies in formal interpreting services, others reported situations in which they were used by choice. Young people were used for preference, either because the family trusted their interpreting skills or because they had a particularly good understanding of their parent's illness and how it affected their life.
>
> *Free et al. 2003: 531*

Most studies focusing on CLB in healthcare detect the contingent and unplanned nature of this phenomenon and ascribe the involvement of children to the lack of funding or to a missing legal framework preventing the practice. However, they all show that CLB in healthcare is ultimately considered to be more convenient than professional alternatives (perceived as missing or more difficult to arrange) to help families with an immigrant background in overcoming communication barriers.

One of the most cited studies on CLB in healthcare by Cohen, Moran-Ellis and Smaje (1999) shows that for general practitioners (GPs) in the UK, CLB is often the only viable and contingent option. However, GPs also express their opposition to this practice by arguing that children should be protected from 'taboo' subjects for which they are not mentally prepared, and that might be part of the consultation. They state that they accepted children as informal interpreters, provided that the consultation was 'straightforward' (Cohen, Moran-Ellis and Smaje 1999: 173), but they were less willing to have children translate in those consultations that they deemed 'complex' (Cohen, Moran-Ellis and Smaje 1999: 173) or 'sensitive' (Cohen, Moran-Ellis and Smaje 1999: 175). Free *et al.* (2003) analysed young people's accounts of interpreting for family or friends in primary care settings in the UK and confirmed the necessity of child language brokers due to deficiencies in services, but also because patients prefer to have their children interpret for them.

In terms of prevalence, the data available have been collected by focusing on specific ethnic and linguistic groups and from different populations (e.g. GPs, immigrant adults, children) and thus cannot be considered as representative of the diverse nature of the population with an immigrant background residing in different countries. One of the few exceptions is a US-wide survey aimed at assessing resident physicians' use of professional and non-professional interpreters, showing that 22 per cent of resident physicians in the United States use children as interpreters (Lee *et al.* 2006). Likewise, in 2011, the TRICC Project (Training in Intercultural and Bilingual Competencies in Health and Social Care) surveyed the official policy on interpreting in healthcare in its five European partners (Germany, Italy, the Netherlands, Turkey and the UK) and found that the use of *ad hoc* and informal interpreters (including children) is widespread in all five countries, even though these countries' policies make the use of professional interpreters mandatory (Meeuwesen and Twilt 2011). In a more recent study (Banas *et al.* 2016), 54.1 per cent of the sample comprising 159 adolescents of Hispanic/Latino origin, all attending the same high school in the Midwest of the United States, indicated that they assist family members with healthcare tasks, which included 'talking to the doctor or nurse, reading prescription labels, looking up health information on the Internet, talking to the pharmacist, and filling in medical insurance forms. Less common were talking to the insurance company or finding a doctor' (Banas *et al.* 2016: 900). These studies, although limited to a few specific countries, give an idea of the attitude towards a phenomenon that is generally frowned upon but still tolerated and which, in the absence of more stringent regulations, is becoming normalised.

The review of literature on CLB in healthcare settings shows that researchers have identified advantages and disadvantages associated with having children interpret/translate in this specific context, with the cons far outweighing the pros. The advantages include the fact that child language brokers develop health knowledge and linguistic abilities (Angelelli 2010), as they are exposed to advanced vocabulary and health-related concepts when interpreting (Valdés 2003). They also learn to work together with their parents to contribute to the success of language brokered interactions with healthcare professionals, so that they can actively team up to understand and comprehend health information (Katz 2014). Other advantages include the 'emotional benefits in enjoying helping the family, and benefits to self-esteem in being able to take on a responsible role' (Free *et al.* 2003: 531) as well as an opportunity for young people 'to speak their own language and demonstrate and practice their skills' (Free *et al.* 2003: 531).

The main disadvantages can be subsumed under three main issues: (1) children may not translate information in an accurate way; (2) the translation of legal and medical information may have a negative effect on the parent-child relationship; and (3) the child may be traumatised by the delivery of information about a serious medical condition concerning the child or a person they love. According to the general practitioners involved in Cohen *et al.*'s study, children in their role as language brokers may acquire precocious knowledge of sensitive and delicate topics that may negatively impact on their psychological stability;

the regular dynamics of the family may also be impacted, contributing to the reversal of the traditional adult-child distribution of knowledge and authority (Cohen, Moran-Ellis and Smaje 1999: 183–184). Other studies (e.g. Corona *et al.* 2012; Free *et al.* 2003; Hsieh 2006) describe issues linked to the fact that child language brokers are untrained as interpreters in general and as medical interpreters in particular. Their ages vary. They may not have the necessary linguistic competence in one or both languages involved, and they are also likely to lack the necessary health literacy and the relevant vocabulary (Green *et al.* 2005). All of these could lead the children to 'alter or selectively interpret information instead of interpreting all aspects of the conversation verbatim' (Guntzviller, Jakob and Carreno 2017: 144). Some child language brokers in the Free *et al.* study (2003) also described interpreting in healthcare settings as 'bothering and boring', and noted that it 'could be hard work and could take time away from preferred activities' (Free *et al.* 2003: 531) as well as from school commitments.

One of the dimensions that has recently been the focus of research is the emotional experience of CLB in healthcare. Studies on feelings associated with CLB have yielded mixed or contradictory results and have shown that children are likely to experience varying degrees of stress, and that the feelings attached to their role as language brokers can be both positive and negative (Hall and Guéry 2010), especially depending on the setting (Banas *et al.* 2016). In their study with 76 young bilingual individuals, Green *et al.* (2005) showed that they associated healthcare interpreting with feelings of pride but also unease. For instance, one adolescent explained that he was embarrassed when he had to talk about intimate topics: 'If it's a woman's problem then I can't speak, and it's difficult for my mother and for me, because I feel bad inside that I can't speak for that problem. I am the son, so it's like embarrassment' (Green *et al.* 2005: 2106). However, this study also emphasised how the interviewees 'rarely saw themselves as "inadequate translators" or exploited children, but as skilled mediators, helping to bridge misunderstandings between family members and the public sector' (Green *et al.* 2005: 2108).

However, when CLB occurs in healthcare settings, studies seem to point more towards negative emotional consequences. More specifically, children associated their language brokering activities with feeling awkward and angry when they were caught in the crossfire of disagreements, and by the frustration of not being able to interpret properly. Moreover, they also described feeling embarrassed when they acquired sensitive information about their parents or had to tell parents what to do, and the difficulty of accepting and repeating bad news about their relatives (Free *et al.* 2003: 532).

Antonini's 2015 research demonstrated dramatic differences between how GPs and children perceive CLB situations. While Italian doctors described children as 'natural', 'spontaneous', 'at ease' and 'in their element' when interpreting during a consultation, children more often described that they were embarrassed, scared and worried. Some studies have confirmed that interpreting in situations involving sensitive issues and/or situations with a heavy emotional load due to the broker's attachment to the patients may be traumatic for the child (Meeuwesen and Twilt 2011). As Jacobs *et al.* (1995) report, a 10-year-old girl who interpreted between the medical staff and her parents when her baby brother was being treated later suffered an emotional trauma when her brother died. According to the authors, this trauma was caused by 'the very close involvement that this young child had in the care of her dying younger brother, including her being used as interpreter between her family and the medical staff' (Meeuwesen and Twilt 2011: 474). These studies show that while the communicative challenges of adult discourse may improve children's linguistic and cognitive abilities, the children also run the risk of being overwhelmed by painful experiences and sensitive matters that are inappropriate for them, particularly in highly challenging or emotionally charged situations. The following case study of the In MedIO PUER(I) research group describes both the healthcare professionals' perception of CLB and the personal experiences of children who broker in healthcare (similar to Cohen, Moran-Ellis and Smaje 1999), and as such provides a detailed example of a multi-method research project into the specific matter of CLB and healthcare.

4 Case study: In MedIO PUER(I) research group in Italy

In MedIO PUER(I) was a multi-method study that pioneered CLB research in Italy (described in Antonini 2010: 8–10 and Antonini 2015: 97–98). Aimed at investigating child-mediated exchanges between migrants and the host country, the project gave visibility to a variety of institutions as active participants in triadic exchanges between two monolingual speakers and a bilingual speaker. Previous CLB research mainly dealt with the impact of brokering practices on the psychology and development of children and adolescents, relegating institutions to the background and equating them with the contextual variable of 'setting' (with a few notable exceptions, such as Cohen, Moran-Ellis and Smaje 1999 mentioned in Section 3). The In MedIO PUER(I) study sought to address this imbalance by collecting institutional perceptions, opinions and perspectives on CLB alongside those of children and their families.

During its initial stage, In MedIO PUER(I) focused on the collection of interviews in the Italian city of Forlì in the Emilia-Romagna region. The first goal of that early part of the research was to confirm whether CLB occurred during encounters between migrants and Italian institutions. Second, it aimed to explore whether civil servants or community service providers had, or were aware of, any formal or informal guidelines on how to conduct child-mediated encounters. The third purpose was to collect the service providers' perceptions and impressions about CLB, including any first- or second-hand anecdotes of events that had occurred within their institutions. These questions were asked in the form of in-depth semi-structured interviews and addressed to 10 senior officers from various public institutions or community services that might be approached by migrant citizens in their daily lives, including two schools, two social cooperatives, a trade union, a charity, the municipal registry, a municipal family support centre, and the police office that issued residence permits. In the following paragraphs, we will summarise the data collected specifically from one senior manager of the local hospital, whom we interviewed in the first stage of the project. We will then discuss the results of later interviews with 10 medical practitioners and nurses, and brokering children's perceptions specifically connected with CLB in healthcare settings (collected through questionnaires and a contest).

The interviewed senior manager was part of the Forlì local health unit (*AUSL*) (Cirillo, Torresi and Valentini 2010, Torresi 2014). Contrary to what was reported by all other interviewees working in institutions unrelated to healthcare, the Forlì local health unit could rely on professional interpreting services provided by a local cooperative through a special convention funded by the region Emilia-Romagna. At the time of the interview (2007), the convention covered 2,200 hours of interpreting per year that could be used by all facilities of the Forlì health unit (including general practitioners' offices) according to their needs. Additionally, the local health unit had commissioned a multilingual phrasebook with common questions and answers (such as 'where does it hurt' or 'when did it start'), and GPs and hospital staff could locate the phrase they needed in Italian and then point to the translation in the relevant language. Another significant difference between the interview with the local health unit manager and the rest of the sample of senior service providers was that the health unit manager was not aware of any cases of CLB happening within the local health unit, while acknowledging that the phenomenon probably did occur and could be 'on the increase' (as was later confirmed by interviews with GPs and hospital staff, all of them working for the local health unit).

Spurred by the above-mentioned differences between the healthcare senior officer and the other respondents to the first interviews, the In MedIO PUER(I) group decided to conduct a second round of 10 semi-structured interviews, more specifically aimed at general practitioners and emergency room staff working in the Forlì and Cesena area (Cirillo and Torresi 2013; Cirillo 2014; Antonini 2015: 103–106). The second study focused on the opinions of the GPs and the emergency staff and its aims were as follows: (1) to confirm whether they were aware of the tools mentioned by the local health unit manager (i.e. the free professional interpreting services and the phrasebook); (2) explore their opinions about whether, and to what extent, brokering children contributed to the success of medical encounters with non-Italian-speakers; (3) identify areas or situations in which they thought children should not act as language brokers; and (4) to compare their expectations about professional interpreting versus child language brokering during medical consultations.

After the interview with the local health unit manager, it came as a surprise that the GPs and emergency staff members were evenly split between those who ignored both the option to request professional interpreters and the phrasebook altogether, and those who knew only about the phrasebook (but one of them stated that they had never seen it). Only one GP and one emergency room nurse were aware of the possibility of requesting professional interpreting services through the cooperative mentioned above. However, they both mentioned that such an option was usually neglected because the interpreters were never available on site – they were not supposed to wait on call physically at the hospital, let alone at individual practices, but took appointments that had to be arranged in advance (real-time telephone interpreting was never mentioned as a possibility). The other interviewees seemed to be simply unaware of the convention.

All of the interviewees had witnessed CLB in their own medical practice or hospital ward. Their approach to CLB was generally a pragmatic one. Similar to the doctors who participated in the study by Cohen, Moran-Ellis and Smaje (1999) mentioned in the previous section, they seemed to accept it as a necessary evil, and most highlighted how well child brokers performed, given their young age and lack of training. Three of them considered children and adolescents to be more accurate and trustworthy than adult *ad hoc* interpreters. Those who expressed negative opinions about CLB did not refer to issues related to the brokers' age, but rather to issues related to dialogue interpreting in general, such as 'I'm never sure whether they report what I actually said', or 'it is very time consuming to have them repeat everything I say'.

When asked about particular cases or situations in which they thought CLB should not happen, three interviewees mentioned 'serious illnesses', and another four the sexual and reproductive sphere. One further respondent offered a generic answer that 'it depends on the kind of medical problem'. Interestingly, the remaining two mentioned situations depending on the child's surroundings or subjectivity rather than the nature of the information to be conveyed. One said that children might not understand certain 'nuances' of the medical encounter; the last one stated that CLB should be avoided altogether if the practitioner perceives the child's family to be unsupportive or unable to protect the child from experiences that could prove traumatic.

All 10 interviewees seemed to have higher expectations about professional interpreters than child *ad hoc* brokers, especially in terms of terminological precision and loyalty to the original message. Those values, however, were not acknowledged as the sole or the most important qualities of a medical interpreter – some medical knowledge was also universally mentioned as desirable, perhaps the most important difference between children and professionals. One interviewee stated that she would rather have a child interpret than an adult professional without any training in medicine. Most interviewees mentioned various situations where CLB was preferable to professional interpreting. One interviewee noted that patients might not accept the presence of an unknown adult during the consultation. Another one complained about the additional administrative burden for the doctor whenever a professional is called ('I have to get a special form signed by the patient'), whereas family interpreters are brought in by patients themselves and are their own responsibility. Most interviewees also highlighted the ease, precision and maturity with which child brokers approach their task.

In addition to interviewing the service providers, we also collected children's voices through two main methods – a questionnaire given to young brokers in junior high schools (ages 11–14), and an art contest among primary and junior high school students (ages 6–14). It should be mentioned that the contest was not part of the original design of the In MedIO PUER(I) project, and that its later editions were outside of the project's timeline. However, the research group decided to continue their research after the funded project's official completion, with the idea of progressively expanding and completing the picture on how CLB is practised and perceived in selected Italian locales. In this respect, the data collected through the contest (and all other data collected through the group's subsequent CLB studies) should be considered as a coherent whole.

Although the healthcare setting was not the focus of these parts of the study, several respondents of the questionnaire and participants in the contest did report or recount mediating in healthcare settings or for health emergencies. The broker questionnaire (Cirillo 2017: 297–301) was given in years 2011–2012 to children with a migrant background in seven junior high schools, five of which were in the province of Forlì-Cesena, and two in the nearby city of Bologna. Of the pupils who self-selected as brokers and returned the 277 valid questionnaires of the study, 31 per cent reported having brokered at the doctor's practice or at the hospital, and 27 per cent stated that they had translated doctors' prescriptions and/or medication leaflets.

A deeper insight was provided by the qualitative and subjective data collected through the *Traduttori in Erba* ('Budding translators/interpreters') contest for the best short essay or drawing illustrating the author's experience of brokering (Antonini 2017: 322–324). The first three rounds of the contest, open to all local primary and junior high school students regardless of heritage, were held in 2010, 2011 and 2017. Healthcare-related verbal narratives from the first two editions have already been discussed at length elsewhere (Antonini 2015: 106–109; Antonini 2017), but the overall results suggest that children's first-hand subjective accounts of brokering in medical settings are more adamantly negative than GPs seem to perceive. When children write about their brokering experiences in healthcare, they almost invariably mention feelings of anxiety (mainly for their relatives' health), confusion, inadequacy and fear that the relative's health could get worse due to their poor interpreting. One child reported having to call the emergency number when his grandmother had a heart attack with no one else around. The main feeling associated with that experience – 'scared' – was understandably not focused on the interpreting between his non-Italian-speaking grandmother and the Italian operator, but only on his grandmother's health. Notably, such negative feelings are reported much less frequently in connection with settings unrelated to healthcare. Similarly, of all the drawings submitted for the competition, only two did not depict brokering in bright colours. One of those two portrayed a boy beside a building labelled as the local city hospital, with an ambulance in the background. The drawing is dominated by desaturated cold colours, mainly greys and blues, which are usually associated with sadness and might denote emotional detachment or withdrawal (Torresi 2017: 349–350).

In conclusion, results from the studies conducted by the In MedIO PUER(I) group highlight a dichotomy in the perceptions of CLB in the healthcare setting. Healthcare providers would usually prefer to avoid the practice, but at the same time admit that it can have benefits in certain circumstances and provided that the child is not exposed to harmful or awkward topics. For children who experience CLB in various domains, the healthcare sphere is usually connected with high levels of anxiety and fear that the brokering might be inadequate and lead to serious consequences. This difference in perception highlights the need for more research in order to inform a political and legal framework that is capable of regulating CLB in healthcare settings.

5 Future directions

As illustrated above, brokering children and institutional representatives seem to hold different views and feelings about CLB, especially in the healthcare setting. The very fact that children and adolescents are asked to mediate during medical consultations by their own relatives (most often parents) can create a tension between the concerns for the children's wellbeing and the overriding need for medical consultations. In order to explore this aspect, further research focusing on the perception of families with special regard to healthcare settings is needed. So far, data from families are very limited and emerge from studies with a broader scope on CLB in general.

In those rare cases where such data emerge, they seem to confirm the extremely problematic application of CLB whenever a close relative's health is at stake. When parents have been interviewed alongside their children (Ceccoli 2019: 197), their perceived frequency of CLB occurring at a medical practice or hospital tended to be the reverse of their children's. While 69 per cent of children reported having brokered 'always/often/sometimes' in such contexts (and the remaining 31 per cent 'rarely' or 'never'), 75 per cent of parents reported that the very same children had 'rarely' or 'never' performed CLB in the healthcare settings. It would be useful to replicate Ceccoli's survey with a more specific focus on CLB in healthcare, so as to explore whether the difference in parents' and their children's subjective memories may in any way be related to the phenomena of parent-child role reversal, often referred to in terms of 'adultification' or 'parentification' (Trickett and Jones 2007; Guske 2010; Orellana 2009).

One particularly telling case study, and thus far the only one that acknowledges a parent's feelings and perceptions about CLB's parentification in healthcare, can be found in Vivaldi (2019). Vivaldi interviewed 10 Albanian parents residing in Italy, who had benefited from their own children's brokering at some point of their lives. Healthcare issues emerged only in one account, and were once again associated with strongly negative feelings. The interviewee, an Albanian mother whose baby son had been hospitalised in the local neonatal intensive care unit (NIC), regularly brought her older daughter to the hospital to broker for her. Eventually, the doctors of the NIC ward called a social worker to relieve the girl of some of the full-time brokering she was providing. The social worker assigned the interviewee a professional interpreter, but the mother reported that she still felt dependent on her daughter, psychologically if not linguistically, despite feeling guilty and inadequate as a result of this very dependence. Of course only one interview is not particularly informative, and more ethnographic data needs to be collected among child brokers' families to further explore their experience of CLB in medical and healthcare settings, especially in connection with adultification and parentification issues that have so far been explored from the children's point of view.

Another area where action, rather than research, is urgently necessary is the development of national or super-national guidelines, as well as codes of ethics for healthcare providers working with patients accompanied by children and adolescents acting as brokers. The current legal frameworks described in Section 2 are too often left unheeded, and do not reach beyond the borders of a few countries. Even in those parts of the world where such guidelines are in place, there seems to be little awareness about them and they are frequently obstructed by political decisions. At present, therefore, the decision on whether to accept untrained minors as interpreters in healthcare interactions seems to be universally as unregulated as CLB in all other settings. In this respect, the method of Action Research – a 'collaborative approach to inquiry' that 'seeks to change the social and personal dynamics of the research situation so that the research process enhances the lives of all who participate' (Stringer 2007: 20) would seem particularly promising in terms of both scientific rigour and practical results.

Further reading

Antonini, R. (2015) 'Unseen Forms of Interpreting: Child Language Brokering in Italy', *Cultus: The Journal of Intercultural Mediation and Communication*, 8, pp. 96–112.

The article contains several examples of children's narratives about CLB in healthcare settings, submitted for the *Traduttori in Erba* ('Budding translators/interpreters') school contest briefly described in Section 4.

Cohen, S., Moran-Ellis, J. and Smaje, C. (1999) 'Children as Informal Interpreters in GP Consultations: Pragmatics and Ideology', *Sociology of Health and Illness*, 21(2), pp. 163–186.

The study that broke ground on CLB in healthcare settings, embracing both practical aspects and subjective perceptions. It was also among the first papers to collect the views of institutional representatives on CLB.

Related topics

Healthcare Interpreting Ethics, Dialogue Interpreting in Mental Healthcare, Remote (Telephone) Interpreting in Healthcare Settings

References

Angelelli, C. V. (2010) 'A Professional Ideology in the Making: Bilingual Youngsters Interpreting for Their Communities and the Notion of (No) Choice', *Translation and Interpreting Studies*, 5(1), pp. 94–108.

Antonini, R. (2010) 'The Study of Child Language Brokering: Past, Current and Emerging Research', *mediAzioni*, 10, pp. 1–23.

Antonini, R. (2015) 'Unseen Forms of Interpreting: Child Language Brokering in Italy', *Cultus: The Journal of Intercultural Mediation and Communication*, 8, pp. 96–112.

Antonini, R. (2017) 'Through the Children's Voice: An Analysis of Language Brokering Experiences', in Antonini, R., Cirillo, L., Rossato, L. and Torresi, I. (eds) *Non-professional Interpreting and Translation*. Amsterdam and Philadelphia: John Benjamins, pp. 315–336.
Banas, R. B., Wallis, L. C., Ball, J. W. and Gershon, S. (2016) 'Adolescent Healthcare Brokering: Prevalence, Experience, Impact, and Opportunities', *Journal of School Health*, 86, pp. 898–905.
Ceccoli, F. (2019) 'Parents' and Children's Perspectives on Child Language Brokering: A Comparative Approach', in D'Arcangelo, D., Elefante, C. and Illuminati, V. (eds) *Translating for Children Beyond Stereotypes. Traduire pour la jeunesse au-delà des stéréotypes*. Bologna: Bononia University Press, pp. 189–206.
Cirillo, L. (2014) 'La mediazione linguistica cultura a opera di bambini e adolescenti: lo sguardo degli operatori sanitari della provincia di Forlì-Cesena', in Antonini, R. (ed.) *La mediazione linguistica e culturale non professionale in Italia*. Bologna: Bononia University Press, pp. 117–132.
Cirillo, L. (2017) 'Child Language Brokering in Private and Public Settings: Perspectives from Young Brokers and Their Teachers' in Antonini, R., Cirillo, L., Rossato, L. and Torresi, I. (eds) *Non-professional Interpreting and Translation*. Amsterdam and Philadelphia: John Benjamins, pp. 295–314.
Cirillo, L. and I. Torresi (2013) 'Exploring Institutional Perceptions of Child Language Brokering: Examples from Italian Healthcare settings', in Schäffner, C., Kredens, K. and Fowler, Y. (eds) *Interpreting in a Changing Landscape*. Amsterdam and Philadelphia: John Benjamins, pp. 149–164.
Cirillo, L. Torresi, I. and Valentini, C. (2010) 'Institutional Perceptions of Child Language Brokering in Emilia Romagna', *mediAzioni*, 10, pp. 269–296.
Cohen, S., Moran-Ellis, J. and Smaje, C. (1999) 'Children as Informal Interpreters in GP Consultations: Pragmatics and Ideology', *Sociology of Health and Illness*, 21(2), pp. 163–186.
Corona, R., Stevens, L. F., Halfond, R. W., Shaffer, C. M., Reid-Quiñones, K. and González, T. (2012) 'A Qualitative Analysis of What Latino Parents and Adolescents Think and Feel About Language Brokering', *Journal of Child and Family Studies*, 21, pp. 788–798.
Department of Health and Human Services (2016) 'Nondiscrimination in Health Programs and Activities', *Federal Register*, 81(96), pp. 31376–31473.
Diamond, L. C., Schenker, Y. Curry, L., Bradley, E. H. and Fernández, A. (2008) 'Getting By: Underuse of Interpreters by Resident Physicians', *Journal of General Internal Medicine*, 24(2), pp. 256–262.
European Union Agency for Fundamental Rights (2013) *Inequalities and Multiple Discrimination in Access to and Quality of Healthcare*. Luxembourg: Publications Office of the European Union.
Flores, G. (2006) 'Language Barriers to Healthcare in the United States', *New England Journal of Medicine*, 355, pp. 229–231.
Free C., Green, J., Bhavnani, V. and Newman, A. (2003) 'Bilingual Young People's Experiences of Interpreting in Primary Care: A Qualitative Study', *British Journal of General Practice*, 53(492), pp. 530–535.
Green, J., Free, C., Bhavnani, V. and Newman, T. (2005) 'Translators and Mediators: Bilingual Young People's Accounts of Their Interpreting Work in Healthcare', *Social Science and Medicine*, 60(9), pp. 2097–2110.
Guntzviller, L. M., Jakob, D. J. and Carreno, L. M. (2017) 'Latino Children's Ability to Interpret in Health Settings: A Parent-Child Dyadic Perspective on Child Health Literacy', *Communication Monographs*, 84(2), pp. 143–163.
Guske, I. (2010) 'Familial and Institutional Dependence on Bilingual and Bicultural Go-betweens – Effects on Minority Children', *mediAzioni*, 10, pp. 325–345.
Hall, N. and Sham, S. (2007) 'Language Brokering as Young People's Work: Evidence from Chinese Adolescents in England', *Language and Education*, 21(1), pp. 16–30.
Hall, N. and Guéry, F. (2010) 'Child Language Brokering: Some Considerations', *mediAzioni*, 10, pp. 24–46.
Harris, B. (1976) 'The Importance of Natural Translation', *Working Papers in Bilingualism*, 12, pp. 96–114.
Harris, B. (1980) 'Elicited Translation by a Three-year Old English/French Bilingual, part I', in Ingram, D., Penn, F. and Dale, P. (eds) *Proceedings of the First International Congress for the Study of Child Language*. Lanham, MD: University Press of America, pp. 610–631.

Jacobs, B., Kroll, L., Green, J. and David, T. J. (1995) 'The Hazards of Using a Child as an Interpreter', *Journal of the Royal Society of Medicine*, August 88(8), pp. 474–475.
Hsieh, E. (2006) 'Understanding Medical Interpreters: Reconceptualizing Bilingual Health Communication', *Health Communication*, 20(2), pp. 177–186.
Juckett, G. and Unger, K. (2014) 'Appropriate Use of Medical Interpreters', *American Family Physician*, 90(7), pp. 476–480.
Katz, V. (2014) 'Children as Brokers of Their Immigrant Families' Healthcare Connections', *Social Problems*, 61(2), pp. 194–215.
La Puma, J., Stocking, C., LaVoie, D. and Darling, C. (1991) 'When Physicians Treat Members of Their Own Families', *The New England Journal of Medicine*, 325(18), pp. 1290–1294.
Lee, K. C. *et al.* (2006) 'Resident Physicians' Use of Professional and Nonprofessional Interpreters: A National Survey', *The Journal of the American Medical Association*, 296(9), pp. 1050–1053.
Levetown, M. (2008) 'Communicating with Children and Families: From Everyday Interactions to Skill in Conveying Distressing Information', *Pediatrics*, 121(5), pp. e1441–e1460.
Liu, Y and Zhang, W. (2019) 'Unity in Diversity: Mapping Healthcare Interpreting Studies (2007–2017)', *Medical Education Online*, 24(1), pp. 1–14.
Malakoff, M. and Hakuta, K. (1991) 'Translation Skill and Metalinguistic Awareness in Bilinguals', in Bialystok, E. (ed.) *Language Processing in Bilingual Children*. Cambridge: Cambridge University Press, pp. 141–166.
Meeuwesen, L. and Twilt, S. (2011) *"If You Don't Understand What I Mean…" Interpreting in Health and Social Care*. Utrecht: Centre for Social Policy and Intervention Studies.
Meyer, B., Pawlack, B. and Kliche, O. (2010) 'Family Interpreters in Hospitals: Good Reasons for Bad Practice?', *mediAzioni*, 10, pp. 297–324.
Orellana, M. (2009) *Translating Childhoods: Immigrant Youth, Language, and Culture*. Piscataway, NJ: Rutgers University Press.
Orellana, M., Dorner, M. and Pulido, L. (2003) 'Accessing Assets: Work as Family Translators or "Para-phrasers"', *Social Problems*, 50(4), pp. 505–524.
Orellana, M., Reynolds, J., Dorner, L. and Meza, M. (2003) 'In Other Words: Translating or "Para-phrasing" as a Family Literacy Practice in Immigrant Households', *Reading Research Quarterly*, 38(1), pp. 12–34.
Ozolins, U. (2010) 'Factors That Determine the Provision of Public Service Interpreting: Comparative Perspectives on Government Motivation and Language Service Implementation', *JoSTrans*, 14, pp. 194–215.
Pöchhacker, F. (2008) 'Krankheit, Kultur, Kinder, Kommunikation: Die Nichte als Dolmetscherin', *Curare*, 31(2–3), pp. 133–142.
Rossato, L. (2014) 'Gli insegnanti e la mediazione linguistica nelle scuole italiane: tra interazione e integrazione', in Antonini, R. (ed.) *La mediazione linguistica e culturale non professionale in Italia*. Bologna: Bononia University Press, pp. 33–54.
Rice, S. (2014) 'Language Liabilities. To Avoid Errors, Hospitals Urged To Use Qualified Interpreters for Patients With Limited English', *Modern Healthcare*, 44(35), pp. 16–20.
Rudvin, M. (2006) 'Issues of Culture and Language in the Training of Language Mediators for Public Services in Bologna: Matching Market Needs and Training', in Londei, D., Miller, D. R. and Puccini, P. (eds) *Insegnare le Lingue/Culture Oggi: Il Contributo dell'Interdisciplinarità*. Bologna: Asterisco, pp. 57–72.
Shannon, S. (1990) 'English in the Barrio: The Quality of Contact among Immigrant Children', *Hispanic Journal of Behavioral Sciences*, 12(3), pp. 256–276.
Stringer, E. T. (2007) *Action Research*, 3rd edition. Thousand Oaks, CA: Sage Publications.
Torresi, I. (2014) 'Child Language Brokering: Voce alle istituzioni', in Antonini, R. (ed.) *La mediazione linguistica e culturale non professionale in Italia*. Bologna: Bononia University Press, pp. 56–89.
Torresi, I. (2017) 'Seeing Brokering in Bright Colours: Participatory Artwork Elicitation in CLB Research', in Antonini, R., Cirillo, L., Rossato, L. and Torresi, I. (eds) *Non-professional Interpreting and Translation*. Amsterdam and Philadelphia: John Benjamins, pp. 337–358.
Trickett, E. J. and Jones, C. J. (2007) 'Adolescent Culture Brokering and Family Functioning: A Study of Families from Vietnam', *Cultural Diversity and Ethnic Minority Psychology*, 13(2), pp. 143–150.

Tse, L. (1995) 'Language Brokering Among Latino Students: Prevalence, Attitudes, and School Performance', *Hispanic Journal of Behavioral Sciences*, 17(2): 180–193.
Tse, L. (1996) 'Language Brokering in Linguistic Minority Communities: The Case of Chinese- And Vietnamese-American Students', *The Bilingual Research Journal*, 20(3–4), pp. 485–498.
Valdés, G. (2003) *Expanding Definitions of Giftedness: The Case of Young Interpreters from Immigrant Countries*. Mahwah, NJ: Erlbaum.
Vivaldi, E. (2019) *Il Child Language Brokering in famiglia: La parola ai genitori.* MA dissertation. University of Bologna.
Yee, L., Díaz, M. and Spitzer, T. (2003) *California Assembly Bill 292*. Available at: Info.sen.ca.gov/pub/bill/ASM/ab_0251_0300/ab_292_ bill_20030206_introduced.html (Accessed: 28 June 2019).

12

Healthcare interpreting ethics

A critical review

Robyn K. Dean

1 Introduction

This chapter addresses ethics in medical or healthcare interpreting and specifically focuses on interpreting situations where the patient does not share, or have a sufficient proficiency in, the language of their healthcare providers. Interpreters working in healthcare settings can seek out ethical guidance from multiple sources. All professions have various types of *ethical content material* (Hill 2004: 131), which both compels practitioners to take action and constrains action. The most obvious source of such ethical guidance is a formal code of ethics or code of professional conduct. There are, however, many other types of ethical content material. Normative ethical material can be found in sanctioned ethical documents (e.g. standards of care), prominent textbooks or other written sources, and even the ethical standards set by prominent educators or scholars in a field (Dean 2015: 96). All of these sources collectively have a normative effect (Hill 2004: 140); that is, they provide some guidance on what is effective or ineffective or what is right and wrong in professional practice.

This chapter reviews these sanctioned materials – ethical codes and standards of practice in healthcare settings.[1] Some attention is given to practice norms outlined in research studies, and other discursive items that might have ethical weight for healthcare interpreters. The chapter concludes with suggestions for further movement toward improving healthcare ethics for practicing interpreters.

2 Ethical content material: ethical codes

An ethics review of any profession begins with the normative ethical material that is sanctioned by professional organisations and other such authoritative bodies that oversee the work of its practitioners. The same would be true for the field of translation and interpreting.

Most interpreters (and translators) are trained to work as generalists. That is, they tend to focus on improving their linguistic and translation skills without a significant emphasis on any particular domain, such as law or medicine. As such, it is important to

 DOI: 10.4324/9781003167983-16

consider generalist ethical codes within translation and interpreting as equally intended for healthcare interpreting contexts.

The generalist ethical codes in the field of translation can offer healthcare translators and interpreters some ethical guidance. Codes of professional conduct or codes of ethics (CoE) have been authored by an array of stakeholders. Most commonly, CoE are created for members in a professional organisation. They can also be created by private agencies or by governmental entities. Some CoE have been written for setting-specific purposes such as legal, educational, and medical settings (Mikkelson 2000: 50).

General translation and interpreting CoE tend to cite a broad range of ethical ideals; there does not appear to be too much variability in guidance across various subfields. In their international study, Leneham and Napier (2003: 79) found several key elements emphasised in CoE: *professionalism, confidentiality, competence, impartiality, accuracy, employment, professional development, and professional solidarity*. McDonough Dolmaya (2011) found similar tenets in her investigation of 16 ethical codes: *accuracy, fidelity, professionalism, competence, and broader issues of employment* (see also Kalina 2015: 68).

The overlap between these codes is significant. It has been argued that the subfields of written translation and interpreting (both conference and community interpreting) share the same set of ethical principles (Kalina 2015: 67). Yet, others have suggested that the generalist CoE limit the ethical options for community interpreters and result in insufficient guidance for ethical practice (Angelelli 2004; Dean and Pollard 2018; Leneham and Napier 2003; McDonough Dolmaya 2011). Some have further proposed that setting-specific ethical codes are therefore warranted (Angelelli 2004; Leneham and Napier 2003). Whether or not an ethical code specific to healthcare interpreting would provide significantly greater ethical guidance for interpreters in healthcare is explored next.

The International Medical Interpreters Association (IMIA) is an international organisation with chapters in 15 countries, including Brazil, Canada, China, Costa Rica, Egypt, India, Italy, Japan, Mexico, Russia, South Africa, South Korea, and Spain. The IMIA is based in the United States as is the National Council on Interpreting in Health Care (NCIHC). The IMIA published its ethical code in 2010[2] and the NCIHC in 2004.[3] The Japanese Association of Medical Interpreters (JAMI) established its Code of Ethics for professional medical interpreters in 2011.[4] Table 12.1 compares the ethical tenets of generalist codes with healthcare-specific codes gleaned from these associations' documents.

As is evident in Table 12.1, most ethical tenets specific to healthcare overlap with the tenets from generalist's codes. Ethical tenets that are unique to the healthcare-specific ethics documents include: advocacy, cultural interface/awareness, education and collaboration, interpreter privacy and health, societal contributions, and professional relationships. Further review of these tenets shows that while they use terms associated with healthcare-specific settings and professionals, there is not much offered that would be distinguishable from another setting. In other words, the healthcare terms that are used in these tenets (e.g. *healthcare professionals* or *biomedical culture*) could be readily replaced with their counterparts from another setting and still read as true and applicable. For the healthcare-specific codes to have a substantive application to healthcare, there would need to be additional content on the impact to those service-users in healthcare settings, such as providers' effectiveness and patients' health.

Furthermore, the same tenet may be used differently in different codes. In the NCIHC Code (2004), for instance, the tenet of advocacy is specifically identified as possibly needed for the sake of *good health outcomes*, whereas in the IMIA (2010) advocacy is only noted

Table 12.1 Comparison of ethical tenets of generalist codes with healthcare-specific codes

Generalist CoE (Leneham and Napier, 2003)	*Generalist CoE (McDonough Dolmaya 2001)*	*Healthcare CoE IMIA (International; 15 countries)*	*Healthcare CoE NCIHC (US)*	*Healthcare CoE JAMI (Japan)*
Confidentiality		Confidentiality	Confidentiality	Confidentiality
Accuracy	Accuracy	Accuracy	Accuracy	Accuracy
Impartiality		Impartiality	Impartiality	Impartiality
Competence	Competence			Discretion
Professional development		Professional development	Professional development	Professional development
			Respect	
Professionalism	Professionalism	Professionalism	Professionalism/ Role Boundaries	
		Advocacy	Advocacy	Advocacy
		Cultural interface	Cultural awareness	
Employment	Employment			
Professional solidarity				
	Fidelity			
				Education and Collaboration
				Interpreter privacy and health
				Societal contributions

as potentially necessary *for good communication*. Good health outcomes are unique to medicine whereas good communication is arguably important in any setting.

In other instances, in all three healthcare-specific ethical codes, unique healthcare content (e.g. concerns for the welfare of the patient) is noted. Only those tenets that specifically identify consequences to patients and providers are noted in italics in Table 12.2.

This review of relevant ethical codes raises the question of whether or not healthcare-specific ethical codes offer greater ethical guidance for practitioners or at least, do so in their current form. Standards of practice documents are explored later for their contribution to ethical guidance in interpreting practice. However, before additional ethical content material is explored, it is important to review some terms from the broader field of ethics. These definitions will both clarify and help to frame an examination of other types of ethical material in healthcare interpreting.

3 Common ethical terms defined

The question, 'What is the role of the interpreter?' is often used to begin discussions on the expected behaviours of interpreters. In response, practitioners, researchers, and educators typically respond with behavioural ideals conveyed through the use of metaphor. They might say: 'Think of an interpreter as *a bridge*, *a co-participant*, or *an advocate*.' Conversations in healthcare interpreting have also relied on the use of metaphors (Davidson 2000; Hsieh 2008).

Table 12.2 Unique healthcare ethical material stated in ethical codes

	NCIHC Code of Ethics	*IMIA Code of Ethics*	*JAMI Code of Ethics*
Confidentiality	Recognises the importance of keeping information confidential *except when doing so will result in harm to patients or others.*	Recognises the importance of keeping information confidential *except in the specific instances of self-harm or abuse.*	No unique healthcare ethical content.
Accuracy	Specific concern for the medical interview and the importance of all data being faithfully conveyed due to *clinical consequences.*	Includes the subtopic of *ensuring informed consent.* Interpreters are encouraged to work in concert with the informed consent process.	No unique healthcare ethical content.
Advocacy	All healthcare workers including interpreters are expected to work in ways that avoid harm and advance the *patients' welfare.*	Identified as a derivative of beneficence. Interpreters may need to *raise patients' awareness to laws that prohibit discrimination.*	Professional Medical Interpreters respect the dignity and rights of all people to live a *healthy* cultural life and to *respect patients' independence in pursuing it.*

In past publications, my co-author and I have critiqued the use of rhetorical devices such as 'role' and 'metaphor' as a means of discussing ethics; these terms and constructs fall under the category of *descriptive ethics* and therefore, differ from how other professionals engage in discussions of *normative* ethical behaviour (Dean and Pollard 2018). As such, the question about the role of the interpreter as it is related to ethics is more accurately conveyed through the construct of *responsibility*. In other words, to make the question *normative* is to instead ask, 'What is the interpreter responsible for?' The construct of responsibility is more readily recognised as a normative ethical term (Dean and Pollard 2011). We have further argued that answers to questions of responsibility should be reframed through a catalogue of values and not through a series of metaphors (Dean and Pollard 2018: 57–60). Regarding healthcare interpreting, the question should instead be framed as, 'What are the responsibilities of the healthcare interpreter?'

This shift from the use of metaphors to the use of values is necessary when interpreters engage with other professionals. The latter, e.g. doctors, lawyers, teachers, social workers, to name a few, are taught to evaluate ethical actions through a *normative lens* and would likely be confused by some of the terms the interpreting field uses to talk about *the interpreting role*. The use of metaphors leads interpreters to think of themselves *like something else* (a conduit, a participant, an advocate). It is more effective to assume the responsibility of a particular set of values, as is typical for service-based professions such as doctors and nurses (Dean and Pollard 2018).

Normative ethics are those values, rules, or principles used to evaluate the ethics of a decision. The term descriptive ethics is used in the ethics field to describe actions without any type of evaluative element. The statement, *the interpreter did not interpret the conversation she could hear about another patient* is stated in a descriptive manner. It is also descriptive to say that the interpreter in this case was behaving like a filter, a gatekeeper, or a judge. However, to be normative and to have an element of evaluation within the realm of healthcare, the behaviour should be linked to a value in healthcare. Therefore, the action could also be stated as, the interpreter *respected the privacy* of another patient when she chose not to interpret overheard conversations. Respecting patient privacy is an established healthcare norm. As such, this type of statement would be more recognisable to healthcare professionals.

In professional ethics, the term *normative* should not be confused with the term *prescriptive*. Prescriptive is often used in a negative way to describe pre-determined actions or a type of behavioural rigidity. While it is true that normative ethics *can be* prescriptive, normative ethics can also allow for behavioural flexibility – a flexibility within the parameters set by a catalogue of normative material like values and principles.

Often the deontological or rule-based approach to decisions is perceived of as the prescriptive brand of normative ethics. Teleological or goal-based decisions, while still normative, allow for behavioural flexibility. A deontological approach is characterised by its list of rules whereas a teleological approach is characterised by a list of values. Unlike rules which guide the practitioner to a right and wrong choice, values identify multiple effective and ethical choices (Dean and Pollard 2005: 270). In professional ethics, the consequences of a practitioner's decisions are assessed in terms of which professional values are prioritised by the decision or whether they are prioritised at all. For example, imagine the decision that needs to be made by mental healthcare providers when they are faced with a patient who has suicidal thoughts and intentions but who makes assurances about their safety and asks to be discharged to go home. That provider is facing the choice between two valid but conflicting principles. The first is to maintain the safety of the patient and the other is to respect the individual's autonomy (free from controlling and constraining behaviours). The provider has to uphold one value while forfeiting the other. These are the very same teleological decisions that healthcare interpreters must make about their own practice (Dean and Pollard 2018).

Normative ethics establishes the *shoulds* – how a person *should* act in a given situation. Whether that *should* is best conveyed through rules (deontology) or values (teleology) is determined by many factors. Ethical codes of service professions (such as those professionals who work in healthcare) almost exclusively come to be articulated through values. However, the ethical codes found in community interpreting have traditionally been articulated through rules (Cokely 2000; Dean and Pollard 2011). Many have found rules unhelpful because, like other service professionals, community interpreters encounter highly nuanced contexts. Instead of a list of dos and don'ts, interpreters should instead be taught to apply values to each situation referred to in the ethics field as *specified principlism*[5] (Beauchamp and Childress 2012: 17–24; Dean and Pollard 2011: 157–158). It has yet to be determined or at least stated in overt terms which values interpreters should be responsible for. There are however, established theories that offer possible guidance in how these values might be determined.

Vermeer's (1989/2000) Skopos theory guides the practitioner towards considering the aims, goals, and objectives of the client and/or the expectations of the target audience. In healthcare interpreting, the audience or the clients are providers and patients. The aims and goals of a healthcare provider, and arguably those individuals seeking their services, are governed by the values inherent in biomedical ethics. While biomedical ethics can be traced back to the ancient times of Hippocrates, it was still in its nascent stages throughout most of the 20th century (Raupich and Vollman 2011).

The *Principles of Biomedical Ethics* by Thomas Beauchamp and James Childress (2012/1985), now in its 7th edition, is credited with creating a systematic and standardised analysis of healthcare principles. Beauchamp and Childress (2012) derived the four core principles of biomedical ethics from a series of universal moral ideals (e.g. nurture the young and dependent). While it was originally written in regard to biomedical ethics, others have proposed that these principles undergird all service-based professions (Dean and Pollard 2018: 59; Jonsen 1995: 248). The four core principles are: *respect for autonomy, non-maleficence, beneficence*, and *justice*, and are defined as follows.

Respect for autonomy: Most know the term autonomy to mean allowing individuals to make decisions for themselves – to have the freedom to direct their own destiny by the choices they make. However, in healthcare this principle is operationalised by two types of *obligation*: positive obligation and negative obligation. In this case, the terms positive and negative refer to the presence of something (positive) or the absence of something (negative). These terms are used the same way in medicine (e.g. a positive test result means the presence of something, such as cancerous cells). Therefore, respecting someone's autonomy in a negative obligation manner would be to, for example, allow an individual to make decisions for themselves (i.e. self-determinacy) in the absence of controlling or constraining behaviours (Beauchamp and Childress 2012: 107).

Non-maleficence and beneficence: While these two principles share commonalities and are often identified and discussed in tandem (as in NCIHC 2004: 8), they are not ethically the same. Non-maleficence dictates that practitioners should not inflict harm, where harm is defined as, 'the thwarting, defeating, or setting back of some party's interest' (Beauchamp and Childress 2012: 153). It is the value first articulated by Hippocrates in his 'First, do no harm'. Beneficence carries a greater ethical obligation than non-maleficence. Beneficence is not just avoiding the direct act of inflicting harm, but protecting and removing other potential harms (as cited in Dean 2015: 55–56). It is also characterised by those actions which contribute to the welfare of another (Beauchamp and Childress 2012: 202).

Justice: The final core principle is justice which can be further defined by a particular justice theory. There are many theories of justice: distributive, libertarian, egalitarian, to name a few (Beauchamp and Childress 2012: 253–264). Not in every situation, but certainly in most professional service settings, the conceptualisation of justice is utilitarian in nature. Utilitarian is often described as the greatest good for the greatest number of people.

Seeking ethical guidance from established ethical norms in healthcare and working in accordance with these values is to firmly root healthcare interpreters in a time-honoured ethical foundation. The four core principles are not to supplant ethical norms established by either generalist or setting-specific ethical codes, as discussed above, but to enhance them. These four core principles and the values that grow out of them can be added to the values that healthcare interpreters are responsible for. That is, instead of asking, what is the role of the interpreter in healthcare settings, the normative question could be framed as, 'What values established by the healthcare setting should similarly compel or contain the actions of the interpreter?'

The following illustration demonstrates how the values of the setting dictate patient, provider, and interpreter behaviour: in a psychiatric inpatient unit, the purpose is to keep patients and staff safe. Safety is the main purpose of the setting and this purpose dictates decisions at every level. It dictates the very decision about admitting (or not) suitable patients to the unit – only those who are an imminent harm to themselves or others are admitted (i.e. to keep them and others safe). The unit is almost always locked and patients are not permitted to leave without the supervision or the permission of the staff. Safety also drives the behaviours of individual clinicians. As an example, no jewellery or ties should be worn in the presence of patients who might seek to use them to cause harm. Clinicians are often discouraged from meeting with patients alone in the patient's room and are instructed to never let the patient move between the clinician and the door. Therefore, in this shared values-based approach to interpreting ethics, the interpreter's behaviours *should* reflect a similar concern for patient safety. That is, interpreters should work in collaboration with (or at least not against) the purpose and values of the setting (Dean and Pollard 2013: 56; Pym 2000: 182).

The challenge is that most interpreters are not taught what the setting-specific values are nor how to operationalise them (i.e. how these values might be reflected in their decisions). If an interpreter did not fully appreciate the value of patient safety in the example of a psychiatric unit, they could inadvertently make decisions that compromised patient safety. Not only should interpreters follow the safety lead of the service professionals in the setting (e.g. similar placement in a room with a patient), but should actively apply the safety value in interpreting-specific decisions. As an example, an interpreter may intentionally choose not to interpret something overheard by a patient in another room if they determine that it is likely to cause additional stress and therefore, instigate possible unsafe behaviour. In other words, the decisions that interpreters make in a given setting need to be evaluated based on the values of the setting and not only evidenced in interpreting (such as, accuracy, impartiality, etc.). If they were only evaluated based on the values included in a generalist code of interpreting, then the interpreter might be compelled by the value of fidelity or completeness (e.g. everything is interpreted) and therefore, interpret all material heard, regardless of concerns for safety. Just like the mental healthcare provider in the above example who had to choose between the value of safety and respect for autonomy of a suicidal patient, the interpreter in this example must choose between safety and fidelity.

The preambles to both the International Medical Interpreters Association (IMIA) and the American National Council on Interpreting in Health Care (NCIHC) do include a series of core values. Both the NCIHC (2004: 8–9) and the IMIA (2010: 1–2) directly identify *beneficence* as one of its core values but not the other three (i.e. respect for autonomy, non-maleficence, and justice), at least not in those terms. Instead, they identify: *fidelity*, *respect for the importance of culture and cultural differences* (NCIHC 2004), *transparency, right to equal treatment, confidentiality,* and *informed consent* (IMIA 2010). The four principles put forward by Beauchamp and Childress are deemed *core* or foundational in healthcare because they are intended to generate other related ethical tenets. For example, right to equal treatment is arguably an outgrowth of justice and informed consent, or the intention that all patients understand and choose freely from available treatment options, is an outgrowth of respect for autonomy.

This contribution has thus far focused on ethical content material in biomedical ethics, generalist ethical codes in interpreting, and those ethical codes specific to healthcare interpreting. The next section returns to a review of available ethical content material for healthcare interpreters. This includes other ethical documents such as standards of practice and norms established by practice and discussions about practice.

4 Other ethical content material

4.1 Standards of practice

Standards of care or standards of practice (SoP) documents are another source of sanctioned ethical content that are designed to be more situationally-specific than broad ethical codes. Both the IMIA and the NCIHC have standards of practice documents. The IMIA (2007) and NCIHC (2005) SoP documents are different in length and structure. The NCIHC (2005) SoP document is 12 pages and devotes the majority of the document to listing each ethical tenet and its corresponding standards, with each standard illustrated with an example from healthcare. The IMIA SoP is almost 50 pages. The majority of the document (about 30 pages) serves as an assessment tool for each of the ethical tenets and the accompanying 27 standards using a Likert scale from 5 to 1 to indicate the degree to which an individual demonstrates behaviours that indicate mastery.

In the NCIHC (2005) national standards document, the original nine tenets listed above are illustrated with 32 standards. The nine tenets each have between two to eight separate standards. These standards further illustrate what is meant by each ethical tenet, including an example of such from healthcare. Also included for each tenet is an objective and a related ethical principle. Those interested in investigating these standards in greater detail are encouraged to download these documents from the NCIHC website (also see the Further Reading section).

The IMIA's (2007) SoP breaks their *27 standards* down into categories of three duties: Duty A: Interpretation; Duty B: Cultural Interface; Duty C: Ethical Behaviour. The duty of interpretation is recognised as the primary task of the interpreter and is defined as, 'convert a message uttered in one source language into an equivalent message in the target language so that the intended recipient of the message responds to it as if he or she heard it in the original' (2007: 13). To fully engage in the duty of cultural interface (duty B), interpreters must understand the inextricable nature of language and culture and therefore, 'Interpreting in the health care arena requires the interpreter to understand the ways in which culturally based beliefs affect the presentation, course, and outcomes of illness as well as perceptions of wellness and treatment' (2007: 15). Lastly, under ethical behaviour (duty C), interpreters are discouraged from abusing the power that they have as the only person in the room who understands both languages. They are also encouraged to keep information about the encounter confidential. Each one of these duties is further explained with 27 standards of best practice examples (Duty A = 18 standards; Duty B = 2 standards; and Duty C = 7 standards; a full list of these standards can be found in Appendix A).

After a review of the IMIA's 27 listed standards, it appears that a majority of these ethical items are already identified in generalist ethics. However, new and distinguishable ethical directives relevant to healthcare interpreting are noted in A-4, A-15, A-16, B-2 and C-7. As a reminder, these items are not explained in written text, but instead offered as a series of behaviours that indicate (or not) mastery of this standard – as if this document is intended for assessment use. The behaviours that demonstrate mastery of the standards that identify new ethical material (A-4, A-15, A-16, B-2, and C-7) is included in the appendix for additional review.

These standards, when further defined by the illustrative behaviours, do seem to indicate that healthcare interpreters need to be concerned about values such as patient welfare (non-maleficence, beneficence), continuity of care (perhaps an outgrowth of justice), and discrimination (non-maleficence and justice).

There are a few mental healthcare-specific standards of practice, published by The Association of Sign Language Interpreters in the UK,[6] the Registry of Interpreters for the Deaf in the US,[7] and the Mental Health Interpreting Guidelines for Interpreters in Australia.[8] Of these three standards of practice documents, the Australian document – developed in partnership with Monash University and Language Loop, and endorsed by the Australian Institute of Interpreters and Translators and the Australian Sign Language Interpreters Association – is the most extensive (over 50 pages). Mental Health Interpreting has arguably enjoyed a longer and more extensive discussion on ethical practice. This is due in part to the more pronounced role of communication in the delivery of mental health services. While communication is important in all aspects of healthcare, in mental healthcare, it is the main avenue for both diagnosis and treatment. Therefore, mental health interpreting ethical documents are more likely to reveal an advanced level of ethical expectations than what would be typical in healthcare.

4.2 Practice and professional norms

Beyond sanctioned ethical documents, healthcare interpreters can seek guidance in their colleagues' practice – the patterns of action that seem to convey a practice norm. Toury defined norms as 'values or ideals shared by a certain community as to what is right and wrong, adequate and inadequate' (1980: 57) and proposed that they are deliberately variable in nature (Toury 1998: 12).

Sanctioned ethical documents can be, or at least *can be perceived as* prescriptive. The emergence of descriptive translation studies or DTS (Chesterman 1993; Marzocchi 2005) was driven by this perception and the desire to understand translators' practices irrespective of prescriptive standards (Pym 2001: 129). Like translation, there was evidence of a prescriptive nature in interpreting that was later countered with data that found that interpreters' practice decisions deviated from these rigid expectations. Interpreters were expected to behave in the least intrusive ways possible and to merely transfer the message between interlocutors, and were discouraged from concerning themselves with other aspects of the communication event (e.g. whether or not the patient understands the treatment plan). With DTS, there was a shift in interpreting studies away from *prescription* and toward *description* (see, e.g. the seminal study of Wadensjö 1998).

Studies into the actual behaviours (or norms) of interpreters have been one of the main sources of research in community interpreting, and especially in the healthcare setting. As mentioned above, interpreting scholarship tends to use roles and metaphors for discussing interpreters' behaviours. These role metaphors are distinguishable from one another by the degree of involvement of the interpreter, from the least active/involved (e.g. conduit) to the more active/involved (e.g. advocate).

In a recent and extensive review of the research involving healthcare interpreters, Brisset, Leanza and Laforest (2013) reported principal findings centred on three themes: interpreters' roles and behaviours (e.g. Hsieh 2008); problems associated with working with interpreters (e.g. Davidson 2001); and typical communication characteristics when working with interpreters (e.g. Fatahi *et al.* 2008). The first theme, interpreters' roles is the one most applicable to this discussion since the term role is the apparent mechanism through which the field discusses behaviour and right-action. Below is a list of some of the ways in which the authors of the reviewed studies described interpreters' roles using metaphors or other descriptors:

Hsieh (2008):	Conduit, advocate, manager, and professional
Kaufert and Koolage (1984)	Language interpreter, informant, cultural broker, advocate
Hasselkus (1992)	Facilitator, intermediary and direct source
Hatton and Webb (1993)	Voice box, collaborator, excluder
Drennan (1999)	Language and culture specialist, patient advocate, and institutional therapist
Davidson (2001)	Co-diagnostician, institutional gatekeeper

Similar to many other studies, Brisset and her colleagues (2013) concluded their review to suggest that interpreters' behaviours fell along a continuum. The use of a continuum or a spectrum to describe the behaviours of interpreters is not unique (see Dean and Pollard 2005; Llewellyn-Jones and Lee 2013). Major and Napier (2019) conducted a case study where healthcare interpreters' actions and decisions were plotted along a series of continua. Regardless of whether a series of metaphors or continuum are used, all of these studies conclude in the same way – interpreters behave in flexible ways and that flexibility is based on contextual factors. This is further evidence for what has been repeatedly emphasised in the field of interpreting studies since the 1980s (e.g. Angelelli 2004; Wadensjö 1998).

Research into interpreters' practice decisions is vital to the development of the field – as it was in translation studies with the application of DTS. Investigations into practitioners' actual behaviours is where a profession can identify the *norms of behaviour* and possibly gain ethical guidance to benefit the field at large. Yet, often times the interpreters' behaviours that researchers have identified are abstracted into metaphor or conventions of role. In other words, research studies usually conclude with evidence that interpreters are not behaving according to prescriptive codes. Instead researchers find practitioners engaging in behaviours that reveal a more action-oriented and context-driven manner. These behaviours, instead of being evaluated by how they advance the values of the setting, are left in their descriptive form by reinforcing or inventing a series of new metaphors (as in the above examples). While those metaphors act as descriptions of behaviours, they are not designed to *evaluate* behaviours.

As explained earlier, in the field of ethics, effective and ethical behaviour are not measured by descriptors but through a normative lens – those values, principles, and rules that measure the rightness of an action. Using descriptors to evaluate actions is similar to the analogy of trying to measure a room by a colour instead of through established metrics, like feet or metres. Research into the behaviours of practitioners need not only be descriptive. It can and should make substantive contributions to normative ethical material. Pym argues that this step of evaluation is necessary, stating: 'Translators, teachers, students, critics, policy-makers rightly expect our research to have something to say on the matter [of ethics]' (2000: 181). In other words, there needs to be an additional step beyond merely describing the interpreters' behaviours. That step requires the use of normative ethical material (i.e. values, principles, and rules) to evaluate those behaviours. In the case of healthcare interpreters, this is reasonably done through normative ethical material already existing in healthcare, such as the four core principles discussed above (*respect for autonomy, non-maleficence, beneficence*, and *justice*).

One way in which descriptive terms have been wrongly used as a normative device is the use of the term 'advocate' in healthcare interpreting. It is not uncommon for the term advocacy to be used for and by healthcare interpreters (sign language interpreters might use the term 'ally' instead). Certainly, there are appropriate times when the terms 'advocacy' or 'advocate' are being used – such as in instances of intentional discrimination based on race, ethnicity, gender, etc. It is out of the concern for patients' *just treatment* that likely drives the interpreter to deliberate on whether or not they should intervene. Arguably, such interventions could be seen as a derivative of Beauchamp and Childress's core principle of justice.

What is arguably controversial about interpreters claiming to be advocates is not the calling out of unjust treatment; it is merely the poor word choice of 'advocate'. At least in the United States, the term 'patient advocates' is reserved for those hospital employees who are hired to ensure quality care. It is important to note that patient advocates are almost exclusively called in when a provider has done something wrong. Therefore, when it is stated that an interpreter is *acting as* or *should act* as an advocate, it is likely to put healthcare providers on the defence. That is, stating there is a need for an advocate implicates wrong doing by a healthcare provider. In the mind of providers, it is reasonable to ask how interpreters who are not often trained in healthcare have the expertise to determine whether there was a wrong doing in the first place (unless, as noted above, it is intentional discrimination). This is in part why there is such controversy over the idea that interpreters should in some cases consider themselves as advocates.

Certainly, overt discrimination in healthcare settings is possible and it might be true that interpreters can identify when it has happened. However, this is less typical than the more frequent occurrence when an interpreter speaks up on a patient's behalf (which is not accurately called 'to advocate for', at least not as it is used by healthcare systems). More often than not, what interpreters are responding to when they feel compelled to speak up on the patient's behalf is when they witness a value inadvertently compromised by the provider – a value that provider already holds. For example, imagine that a provider hands a document which explains a treatment procedure to a patient who relies on interpreters for access and is told to review it in time for the provider to return for any questions. While this action may well be *just* and effective for a patient who shares the provider's language, it may not be for a patient who does not. The provider is not likely to catch these types of missteps because, in their mind, it works well in most instances. For the interpreter to bring this possible misstep to the attention of the provider is not to be a *patient advocate*. It is merely an example of a physician being alerted to a compromised value that they *already hold* which may be beyond their awareness. The interpreter might instead say, 'I understand that you're aiming for informed consent with the use of this document, but given the patient's lack of familiarity with the language and the healthcare system [or other such reasons that are specific to that patient], I am concerned that this document will not help in providing informed consent'. If the provider were then to respond by saying 'I don't care about informed consent' (which is not likely to happen), then this would be an example of discrimination and the interpreter might be compelled toward advocacy. However, merely speaking up on behalf of the patient to alert the provider of a compromised, already held value should not be deemed advocacy. The implicit meaning and implication of the term advocate is not shared between provider and interpreter, and therefore appears to cause conflict. Specificity with terms and their meanings between descriptive ethics terms and normative terms would greatly reduce perceived conflict between provider, patient, and interpreter. The field could find forward traction if it did not use descriptors (e.g. advocate) and instead, learnt to speak the same language of values used by healthcare professionals.

This is just one example of steps that need to be taken on a larger scale within the field of interpreting ethics. Instead of instituting rules for healthcare interpreters or relying on sociological constructs (metaphors and role conventions), the field should attempt to take its existing ethical ideals and compare them to those of the four core principles prevalent in healthcare. Further, newer ethical ideals can also emerge as a result of contemplating the implications of the four core principles in the profession. This is not a task to be undertaken by one individual, nor in the context of a single publication; it is outside of the scope of this chapter. Hopefully, this chapter will serve as a prompt for serious consideration of how the profession thinks and talks about healthcare ethics in healthcare interpreting (and translation and interpreting ethics more broadly) and how using the setting-specific values might advance practice and improve collaborative efforts with service providers.

5 Issues and forward advancement

Ethical codes were never intended to be a sufficient source of ethical guidance for practitioners. In the NCIHC's CoE, it states this explicitly (2004: 7). Instead, they are designed to protect service-users from untoward consequences at the hands of service professionals (Solow 1980). Hill (2004) proposed that ethical tenets were codified as a direct result of past practitioners' unethical behaviour. It is understandable therefore, that ethical codes tend to contain a list of prohibitive tenets (*interpreters shall not…*) and are written in a rule-based or deontological manner. For example, interpreters are directed not to accept work that is outside their competency levels (discretion), not to disclose information about their work (confidentiality), not to advise or express opinions (neutrality/impartiality), and not to add or omit source material (fidelity). While the tenets might be stated deontologically, in more rigid terms such as 'dos and don'ts', other ethical material in these same documents frames things in a teleological manner (e.g. a patient's welfare is at stake). Similarly, in the preamble to the IMIA code of ethics, it states that the code is designed to help interpreters with *ethical dilemmas* which is not the same thing as guiding interpreters in moment-to-moment decisions (2010: 3). In the field of translation, practice norms have attempted to guide translators and interpreters in their moment-to-moment decisions. DTS have aimed to identify regularities or norms in translation practice. For Chesterman the study of norms can add 'an empirical account of actual translation behaviour' (1993: 2) which he further suggested could lead to 'general descriptive laws' (1993: 2). Both Chesterman (1993) and Pym (2000: 5) affirmed that some normative element is necessary in DTS (see also Marzocchi 2005). Further, Pym asserted that 'Translators, teachers, students, critics, policy-makers rightly expect our research to have something to say on the matter [of ethics]' (2000: 181).

This is where descriptive *interpreting* studies appears to be struggling for forward movement – unable to translate the research identifying the actual actions of interpreters into saying something *evaluative* about those actions. Most of what is offered at the conclusion of such studies is new and different metaphors or other abstractions such as *role space* (Llewellyn-Jones and Lee 2013), *role fluidity* (Major and Napier 2019), or *role transparency* (Nicodemus, Swabey and Witter-Merithew 2011). In another publication (Dean 2015: 86–87), I noted that in nine separate qualitative studies, the authors offered a full *40 different metaphors* to describe interpreters' behaviours (Davidson 2000 and 2001; Hsieh 2007 and 2008; Leanza 2005; Angelelli 2004 and 2006; Hale 2007; Dysart-Gale 2005). This material can only be helpful if it is operationalised within the ethical framework of healthcare ethics (as demonstrated above in the example of 'advocate').

Roy (1993) proposed that new and different metaphors have not appeared to move interpreters out of the conduit norm. Instead, she concluded that the use of metaphors has, 'limited the profession's own ability to understand the interpreting event itself and the role of the interpreter within the event' (1993: 127). She also suggested that the profession needed to adopt a different paradigm (1993). Perhaps this paradigm can be advanced by constructs from ethics. First, the field of ethics would make a distinction between normative and non-normative ethics (Beauchamp and Childress 2012: 1–2). Descriptive ethics are non-normative. Descriptive ethics *describe* actions taken, i.e. what healthcare interpreters *actually do* in practice (such research has been summarised by Brisset, Leanza and Laforest 2013). Normative ethics attempts to evaluate the ethical nature of those practices (Beauchamp and Childress 2012: 1).

Having a normative or evaluative element in translation and interpreting practice does not automatically lead to rigidity or prescription, as a deontological approach would (Dean and Pollard 2018: 55). Behavioural flexibility *is normative* in the ethical construct of teleology. However, regardless of the approach, deontological or teleological, there needs to be a series of ethical principles by which an action is assessed and measured. While there have been multiple studies on the actions of healthcare interpreters (summarised in Brisset, Leanza and Laforest 2013), very few actually comment on the ethical nature of the decisions made. In cases where evaluation of behaviours *is* offered as ethical or unethical behaviour, normative ethical material was not used (Davidson 2001; Major and Napier 2019: 198). Norms, or regularities of behaviour, 'must be followed up by evaluation, compared to a set of standards, or substantiated with some ethical traction' (Dean 2015: 15). After a decade or more of translation practice *descriptions*, Pym exhorted the field to make 'a return to ethics' (2001: 129). To take this advice would mean an overhaul in how the profession of healthcare interpreting conceives of and talks about ethics.

6 Conclusion

Healthcare interpreting has made significant strides towards documenting and codifying context-specific ethical material. Indeed, advancements in healthcare interpreting ethics are arguably greater than most speciality settings in community or public service interpreting. Not only do some countries have sanctioned ethical codes and documented practice standards, there are even efforts to codify healthcare interpreting standards at an international level.

Many of these ethical content documents illustrate an interest in the ideals already established by the medical field and by healthcare professionals. This effectively aligns the ethics and practice of interpreters with their healthcare colleagues – a justifiably ethical position. Not only does the codifying of shared healthcare values ground interpreters ethically, it can also serve as a practical guide for practitioners' decisions.

What is less known is the degree to which interpreters have the skills necessary to apply these shared values to their practice decisions. Indeed, the use of practice values is not evident in interpreters' discourse. Based on terms and phrases that have been documented in research, it is evident that both participants and researchers employ metaphorical (e.g. team member) or other figurative devices (e.g. role) to describe the actions taken by interpreters. In other words, the field has not fully demonstrated that it knows how to articulate decisions as a reflection of practice values even if there is evidence that standards and codes document some of these same values.

The lack of an articulated understanding of ethical values can be an indication that these values are not compelling practitioners' behaviours. It is also true that the ability to articulate values does not necessarily predict associated behaviours. It is unclear whether or not the values expressed in the field's ethical content material are similarly evident in the decisions of the average healthcare interpreter. This is where the field needs to focus its advancement efforts (for educational efforts in this direction see Marin 2020). The ethical content material of the field, from the ethical codes to the prominent discourse of practitioners, educators, and researchers, needs to be consistent. Practice values and how they are articulated and operationalised within healthcare settings need to be the priorities for practitioners' professional development.

Notes

1 Searching in traditional databases for ethical content material does not often produce complete results. Ethical content material can be documented in ethical codes, standards of practice documents, government policies and protocols, and certainly also in academic articles. For this chapter, the searches were conducted mostly in English. However, several colleagues in other countries were able to conduct a basic search in their specific languages (German, Spanish, French, etc.) and indeed, an array of ethical content material in healthcare ethics was available in these languages. Only a few of those were sanctioned ethical codes specific to healthcare. One ethical code for interpreters offered by the International Organization for Standardization had a section devoted to healthcare interpreting ethics but was not publicly available. The search also produced several standards of practice documents in both medicine and mental health settings (addressed in detail later), a university sponsored report with limited uptake in medical facilities (Finland), a theoretical article on the need for mediators to work with interpreters in medicine (France), and policies and procedures regarding interpreting services designed for medical facilities and healthcare providers (the Netherlands, United Kingdom).

2 www.imiaweb.org/uploads/pages/376.pdf (Accessed: 21 March 2020).

3 www.ncihc.org/assets/documents/publications/NCIHC%20National%20Code%20of%20Ethics.pdf (Accessed: 21 March 2020).

4 English translation available at www.jami-net.jp/htdocs/?action=common_download_main&upload_id=11 (Accessed: 21 March 2020).

5 Specified principlism 'is the process by which a person harmonises a broader principle to a given situation. It is a constant negotiation between what the principle aims for and how that comes to play out in the nuance of circumstance, seeking to maximise the positive outcome and mitigate the negative impact' (Dean 2015: 52).

6 https://asli.org.uk/wp-content/uploads/2018/03/MHIBP.-FINAL.pdf (Accessed: 21 March 2020).

7 https://drive.google.com/file/d/0B3DKvZMflFLdWmFVV2tydVRFTHM/view (Accessed: 21 March 2020).

8 www.naati.com.au/media/1912/mental-health-interpreting-guidelines-for-interpreterspdf.pdf (Accessed: 21 March 2020).

Further reading

Beauchamp, T. L. and Childress, J. F. ([2012] 1985) *Principles of Biomedical Ethics*, 7th ed. New York: Oxford University Press.

This text is seminal to the field of medicine; the impact that this text has had on ethics in healthcare and professional ethics in general cannot be overstated. For healthcare interpreters, the first chapter would be a good introduction to medical ethics.

Dean, R. K. and Pollard, R. Q. (2018) 'Promoting the Use of Normative Ethics in the Practice Profession of Community Interpreting', in Roberson, L. and Shaw, S. (eds) *Signed Language Interpreting in the 21st Century: An Overview of the Profession*. Washington, DC: Gallaudet University Press, pp. 37–64.

This chapter addresses the use of descriptive ethics and normative ethics in community interpreting and the associated concerns. It also proposes a list of values that could be used in community interpreting (including the four core principles). This list is derived from ethical codes as well as other ethical content material in the profession.

Brisset, C., Leanza, Y. and Laforest, K. (2013) 'Working with Interpreters in Health Care: A Systematic Review and Meta-Ethnography of Qualitative Studies', *Patient Education and Counseling*, 91(2), pp. 131–140.

This review article examined 66 qualitative studies of interpreters in healthcare. It provides an overview of research into healthcare interpreting over the last 30 years. The authors reported three principal findings: interpreters' roles and behaviours; problems associated with working with interpreters; and typical communication characteristics working with interpreters.

Related topics

Dialogue Interpreting in Mental Healthcare, Community/Liaison Interpreting in Healthcare Settings, Child Language Brokering in Healthcare Settings

References

Angelelli, C. V. (2004) *Revisiting the Interpreter's Role: A Study of Conference, Court, and Medical Interpreters in Canada, Mexico, and the United States*. Amsterdam and Philadelphia: John Benjamins.

Angelelli, C. V. (2006) 'Validating Professional Standards and Codes: Challenges and Opportunities', *Interpreting*, 8(2), pp. 175–193.

Beauchamp, T. L. and Childress, J. F. (2012) *Principles of Biomedical Ethics*, 7th ed. New York: Oxford University Press.

Brisset, C., Leanza, Y. and Laforest, K. (2013) 'Working with Interpreters in Health Care: A Systematic Review and Meta-Ethnography of Qualitative Studies', *Patient Education and Counseling*, 91(2), pp. 131–140.

Chesterman, A. (1993) 'From "Is" to "Ought": Laws, Norms and Strategies in Translation Studies', *Target*, 5(1), pp. 1–20.

Cokely, D. (2000) 'Exploring Ethics: A Case for Revising the Code of Ethics', *Journal of Interpretation*, pp. 25–60. Available at: www.routledgehandbooks.com/doi/10.4324/9781315745381.ch2 (Accessed: 6 January 2021).

Davidson, B. (2000) 'The Interpreter as Institutional Gatekeeper: The Social-Linguistic Role of Interpreters in Spanish-English Medical Discourse', *Journal of Sociolinguistics*, 4(3), pp. 379–405.

Davidson, B. (2001) 'Questions in Cross-Linguistic Medical Encounters: The Role of the Hospital Interpreter', *Anthropological Quarterly*, 74(4), pp. 170–178.

Dean, R. K. (2015) *Sign Language Interpreters' Ethical Discourse and Moral Reasoning Patterns*. PhD thesis. Heriot-Watt University.

Dean, R. K. and Pollard Jr, R. Q (2005) 'Consumers and Service Effectiveness in Interpreting Work: A Practice Profession Perspective', in: Marschark, M., Peterson, R. and Winston, E. A. (eds) *Interpreting and Interpreter Education: Directions for Research and Practice*, New York: Oxford University Press, pp. 259–282.

Dean, R. K. and Pollard Jr, R. Q (2011) 'Context-Based Ethical Reasoning in Interpreting: A Demand Control Schema Perspective', *Interpreter and Translator Trainer*, 5(1), pp. 155–182.

Dean, R. K. and Pollard Jr, R. Q (2013) *The Demand Control Schema: Interpreting as a Practice Profession*. North Charleston, SC: CreateSpace Independent Publishing Platform.

Dean, R. K. and Pollard Jr, R. Q (2018) 'Promoting the Use of Normative Ethics in the Practice Profession of Community Interpreting', in Roberson, L. and Shaw, S. (eds) *Signed Language*

Interpreting in the 21st Century: An Overview of the Profession. Washington, DC: Gallaudet University Press, pp. 37–64.
Drennan, G. (1999) 'Post-Apartheid Integration and the Neglected Role of Language in South African Institutional Contexts', *Transcultural Psychiatry*, 36(1), pp. 5–22.
Dysart-Gale, D. (2005) 'Communication Models, Professionalization, and the Work of Medical Interpreters', *Health Communication*, 17(1), pp. 91–103.
Fatahi, N., Hellström, M., Skott, C. and Mattsson, B. (2008) 'General Practitioners' Views on Consultations with Interpreters: A Triad Situation with Complex Issues', *Scandinavian Journal of Primary Health Care*, 26(1), pp. 40–45.
Hale, S. (2007) *Community Interpreting*. Basingstoke and New York: Palgrave Macmillan.
Hasselkus, B. R. (1992) 'The Family Caregiver as Interpreter in the Geriatric Medical Interview', *Medical Anthropology Quarterly*, 6(3), pp. 288–304.
Hatton, D. C. and Webb, T. (1993) 'Information Transmission in Bilingual, Bicultural Contexts: A Field Study of Community Health Nurses and Interpreters', *Journal of Community Health Nursing*, 10(3), pp. 137–147.
Hill, A. L. (2004) 'Ethical Analysis in Counseling: A Case for Narrative Ethics, Moral Visions, and Virtue Ethics', *Counseling and Values*, 48(2), pp. 131–148.
Hsieh, E. (2007) 'Interpreters as Co-Diagnosticians: Overlapping Roles and Services Between Providers and Interpreters', *Social Science and Medicine*, 64(4), pp. 924–937.
Hsieh, E. (2008) '"I Am Not a Robot!" Interpreters' Views of Their Roles in Health Care Settings', *Qualitative Health Research*, 18(10), pp. 1367–1383.
International Medical Interpreters Association (2007) *Medical Interpreting Standards of Practice*. Available at: www.imiaweb.org (Accessed: 24 March 2019).
International Medical Interpreters Association (2010) *IMIA Guide on Medical Interpreter Conduct*. Available at: www.imiaweb.org (Accessed: 24 March 2019).
Japan Association of Medical Interpreters (2011) *The Code of Ethics for Professional Medical Interpreters*. Available at: www.jami-net.jp/htdocs/?action=common_download_mainandupload_id=11 (Accessed: 31 January 2020).
Jonsen, A. R. (1995) 'Casuistry: An Alternative or Complement to Principles?', *Kennedy Institute of Ethics Journal*, 5(3), pp. 237–251.
Kalina, S. (2015) 'Ethical Challenges in Different Interpreting Settings', *MonTI*, 2, pp. 63–86.
Kaufert, J. M. and Koolage, W. W. (1984) 'Role Conflict Among "Culture Brokers": The Experience of Native Canadian Medical Interpreters', *Social Science and Medicine*, 18(3), pp. 283–286.
Leanza, Y. (2005) 'Roles of Community Interpreters in Pediatrics as Seen by Interpreters, Physicians and Researchers', *Interpreting*, 7(2), pp. 167–192.
Leneham, M. and Napier, J. (2003) 'Sign Language Interpreters' Codes of Ethics: Should We Maintain the Status Quo?', *Deaf Worlds*, 19(2), pp. 78–98.
Llewellyn-Jones, P. and Lee, R. G. (2013) 'Getting to the Core of Role: Defining Interpreters' Role-Space', *International Journal of Interpreter Education*, 5(2), pp. 54–72.
Major, G. and Napier, J. (2019) '"I'm There Sometimes as a Just in Case": Exploring Role Fluidity in Healthcare Interpreting', in Meng, J., Taibi, M. and Crezee, I. (eds) *Multicultural Health Translation Interpreting and Communication*. London and New York, Routledge, pp. 183–204.
Marin, J. (2020) 'A Medical Interpreter Training Program and Signed Language Interpreters' Decision Latitude: Exploring the Impact of Specialized Training', in Souza, I. and Fragkou, E. E. (eds), *Handbook of Research on Medical Interpreting*. Hershey, PA: IGI Global, pp. 421–455.
Marzocchi, C. (2005) 'On Norms and Ethics in the Discourse on Interpreting', *The Interpreters' Newsletter*, 13, pp. 87–107.
McDonough Dolmaya, J. (2011) 'Moral Ambiguity: Some Shortcomings of Professional Codes of Ethics for Translators', *The Journal of Specialised Translation*, 15, pp. 28–49.
Mikkelson, H. (2000) 'Interpreter Ethics: A Review of the Traditional and Electronic Literature', *Interpreting*, 5, pp. 49–56.
National Council on Interpreters in Healthcare (2004) *National Code of Ethics for Interpreters in Health Care*. Available at: www.ncihc.org (Accessed: 24 March 2019).
National Council on Interpreters in Healthcare (2005) *National Standards of Practice for Interpreters in Health Care*. Available at: www.ncihc.org (Accessed: 24 March 2019).

Nicodemus, B., Swabey, L. and Witter-Merithew, A. (2011) 'Establishing Presence and Role Transparency in Healthcare Interpreting: A Pedagogical Approach for Developing Effective Practice', *Rivista di Psicolinguistica Applicata,* 11(3), pp. 69–83.
Pym, A. (2000) 'On Cooperation', in Olohan, M. (ed.) *Intercultural Faultlines: Research Models in Translation Studies I: Textual and Cognitive Aspects.* Manchester: St. Jerome Publishing, pp. 181–192.
Pym, A. (2001) 'Introduction: The Return to Ethics in Translation Studies', *The Translator,* 7(2), pp. 129–138.
Raupich, O. and Vollmann, J. (2011) '30 Years of Biomedical Ethics: Introduction to a Symposium on the 6th Edition of Beauchamp and Childress' Seminal Work', *Journal of Medical Ethics,* 37(8), pp. 582–583.
Roy, C. B. (1993) 'The Problem with Definitions, Descriptions, and the Role Metaphors of Interpreters', *Journal of Interpretation,* 6(1), pp. 127–154.
Solow, S. N. (1980) *Sign Language Interpreting: A Basic Resource Book.* Washington, DC: National Association of the Deaf.
Toury, G. (1980) *In Search of a Theory of Translation.* Tel Aviv: Porter Institute for Poetics and Semiotics.
Toury, G. (1998) 'A Handful of Paragraphs on "Translation" and "Norms"', *Current Issues in Language and Society,* 5(1–2), pp. 10–32.
Vermeer, H. ([1989] 2000) 'Skopos and Commission in Translational Action' in Venuti, L. (ed.) *The Translation Studied Reader.* London and New York: Routledge, pp. 191–202.
Wadensjö, C. (1998) *Interpreting as Interaction.* London and New York: Routledge.

Appendix A

Appendix A 27 Standards of Best Practice

Item	*Standard*	*Demonstrated Behaviour*
A-4	Address the 'comfort needs' of the patient...	• When the issue arises, assesses potential areas of discomfort for the patient (e.g. gender or age of the interpreter) and discusses them with the patient • Is cognisant of body language and/or specific verbalisation suggesting discomfort • Checks to identify the source of distress • Reassures the patient by providing information about credentials, professionalism, and the ethics of confidentiality • Explains the reality of the situation (e.g. perhaps only one interpreter is available) and tries to put the patient at ease • Offers options to address the discomfort, when available
A-15	Assist the provider with interview closure activities	• Encourages the provider to give appropriate instructions, making sure the patient is clear about next steps and has asked any questions they may still have • Checks with the patient on the need for an interpreter at any of the follow-up appointments • Observes 'closure etiquette' by making closing remarks appropriate to each party

Item	*Standard*	*Demonstrated Behaviour*
A-16	Ensure that concerns raised during or after the interview are addressed and referred to the appropriate resources	• Encourages the provider to make the appropriate referrals • Understands or asks about the institution's system of service delivery • Makes sure patient gets appointment with the appropriate resources and with an interpreter if needed
B-2	Recognise and address instances that require intercultural inquiry to ensure accurate and complete understanding	Pays attention to verbal and nonverbal cues that may indicate implicit cultural content or culturally based miscommunication (e.g. responses that do not fit the transmitted message; display of discomfort or distress when certain topics are brought up) Assesses the urgency/centrality of the issue, at that point in time in that particular exchange, to the goals and outcomes of the encounter: • Assesses the best time and method by which to raise the issue • Interjects and makes explicit to both parties what the problem might be • Prompts the provider and patient to search for clarity Shares cultural information with both parties that may be relevant and may help clarify the problem (e.g. says, 'It's possible this is what is happening, because often people from... believe that...') In cases where 'untranslatable' terms are used, assists the speaker in developing an explanation that can be understood by the listener
C-7	Deal with discrimination	On occasions where the interpreter feels strongly that either party's behaviour is affecting access to or quality of service, or compromising either party's dignity, uses effective strategies to address the situation If the problem persists, knows and uses institutional policies and procedures relevant to discrimination

13

Remote (telephone) interpreting in healthcare settings

Raquel Lázaro Gutiérrez

1 Introduction

Remote interpreting can take different shapes and forms. Ruiz Mezcua (2018: 10) defines remote interpreting as the interpreting that 'happens when the interpreter is not in the same room with the rest of the participants. This means that the interpreter needs a piece of equipment or tool to be connected to the speakers.' Braun and Taylor (2011: 352) note that '[r]emote interpreting by telephone is nowadays often called *telephone interpreting* or *over-the-phone interpreting*'. Remote interpreting implies that the primary participants in a conversation who are together at one site connect with an interpreter in another location through a video or audio link, and the interpreting services are provided simultaneously, consecutively and/or bilaterally in dialogue mode.

When the main participants are not at the same site and connect to one another through a three-way telephone or video call, the method of interpreting is called, following Braun and Taylor (2011: 352), 'teleconference interpreting'. Although the authors prefer 'telephone-based interpreting' as an umbrella term for these two modalities, they also acknowledge that 'telephone interpreting' is used widely as a shortcut. Following Ruiz Mezcua (2018: 10), in a three-way telephone call 'interpretation [...] takes place in consecutive mode or dialogue mode, which means that the interpreter waits until the speaker finishes their statement before rendering the interpretation into the target language'.

In medical settings, both remote telephone interpreting (when service provider and patient are physically together and connect via telephone with an interpreter) and interpreter-mediated phone calls (three-way phone call) occur. The first modality is used, for instance, during onsite doctor-patient consultations or when allophone patients (those who do not speak the language of the host country) need to communicate onsite with healthcare staff, whereas the second one is needed, for example, when patients call a medical emergency number or when they are contacted by clinics to schedule medical appointments.

The first known reference to telephone interpreting in academic literature is that by Paneth, who characterised this modality as a 'very neat and obvious use of interpreters'

 DOI: 10.4324/9781003167983-17

(Paneth 2000: 39) and foretold its future development. The first service for telephone interpreting was set up in Australia already in 1947 by TIS National (Translating and Interpreting Service). At the time, telephone interpreting services were offered thanks to joint efforts by Red Cross and the Commonwealth; they came to be offered nationally and for free under the auspices of the Australian Government from 1973 onwards (Cabrera Méndez 2016). Around 40 years later, telephone interpreting reached the United States, where Jeff Munks (a policeman) and Michael McFerrin (a former marine) joined forces to set up the company Language Line (Kelly 2008b). Ten years later, telephone interpreting arrived in Japan and the United Kingdom (Phelan 2001). Nowadays, as Ruiz Mezcua (2018: 11) mentions, '[t]elephone interpretation is becoming increasingly common [...], as it provides a professional interpreting service almost instantaneously, saving time and money, and with successful outcomes'.

Within the wider field of public service interpreting, telephone interpreting is particularly popular in healthcare settings (Braun 2015: 353). The reasons for this are varied and usually revolve around interpreters' availability (Phillips 2013; Gracia-García 2002; Mintz 1998; Fors 1999; Hewitt 1995, Jones and Gill 1998; Wadensjö 1999) and cost-effectiveness of the interpreting provided (Ko 2006; Phelan 2001; Rosenberg 2004).

In healthcare settings, the number of language combinations in demand is high; it is also often difficult to predict which language is going to be needed and when. Although many medical consultations are scheduled beforehand, patients' registers do not include information on the languages they speak and, consequently, whether they will need an interpreter to be able to communicate. Furthermore, many interactions in the healthcare settings are unplanned, not only in emergency situations, but also in face-to-face encounters with administrative services (for example, when patients try to arrange an appointment) or in telephone calls when patients phone a doctor's surgery or hotline, or receive calls about their appointments or test results.

Telephone interpreting services can be provided by governmental organisations, private agencies and non-profit organisations (Ruiz Mezcua 2018). In public healthcare settings, public institutions (hospitals and healthcare services) launch calls for tenders, and telephone interpreting agencies bid to provide services. Private hospitals and clinics can either contact interpreters directly or through agencies which offer telephone interpreting. Recently, mobile applications made telephone interpreting even more popular, as patients themselves or anyone else acting on their behalf can now contact an interpreter directly without having to rely on healthcare institutions or private practices, which also implies that the payment of interpreting services is assumed by patients themselves (Jaime Pérez 2015).

As interpreting assignments in healthcare settings are often short (compared to e.g. conference interpreting), telephone interpreting emerges as a convenient option, as it cuts the cost of travel for interpreters, and consequently, for the clients. Waiting times are usually difficult to predict, as it is not uncommon for medical appointments to be delayed, which adds on to the costs of an interpreter onsite. Telephone interpreters, on the other hand, are not contacted until the conversation actually starts. Although these are the most commonly stated reasons for the popularity of telephone interpreting in healthcare settings, this interpreting modality has other advantages that will be commented on in the following sections.

2 Critical issues in telephone interpreting

Telephone interpreters require specific skills to perform effectively without being physically present during the interaction. They usually do not have access to contextual information, including the individuals who are present, their roles, body language, movements, as well as other relevant elements which can provide contextual information, such as clothes, furniture, instruments, signs, etc. Furthermore, difficulties may arise due to the use of a telephone, such as lack of coverage, damaged or old equipment, its incorrect use, etc. (Pertusa Elorriaga 2012). Telephone interpreting therefore has a set of characteristics and peculiarities which will be explored in this section under the following subheadings: lack of visual context, coordination of discourse, use of technology, working conditions, stress and emotional impact, training, and ethics.

2.1 Lack of visual context

One of the most critical issues concerning telephone interpreting is the lack of visual context. It has been singled out by researchers and practitioners as one of the most notable difficulties of this modality of interpreting and has been frequently targeted as a research topic and described as both an advantage and a disadvantage (Heh and Qian 1997; Phelan 2001; Gracia-García 2002).

Visual cues help onsite interpreters to gain a clearer understanding of the communicative situation and to make interpreting decisions. Telephone interpreters, however, miss out on gestures, postures and facial expressions (Gentile, Ozolins and Vasilakakos 1996; Roy 2000; Wadensjö 1998, 1999; Oviatt and Cohen 1992; Fors 1999; Kurz 1999; Mack 2001; Vidal 1998; Lee 2007) and they have to develop coping skills to address this (Lázaro Gutiérrez and Cabrera Méndez 2019). Interpreters themselves have stated that the lack of visual cues results in additional effort. For example, David Mintz, former President of NAJIT (National Association of Judicial Interpreters and Translators) sent a letter to the journal *Proteus* after having visited the US Court Telephone Interpreting Project together with other interpreters. Experienced interpreters reported having had to struggle with the insecurity that the lack of visual information provoked in them (Mintz 1998).

Lázaro Gutiérrez and Cabrera Méndez (2019) argue that telephone interpreters' lack of visual context in healthcare emergency settings has a high impact on interpreters' performance. They may, for instance, have no information on the number of people present in an emergency setting or on their particular roles (e.g. paramedic, nurse, doctor, etc.). The impossibility of proper briefing prior to an emergency aggravates the situation.

Other researchers state that lack of visual context does not necessarily impair communication (Braun 2006) or affect the interpreter's performance, as skilled interpreters are usually able to overcome these difficulties (Ko 2006), providing sound is clear and assignments are not long (Mintz 1998). They argue that interpreters are still able to perceive paralanguage and other auditory cues, such as tone of voice, breathing patterns, inflection, pitch, or volume (Kelly 2008b; Crezee 2013; Cheng 2015). In fact, non-verbal communication cues have even been considered a distraction by some researchers (Mikkelson 2003, Lee 2007) and some interpreters prefer interpreting remotely because they can allegedly remain more neutral (Lee 2007) and/or avoid being in close physical proximity to unpleasant and/or traumatic situations (blood, vomit, injuries, etc.). Interpreting over the phone in healthcare settings may also ensure less interference with patients' privacy.

Nevertheless, several authors agree on the unsuitability of telephone interpreting for particular situations. For example, Wadensjö (1998) discourages this modality when many participants are involved in a communication, and Kelly (2008a: 9) specifically suggests that telephone interpreting is not a good choice for those doctor-patient interviews in which visual information is especially important, such as patient education and teaching scenarios. In the same vein, patients who have to undergo mental health evaluations or have suffered from trauma might not be in a condition to communicate over the phone (see e.g. Lázaro Gutiérrez and Cabrera Méndez 2019, describing an interpreter-mediated consultation with a drunk patient). Lázaro Gutiérrez and Cabrera Méndez (2019) describe the most common challenges a telephone interpreter faces in healthcare settings and state that they often occur at the beginning of the interaction, as that is the moment when most information is missing. In their research, they found out that the interpreter repeatedly sought to collect contextual information by leaving aside an invisible role and interacting with healthcare providers and patients by means of questions and requests for repetitions.

2.2 Coordination of discourse

Discourse coordination is a typical concern in bilateral onsite interpreting but presents a set of particular challenges when performed over the phone. One of the main issues related to discourse management and coordination is the use of first- or third-person pronouns. Although interpreters are strongly encouraged to use the first person (Bot 2005; Kelly 2008b), it has been found out that telephone interpreters need to use the third person more often, particularly when difficulties and misunderstandings arise and interventions become necessary to provide clarification (Lee 2007; Hsieh 2006; Oviatt and Cohen 1992; Rosenberg 2004). This practice has also been reported as a means through which interpreters distance themselves from the interpreted information. For instance, Gracia-García (2002: 8) states that telephone interpreters in medical settings can more easily avoid situations in which they have to act as an advisor, such as culturally marked situations, episodes in which interpreters feel identified with or emotionally attached to patients, or cases when they are asked questions they are not prepared or qualified to answer.

Wadensjö (1999) studied coordination in telephone-interpreted conversations in depth and observed that inaccuracies arise for three main reasons: interpreters may fail to control turn-taking; they may not be able to retain long utterances in memory; or they may need to interrupt the participants to ask for clarification. Wadensjö also found out that it is more difficult to control turn-taking when the interpreter is not physically present and that this necessitates the interpreter to take a more active role; other authors such as Hsieh (2006) and Oviatt and Cohen (1992) also make the same observation. Similarly, as interpreters lack visual information, they may attribute any silence or naturally occurring pauses between turns in a conversation to a connection breakdown (Mikkelson 2003; Oviatt and Cohen 1992).

Fernández Pérez (2015, 2017) also identified coordination of discourse amongst the specific skills telephone interpreters must possess. The interpreters' coordination role involves managing the beginning and ending of the encounter, organising turn-taking, and interrupting the speakers at appropriate times. Lázaro Gutiérrez and Cabrera Méndez (2019) indicate that a good way to make this coordination task possible is to allow the interpreters to properly introduce themselves to all participants in the conversation. In this way, interpreters are able to explain their role and code of ethics, and suggest basic guidelines for successful communication. These guidelines may include avoiding speaking over each other, speaking directly to the interlocutor using the first person, not addressing the interpreter directly unless it is necessary to transmit situational information, or to correct a misunderstanding. The interpreter may also wish to emphasise at the start that they will translate everything that is said and will keep the interaction confidential, and that they may have to speak on their own behalf if they feel there is a misunderstanding or a need to clarify information.

2.3 Use of technology

The increasing prevalence of mobile phones and videoconferencing, the decreasing price of telecommunication costs, and the almost instant availability of large teams of interpreters through agencies have made telephone interpreting highly popular in recent years. These interpreters can receive calls from any part of the world, cover a wide range of languages and can commit to work over many hours a day, thus making it unnecessary to spend money on interpreters' transportation to the location of the interaction.

Although technological improvements allow for more frequent and better communication, sound quality is still a concern. Several researchers have focused on technological needs of telephone interpreters and have emphasised the importance of the sound quality of the phone and connectivity of the line (Kelly 2008b; Lee 2007), particularly since the increased use of mobile phones. Mobile phones' hands-free equipment is highly popular amongst clients, preferred over the passing of the handset back and forth, but have proved to cause difficulties for interpreters, as their use impacts on the sound quality and, consequently, the interpreters' performance (Kelly 2008b; Rosenberg 2004). For instance, in the study carried out by Lázaro Gutiérrez and Cabrera Méndez (2019: 57–58), sound quality was not checked at the beginning of the interaction, and it took up to six minutes for the interpreter to be able to hear properly during a telephone call made from an emergency department. This prevented the interpreter from collecting essential details about the communicative event that would have helped her to subsequently build up the meaning in the interaction.

The main telephone interpreting agencies usually offer their clients telephone devices with dual handsets (landline) or headsets (mobile phone). However, healthcare providers have reported the unavailability of these devices (usually located in particular rooms or units) when they needed them and have expressed a clear preference for their own mobile phones. In three-way conversations, when patients are also in remote locations, it is impossible to control the quality of their devices or connectivity; therefore, it is not uncommon that connections break down or the sound quality is too poor for effective communication.

The appearance of smartphones allowed for further developments in telephone interpreting practice and accessibility. For example, in 2005, a Spanish company, Migralingua, developed an application called Voze, which popularised the use of telephone interpreting in Spain, as it was made available to any user with an Android-operating mobile phone. Before Voze, telephone interpreting services did not reach all users in Spain, since it was usually the public institutions that decided whether or not to offer this service, depending on their financial budgets and levels of awareness of the patients' needs. This application has also become a platform for data collection that allowed for the evaluation of issues such as frequency of use, areas where the service was most requested, languages required and average length of calls. It also allowed random recordings of interpreting sessions for subsequent assessment of their quality (Jaime Pérez 2015).[1] The user of this application may access telephone interpreting services anywhere in the world through virtual geographic numbering and they can do so through an app for Android phones, the system's website, or prepaid cards for use with any kind of mobile phone or landline. Apart from telephone interpreting, the application includes additional services, such as general, sworn, and express translations of short texts and pictures (of, for instance, handwritten texts or diagrams and images that contain text).

2.4 Working conditions

Professional interpreters and associations have often discussed telephone interpreters' working conditions, as performance over phone implies a new understanding of interpreting assignments. One of the most discussed issues is the lack of briefing, particularly in emergency situations. The immediacy of telephone interpreting is both a great advantage and a great challenge for interpreters, as they often have to deal with unpredictable content (Lee 2007). Kelly (2008b) suggests that terminology frequently used in emergency situations should be provided for interpreters in advance. Some telephone interpreting agencies currently try and put together protocols and glossaries for their workers, however these efforts are not yet sufficient or widespread. Lázaro Gutiérrez and Cabrera Méndez (2019) suggest that service providers offer interpreters basic information about the setting, such as how many people are present and who is going to speak in which language, in order to avoid misunderstandings and render the conversation more fluent. Background information about the patient is also desirable.

It has also been mentioned that telephone interpreters are not able to specialise as much as onsite interpreters (Heh and Qian 1997; Gracia-García 2002) because they are subject to the contracts signed by the agencies they work for. This means that agencies may offer interpreting for regional healthcare services on the one hand, and for an insurance company on the other, hiring the same interpreters for both contracts.

One of the main advantages of telephone interpreting is its near constant availability. Agencies provide interpreting services round the clock in a wide range of languages. This can be achieved either through hiring interpreters from different time zones or by using local interpreters who prefer the flexibility of interpreting outside typical working hours (Kelly 2008b). Some agencies have developed online systems that allow interpreters to avoid being called outside their chosen working hours.

Interpreters are usually not paid for 'being on-call', although some agencies do make additional payments on a monthly basis for overnight and weekend shifts. The majority of telephone interpreters receive payment according to the number of minutes they are on the phone; some agencies may have a minimum amount of minutes paid to the interpreters for each call. As the interpreters can choose their working locations, they can combine their work as telephone interpreters with other occupations, such as freelance translation.

2.5 Stress and emotional impact

Most telephone interpreters work part-time and as freelancers (Crezee, Jülich and Hayward 2013; Iglesias Fernández and Ouellet 2018). It has been reported that the unpredictability and irregularity of their assignments, together with lower pay rates compared to other forms of interpreting, may cause stress and impact on work-life balance.

Crezee *et al.* (2015) argue that there are many factors that can cause stress for healthcare interpreters. Lower working rates, instability and unpredictability have already been mentioned as examples, but other personal factors, such as life experiences, their level of resilience and their psychological skills naturally also play a part (Crezee *et al.* 2015; Cheng 2015). Besides these factors, some authors mention that remote interpreters suffer more stress than onsite interpreters. For instance, Andres and Falk (2009: 21–22) point, on the one hand, to the lack of non-verbal information, which could lead to confusion and misunderstandings, causing stress, particularly in healthcare settings where human lives are at stake. On the other hand, they mention that telephone interpreters may also have to deal with many different topics over a short period of time, which can lead to stress and a higher risk of quality loss. However, some authors, like Gracia-García (2002) point out that interpreters' remoteness can allow them some detachment from the patients' suffering and a relatively lower level of emotional involvement.

Generally speaking, public service interpreters and, in particular, healthcare interpreters, tend to empathise with their clients. It is hard for them to control their feelings when they hear traumatic experiences and have to recount them using the first person (Costa, Lázaro Gutiérrez and Rausch 2020; Hale 2007; Wadensjö 1999; Wilson 2010). Some situations, like end-of-life care, can be more emotionally-loaded (Schenker *et al.* 2012). Telephone interpreters find debriefing even more difficult, as most of the time they are not contacted prior to an assignment and miss the opportunity to obtain information and get ready, if needed, for an emotionally challenging situation (Wilson 2010), and sometimes they move too quickly to their following phone call, even before being able to recover from the emotional impact of a previous traumatic assignment (Kelly 2008b).

2.6 Training

Training provided to telephone interpreters is relatively scarce, even though it is crucial for high-quality telephone interpreting (Kelly 2008b). In Spain, for instance, the results of the investigations conducted by Luque (2008), Murgu and Jiménez (2011), Prieto (2008) and Martínez-Gómez (2008) point to a general lack of knowledge on telephone interpreting and, consequently, a lack of educational resources for both community interpreters and public service providers that use telephone interpreting systems. Kelly (2008b) mentions the need for specific protocols and training for telephone interpreting and contributes with a comprehensive guide for telephone interpreters which includes guidelines for working as a telephone interpreter, a full chapter on ethics, and scenarios for practice (2008b), as well as an abridged version specifically aimed at telephone interpreters working in healthcare settings (2008a). Verrept (2011), in his study of remote interpreters in four Belgian hospitals, signals that interpreters need supplementary training to make adequate use of equipment. Ozolins (2011) suggests that further research is needed in this field so that technological issues can be resolved and the performance of interpreters improved. Although Hlavac (2013) does not endow technology with a prominent position in the interlingual transfer, he acknowledges that telephone and video-link interpreting should be included in both training and testing interpreting programmes. Fernández Pérez (2012), another scholar insisting on the need for training specifically for telephone interpreters, first identifies the characteristics of this type of interpreting (lack of visual information, increased access to interpreters in a short period of time by a larger number of users from different backgrounds, use of technical equipment) and later establishes a classification of particular skills telephone interpreters need to acquire according to their two main roles: the discourse coordination role, as discussed above, and the translation role (e.g. adapting note taking to the use of telephone). Command of prosodic elements and direct/

indirect speech are two further skills which relate to both roles. Fernández Pérez also designed a set of training activities based on role-play (2015).

Although when compared to onsite interpreting, remote and telephone interpreting involve some new skills that must be acquired, training in telephone interpreting at university level remains scarce for many reasons. First of all, the field of practice is relatively new. Second, in order to achieve optimum learning, a certain amount of technology is needed for its practice, which means that the little training that is offered at university level remains theoretical. Finally, it is a highly specialised field that does not fit easily into undergraduate programmes, and graduate programmes usually already have full course loads. University training usually consists of intensive workshops and seminars that take place over the course of a day or two and are not normally mandatory for undergraduate or graduate students. It is not rare for telephone interpreting agencies to be called upon to offer this kind of training to postgraduate programmes or in the form of professional development courses.

Therefore, the bulk of training available is provided by agencies that offer telephone interpreting services. Besides entry training for new workers (both members of staff and freelancers), telephone interpreting agencies have significant quality control and continuous professional development programmes. Training usually includes the use of specific protocols, basic information about the field in which work will be conducted (for instance, healthcare interpreting), and ethical issues. They also incorporate new content into their training programmes as needed for latest technological advances or new clients. Ongoing training is also usually provided as part of quality assurance programmes, and it is informed by the changing needs and emerging challenges.

In addition to the necessary general training in telephone interpreting, interpreters need training in the specific field they are working in – in this case, healthcare. To this end, interpreters need to gain knowledge of healthcare topics, awareness of typical procedures and communicative situations, linguistic and cultural knowledge, an understanding of terminology, as well as stress management skills for tense situations. In this field, it is also very important to know that a specific protocol is designed and established for each client institution (for example, some protocols for emergency hotlines require interpreters to ask themselves about personal data and location in order to gain time), and telephone interpreters must have a solid knowledge of these protocols and be aware of the motivation behind certain procedures and questions.

2.7 Ethics

Telephone interpreting can contribute to maintaining confidentiality and privacy (Hewitt 1995; Kelly 2008b; Wadensjö 1999; Rosenberg 2004; Phillips 2013; Ko 2006; Mikkelson 2003). During onsite interpreted medical consultations, it is common that interpreters have to remain behind a curtain or turn around when patients are asked to get undressed, whereas over the phone, the interpreters cannot see the patients. Telephone interpreting also cuts down on cases where onsite interpreters are asked to stay with the patients in waiting rooms until the actual consultation starts; this reduces instances of personal conversation with patients (see Lázaro Gutiérrez 2018 for examples in which patients disclose information to interpreters when members of medical staff are absent).

A recurrent topic within interpreting ethics is role boundaries. In the healthcare domain, interpreters are considered part of the healthcare team that assist the patients, as dictated by medical protocols,[2] and usually have some general knowledge of the medical field. In Gracia-García's words, '[...] guidelines on interpreter professionalism and ethics affirm [...] interpreters are professional mediators and, therefore, both parties [medical staff, on the one hand, and interpreters on the other] should be present to discuss anything that is relevant to the medical case' (Gracia-García 2002: 202). However, it must be remembered that interpreters are not medical staff and may lack information about particular protocols and procedures. The best practice would be to inform interpreters of the reasoning behind the questions and procedures so that they can better adapt their interpreted discourse to the situation (Lázaro Gutiérrez and Cabrera Méndez 2019). When the healthcare professionals ask interpreters for advice, for example on cultural matters, all parties should be conscious of the limitations of the interpreter's knowledge and only base their exchanges on the information that is mastered by the interpreter.

3 Research on telephone interpreting

Six decades after the first mention of telephone interpreting by Paneth in 1957 (2002), research about this interpreting modality is still scarce (Ruiz Mezcua 2018). However, the increasing use of telephone interpreting in more diverse settings has stimulated the curiosity of researchers around the world, who have begun to study this modality either for academic purposes or in order to develop policy recommendations and training materials.

Among the first studies carried out on telephone interpreting, Oviatt and Cohen (1992) compared telephone conversations with and without an interpreter, and Wadensjö (1999) compared an onsite interpreter-mediated conversation with a telephone-interpreted one. A few years later, telephone interpreter-mediated conversations became a subject of enquiry on their own, distinct from onsite interpreting, and studies using large amounts of data were produced, such as that by Rosenberg (2002), who analysed 1876 telephone interpreter-mediated conversations in healthcare settings.

Although research about telephone interpreting that focuses on healthcare settings is limited, in recent years, several projects have focused on telephone and remote interpreting. For instance, the Department of Justice of the European Commission, within the framework of the Criminal Justice programme, funded the *Avidicus project* (www.videoconference-interpreting.net/index.html) from 2008 to 2016. It was coordinated by the University of Surrey and its main objectives were to identify situations where remote interpreting and videoconference interpreting are most useful within the legal field, to compare remote interpreting and face-to-face interpreting, and to elaborate on training courses for interpreting students, interpreters and legal professionals.

The group FITISPos-UAH, based in Madrid (Spain) and active since 1998, is also carrying out research in the field of telephone interpreting.[3] Among the main outcomes of their latest research activities are the creation and improvement of performance protocols, description of typical interactions between patients and healthcare professionals, identification of the most frequently used vocabulary and sentence patterns, selection of real examples for training, translation of terms, and some guidelines for stress management and coordination of interaction. These projects also contributed to the improvement of mutual understanding between university researchers and agencies, and the adoption of a more informed approach to the elaboration and use of protocols, as transgressions have been analysed in a more systematic and scientific way.

Most of the available research on telephone interpreting deals with quality issues, comparing it with onsite interpreting (Martínez-Gómez 2008; Jaime Pérez 2015). For example,

Azarmina and Wallace (2005) review publications on remote interpreting in healthcare settings and conclude that 'remote interpretation is at least as acceptable as physically present interpretation to patients, doctors and (to a lesser extent) interpreters themselves' (2005: 44). Verrept (2011), in his study about videoconference interpreting in Belgian hospitals, states that this modality poses further difficulties (the need to check sound and image quality, the moderate use of gestures, note taking, and the coordination of turn-taking) when compared to face-to-face interpreting. Other studies carried out in this field focus on assessing the quality of the service through the collection of user feedback (Jaime Pérez 2015).

A very prominent contribution to the research into telephone interpreting is the European Research project SHIFT in Orality, an Erasmus+ 3-year project funded by the European Commission in 2015, within Key Action 2: Strategic Partnership in Higher Education and led by the University of Bologna,[4] which aims at contributing to the provision of training solutions for remote interpreting and to bridge the gap between academia and the telephone interpreting industry (Russo *et al.* 2012; González Rodríguez and Spinolo 2017; Spinolo, Bertozzi and Russo 2018). One of their objectives is defining the telephone interpreter's profile. Iglesias Fernández and Ouellet (2018) compare experienced and novice telephone interpreters to find out about the issues they encounter and how they grapple with various difficulties, in order to feed this information into pedagogical material. They have done so through an online survey addressed to Spanish and Swedish telephone interpreters, which highlighted the contrasting perceptions of difficulty and degree of experience on the phone.

4 Further directions in research

Further directions in research on telephone interpreting in healthcare settings must be based on cooperation among research bodies, healthcare authorities, and telephone interpreting providers (both agencies and interpreters). For instance, the research group FITISPos-UAH signed cooperation agreements with the most prominent agencies providing telephone interpreting services in Spain. It is thanks to these joint efforts between the academia and the industry that larger projects about telephone interpreting are becoming possible. The research group is interested in developing training materials for postgraduate and university-based continuous education programmes. The agencies, on the other hand, are keen on attracting graduates from these university programmes, as they will enter the labour market with sufficient knowledge to perform telephone interpreting. The agencies also benefit from the elaboration of training materials, because these can then be used for in-house training. The results of the research projects can also yield protocols, performance guidelines, glossaries, etc. which can ultimately improve the services these agencies provide.

There are three main lines along which the Group FITISPos-UAH is currently working; these could be considered as possible further directions in telephone interpreting research in healthcare settings. The first of them addresses telephone interpreting in medical emergencies from a pragmatic point of view. It uses (Im)Politeness Theories (Culpeper 1996) to explore, among other aspects, face threatening acts (Lázaro Gutiérrez 2017b; Lázaro Gutiérrez and Cabrera Méndez 2018). It has been discovered that telephone interpreter-mediated conversations are more prone to contain face threatening acts than standard and onsite mediated encounters because of their asynchronous and indirect nature, and face threatening acts have proved to be very challenging for interpreters to deal with.

The second area of innovation of the Group deals with the setting where the interpreted conversations take place. Instead of focusing on telephone interpreting in general, some particularisation has been introduced according to current research trends (Cox and Lázaro Gutiérrez 2016), and the setting has been restricted to specific areas, such as healthcare emergency services, where telephone interpreting is popular. For instance, Lázaro Gutiérrez and Cabrera Méndez (2019) found out that many of the conversations telephone interpreters have to mediate take place in the Accident and Emergency Departments or are related to other kinds of health emergencies (telephone calls to emergency services). These conversations follow generalisable patterns and characteristics, such as their asymmetry – understood as the different levels of knowledge about the topic, setting and situation and the unequal participation of interactants (Lázaro Gutiérrez 2012) – or their urgent nature, and could be classified as an 'activity type' (Levinson 1979) or even a 'genre' (Briggs and Bauman 1992). The classification of the conversations and their description provide useful contextual information, which compensates for the lack of visual cues. For instance, the urgent nature of these encounters greatly influences how the interaction is going to develop, as the speakers usually want to communicate essential information as quickly as possible.

Finally, some innovation has been introduced regarding the methodology of the studies. The cooperation with telephone interpreting agencies has allowed the researchers to compile a great number of real conversations, which can be analysed in a variety of ways. Apart from the classic discourse analysis methodology, research methods from corpus-based studies have been used to allow for the extraction of recurrent terminology and discourse patterns. According to Flowerdew (1993), the main advantages for using corpora together with concordance programmes are that they give us linguistic information, and that they are a basis for creating teaching materials, including the use of real-life examples of text or discourse. Besides, sociological methods such as focus groups or Delphi questionnaires have been applied to complement quantitative and qualitative analyses (Lázaro Gutiérrez 2017a).

Other research groups are looking into similar aspects. In Australia, the University of Queensland, currently working on data extracted from surveys distributed amongst telephone interpreters, aims at completing information by introducing opinions and insights from end-users and interpreting agencies (Wang 2018). Another major concern for them is to analyse authentic telephone interpreting, focusing on performance quality and turn-taking techniques, for the purpose of contributing to the elaboration of national protocols (*ibid.*).

SHIFT researchers, on the other hand, after having developed training materials for remote interpreting, are now focusing on their piloting and testing. These materials include a remote interpreting handbook for trainers, trainees and professionals, a set of training materials to be used in class (role-plays and preparatory activities in English/Italian, Spanish/Italian and Spanish/English), and a glossary of remote interpreting terms in English, Spanish and Italian.

5 Conclusion

In this chapter, the main characteristics of remote (telephone) interpreting in healthcare settings have been described. Healthcare professionals and patients can connect to a remote interpreter when they need to communicate during a visit. Alternatively, healthcare telephone conversations can be interpreted in a three-way call. Telephone interpreting presents many advantages, such as its immediacy, cost-effectiveness and availability. However, in healthcare settings, interpreters have to face some challenges, such as the lack of visual context, the use of technology, difficulties in the coordination of talk, poor working conditions, stress and emotional impact, ethical dilemmas and lack of training. Research on telephone interpreting in healthcare settings mainly deals with quality and the different roles of the interpreter, but is also evolving to address the evaluation and testing of training materials and to provide deeper analyses of performance and discourse in real-life, recorded conversations. Telephone interpreting is definitely a flourishing field both in research and practice.

Notes

1 Consent to being recorded is provided by interpreters through the contract they sign to work for the telephone interpreting company. Telephone interpreting companies and healthcare institutions sign an agreement that regulates the conditions under which the quality control and assurance process is carried out, including the way in which conversations are recorded and processed. Service providers (healthcare staff) are informed about the fact that telephone interpreted conversations might be recorded by their institutions in training courses about how to work with telephone interpreters or through guidelines and instruction packs. Finally, before the conversation with healthcare staff starts, patients are presented with a recorded message that explains that conversations might be recorded for security and quality purposes. If they proceed to use the telephone interpreting service, they consent to the recording.
2 Medical protocols state that everybody who assists a patient is part of the medical assistance team and must abide by the medical codes of beneficence and non-maleficence.
3 http://www3.uah.es/traduccion/en/fitispos-ingles/ (Accessed: 3 February 2021).
4 http://www.shiftinorality.eu/en (Accessed: 3 February 2021).

Further reading

Fernández-Pérez, M. (2017) 'Interaction Management Skills in Telephone Interpreting', *Revista Canaria de Estudios Ingleses,* 75, pp.103–117.

This article discusses some of the specifics of telephone interpreting and particularly focuses on the interpreter's coordination skills needed to manage the interaction between the participants in conversations.

González Rodríguez, M. J. and Spinolo, N. (2017) 'Telephonic Dialogue Interpreting. A Short Teaching Course', in Cirillo, L. and Niemants, N. (eds) *Teaching Dialogue Interpreting. Research-Based Proposals for Higher Education.* Amsterdam and Philadelphia: John Benjamins, pp. 242–257.

This chapter offers a specific short course for telephone interpreters which includes five practical units in increasing difficulty to be used for various language combinations.

Kelly, N. (2008a) *A Medical Interpreter's Guide to Telephone Interpreting.* Available at: www.imiaweb.org/uploads/pages/380.pdf (Accessed 15 December 2020).

This is a short guide about telephone interpreting for medical interpreters. It is presented as a list of questions and answers and is the IMIA's (International Medical Interpreters Association) response to its members' doubts about telephone interpreting in healthcare settings, which had been previously submitted to the association.

Ozolins, U. (2011) 'Telephone Interpreting: Understanding Practice and Identifying Research Needs', *Translation and Interpreting*, 3(2), pp. 33–47.

This article sums up the history of telephone interpreting provision and research, and identifies future trends which revolve around technological issues, interpreting techniques, ethics and the interpreters' role.

Ruiz Mezcua, A. (ed.) (2018) *Approaches to Telephone Interpretation. Research, Innovation, Teaching and Transference*. Bern: Peter Lang.

This volume contains 14 chapters organised in three sections about research carried out both by telephone interpreting companies and academia, pedagogical approaches and proposals, and sociological and professional aspects.

Related topics

Healthcare Interpreting Ethics, Dialogue Interpreting in Mental Healthcare, Child Language Brokering in Healthcare Settings

References

Andres, D. and Falk, S. (2009) 'Information and Communication Technologies (ICT) in Interpreting-Remote and Telephone Interpreting', in Andres, D. and Pöllabauer, S. (eds) *Spürst Du wie der Bauch rauf runter? Fachdolmetschen im Gesundheitsbereich / Is Everything All Topsy Turvy in Your Tummy? Health Care Interpreting*. Munich: Martin Meidenbauer, pp. 9–27.

Azarmina, P. and Wallace, P. (2005) 'Remote Interpretation in Medical Encounters: A Systematic Review', *Journal of Telemedicine and Telecare*, 11(3), pp. 140–145.

Bot, H. (2005) 'Dialogue Interpreting as a Specific Case of Reported Speech', *Interpreting*, 7(2), pp. 237–261.

Braun, S. (2006) 'Multimedia Communication Technologies and Their Impact on Interpreting', in Gerzymisch-Arbogast, H. (ed.), *Proceedings of the Marie Curie Euroconferences Mutra: Audiovisual Translation Scenarios, Copenhagen, 1–5 May 2006*.

Braun, S. (2015) 'Remote Interpreting', in Mikkelson, H., and Jourdenais, R. (eds) *The Routledge Handbook of Interpreting*. London and New York: Routledge, pp. 352–367.

Braun, S. and Taylor, J. L. (2011) 'Video-Mediated Interpreting: An Overview of Current Practice and Research', in Braun, S. and Taylor, J. L. (eds.) *Videoconference and Remote Interpreting in Criminal Proceedings*. Guildford: University of Surrey, pp. 27–57.

Briggs, C. and Bauman, R. (1992) 'Genre, Intertextuality, and Social Power', *Journal of Linguistic Anthropology*, 2(2), pp. 131–172.

Cabrera Méndez, G. (2016) *La interpretación a distancia: nacimiento, maduración y proyección de futuro*. Technical report submitted to VIU-Valencia International University. Valencia: Universidad Internacional de Valencia.

Cheng, Q. (2015) *Examining the Challenges for Telephone Interpreters in New Zealand*. Master's Thesis. Auckland University of Technology.

Costa, B., Lázaro Gutiérrez, R. and Rausch, T. (2020) 'Self-Care as an Ethical Responsibility. A Pilot Study on Support Provision for Interpreters in Human Crises', *Translation and Interpreting Studies*, 15(1), pp. 36–56.

Cox, A. and Lázaro Gutiérrez, R. (2016) 'Interpreting in the Emergency Department. How Context Matters for Practice', in Federici, F. (ed.), *Mediating Emergencies and Conflicts: Frontline Translating and Interpreting*. London: Palgrave Macmillan, pp. 33–58.

Crezee, I. (2013) *Introduction to Healthcare for Interpreters and Translators*. Amsterdam and Philadelphia: John Benjamins.

Crezee, I., Atkinson, D., Robyn, P., Au, P., and Wong, S. (2015) 'Teaching Interpreters About Self-Care', *International Journal of Interpreter Education*, 7(1), pp. 74–83.

Crezee, I., Jülich, S. and Hayward, M. (2013) 'Issues for Interpreters and Professionals Working in Refugee Settings', *Journal of Applied Linguistics and Professional Practice*, 8(3), pp. 253–273.

Culpeper, J. (1996) 'Towards an Anatomy of Impoliteness', *Journal of Pragmatics*, 25, pp. 349–367.

Fernández Pérez, M. M. (2012) *Identificación de las destrezas de la interpretación telefónica*. La Laguna: Universidad de La Laguna.

Fernández Pérez, M. M. (2015) 'Propuestas de ejercicios de simulación para la didáctica de la interpretación telefónica', *MonTI Special Issue*, 2, pp. 259–279.

Fernández-Pérez, M. M. (2017) 'Interaction Management Skills in Telephone Interpreting', *Revista Canaria de Estudios Ingleses*, 75, pp. 103–117.

Flowerdew, J. (1993) 'Concordancing as a Tool in Course Design', *System*, 21(2), pp. 231–244.

Fors, J. (1999) 'Perspectives on Remote Public Service Interpreting', *Anovar/anosar estudios de traducción e interpretación,* I, pp. 119–121.

Gentile, A., Ozolins, U. and Vasilakakos, M. (1996). *Liaison Interpreting: A Handbook*. Melbourne: Melbourne University Press.

González Rodríguez, M. J. and Spinolo, N. (2017) 'Telephonic Dialogue Interpreting. A Short Teaching Course', in Cirillo, L. and Niemants, N. (eds) *Teaching Dialogue Interpreting. Research-Based Proposals for Higher Education.* Amsterdam and Philadelphia: John Benjamins, pp. 242–257.

Gracia-García, R. A. (2002) 'Telephone Interpreting: A Review of Pros and Cons', in S. Brennan (ed.), *Proceedings of the 43rd Annual Conference,* Alexandria, VA: American Translators Association, pp. 195–216.

Hale, S. (2007) *Community Interpreting*. New York: Palgrave Macmillan.

Heh, Y. and Qian, H. (1997) 'Over-The-Phone Interpretation: A New Way of Communication Between Speech Communities', in Jérôme-O'Keeffe, M. (ed.), *Proceedings of the 38th Annual Conference.* Alexandria, VA: American Translators Association, pp. 51–62.

Hewitt, W. E. (1995) *Court Interpretation: Model Guides for Policy and Practice in the State Courts.* Williamsburg, VA: National Center for State Courts.

Hlavac, J. (2013) 'Should Interpreters Be Trained and Tested in Telephone and Video-Link Interpreting? Responses from Practitioners and Examiners', *International Journal of Interpreter Education (IJIE)*, 5(1), pp. 34–50.

Hsieh, H. (2006) 'Understanding Medical Interpreters: Reconceptualizing Bilingual Health Communication', *Health Communication,* 20(2), pp. 177–186.

Iglesias Fernández, E. and Ouellet, M. (2018) 'From the Phone to the Classroom: Categories of Problems for Telephone Interpreting Training', *The Interpreters' Newsletter* 2018, 23, pp. 19–44.

Jaime Pérez, A. (2015) 'Remote Interpreting in Public Services. Developing a 3G Phone Interpreting Application', in Lázaro Gutiérrez, R., Vigier Moreno, F. and Sánchez Ramos, M. M. (eds.) *Investigación emergente en traducción e interpretación*. Granada: Comares, pp. 73–82.

Jones, D. and Gill, P. (1998) 'Breaking Down Language Barriers', *British Medical Journal,* 316(7143), pp. 1476–1480.

Kelly, N. (2008a) *A Medical Interpreter's Guide to Telephone Interpreting.* Available at: www.imiaweb.org/uploads/pages/380.pdf (Accessed: 15 December 2020).

Kelly, N. (2008b) *Telephone Interpreting: A Comprehensive Guide to the Profession*. Victoria, BC: Trafford.

Ko, L. (2006) 'The Need for Long-Term Empirical Studies in Remote Interpreting Research: A Case Study of Telephone Interpreting', *Linguistica Antverpiensia,* 5, pp. 325–338.

Kurz, I. (1999) 'Remote Conference Interpreting: Assessing the Technology', *Anovar/anosar estudios de traducción e interpretación,* I, pp. 114–116.

Lázaro Gutiérrez, R. (2009) 'Dilemas éticos del traductor / intérprete en los servicios públicos', *Translation, Interpreting and Social Activisim.*

Lázaro Gutiérrez, R. (2012) *La Interpretación en el Ámbito Sanitario. Estudio de la Asimetría en Consultas Médicas.* Saarbrücken: Editorial Académica Española.

Lázaro Gutiérrez, R. (2017a) 'Research into the Practice of Telephone Interpreting in Spain', in Valero Garcés, C., and Pena Díaz, C. (eds.) *Superando límites en traducción e interpretación.* Geneva: Editions Tradulex, pp. 159–164.

Lázaro Gutiérrez, R. (2017b) 'El estudio de la cortesía en conversaciones mediadas por un intérprete sanitario', in Ortega Arjonilla, E. (ed.) *Sobre la práctica de la traducción y la interpretación en la actualidad* (vol. 2 Barceló Martínez, T., and Delgado Pugés, I., *De traducción jurídica y socioeconómica e interpretación para los servicios públicos*). Granada: Comares, pp. 265–276.

Lázaro Gutiérrez, R. (2018) 'Interpretación sanitaria para víctimas de violencia de género', *Panace@*, XIX(47), pp. 96–105.

Lázaro Gutiérrez, R. and Cabrera Méndez, G. (2018) 'Pragmática e interpretación telefónica: un estudio sobre ataques contra la imagen de los intérpretes (FTA, Face threatening acts)', in Curado, A. (ed.) *LSP in Multi-disciplinary Contexts of Teaching and Research. EPiC Series in Language and Linguistics*, 3, pp. 85–90.

Lázaro Gutiérrez, R. and Cabrera Méndez, G. (2019) 'Context and Pragmatic Meaning in Telephone Interpreting', in Garcés-Conejos Blitvich, P., Fernández-Amaya, L. and Hernández-López, M. O. (eds) *Technology Mediated Service Encounters.* Amsterdam: John Benjamins, pp. 45–68.
Lee, J. (2007) 'Telephone Interpreting Seen from the Interpreters' Perspective', *Interpreting*, 9(2), pp. 231–252.
Levinson, S. (1979) 'Activity Types and Language', *Linguistics*, 17, pp. 356–399.
Luque Martín, M. (2008) 'La interpretación telefónica en España', *Hermeneus*, 10, pp. 313–320.
Mack, G. (2001) 'Conference Interpreters on the Air: Live Simultaneous Interpreting on Italian Television', in Gambier, Y., and Gottlieb, H. (eds.) *(Multi)Media Translation: Concepts, Practices, and Research.* Amsterdam and Philadelphia: John Benjamins, pp. 125–132.
Martínez-Gómez, A. (2008) 'La interpretación telefónica en los servicios de atención al inmigrante de Castilla-La Mancha', in Valero Garcés, C., Pena Díaz, C. and Lázaro Gutiérrez, R. (eds) *Investigación y práctica en traducción e interpretación en los servicios públicos: desafíos y alianza.* Alcalá de Henares: Servicio de Publicaciones de la Universidad de Alcalá, pp. 339–354.
Mikkelson, H. (2003) 'Telephone Interpreting: Boon or Bane?', in González, L. P. (ed.), *Speaking in Tongues: Language Across Contexts and Users.* Valencia: Universitat de València, pp. 251–269.
Mintz, D. (1998) 'Hold the Phone: Telephone Interpreting Scrutinized', *Proteus,* 7(1), pp. 1–5.
Murgu, D. and Jiménez, S. (2011) 'La formación de un intérprete telefónico', in Valero Garcés, C., Bodzer, A., Vitalaru, B. and Lázaro Gutiérrez, R. (eds.) *Traducción e interpretación en los servicios públicos en un mundo INTERcoNEcTado (TISP en INTERNET).* Alcalá de Henares: Servicio de publicaciones de la Universidad de Alcalá, pp. 214–219.
Oviatt, S. and Cohen, P. (1992) 'Spoken Language in Interpreted Telephone Dialogues', *Computer Speech and Language,* 6, pp. 277–302.
Ozolins, U. (2011) 'Telephone Interpreting: Understanding Practice and Identifying Research Needs', *Translation and Interpreting*, 3(2), pp. 33–47.
Paneth, E. (2002) 'An Investigation into Conference Interpreting', in Pöchhacker, F. and Shlesinger, M. (eds), *The Interpreting Studies Reader*. London and New York: Routledge, pp. 31–41.
Pertusa Elorriaga, I. (2012) 'La interpretación en la distancia', *Suplemento: la traducción y la interpretación en los servicios públicos. Revista Traditori*, 3, pp. 25–29.
Phelan, M. (2001) *The Interpreter's Resource.* Manchester: Multilingual Matters.
Phillips, C. (2013) 'Remote Telephone Interpretation in Medical Consultations with Refugees: Meta-Communication About Care, Survival and Selfhood', *Journal of Refugee Studies,* 26(4), pp. 505–523.
Prieto, M. N. (2008) 'La interpretación telefónica en los servicios sanitarios públicos. Estudio de caso: el servicio de 'conversación a tres' del Hospital Carlos Haya de Málaga', in Valero Garcés, C., Pena Díaz, C. and Lázaro Gutiérrez, R. (eds.) *Investigación y práctica en traducción e intepretación en los servicios públicos: desafíos y alianza*. Alcalá de Henares: Servicio de Publicaciones de la Universidad de Alcalá, pp. 369–384.
Rosenberg, B. A. (2002) 'Un análisis de la interpretación telefónica', in Valero Garcés, C. (ed.) *Traducción como mediación entre lenguas y culturas*. Alcalá de Henares: Servicio de Publicaciones de la Universidad de Alcalá, pp. 243–249.
Rosenberg, B. A. (2004) 'A Data Driven Analysis of Telephone Interpreting', in Wadensjö, C., Dimitrova, B. E. and Nilsson, A. (eds.) *The Critical Link 4: Professionalisation of Interpreting in the Community.* Amsterdam and Philadelphia: John Benjamins, pp. 65–77.
Roy, C. (2000) *Interpreting as a Discourse Process*. Oxford: Oxford University Press.
Ruiz Mezcua, A. (2018) 'General Overview of Telephone Interpretation (TI): A State of the Art', in Ruiz Mezcua, A. (ed.) *Approaches to Telephone Interpretation. Research, Innovation, Teaching and Transference*. Bern: Peter Lang, pp. 7–17.
Russo, M., Bendazzoli, C., Sandrelli, A. and Spinolo, N. (2012) 'The European Parliament Interpreting Corpus (EPIC): Implementation and Developments', in Straniero Sergio, F. and Falbo, C. (eds.) *Breaking the Ground in Corpus-Based Interpreting Studies*. Bern: Peter Lang, pp. 53–90.
Schenker, Y., Fernández, A., Kerr, K., O'Riordan, D. and Pantilat, S. Z. (2012) 'Interpretation for Discussions About End-Of-Life Issues: Results From a National Survey of Health Care Interpreters', *Journal of Palliative Medicine,* 15(9), pp. 1019–1026.
Spinolo, N., Bertozzi, M. and Russo, M. (2018) 'Shaping the Interpreters of the Future and of Today: Preliminary Results of the SHIFT Project', *The Interpreters' Newsletter*, 23, pp. 45–61.

Verrept, H. (2011) 'Intercultural Mediation Through the Internet in Belgian Hospitals', *4th International Conference on Public Service Interpreting and Translation*, Madrid, 13–15 April 2011. Available at: http://tisp2011.tucongreso.es/ti2011/files/book-abstracts.pdf (Accessed: 15 December 2020).

Vidal, M. (1998) 'Telephone Interpreting: Technological Advance or Due Process Impediment?' *Proteus,* 7(3), pp. 1–6.

Wadensjö, C. (1998) *Interpreting as Interaction*. London and New York: Addison Wesley Longman.

Wadensjö, C. (1999) 'Telephone Interpreting and the Synchronization of Talk in Social Interaction', *The Translator*, 5(2), pp. 247–264.

Wilson, C. W. (2010) 'Working Through, With or Despite Technology? A Study of Interpreter-Mediated Encounters When Interpreting Is Provided by Video Conferencing Link', *Critical Link 6: Interpreting in a Changing Landscape*, Birmingham, July 2010.

14

Reducing health disparities in the Deaf community

The impact of interpreters and the rise of deaf healthcare professionals

Christopher J. Moreland and Laurie Swabey

1 Introduction

Deaf communities are as diverse as any other patient population – culturally, linguistically, and socially – and there are many important factors to consider related to their healthcare and communication. As with other underserved healthcare minority groups, deaf people are at higher risk for experiencing serious healthcare disparities as compared to the general population. Signed language interpreters with specialised training in healthcare can contribute to reducing those disparities through multiple channels. It should be noted that interpreters are not the only avenue available to deaf patients seeking healthcare and, in many cases, using a language-concordant provider or a healthcare programme that is run by and for deaf people, may be the preferred choice for the patient. However, in this chapter we will explore the systems within which qualified healthcare interpreters work and their impacts on the health of the Deaf and Hard of Hearing (DHH) community.

We begin this chapter by briefly defining concepts fundamental to signed language interpreting and summarising the relevant similarities and differences between signed language and spoken language interpreting in healthcare settings. From there, we describe historical perspectives on and critical issues in healthcare interpreting. We then explore the health disparities affecting the deaf population, followed by the means through which professional interpreting can impact deaf health outcomes. We will also address the significance of interpreters for deaf professionals seeking training and practice as clinicians, leading to critically important language concordance between deaf clinicians and deaf patients.

2 Definitions and comparisons

Signed languages are naturally occurring languages that have been in existence for as long as there have been deaf people in contact with each other. Although many people assume

 DOI: 10.4324/9781003167983-18

that signed language is universal, it is not. Another common misconception is that if regions or countries share a common spoken language, they will also share a common signed language. As an example, although English is spoken in the United States, the United Kingdom, Ireland and Australia, each country, or sometimes region, has its own signed language. Some countries, such as Mexico, have more than one signed language. Most signed languages are referred to by acronyms, e.g. Nederlandse Gebarentaal, NGT (Netherlands); Lengua de Signos Española, LSE (one of the signed languages used in Spain); American Sign Language, ASL (used in the United States and parts of Canada); and Polski Język Migowy, PJM (Poland). It is also worth mentioning that the DHH community comprises a widely heterogeneous range of linguistic, communicative and adaptive preferences and skills, and that signed language is only one of the various forms of communication. Other forms include spoken and written language (e.g. English, Japanese), signed communication apart from formal languages (e.g. cued speech, Signed Exact English), speech-reading, and the use of hearing aids, cochlear implants, or other adaptive technologies.

Signed language interpreting is often described as bimodal because interpreters frequently work between a language that is signed – produced by the hands, face, and body and perceived by the eyes – and a language that is spoken, that is produced through vocalisation and perceived auditorily. However, signed language interpreters also work between different signed languages (e.g. between ASL and LSE). In contrast, the work of spoken language interpreters is usually unimodal, working between languages that are conveyed in a spoken mode (e.g. spoken English and spoken Spanish).

In dialogic medical settings, such as doctor-patient interviews, spoken language interpreters will often use a consecutive mode for a variety of reasons, including the avoidance of interference that may occur when two people speak at the same time. Signed language interpreters have traditionally been taught to interpret primarily in the simultaneous mode, despite studies indicating benefits of consecutive interpreting (Russell 2005). A professional signed language interpreter considers several factors when determining whether consecutive interpreting, simultaneous interpreting, or moving between both formats is most effective for communication in a given situation. If a patient is telling an emotional story that they have been reticent to reveal, simultaneous interpreting may be preferable. If a series of questions is being asked or when an interpreting team is being used (trilingual and/or deaf-hearing team), consecutive interpreting may be preferable. Whatever the mode, healthcare providers need to remain cognisant of non-verbal interactional behaviours that establish therapeutic rapport with the patient even in the presence of an interpreter (e.g. producing emotionally appropriate expressions, looking directly at the DHH patient).

Healthcare interpreting may be carried out through several different types of interpreting teams. In areas with high numbers of immigrants and refugees, it is becoming more common for signed language interpreters to work with three languages (trilingual interpreting). This is illustrated by an example from the United States in which the physician speaks only English, the mother of a deaf teenage patient speaks only Spanish, and the patient uses only ASL. In this case, the trilingual interpreter goes between spoken English, spoken Spanish, and ASL. If a trilingual interpreter with fluency in these three languages is not available, the services of two interpreters would be required: a Spanish/English interpreter and an ASL/English interpreter.

Increasing evidence suggests that teams consisting of an interpreter who is deaf and an interpreter who can hear may be an effective option in healthcare. In medical contexts, there is often a lack of lexical correspondence between a signed language (e.g. ASL) and the spoken language (e.g. English) for specialised terminology, an issue often complicated by regional variations (or dialects) in sign use. Standard signs may exist for concepts such as diabetes and blood pressure but not for glaucoma, osteoporosis or hormones. Signed languages have a rich array of linguistic features for expressing medical concepts and deaf interpreters, as native or near-native users of ASL, may be more effective in using these linguistic features in interpreting than hearing interpreters who learn signed language as an adult. Furthermore, deaf interpreters have cultural competencies that may not be as deeply developed in hearing interpreters; those competencies may positively inform the development of strong therapeutic rapports between the patient and clinician in the context of potentially stressful medical issues. The following are examples when a deaf interpreter or a deaf clinician fluent in sign language may best serve the needs of the patient:

- A deaf patient who is an immigrant or refugee
- A deaf patient with limited health literacy
- Situations that involve deaf children or elderly patients (or others) with idiosyncratic ways of signing, and
- A deaf patient with mental health or cognitive issues

Some clinics and hospitals have common medical forms translated into multiple languages. For deaf patients, these forms are translated into the local signed language and presented in a video format. Translation work from written language to the signed language of the local deaf community (or vice versa), is frequently done by translators who are deaf and often performed by teams. Since signed languages do not have written forms, a translation is usually done from a printed document (the written form of the local spoken language) to a video-recorded translation in the patient's signed language or from a video recording in a signed language to a written document.

Some signed language interpreters specialise in working with people who are DeafBlind. People who are DeafBlind prefer different types of interpreting and may use a signed language interpreter at close visual range or tactile interpreting which is received by the DeafBlind person by touch with one or two hands. ProTactile is a newer approach that began in 2007 and has since gained momentum. Developed by DeafBlind people, ProTactile supports access to the world through touch, providing signers with rich information about the environment, non-verbal responses of interlocutors, and other critical information. One of the central ideas behind the philosophy of ProTactile is that DeafBlind people can achieve all human activities – learning, communicating, building, navigating – by touch. Vision and hearing are not required. According to two leaders of the ProTactile movement, Jelica Nuccio and aj granda, 'Protactile philosophy has grown out of the realisation that DeafBlind people's intuitions about tactile communication are stronger than the intuitions sighted people have. This realisation has changed the way we communicate with each other, the way we work with interpreters, and more generally, the way we live' (DeafBlind Interpreting National Training and Resource Center). Increasingly, interpreters are being trained by DeafBlind ProTactile experts in the philosophy and use of ProTactile. Recent research from Edwards (2014) documents some of the differences between visual ASL and ProTactile ASL.

Signed language interpreters who grew up in deaf families, often referred to as heritage signers, are recognised as having cultural and linguistic knowledge that makes them suitable for developing professional interpreting competencies. In many countries, these individuals may also be referred to as Codas. Originally this stood for 'children of deaf adults' and now refers to a hearing person with one deaf parent. CODA International is a worldwide organisation with a presence in many places including Ireland, Hong Kong, Germany, France and Italy. Although some deaf people may want trusted family members or friends who sign to be part of the medical interview, care should be taken to not confuse a relative, family member or friend who signs with a professionally prepared interpreter. Family members and friends have a different role in healthcare interpreted interactions than a professionally trained interpreter; as *ad hoc* interpreters with roles influenced by emotional and other factors, they may adversely impact the accuracy of the interpreted message.

2.1 Areas of similarity and difference for signed language interpreters and spoken language interpreters

There are many similarities between signed language and spoken language interpreters in healthcare settings. Both spoken and signed language interpreters may interpret consecutively or simultaneously, as well as perform sight translations. Both signed language and spoken language interpreting have also undergone a process of professionalisation in the last 40 years, including healthcare interpreting. As part of this professionalisation, interpreters of any language pair are expected to understand and apply ethical principles in their decision-making, and be able to accurately monitor their own work. All interpreters must be aware that a purely lexical or phrasal approach – literally trying to match words/signs – does not allow a patient to have meaningful access to the interaction. In some parts of the world, education and training programmes for signed language interpreters and spoken language interpreters have evolved over the years from very short training courses (40 hours or less) to bachelor's and master's degree programmes, and have embraced approaches that focus on discourse and interaction. In order to interpret effectively, interpreters need to know something about the purpose and goals of the medical encounter before interpreting. Furthermore, the healthcare encounter is likely to be most successful when the clinician, patient and interpreter all share an understanding of the interpreter's role and when the healthcare providers have had training in working with an interpreter. For example, the clinician's use of visual aids, such as anatomical models or diagrams, is often beneficial for communication for all parties.

In addition to generalist competencies, interpreters working in healthcare settings need expertise related to the healthcare context. As an example, below are qualifications for ASL/English medical interpreters, developed by a national expert panel (Swabey and Craft Farber 2012):

- Bilingual fluency in English and ASL, including the ability to produce and comprehend sociolinguistic variation
- Understanding of linguistic, social and cultural influences that impact healthcare interactions (e.g. specialised vocabulary, discourse styles, language register, dynamics of power and prestige between interlocutors, and triadic communication)
- Adhering to the Registry of Interpreters for the Deaf and the National Association of the Deaf Code of Professional Conduct and familiarity with the National Council on Interpreting in Health Care code of ethics
- Balancing the need for maintaining professional distance with empathy and flexibility

- Knowing the laws and policies related to healthcare settings (e.g. liability, Americans with Disabilities Act, state-specific human rights laws, hospital policies)
- Knowing the general physiological and psychological implications of healthcare
- Understanding of various health care approaches (e.g. Chinese medicine, ayurvedic, holistic, homeopathic, Western medicine, hospice)
- Understanding underlying practices of various health care delivery systems and the role of self and others on the health care team (e.g. employing CDIs, Deaf Community Healthcare Workers [CHWs] and advocates when they can enhance the communication)
- Sharing information and resources about communication through advocacy, leadership and education in healthcare settings

Preparation, reflection and professional development are important for all interpreters; and where available, interpreters who work in healthcare should pursue advanced training and credentialing in healthcare interpreting.

Although both spoken language interpreters and signed language interpreters provide valuable and needed services in healthcare settings, the phrase 'the illusion of inclusion' is used more frequently as the population that uses interpreting becomes increasingly diverse. The assumption that providing a patient with an interpreter automatically means equal access is a notion that needs to be examined. There are many factors in play – for example, the skills and knowledge of the interpreter, including the ability to convey discourse functions, the communication needs and preferences of the interlocuters, the background/contextual knowledge about the topic/situation, and the demands of the particular interaction. Related to signed language interpreting across all settings, De Meulder and Haualand (2019) make the case that the provision of interpreting services should not be synonymous with access.

Regarding the differences between spoken language and signed language interpreting in healthcare settings, interpreting with deaf patients or deaf healthcare providers requires attention to placement of people and equipment that differ from the requirements for interactions between non-deaf patients and providers. Spoken language interpreting can occur via telephone/audio conferencing or with the interpreter behind a privacy screen. However, deaf people and signed language interpreters must be able to see each other in order to communicate, thus neither audio conferencing nor interpreting behind a screen are available options. Video relay and video remote interpreting may be used in healthcare situations with deaf patients. However, in many situations, an onsite interpreter is preferable and a video interpreter is used only until the onsite interpreter arrives. Some of the challenges include technical inadequacies (e.g. the strength of the internet connection in order to have a clear and consistent video of the interpretation), the inability of the patient to see the video screen due to musculoskeletal or other clinical hindrances, and the ability to move the video interpreting technology quickly and efficiently with the patient into different rooms/areas (which can lead to frequently dropped connections).

There are other settings in which consideration needs to be given to how the patient will have visual access to the situation, including the ability to see the interpretation clearly. Examples include:

- When the patient is face down for an examination or treatment
- A room for an eye examination where the lights are turned down or out
- When the doctor is speaking to a patient who cannot keep their eyes open

The interpreter must also be well prepared to interpret for deaf patients who have limited use of their hands and arms due to illness, injury, or IVs. For patients who have back, head or neck injuries, finding a position that allows for effective visual communication can be challenging. Ideally, the patient, the provider and the interpreter should be able to see each other, as this is one component of rapport building which is crucial for the patient-clinician relationship.

Another difference between signed language and spoken language interpreters is that, as mentioned earlier, signed language interpreters are not always trained in consecutive interpreting and notetaking, although these are competencies commonly incorporated into spoken language community interpreting programmes. Spoken language interpreters have a long history in the areas of translation and conference interpreting. In comparison, these are relatively new fields of professional study and training for signed language interpreters. Interpreting services for refugees and immigrants reveal further differences between spoken and signed languages. While it is sometimes assumed or expected that people from these groups will learn the language of the area and not need interpreting services across their lifespan, deaf people use interpreters across all ages and stages of life. The laws for providing interpreting services for non-deaf immigrants and refugees are different in many countries form what they are for deaf people; for the latter, legal requirements often focus on the framework of disability. Finally, for immigrants and refugees who are patients in healthcare systems and use interpreters to communicate with healthcare providers, there is an imbalance of power. Although this is true for many patients who are deaf, as this chapter later points out, deaf physicians and other healthcare providers who are deaf can be the ones using an interpreter in their professional role in a clinic or hospital, reinforcing the aforementioned concept of deaf people often working with interpreters through different times and in varying roles across their lives. As will be described later in this chapter, interpreters working with deaf healthcare providers need specialised training, education and skills.

In order to interpret effectively between deaf patients and hearing clinicians, it is important for interpreters to explore the deaf perspective of the inequities and challenges many deaf people experience when they try to access healthcare services and the impact that the historical oppression of deaf people has had on health. The next section therefore provides foundational information that is crucial for signed language interpreters working in healthcare settings.

2.2 Healthcare disparities in the Deaf community

People in the DHH community experience significant health disparities, as compared to the general population. A health disparity occurs when a particular health outcome (such as the incidence of diabetes, smoking prevalence, or death) occurs significantly more often in a certain subpopulation than another. Healthy People 2020 defines health disparity as 'a particular type of health difference that is closely linked with social, economic, and/or environmental disadvantage'. The means by which health disparities arise are numerous and complex, ranging from nutrition to racism. Among the factors contributing to health disparities is deafness, and poor access to communication has been identified as a major cause of this disparity.

When growing up, people can learn about health issues through formal and incidental pathways. Formal pathways include health education classes, receiving advice from one's physician, and reading about health information. Incidental learning, on the other hand, occurs by picking up cues and information in one's environment. These can include listening to one's parents while they discuss their own health information (or that of other family members) with their physicians, with friends in person, or over the phone; this learning can even take place when listening to television commercials about medications. The process of naming and describing one's own health issues can be acquired in similar fashion. The DHH child with one or more DHH parents is more likely to have mutual access to communication and thus incidentally learn, a statement which has been supported in early retrospective work (Hall *et al.* 2018). When one is DHH with hearing parents, which is estimated to occur among 90 per cent of the DHH population, one frequently cannot overhear such comments, and thus must rely dominantly, if not fully, on formal learning mechanisms about healthcare.

What barriers then exist with formal learning mechanisms? For the written word, health information in the United States is often published above approximately the reading level of the average 11- to 12-year old, while the data suggest that the average DHH American's reading level is notably lower. If a DHH person were to seek information published in a signed language format, such as a video online or via social media, few well developed or validated resources exist, even though it has been shown that such sign-based resources are effective in improving DHH people's health knowledge (Zazove 2012).

Although visits to one's physician are frequently seen as the primary resource of individualised health care and education, this is not always the case for the DHH community. In multiple studies, deaf people have identified inadequate communication as a dominant barrier to fully accessing and optimising their healthcare (O'Day *et al.* 2004). Many people think first of face-to-face communication; in this situation, DHH patients have reported experiencing providers' inaccurate assumptions without first engaging the DHH person. For those who rely on spoken language and speech-reading, more time is often needed to understand others' speech, yet providers and clinical staff may speak too quickly or without looking directly at the DHH person. The limited literacy of some DHH people precludes note-writing as an effective means of discussing complex health-related information, from symptomatology to possible diagnoses to complex health management planning. Some have reported that, if their English proficiency is limited, they perceive that physicians underestimate their intelligence and may not fully engage the DHH person during interviews, physical examinations, or even medical procedures, increasing the risk of patient discomfort, confusion and fear. Such barriers impact DHH people internationally; in a survey of deaf adolescents in Ghana, many reported struggling to access healthcare communication effectively due to the absence of resources available for those who sign (Senayah *et al.* 2018). Similarly, a focus group study of hospitalised Italian deaf people sustained the theme of communicative disempowerment (Sirch, Salvador and Palese 2017).

What specific health disparities impact the DHH population as a result of these barriers and challenges? Research thus far has identified a number of areas, mostly via surveys. Health knowledge comprises the largest domain for disparities studied in the literature, particularly among DHH people who use primarily signed language. A study in the 1990s of DHH people's health literacy showed less understanding of risk factors for acquiring HIV (Human Immunodeficiency Virus); these results persisted in studies in the 2000s, suggesting little progress over that decade in the United States (Heuttel 2001; Bat-Chava, Martin and Kosciw 2005). Similar findings have been reported in Swaziland and Brazil (Groce *et al.* 2006; Bisol *et al.* 2008). Deaf women in focus groups reflected lower understanding of the value of mammograms and Pap smears in cancer surveillance

(Steinberg *et al.* 2002); a survey of DHH women and men published in 2018 showed similarly low understanding of HPV's relevance to cervical cancer and whether HPV vaccination would reduce the risk of cervical cancer (Spellun, Moreland and Kushalnagar 2018). Orsi *et al.* found persisting low knowledge of Pap smear value (2007). Fewer than half of a study's respondents recognised chest discomfort as a potential sign of a heart attack (Margellos-Anast, Estarziau and Kaufman 2006). Overall knowledge about cancer prevention intervention knowledge has been noted to be low as well (Zazove *et al.* 2009). Such disparities extend beyond the domain of clinical knowledge and impact DHH people's physical health, the use of healthcare services, and even healthcare outcomes. For instance, marked food insecurity has been reported by DHH people at higher rates than the general US population; such food insecurity correlates with having worse overall health (Kushalnagar *et al.* (2018). DHH people might use the emergency departments more often than the general population (McKee *et al.* 2015), and Mitra *et al.* (2016) identified worse perinatal outcomes for pregnant women with hearing loss.

3 Historical perspectives

Signed languages have existed throughout time in all parts of the world in which there have been deaf people living within a community. Just as long, members of these communities have been called upon to act as (*ad hoc*, or untrained) interpreters (Stone 2009). Although the documentation to date is sparse, there are records of signed language interpreters being utilised in Europe in the 16th century and in the United States from the beginning of the 19th century. Without training or educational programmes, those who acted as interpreters or translators were often members of a Deaf community, having learned how to sign from deaf family members. In addition, those who worked with deaf individuals as teachers, social workers or clergy often knew some signed language and acted as interpreters. Stone (2009) documented that bilingual deaf members of communities (fluent in the written language of the country as well as the signed language of the country) often functioned as translators. The professionalisation of signed language interpreting – including training programmes, degrees and credentialing – only began in the 1960s and is still in its infancy in many countries. The United States is often recognised as leading the world in the development of signed language research and signed language interpreter training programmes. The civil rights movement that began in the mid-20th century fuelled some of these changes, as well as the recognition of American Sign Language as a naturally occurring language, separate from English. Registry of Interpreters for the Deaf (RID), the national organisation of interpreters in the United States, was established in 1964.

Professional publications and research on signed language interpreting began in the early 1960s, with most of the publications in the 1960s and 1970s coming from the United States and written in English (Metzger 2006; Grbic 2007). In 1978, a conference in Venice brought together spoken and signed language interpreters. At that conference Robert M. Ingram, a pioneer in promoting linguistic research of signed language interpreting, made the argument that 'no description (practical or theoretical) of interpretation which fails to take account of sign language interpretation can be regarded as complete' (Ingram 1978: 109). Although this viewpoint was not immediately adopted, the number of signed language interpreting publications increased by the mid- to late 1990s, both in number and country of origin. Initially, signed language and spoken language interpreting developed separately in education, research, publications and conference programming. Some notable changes to this began in 1995, with the series of Critical Link Conferences which brought together stakeholders from different countries involved in community interpreting in both spoken languages and signed languages, including programme administrators, language planners, educators, researchers and interpreters from across the world. *Introducing Interpreting Studies* (Pöchhacker 2004) was one of the first interpreting studies textbooks to integrate signed language interpreting. Since that time, journals, books, conferences and educational programmes have integrated signed language interpreting as part of interpreting studies, a subfield of the larger academic discipline of translation studies.

In most countries, signed language interpreting was initially a field of 'generalists'. In other words, those who were fluent in a signed language and spoken language and had well-honed interpreting skills functioned as interpreters in all settings, including medical settings. In the United States, RID began testing and certifying generalist interpreters in 1972. To date, there is not a national certification in healthcare interpreting offered by RID, although some states have certificates or licences for medical interpreting. In the United States, lawsuits filed against hospitals for not providing adequate communication access have also ignited some healthcare systems to institute better policies for providing qualified medical interpreters.

Training and credentialing for signed language interpreters in the United Kingdom and Europe began in the 1970s and in Australia in the 1980s. In contrast to the United States, Australia has a certification system that recognises the specialisation of medical interpreting. However, in many countries, there still are no organised programmes for teaching signed language or signed language interpreting, let alone a specialty such as medical interpreting. Some countries, such as Scotland, New Zealand, Canada and Germany, do have signed language interpreting programmes at the undergraduate or graduate levels. However, many countries in Latin America, Africa and Asia do not have degree programmes in signed language interpreting. Overall, 'developing' countries often have no organised training for signed language interpreters. 'Developed' countries may have only general training (e.g. workshops, short courses) or full degree programmes at the undergraduate or graduate levels. Few countries have in-depth, specialised training in healthcare interpreting. Even in countries with qualified, trained healthcare interpreters, a request for a qualified healthcare interpreter at a specific time and place often cannot be fulfilled due to the imbalance between supply and demand, particularly in rural areas.

Even with the advancements in the last 40 years to professionalise signed language interpreting, and more recently to provide specialised training in healthcare interpreting, access to interpreting services is still a challenge for many deaf patients. As interpreters gained education and credentials, they also expected to be compensated for their services, just as other professionals are in health settings. However, the responsibility of paying for a signed language interpreter in healthcare settings varies, depending on many factors. In the United States, legislation requires that hospitals and clinics provide access to people with disabilities, including the provision of interpreters for deaf people. However, deaf people still identify healthcare as one of the most difficult settings in which to attain a qualified interpreter. In most European countries, the government is responsible for funding the cost of interpreters in medical settings, although there are restrictions. For example, in the Netherlands, deaf people have a right to an interpreter at no cost for 15 per cent of their work time, 100 per cent of their education, and then only 30 hours a year for other situations (De Wit 2016). Further, even if the government is responsible for the expense of an interpreter, there may not be an interpreter or a reliable service that connects deaf patients with qualified interpreters available at the time they are needed. In two European countries, Kosovo and Albania, no payment is available for medical interpreters (De Wit 2016). Similarly, although Uganda has more than 200 certified interpreters, interpreting services remain unfunded by the government. In Albania, Cyprus, France, Germany, Luxembourg, and Turkey, deaf people cannot choose or request a preferred interpreter. Even in countries where this is an option, the preferred interpreter may not be available. Thus, even in very personal, intimate or painful encounters, deaf people may have no control over who will interpret. Specifically, men who prefer a male interpreter may not have that option, even in countries where that request can be made. In the United States and Europe, signed language interpreting is a highly female profession with approximately 87 per cent female (self-reported) in the United States (RID, 2018) and 87 per cent in Europe (De Wit 2016).

4 Current contributions and research

Interpreting has been described by Roy and Metzger (2014) as both interdisciplinary and cross-disciplinary. In the former case, this means that interpreting can be studied from a variety of disciplines including, but not limited to: linguistics, psychology, anthropology and sociology. In the latter case, it means that methodologies, frameworks, and theories from more than one discipline can be used to pursue research questions about interpreting. Following this, it is not surprising that qualitative, quantitative and mixed methods are all used in interpreting research. As a snapshot, Liu (2012) analysed the methodologies used in a sample of 48 articles published in the journal *Interpreting* during the period of 2004–2009, with three special issues on the topic of healthcare. Twenty-six of the 48 studies used a qualitative approach, including grounded theory, action research, and case study. Of the 22 studies that used a quantitative approach as the main method, approaches included descriptive quantitative studies, survey studies, correlational studies and experiments. The methodologies utilised in signed language interpreting research are similar to those used in studies of spoken language interpreting. One major variation exists because of the visual nature of signed language interpreting. To adequately measure, code and analyse signed language, researchers must employ video recording, which can lead to longer timeframes for data processing and analysis. Interpreting in public services settings, including healthcare interpreting, has been a major strand of research in interpreting studies. Signed language interpreting is part of the 'sociological turn' that is often described as occurring in interpreting and translation studies over the past 30 years (Angelelli 2012). This 'turn' is reflected in the increasing attention in research studies to the agency of interpreters and translators as well as social factors that influence the work of practitioners across all settings, including healthcare.

As recognition for the human rights of deaf citizens to have language and communication access has increased, so has the research that continues to investigate the complexity of bimodal interpreting and communication between deaf and non-deaf patient providers in healthcare settings. Of particular importance is the increase in contributions by interpreters, translators, interpreter educators, and healthcare professionals who are themselves deaf. Similarly, the number of educational programmes that focus on mental and medical healthcare interpreting is slowly increasing, providing much needed education to those who work in these settings. Understanding of the role and decision-making processes of a bimodal interpreter continues to evolve, with important contributions from Metzger (1999) on deconstructing the myth of neutrality, Llewellyn-Jones and Lee

(2014) redefining the role of the interpreter as having multiple dimensions and fluidity, and Dean and Pollard (2014) on demand control schema and observation and supervision. The need to recognise the importance of interpreters who are deaf and the lived experiences of deaf people has also increased, including the work of Forestal and Cole (2018) who provide a socio-cultural perspective on deaf translation. Interpreting as a social institution, as well as inclusion and access for deaf people, is critically analysed by De Meulder and Haualand (2019). Foundational work regarding the domains and competencies of healthcare interpreters (Swabey and Craft Faber 2012); the identification of task categories and tasks for describing the work of ASL healthcare interpreters, indicating the complexity and multidimensionality of the job (Olson and Swabey 2016), and the development of a career lattice for healthcare interpreters (Swabey *et al.* 2016) have contributed to the development of education in the United States. The European Union funded the *Medisigns* project in 2013, which had multiple goals, including the provision of training for interpreters, deaf people and medical professionals to interact more effectively in healthcare encounters. In Australia, Napier and Major have been prolific contributors to healthcare interpreting research (e.g. Major and Napier 2012 and 2019; Major 2014; Major, Napier and Stubbe 2012 and Major *et al.* 2012). The project *Medical Sign Bank: Sign Language Planning and Development in Interpreter-mediated Medical Health Care Delivery for Deaf Australians* (Johnston and Napier 2010) is breaking new ground by bringing together stakeholders, including interpreters, linguists, healthcare professionals and members of the deaf community, to create an effective and shared sign language vocabulary for healthcare encounters mediated by interpreters.

De Wit's (2016) documentation of interpreting services, costs and access helps to build an understanding of the availability of healthcare interpreting services for deaf people in Europe. Studies in Haiti (Hochgesang and McAuliff 2016), Kenya (Mweri, Akaranga and Okomo 2009), and Ghana (Maroney *et al.* 2018) document the development of signed language interpreting services and interpreting education. Video relay interpreting and video remote interpreting continue to be examined, both for increasing access to healthcare when used appropriately and denying access when used inappropriately (NAD-DSA 2016). It has become increasingly evident that there is a need in most parts of the world for interpreters who are well prepared to work in behavioural health and mental settings. An example of a programme that prepares experienced generalist interpreters in behavioural and mental health settings consists of a week-long intensive programme followed by observation and case study work, and finally a practicum. If all of these components are completed successfully, there is an eight-hour exam that, if passed, leads to the credential of Qualified Mental Health Interpreter. This programme was developed by the Deaf Services Division of the State of Alabama (Crump 2012) and has resulted in over 125 credentialed mental health interpreters in the United States.

However, it needs to be pointed out that while existing literature reflects significant advances in signed language interpreter education and research, as well as the benefits of clinicians' working with professional interpreters, many clinicians do not engage interpreters with appropriate training, even to the extent of normalising such behaviour in the context of time and other pressures (Ebert and Heckerling 1995; Diamond 2009). These behaviours have been identified in various places including the United States and Switzerland (Würth *et al.* 2018). Physicians acknowledge utilising *ad hoc* interpreters (e.g. family members), recognising the convenience of someone already present and familiar with the patient. Interpreting can also occur via video-based technologies, with the interpreters located off-site; these situations, while often serving when in-person interpreters are not available, are dependent on intact technology, Internet connections, and appropriate use. Video relay services, for example, may be challenging for the visually impaired or severely ill DHH person. In one national survey, over one-third of DHH respondents reported being dissatisfied with VRI services (Kushalnagar 2019). In one study in South Africa, signed language interpreting use was thought to contribute to more equivalent health care utilisation as compared to the general population (Zulu, Heap and Sinanovic 2017).

4.1 Language-concordant care and the Deaf community

While signed language interpreting is a critical means of reducing health disparities, another increasingly important approach exists in the form of language and deafness concordance. Patient-physician concordance occurs when people seeking healthcare share one or more important characteristics with their healthcare providers. Those characteristics can include race, ethnicity, military veteran status, sex, and gender, among others. Patient-physician concordance in various forms has been shown to improve patient satisfaction and health measures, although the quality and results of studies are heterogeneous. For example, evidence suggests that people with language-concordant physicians have better diabetes control (Parker 2017) and are more likely to discuss dietary and exercise modifications (Eamranond 2009). Race concordance has been linked with more positive patient affect and satisfaction (Cooper 2003) and with generally improved health communication and patient engagement (Shen 2018). Gender concordance may have some effect on cardiovascular disease risk factor control (Schmittdiel 2009). While not uniform, these findings suggest that patient-physician concordance has viable effects on patient care.

Discrimination in healthcare has been well described in the forms of racism and sexism and forms directed at other underserved healthcare minorities; in line with these descriptions, audism is a term coined by a deaf scholar, Tom Humphries, in 1975. It refers to the discrimination of deaf people and parallels other terms that are part of discussions on human rights and oppression, such as racism and classism. Bauman (2004) suggested the following three definitions of audism: 'The notion that one is superior based on one's ability to hear or behave in the manner of one who hears; a system of advantage based on hearing ability; a metaphysical orientation that links human identity with speech (p. 245).' The first definition is the initial seed planted by Tom Humphries (1975). The second is adapted from Wellman's (1993) definition of racism and is mindful of Lane's (1992) discussion of institutionalised audism. The third definition was presented at the Deaf Studies VI conference by Bahan and Bauman (2000). It is vital that interpreters are aware of audism, as it permeates almost every situation in which deaf people interact with hearing people.

Research on DHH patient concordance with clinicians, whether through deafness (i.e. with DHH clinicians) or signed communication (i.e. with clinicians who sign fluently) has findings similar to race- and language concordance as described above, though this particular form of deafness concordance has been less explored. In one study, DHH patients with providers who signed were more likely to have received preventive health services (McKee *et al.* 2011), although no reliable estimate exists to quantify how many physicians sign fluently. Beyond deafness alone, rising numbers of physicians with disabilities have been discussed as a means of improving patient care for those with disabilities, yet another form of concordance (Iezzoni 2016). This can occur by direct care concordance as well as via the impact on social awareness and education of colleagues working with those clinicians with disabilities. The University of Rochester Medical Center's School of

Medicine is situated in Rochester, NY, where a highly concentrated DHH community resides. To foster greater understanding of the DHH experience, all medical students at this university undergo a simulated exercise in which they take on the role of patients navigating a simulated medical centre, one that functions fully in ASL with DHH community members playing staff and provider roles, with positive feedback from hearing participants (Thew 2012).

4.2 Deaf people as part of the healthcare workforce

Over the last two decades, the numbers of DHH people entering medical and other healthcare professional schools and completing training to become practitioners have rapidly risen. While we have yet to get a sense of the United States' DHH healthcare workforce as a whole (e.g. nurses, dentists), a 2013 study identified 86 people who identified as DHH physicians or medical students (Moreland *et al.* 2013). Owing to the snowball sampling approach used, this study did not provide a complete picture of DHH clinicians across the country. No parallel data yet exist in the literature to describe the DHH healthcare workforce in other countries.

In the late 1990s, a small group of DHH physicians formed the Society of Hearing Impaired Physicians; this organisation, along with an email listserv named NOISE created by Dr Danielle Rastetter, facilitated colleagues' connections with one another on thriving as DHH professionals. Shortly thereafter, in 2000, a small group of DHH veterinarians and physicians formally founded the Association of Healthcare Professionals with Hearing Loss (AMPHL), a group that has grown in size since then and now holds biennial conferences for DHH healthcare professionals, students, and allies focusing on skill development, technological adaptations, and innovations with the aim of supporting the organisation's mission of advocacy, networking and mentorship.

Along with this growing group has come the need for newly specialised accommodations, including signed language and oral interpreters, in the United States. In the previously mentioned survey (Moreland *et al.* 2013), DHH physicians and medical students reported using a wide range of accommodations, including signed (23 per cent) and oral (14 per cent) interpreters, and computer-assisted real-time captioning (CART, 21 per cent). While some of those accommodations were reportedly used more often in particular situations (e.g. CART for lectures), interpreters' skills were employed across the board, from lectures and small group work to clinical administration and teaching. Indeed, DHH physicians utilised interpreters throughout their career stages, from school to residency training to independent practice. The same study reported evidence that physicians' satisfaction with accommodations correlated positively with career satisfaction and with the likelihood they would recommend a career in medicine to other DHH people. In other words, working well with interpreters seems to correlate with DHH physicians continuing to work in their careers and even potentially recruiting other DHH people into healthcare.

Interpreters have adapted to work effectively with DHH healthcare professionals (DHPs). Many interpreters have adopted more traditional approaches, often working intermittently as contractors when needed by the DHP, and rotating among a pool of other interpreters, dependent on scheduling decisions made by an interpreting agency or other organisation. Over time, in healthcare and in other fields, many deaf professionals (DPs, when used to describe professionals in fields not limited to healthcare) and interpreters formed and maintained long-lasting professional relationships, with numerous benefits noted by both as those longitudinal interpreters became their DPs' primary and preferred interpreters. This concept has been called the 'designated interpreter' (DI), a term first coined and explored by Hauser, Finch and Hauser (2008), with one chapter focusing on one DP/DI team's healthcare experience (Earhart and Hauser 2008).

In healthcare, the rapid expansion of the DI concept, in parallel with DHPs' larger presence, has led to changes in interprofessional dynamics, with the DHP often holding a higher-level degree than the interpreter (Swabey *et al.* 2016). In these situations, the DI becomes deeply familiar with the terminology, clinical situations, healthcare system and workflow within which the DHP functions. Relatively unusual situations may include frequent medical interpreting over the phone, working night or even 24-hour shifts, interpreting during critical care ('code blue') medical emergencies, and functioning in the sterile environment of the operating room. They may have to interpret for hearing clinicians who have a combination of rapid speech, strong accents, and complex terminology with rare pauses (Moreland and Agan 2012). In the case of the DHP who is in training, the DHP and DI often find themselves in a wide range of clinical situations, since students are often expected to learn about and work briefly in a multitude of subspecialties where they may practise after training is completed. DIs, like their DHPs, then face the challenge of regularly acclimatising to new team members as the DHP students rotate from one environment to another.

While many interpreters and DHPs have discussed what constitutes the most appropriate parameters for the DHP/DI relationship, one element with increasing emphasis seems to be the relationship of DHP to DI, and how they explicitly or unintentionally determine the boundaries of their professional spaces and relationships. Examples range from more concrete decisions such as where the DHI should stand, to broader concepts such as what channels and modes of feedback the team will use with one another (Agan 2018).

The opportunities for further exploration are rich. The very definition of a DI may have evolved. Some see the DHP-DI relationship as one shaped primarily by the DHP's values and preferences in their clinical role, while others may perceive it as a mutual partnership (Agan 2018; personal communication, Featherstone 2019, Moreland *et al.* 2013). Delineating the factors underlying the optimisation of an effective relationship will be critical, possibly drawing from other disciplines relevant to interprofessional communication, including in training environments. Training opportunities as a DI are in their infancy, with some content as part of a larger programme being developed (Hall, Elliott and Cullen 2019), and their experiences only beginning to be described in innovative fashion (Argenyi 2019, Moreland and Agan, 2012).

Finally, the DHH healthcare workforce needs to be more fully explored. Our understanding is currently limited to the workforce subset of physicians, physician trainees and medical students; a deeper understanding of other DHH workforce members (e.g. nurses, physical therapists) would paint a broader picture of potential routes of service to the DHH population as well as means of effectively recruiting and retaining DHH people into healthcare careers.

5 Conclusion

Rich in cultural, linguistic, communicative and clinical diversity, deaf and hard of hearing communities across the world face significant health care disparities, in large part due to systemic barriers to communication access; those disparities result in less understanding of one's own health as well as poorer health outcomes. Signed language interpreters can play powerful roles in facilitating effective communication between DHH patients. Over the past decades, signed language interpreting as a professionally generalised field has begun to incorporate specialised training in healthcare concepts, terminology and systems, allowing interpreters to function optimally in healthcare climates. That evolution has seen shifts in how signed language interpreters frame decision-making and other aspects of their work, including the inclusion of deaf people as professional interpreters. Another major emergence has been that of DHH people now practising as healthcare professionals, such as physicians and nurses, who likewise may see interpreting services and thus have spurred interpreters' further specialisation in working with clinicians. Those clinicians and interpreters provide a potent source of communication- and culture-concordant care for DHH people. Along with the increasing inclusion of DHH people as professionals, the education and practice of signed language interpreters continues to evolve, creating multiple potent pathways to improve healthcare outcomes for DHH people.

Further reading

Forestal, E. (2005) 'The Emerging Professionals: Deaf Interpreters and Their Views and Experiences of Training', in Marsharck, M., Peterson, R., Winston, E. A. and Sapere, P. (eds.) *Sign Language Interpreting and Interpreter Education: Directions for Research and Practice*. Oxford: Oxford University Press, pp. 235–258.

This chapter provides readers with a perspective from interpreters and interpreter educators who themselves are deaf, an important viewpoint that previously has often been missing from the literature.

Major, G. and Napier, J. (2012) 'Interpreting and Knowledge Medication in the Healthcare Setting. What Do We Really Mean by "Accuracy"?', *Linguistica Antverpiensia*, 11(11), pp. 207–225.

This chapter provides an in-depth look at what is meant by the concept of 'accuracy' when interpreting in the healthcare setting by two prominent scholars in signed language interpreting and translation.

McKee, M. M., Barnett, S., Block, R. C., and Pearson, T. A. (2011) 'Impact of Communication on Preventive Services Among Deaf American Sign Language Users', *American Journal of Preventive Medicine*, 41(1), pp. 75–79.

This chapter is written for healthcare clinicians and focuses on language concordance between deaf patients and ASL-skilled clinicians.

Metzger, M. (1999) *Sign Language Interpreting: Deconstructing the Myth of Neutrality*. Washington, DC: Gallaudet University Press.

This seminal book dispels the pervasive myth of neutrality in signed language interpreting, and includes examples and analyses related to the healthcare context.

Swabey, L., and Nicodemus, B. (2011) 'Bimodal Bilingual Interpreting in the U.S. Healthcare System: A Critical Linguistic Activity in Need of Investigation', in Nicodemus, B. and Swabey, L. (eds) *Advances in Interpreting Research: Inquiry in Action*. Amsterdam and Philadelphia: John Benjamins, pp. 241–260.

This chapter provides an overview of healthcare interpreting in the United States.

Related topics

Community/Liaison Interpreting in Healthcare Settings, Disability in Translation, Healthcare Interpreting Ethics

References

Agan, T. S. K. (2018) *Exploring Deaf Physicians' and Physician Trainees' Experiences with Designated Interpreters.* Unpublished Thesis. St. Catherine University, Minnesota.

Angelelli, C. (2012) 'The Sociological Turn in Translation and Interpreting Studies', *Translation and Interpreting Studies,* 7(2), pp. 125–128.

Argenyi, M. (2019) 'Beyond Facilitating Communication: The Value of Designated Interpreters. Am Rounds', *Academic Medicine*. Available at: http://academicmedicineblog.org/beyond-facilitating-communication-the-value-of-designated-interpreters/ (Accessed: 15 December 2020).

Bat-Chava, Y., Martin, D. and Kosciw, J. G. (2005) 'Barriers to HIV/Aids Knowledge and Prevention Among Deaf and Hard of Hearing People', *AIDS Care: Psychological and Socio-Medical Aspects of AIDS/HIV*, 17(5), pp. 623–634.

Bahan, B. and Bauman, H.-D. L. (2000) 'Audism: Toward a Postmodern Theory of Deaf Studies', *Deaf Studies VI Conference*, Orlando, FL.

Bauman, H.-D. L. (2004) 'Audism: Exploring the Metaphysics of Oppression', *The Journal of Deaf Studies and Deaf Education*, 9(2), pp. 239–246. DOI:https://doi-org.pearl.stkate.edu/10.1093/deafed/enh025

Bisol, C. A., Sperb, T. M., Brewer, T. H., Kato, S. K. and Shor-Posner, G. (2008) 'HIV/AIDS Knowledge and Health-Related Attitudes and Behaviors Among Deaf and Hearing Adolescents in Southern Brazil', *American Annals of the Deaf*, 153(4), pp. 349–356.

Cooper, L. A., Roter, D. L., Johnson, R. L., Ford, D. E., Steinwachs, D. M. and Powe, N. R. (2003) 'Patient-Centered Communication, Ratings of Care, and Concordance of Patient and Physician Race', *Annals of Internal Medicine*, 139(11), pp. 907–915.

Crump. C. (2012) 'Mental Health Interpreting Training, Standards, and Certification', in Malcolm, K. and Swabey, L. A. (eds) *In Our Hands: Educating Healthcare Interpreters.* Washington, DC: Gallaudet University Press, pp. 54–76.

Dean, R. and Pollard Jr, R. (2014) Context-based Ethical Reasoning in Interpreting. *The Interpreter and Translator Trainer*, 5, pp. 155–182. DOI:10.1080/13556509.2011.10798816.

De Meulder, M. and Haualand, H. (2019) 'Sign Language Interpreting Services: A Quick Fix for Inclusion?', *Translation and Interpreting Studies. The Journal of the American Translation and Interpreting Studies Association*. DOI:https://doi.org/10.1075/tis.18008.dem.

De Wit, M. (2016) *Sign Language Interpreting in Europe*. Baarn: Create Space.

Diamond, L. C., Schenker, Y., Curry, L., Bradley, E. H. and Fernandez, A. (2009) 'Getting By: Underuse of Interpreters by Resident Physicians', Journal of General Internal Medicine, 24(2), pp. 256–262. DOI:10.1007/s11606-008-0875-7.

Eamranond, P. P., Davis, R. B., Phillips, R. S. and Wee, C. C. (2009) 'Patient-Physician Language Concordance and Lifestyle Counseling Among Spanish-Speaking Patients', *Journal of Immigrant and Minority Health* 11(6), pp. 494–498. DOI:http://doi.org/10.1007/s10903-008-9222-7.

Earhart, A. and Hauser, A. (2008) 'The Other Side of the Curtain', in Hauser, P., Finch, K. and Hauser, A. (eds.) *Deaf Professionals and Designated Interpreters: A New Paradigm.* Washington, D.C: Gallaudet University Press, pp. 143–164.

Ebert, D. A. and Heckerling, P. S. (1995) 'Communication with Deaf Patients: Knowledge, Beliefs, and Practices of Physicians', *JAMA*, 273(3), pp. 227–229.

Edwards, T. (2014) 'From Compensation to Integration: Effects of the Pro-tactile Movement on the Sublexical Structure of Tactile American Sign Language', *Journal of Pragmatics*, 69, pp. 22–41. DOI:10.1016/j.pragma.2014.05.005.

Featherstone, Z. (2019). 'Medical Interpreting Roundtable', *Registry of Interpreters for the Deaf.* Available at: https://rid.org/medical-interpreting-roundtable/ (Accessed: 15 December 2020).

Forestal, E. and Cole, J. (2018) 'Deaf Translation: Socio-cultural Perspective', in Winston, B., Monikowski, C. and Lee, R. G. (eds) 'Reaching New Heights in Interpreter Education: Mentoring, Teaching and Leadership', *Proceedings from CIT '18*, Salt Lake City, Conference of Interpreter Trainers.

Grbic. N. (2007) 'Where Do We Come From? What Are We? Where Are We Going? A Bibliometrical Analysis of Writings and Research on Sign Language Interpreting', *The Sign Language Translator and Interpreter (SLTI)*, 1(1), pp. 15–51.

Groce, N., Yousafzai, A., Dlamini, P., Zalud, S. and Wirz, S. (2006) 'HIV/Aids and Disability: A Pilot Survey of HIV/Aids Knowledge Among a Deaf Population in Swaziland', *International Journal of Rehabilitation Research*, 29(4), pp. 319–324.
Hall, W. C. Elliott, M. and Cullen, J. P. P. (2019) 'Designated Interpreters: A Model to Promote the Diversity and Inclusion of Deaf Professionals', *Academic Medicine*, 94(5) DOI:10.1097/ACM.0000000000002570.
Hall, W. C., Smith, S. R., Sutter, E. J., DeWindt, L. A., and Dye, T. (2018) 'Considering Parental Hearing Status as a Social Determinant of Deaf Population Health: Insights From Experiences of the "Dinner Table Syndrome"', *PLoS One*, 13(9), e0202169. DOI:10.1371/journal.pone.0202169.
Hauser, P., Finch, K. and Hauser, A. (2008) *Deaf Professionals and Designated Interpreters*. Washington, DC: Gallaudet University Press.
Healthy People. (2020) *Disparities*. Available at: www.healthypeople.gov/2020/about/foundation-health-measures/Disparities (Accessed: 15 December 2020).
Heuttel, K. L. and Rothstein, W. G. (2001) 'HIV/ AIDS Knowledge and Information Sources Among Deaf and Hearing College Students', *American Annals of the Deaf*, 146(3), pp. 280–286.
Hochgesang, J. A. and McAuliff, K. (2016). 'An Initial Description of the Deaf Community in Haiti and Haitian Sign Language (LSH)', *Sign Language* Studies, 16(2), pp. 227–294.
Humphries, T. (1975) *Audism: The Making of a Word*. Unpublished essay.
Iezzoni, L. (2016) 'Why Increasing Numbers of Physicians with Disability Could Improve Care for Patients with Disability', *AMA Journal of Ethics*, 18(10), 1041–1049. DOI:10.1001/journalofethics.2016.18.10.msoc2-1610.
Ingram. R. (1978) 'Sign Language Interpretation and General Theories of Language, Interpretation and Communication', in Gerver, D. and Sinaiko, H. (eds) *Language Interpretation and Communication*. New York: Springer, pp. 109–118.
Johnston, T. and Napier, J. (2010) 'Medical Signbank: Bringing Deaf People and Linguists Together in the Process of Language Development', *Sign Language Studies*, 10(2), pp. 258–275.
Kushalnagar, P., Moreland, C., Simons, A., and Holcomb, T. (2018) 'Communication Barrier in Family Linked to Increased Risks for Food Insecurity Among Deaf People Who Use American Sign Language', *Public Health Nutrition*, 21(5), pp. 912–916. DOI:10.1017/S1368980017002865.
Lane, H. (1992) *Masks of Benevolence: Disabling the Deaf Community*. New York: Alfred Knopf.
Liu, M. (2012) 'Methodology in Interpreting Studies: A Methodological Review of Evidence-Based Research', in Nicodemus, B. and Swabey, L. (eds) *Advances in Interpreting Research*. Amsterdam: John Benjamins, pp. 85–120.
Llewellyn-Jones, P. and Lee, R. G. (2014) *Redefining the Role of the Community Interpreter: The Concept of Role-Space*. Lincoln: SLI Press.
Margellos-Anast, H., Estarziau, M. and Kaufman, G. (2006) 'Cardiovascular Disease Knowledge Among Culturally Deaf Patients in Chicago', *Preventive Medicine*, 42(3), pp. 235–239.
Maroney, E. *et al.* (2018) 'Reaching Ghanaian Interpreters through Ongoing Short-Term Training', in Winston, B., Monikowski, C. and Lee, R. G. (eds) 'Reaching New Heights in Interpreter Education: Mentoring, Teaching and Leadership', *Proceedings from CIT'18*, Salt Lake City, Conference of Interpreter Trainers.
Major, G. (2014) '"Sorry, Could You Explain That"? Clarification Requests in Interpreted Healthcare Interaction', in Nicodemus, B. and Metzger, M. (eds) *Investigations in Healthcare Interpreting*. Washington. DC: Gallaudet University Press, pp. 32–69.
Major, G. and Napier, J. (2012) 'Interpreting and Knowledge Medication in the Healthcare Setting. What Do We Really Mean by "Accuracy"?' *Linguistica Antverpiensia*, 11(11), pp. 207–225.
Major, G. and Napier, J. (2019) '"I'm There Sometimes as a Just in Case": Examining Role Fluidity in Healthcare Interpreting', in Ji, M. Taibi, M. and Crezee, I. (eds) *Multicultural Health Translation, Interpreting and Communication*. London and New York: Routledge, pp. 183–204.
Major, G., Napier, J., Ferrara L. and Johnston, T. (2012) 'Exploring Lexical Gaps in Australian Sign Language for the Purposes of Health Communication', *Communication and Medicine*, 9(1), pp. 37–47.
Major, G., Napier, J. and Stubbe, M. (2012) '"What Happens Truly, Not Text Book!": Using Authentic Interactions in Discourse Training for Healthcare Interpreters', in Swabey, L. and Malcolm, K. (eds) *In Our Hands – Educating Healthcare Interpreters*. Washington, DC: Gallaudet University Press, pp. 27–53.

McKee, M. M., Winters, P. C., Sen, A, Zazove, P. and Fiscella, K. (2015) 'Emergency Department Utilization Among Deaf American Sign Language Users', *Disability and Health Journal* 8(4), pp. 573–578. DOI:10.1016/j.dhjo.2015.05.004.
Metzger, M. (1999) *Sign Language Interpreting: Deconstructing the Myth of Neutrality*. Washington, DC: Gallaudet University Press.
Metzger, M. (2006) 'Salient Studies of Signed Language Interpreting in the Context of Community Interpreting Scholarship', *Linguistica Antverpiensia, New Series – Themes in Translation Studies*, special issue 'Taking Stock: Research and Methodology in Community Interpreting', 5, pp. 263–291.
Mitra, M., Akobirshoev, I., McKee, M. M. and Iezzoni, L. I. (2016) 'Birth Outcomes Among U.S. Women with Hearing Loss', *American Journal of Preventive Medicine*, 51(6), pp. 865–873. DOI:10.1016/j.amepre.2016.08.001.
Moreland, C. and Agan, T. (2012) 'Educating Interpreters as Medical Specialists with Deaf Health Professionals', in Swabey, L. and Malcolm, K. (eds) *In Our Hands – Educating Healthcare Interpreters.* Washington, DC: Gallaudet University Press, pp. 147–163.
Moreland, C. J., Latimore, D., Sen, A., Arato, N. and Zazove, P. (2013) 'Deafness Among Physicians and Trainees: A National Survey' (2013). *Academic Medicine*, 88(2), pp. 224–232. DOI:10.1097/ACM.0b013e31827c0d60.
Mweri, J. G., Akaranga, W. and Okomo, O. (2009) 'Sign Language Interpreter Training in Kenya', in Napier, J. (ed.) *International Perspectives on Sign Language Interpreter Education*. Washington, DC. Gallaudet University Press, pp. 295–300.
NAD-DSA VRI Task Force (2016) 'Minimum Standards for Video Remote Interpreting Services in Medical Settings', *National Association of the Deaf.* Available at: www.nad.org/about-us/position-statements/minimum-standards-for-video-remote-interpreting-services-in-medical-settings/ (Accessed: 15 December 2020).
O'Day, B. L., Killeen, M., Harker, H. and Iezzoni, L. I. (2004) 'Communicating About Health Care: Observations From Persons Who Are Deaf or Hard of Hearing', *Annals of Internal Medicine*, 140(5), pp. 356–362.
Olson, A. M. and Swabey, L. (2016) 'Communication Access for Deaf People in Healthcare Settings: Understanding the Work of American Sign Language Interpreters', *Journal of Healthcare Quality*, 39(4), pp. 191–199. DOI:10.1097/JHQ.0000000000000038.
Orsi, J. M., Margellos-Anast, H., Perlman, T. S., Giloth, B. E and Whitman, S. (2007) 'Cancer Screening Knowledge, Attitudes, and Behaviors Among Culturally Deaf Adults: Implications for Informed Decision Making', *Cancer Detection and Prevention*, 31(6), pp. 474–479. DOI:10.1016/j.cdp.2007.10.008.
Parker, M. M. (2017) 'Association of Patient-Physician Language Concordance and Glycemic Control for Limited-English Proficiency Latinos With Type 2 Diabetes', *JAMA Internal Medicine*, 177(3), pp. 380–387. DOI:http://doi.org/10.1001/jamainternmed.2016.8648.
Pöchhacker, F. (2004). *Introducing Interpreting Studies.* London and New York: Routledge.
RID Annual Report (2018) *2018 Annual Report of the Registry of Interpreters for the Deaf.* Available at: https://rid.org/2018-annual-report/ (Accessed: 15 December 2020).
Roy, C. and Metzger, M. (2014) 'Researching Signed Language Interpreting Through a Sociolinguistic Lens', *The International Journal for Translation and Interpreting Research*, 6(1), pp. 158–176. DOI:10.12807/ti.106201.2014.a09.
Russell, D. (2005) 'Consecutive and Simultaneous Interpretation', in Janzen, T. (ed.) *Topics in Signed Language Interpreting*. Amsterdam and Philadelphia: John Benjamins, pp. 135–164.
Schmittdiel J. A. *et al.* (2009) 'The Association of Patient-Physician Gender Concordance with Cardiovascular Disease Risk Factor Control and Treatment in Diabetes', *Journal of Women's Health*, 8(12), pp. 2065–2070. DOI:10.1089/jwh.2009.1406.
Senayah, E., Mprah, W., Opoku, M., Edusei, A. and Torgbenu, E. (2018) 'The Accessibility of Health Services to Young Deaf Adolescents in Ghana', *International Journal of Health Planning and Management*, 34(1), pp. e634–e645. DOI:10.1002/hpm.2679.
Shen, M. J. *et al.* (2018) 'The Effects of Race and Racial Concordance on Patient-Physician Communication: A Systematic Review of the Literature', *Journal of Racial and Ethnic Health Disparities*, 5(1), pp. 117–140.
Spellun, A., Moreland, C. J. and Kushalnagar, P. (2018) 'Young Deaf Adults' Knowledge of Human Papillomavirus (HPV) and Perceived Risk of Vaccine in Preventing Cervical, Anal, Penile, and

Oral Cancer', *Journal of Pediatric and Adolescent Gynecology*, 32(3), pp. 293–299. DOI:10.1016/j.jpag.2018.11.013.

Sirch, L., Salvador, L. and Palese, A. (2017) 'Communication Difficulties Experienced by Deaf Male Patients During Their In-Hospital Stay: Findings from a Qualitative Descriptive Study', *Scandinavian Journal of Caring Sciences*, 31(2), pp. 368–377. DOI:10.1111/scs.12356.

Steinberg, A. *et al.* (2002) 'Deaf Women: Experiences and Perceptions of Healthcare System Access', *Journal of Women's Health*, 11(8), pp. 729–741.

Stone, C. (2009) *Towards a Deaf Translation Norm*. Washington, DC: Gallaudet University Press.

Swabey, L., Agan, T., Moreland, C. J. and Olson, A. (2016) 'Understanding the Work of Designated Healthcare Interpreters', *International Journal of Interpreter Education*, 8(1), pp. 40–56.

Swabey, L. and Craft Faber, Q. (2012) 'Domains and Competencies for Healthcare Interpreting: Applications and Implications for Educators', in Swabey, L. and Malcolm, K. (eds) *In Our Hands – Educating Healthcare Interpreters*. Washington, DC: Gallaudet University Press, pp. 1–26.

Swabey, L., Laurion, R., Patrie, C. and Ramírez, R. (2016) 'Using a Career Lattice to Chart a Path to Competency in Healthcare Interpreting', in Rankin, M., Shaw, R. and Thumann, M. (eds) *Out of the Gate: Towards the Triple Crown*. Lexington, KY: CIT, pp. 1–16.

Thew, D., Smith, S. R., Chang, C. and Starr, M. (2012) 'The Deaf Strong Hospital Program: A Model of Diversity and Inclusion Training for First-Year Medical Students', *Academic Medicine*, 87(11), pp. 1496–1500. DOI:http://doi.org/10.1097/ACM.0b013e31826d322d.

Wellman, D. (1993) *Portraits of White Racism*. Cambridge: Cambridge University Press.

Würth, K. M., Reiter-Theil, S. Langewitz, W. and Schuster, S. (2018) '"Getting by" in a Swiss Tertiary Hospital: The Inconspicuous Complexity of Decision-making Around Patients' Limited Language Proficiency', *Journal of General Internal Medicine*, 33(11), pp. 1885–1891. DOI:10.1007/s11606-018-4618-0.

Zazove, P., Meador, H. E., Reed, B. D., Sen, A. and Gorenflo, D. W (2009) 'Cancer Prevention Knowledge of People with Profound Hearing Loss', *Journal of General Internal Medicine*, 24(3), pp. 320–326. DOI:http://doi.org/10.1007/s11606-008-0895-3.

Zazove, P., Meador, H. E., Reed, B. D., Sen, A. and Gorenflo, D. (2012) 'Effectiveness of Videos Improving Cancer Prevention Knowledge in People With Profound Hearing Loss', *Journal of Cancer Education*, 27(2), pp. 327–337. DOI:http://doi.org/10.1007/s13187-011-0292-1.

Zulu, T., Heap, M., Sinanovic, E. (2017) 'The Cost and Utilisation Patterns of a Pilot Sign Language Interpreter Service for Primary Health Care Services in South Africa', *PLoS One*, 12(12), e0189983. DOI:http://doi.org/10.1371/journal.pone.0189983.

Part IV

Areas of health

15

Translation and interpreting in disaster situations

Patrick Cadwell

1 Introduction and definitions

Disasters affect the health and wellbeing of many people simultaneously in many different ways. People in a disaster may face life-threatening situations, become injured or disabled, lack essentials such as water, food and shelter, become exposed to environmental pollution, or experience elevated psychosocial stress (Abrahams and Murray 2017). In order to respond to and recover from these effects and to reduce the future impact of similar situations, people need to communicate with each other (Coppola 2011). In a context of linguistic and cultural diversity, this communication may involve translation and interpreting (Federici 2016). Therefore, disaster settings can help us to understand more about translation and interpreting for global health.

Presenting a definition of disaster that is widely agreed upon is challenging; researchers and practitioners across various disciplines and occupations in the sciences, social sciences, humanities and humanitarian sector adopt different perspectives on the concept (Perry 2007). Some have focused their definitions on scale – such as lives lost or damage incurred – and on the idea that the scale of a disaster must overwhelm those affected by it (Coppola 2011). Others have focused on hazards – events or conditions that have the potential to cause harm – and on associated risks and vulnerabilities, arguing that a risk of disaster exists only when someone or something that is vulnerable becomes exposed to a hazard (Birkmann 2013). Nowadays, scale or hazard alone are not considered sufficient to define disasters. There is broad agreement among researchers and practitioners that disasters should be defined as social phenomena (Perry 2007). Incidents such as disease outbreaks or tsunamis are not disasters in and of themselves; we consider them disasters only once the extent to which they disrupt the social world becomes clear. Consider the difference between a massive earthquake occurring in an isolated, uninhabited rural area and an earthquake of the same intensity occurring in an urban setting; the risk of disaster is higher in the latter because of the vulnerable people and property exposed to severe

DOI: 10.4324/9781003167983-20

shaking. The United Nations Office for Disaster Risk Reduction or UNDRR (2017) foregrounds social aspects in its comprehensive definition of a disaster:

> A serious disruption of the functioning of a community or a society at any scale due to hazardous events interacting with conditions of exposure, vulnerability and capacity, leading to one or more of the following: human, material, economic and environmental losses and impacts [...] The effect of the disaster can be immediate and localized, but is often widespread and could last for a long period of time. The effect may test or exceed the capacity of a community or society to cope using its own resources, and therefore may require assistance from external sources, which could include neighbouring jurisdictions, or those at the national or international levels.
>
> *UNDRR 2017: n.p.*

Researchers and practitioners sometimes use terms such as disaster, emergency and crisis interchangeably; the conceptual field is somewhat unclear. For instance, the mission statement of the US Federal *Emergency* Management Agency involves '[h]elping people before, during, and after *disasters*' (see Department of Homeland Security 2019: n.p., my emphasis). Similarly, a recent *emergency* policy of the United Nations High Commissioner for Refugees or UNHCR is set down to deal with the onset of a *crisis* (see UNHCR 2017: n.p.).

Prominent definitions of crisis, disaster and emergency indicate that these concepts share some common characteristics and that their interchangeable use may be justified at times. Sellnow and Seeger (2013: 4–20) identify three primary characteristics of a crisis: violated expectations, posed threats and required responses. The definition of a disaster from UNDRR (2017) above is also based on response to a posed threat or hazard, however, it emphasises the severity of societal disruption that a disaster causes and does not limit the concept to unforeseen circumstances. Alexander's (2005) definition of an emergency is equally centred on responding to a threat. An emergency here is similar to a crisis in that it is usually unanticipated, but it is different from both a crisis and a disaster in that the rapidity of response required is worth noting. In short, when circumstances involve responding to a threat, the situation can be called a crisis, a disaster, or an emergency. Additionally, though, to emphasise the urgency and immediacy of the required response, use of the term emergency might be preferred, or to emphasise the scale and severity of societal disruption caused, use of the term disaster could be more effective.

At other times, some researchers and practitioners find it useful to more clearly differentiate types of disaster, emergency and crisis. They use expressions such as natural or technological disaster, humanitarian crisis, or health emergency and define each one by the triggering hazard or potential effect involved (Coppola 2011; Perry 2007; UNDRR 2017). For instance, disasters arising from geological or meteorological processes, such as volcanic eruptions or hurricanes, are sometimes called natural disasters. Those triggered by circumstances other than natural processes, such as large-scale transport accidents or chemical explosions, may be identified as technological disasters. Mass social disruptions arising from biological processes – such as Ebola or swine flu – can be categorised as health emergencies, while those triggered by conflict, insecurity, famine, drought or mass migration may be labelled as humanitarian crises.

It is now less common to differentiate categories of disaster, and especially to separate natural from human-made disasters (Quarantelli 2000). This is to recognise the ways in which human decisions and activities influence and exacerbate geological, meteorological, biological, or migratory processes. The relationship between climate change and disaster is an issue of particular concern (Eiser *et al.* 2012). It is argued that all disasters are ultimately human-made. In addition, there continues to be debate over the extent to which intentional disruption to society brought about in situations of deliberate conflict should be included in conceptualisations of disaster (Quarantelli 2000). For instance, the UNDRR – an influential stakeholder – does not include armed conflict or social instability in its conceptualisation of the hazards that can lead to disaster (UNDRR 2017). Nevertheless, others acknowledge the place of conflict at the root of some disasters, labelling them complex emergencies (Coppola 2011). In short, this chapter focuses on disasters, however, the conceptual field in Disaster Studies is somewhat unclear, and circumstances that could be categorised as emergencies or crises may also be relevant.

Another terminological convention when discussing a disaster is to refer to its stakeholders using variations of two broadly encompassing terms: those 'affected' by the disaster and those 'responding' to it. At the same time, these concepts should not be separated rigidly, as the very first responders in a disaster are likely to be those directly affected as well, such as family, neighbours, or passers-by (Harvard Humanitarian Initiative 2011). In large-scale, international disasters, stakeholders involved in response and management can include: the state, civil institutions, and the military; non-governmental and international governmental organisations, such as UN agencies and the International Federation of Red Cross and Red Crescent Societies; private sector organisations; *ad hoc* humanitarian groups; and diaspora communities living outside the affected state (UNDAC, 2018). It is also common in the study of disasters to specify a number of phases to anchor discussion, typically in a cyclical pattern along short-, medium- and long-term timelines. Various models describe and explain these disaster timelines (Coppola 2011). Alexander (2002: 5) proposed a frequently-cited version comprising four phases: mitigation (to minimise future impacts of a disaster, e.g. through the formulation of particular building codes); preparedness (to reduce impending impacts of a disaster, e.g. through training populations at risk and other key stakeholders); response (to deal with the immediate aftermath of a disaster, e.g. through search and rescue activities); and recovery (to restore affected populations to normal life following a disaster, e.g. through the provision of temporary housing). This model represents a shift in thinking in Disaster Studies away from a reactive approach (where the timeline of a disaster starts at the onset of an event) to a proactive approach (where disasters are considered before the need to respond arises and the focus is on mitigating and preparing).

The conceptual perspective on disaster adopted in this chapter is broad. The term disaster is used here to refer to any overwhelming social disruption – whatever the triggering hazard – with potential for serious, negative consequences, especially for the health and wellbeing of those affected. In addition, the terms 'stakeholder', 'mitigation', 'preparedness', 'response' and 'recovery' will all assist in the discussion that follows.

2 Importance of language and culture in disaster situations

Many researchers who examine disasters, including those with a particular interest in health, argue for the importance of communication in disaster settings (see, e.g. Altay and Labonte 2014; Coombs 2012; Henrich and Holmes 2011; Holmes *et al.* 2009; Longstaff and Yang 2008; Tanner *et al.* 2009). Practitioners also recognise the operational and strategic importance of information and communication (see, e.g. ActionAid 2012; Slade 2011; World Health Organisation 2012), especially through wide-ranging, international agreements and structures, such as the Sendai Framework for Disaster Risk Reduction 2015–2030 (Aitsi-Selmi *et al.* 2016) or the European Union's General Guidelines for Operational Priorities on Humanitarian Aid (European Commission 2018). While it is clear that communication in disasters is a valued object of enquiry, can the same be said of languages and cultures through which disaster-related communication is mediated?

The likelihood of disasters striking culturally and linguistically diverse populations is increasing, and those involved in disaster communication need to account for this diversity. Recent studies of disaster management indicate that, while fewer lives are being lost each year to disaster, the number of disasters and the number of people affected by them annually are both rising, with the world's poorest citizens being disproportionately affected (Coppola 2011). Human societies are becoming concentrated around large-scale urban environments (Smith 2013), and long-term displacement of populations – driven especially by political insecurity and conflict – add increasing complexity to disaster settings (IDMC 2018). In the future, therefore, there will be more disasters forcing large-scale movements of diverse groups to and from already-diverse mega-cities.

Clear, timely, accurate and reliable information is essential for communication in a disaster to succeed (Coyle and Meier 2009). Despite recognition of the importance of these features of communication in research on disasters (see, e.g. Fischer 2008; Haddow, Bullock and Coppola 2017; Tierney and Waugh 2007), and despite acknowledgement in the literature of the need for effective communication throughout all phases of disaster situations (Comfort 2007; Kapucu 2006; Kendra and Wachtendorf 2003), researchers and practitioners have so far overlooked or downplayed the potential negative consequences when those involved in a disaster have limited or no understanding of each other's languages and cultures (Moser-Mercer, Kherbiche and Class 2014; Nepal *et al.* 2012; O'Brien *et al.* 2018). Moreover, core texts in Disaster Studies mention language, culture, translation or interpreting either only briefly and without critical discussion (e.g. Rodríguez, Quarantelli and Dynes 2006) or not at all (e.g. Drabek 2003, 2010; Quarantelli 1987).

Recent research has begun to affirm that the effectiveness of disaster operations is reduced when diverse language needs are not considered and that benefits accrue when linguistic and cultural issues are taken into account. Research has indicated that those affected by a disaster can misunderstand risks and make poor decisions when communicating in a language they do not understand well (McKee 2014; Santos-Hernández and Hearn Morrow 2013). The accessibility and effectiveness of information throughout all phases of a disaster are contingent on the information being provided in an appropriate linguistic and cultural frame (Nsiah-Kumi 2008; Purtle, Siddiqui and Andrulis 2011). Linguistic and cultural barriers can hinder participation in response and recovery as well as mitigation and preparedness efforts (see, e.g. Kirsch, Sauer and Sapir 2012; Koenig 2013). In particular, linguistic and cultural barriers risk excluding disaster-affected communities from these efforts, cutting off valuable sources of in-depth local knowledge and information (Munro 2013). Some researchers and practitioners have identified lack of translation as a perennial hidden issue in disaster-related communication (Harvard Humanitarian Initiative 2011). Influential stakeholders, such as the International Federation of Red Cross and Red Crescent Societies, acknowledge that multilingual communication strategies in disaster situations around the world – where they exist – are limited and rarely based on appropriate evidence concerning real language needs:

> However linguistically diverse the affected population, humanitarian responses are usually coordinated in international lingua francas and delivered in a narrow range

> of national languages. Basic data on the languages and literacy levels of the affected population is not systematically collected and shared in the way that other fundamental characteristics such as gender and age might be. As a result, evidence-based multilingual communication strategies are rarely developed.
>
> *Fisher et al. 2018: 103*

An incapacity to understand the language in which disaster-related information is disseminated is a key marker of social vulnerability and is often accompanied by a lack of established social networks, lack of experience of disaster events, inability to access key resources due to physical and social isolation, and poor socio-economic conditions (Ogie *et al.* 2018).

Operational effectiveness is not the only reason to argue for consideration of language, culture, and their mediation in disaster situations. Rights-based or ethics-based arguments can also be made. Greenwood *et al.* (2017) assert that information and the methods of its communication are basic humanitarian rights that should constitute – alongside other rights, such as the right to protection, privacy, or security – the foundation of humanitarian activities before, during and after a disaster. O'Brien *et al.* (2018) acknowledge this and further argue that language, as a trait, should not prevent entitlement to other fundamental rights or be a cause for discrimination. They apply this claim to the provision of translation and interpreting in disaster communication and find support for it in milestone documents, such as the United Nations' Universal Declaration of Human Rights (United Nations 1948) and the European Union Charter of Fundamental Rights (Council of the European Union 2008). Moreover, Geale (2012) argues that consideration of language and culture in disasters, especially the languages and cultures of those directly affected, are central to achieving the ethical principles of equity, justice, dignity and fairness that should guide disaster management.

3 Views on translation and interpreting in disasters

Various communicative strategies could be adopted to respond to the linguistic and cultural needs outlined above. For instance, an approach based on plurilingualism could encourage the learning and use of multiple languages by key stakeholders (see, e.g. Clerveaux, Spence and Katada 2010 for an introduction to this idea). This approach could range from learning key vocabulary or phrases to undertaking more comprehensive language instruction. Given the time, resources and motivation required to learn another language, researchers are focusing on creative, targeted, flexible and low-resource acquisition methods, for instance, through gamification. Allied to language learning could be the use of a small number of vehicular languages – such as English, French or a dominant regional language – in disaster situations (see, e.g. Fisher *et al.* 2018 for discussion of this phenomenon). Additionally, a lingua franca or dominant language in a disaster setting could be simplified and controlled to make it more accessible to greater numbers of people with some grasp of the language (see, e.g. Carroll 2012 for debates around simplification). Alternatively, conventional language could be abandoned, and pictographs or symbols could be used to satisfy the communicative needs of diverse groups (see, e.g. Sahana Software Foundation 2019 for an outline of preliminary research). These are all valid communicative strategies; however, they do not entail interlingual translation and interpreting. Nevertheless, as the following will show, interlingual and intercultural translation and interpreting have been used to respond to diverse communicative needs in many disaster situations.

Researchers in Turkey – a country with significant exposure to hazards including earthquakes, floods and landslides – carried out pioneering work on the experiences, needs and training of interpreters in disasters there (Bulut and Kurultay 2001; Doğan 2016; Doğan and Kahraman 2011; Kurultay and Bulut 2012). The 2010 Haiti Earthquake was another turning point in the study of translation and interpreting in disasters. At the time, Haitian diaspora, along with technologically-proficient volunteer organisations based outside of Haiti, translated text messages, created maps and person-finder tools and built machine translation engines (Lewis 2010; Lewis, Munro and Vogel 2011; Munro 2013). Successive disasters in New Zealand and Japan in 2010–2011 formed the basis of further research. Studies centred on: the lived experience of translation and interpreting (Cadwell 2015); the work of community interpreters (Naito 2012); best practice guidelines highlighting the value of training and skill (Wylie 2012); interpreting services on television in the aftermath of these disasters (McKee 2014); and the use of information and communication technology for translation and interpreting (Cadwell and O'Brien 2016). Translation and interpreting in conflict zones and military operations have also been objects of considerable enquiry (see, e.g. Kelly and Footitt 2012; Moser-Mercer, Kherbiche and Class 2014; Salama-Carr 2007; Snellman 2016). Moreover, practitioners have conducted valuable research to illustrate the contributions and challenges of translation and interpreting in disaster settings. Chief among these is Translators without Borders, a non-profit organisation whose goal is to ensure the appropriateness and availability of understandable humanitarian content. The organisation achieves this goal by providing translations and language technology solutions in areas of crisis relief, health and education to other non-profit and aid organisations (Translators without Borders 2019). It also trains translators and interpreters and promotes the importance of language in humanitarian work (*ibid.*). It has produced a number of detailed reports on its crisis relief operations in various earthquakes, conflicts and disease outbreaks (*ibid.*).

Researchers and practitioners particularly interested in health have also carried out studies involving translation and interpreting in disasters. A body of research presents recommendations on how medical teams can work effectively with translators and interpreters (e.g. Bolton and Weiss 2001; Powell and Pagliara-Miller 2012) and on how parties involved can manage the physical and mental health risks and ethical dilemmas associated with disaster settings (e.g. Athey and Moody-Williams 2003; Greenstone 2010; Shiu-Thornton *et al.* 2007). These studies tend to focus on the responder side – the health professionals or the interpreters and translators – and only a limited number of studies approach issues of health, disaster and translation or interpreting from the side of the disaster-affected population (e.g. Hanson-Easey *et al.* 2018; O'Brien and Cadwell 2017). This means that existing research findings related to disaster may not encourage healthcare decisions that respect the needs, preferences and values of patients sufficiently.

Much of the research cited above consists of small studies supported by relatively small amounts of empirical data. It is therefore difficult to draw broad, generalised conclusions based on these studies. Nonetheless, certain features of translation and interpreting can be discerned that are common across many of the research contexts involved. These include the *ad hoc*, local, and voluntary nature of the activities and the importance of cultural issues to the communication.

3.1 Ad hoc, local, voluntary and culture-centred

In many disaster contexts, translation and interpreting were carried out in an *ad hoc*, uncoordinated manner and on a voluntary basis by local groups of affected people who had linguistic proficiency and cultural knowledge, and often not any formal training (Bulut and Kurultay 2001; Cadwell 2015; Federici and Cadwell 2018; Lewis, Munro and Vogel 2011; Moser-Mercer, Kherbiche and Class 2014; Munro 2013; Wylie 2012). One reason proposed for the *ad hoc*, bottom-up nature of these efforts is that the pool of trained translators and interpreters in the languages required in contemporary disaster situations is limited (Fisher *et al.* 2018). Translation and interpreting efforts required in disaster situations at the time of writing include, for instance, Rohingya, Tamasheq or Tigrinya (ICRC 2019), none of which is available as a search option on the widely used database of language professionals, ProZ.com (www.proz.com/). Therefore, structures for the systematic and professional provision of services in and out of the required languages and cultures are already un- or underdeveloped before a disaster strikes.

Local grassroots endeavours can sometimes hold high personal stakes for the translators and interpreters concerned; as members of the disaster-affected population, they may have a special interest in some of the disaster-related information they mediate. While this can lead to feelings of stress and potential traumatisation, translators and interpreters in disaster settings also report positive psychological effects through engaging proactively and communally with disaster-related information (McKee 2014).

The voluntary basis of much disaster translation and interpreting is taken here to mean that the individuals concerned offer their time and effort to help others without compensation (Erickson 2012). However, compensated, trained professionals also contribute to disaster translation and interpreting activities. It should be remembered that acting as a volunteer does not preclude being a professional (O'Hagan 2011), and professional interpreters and translators volunteered their time in many disaster settings (see, e.g. Bulut and Kurultay 2001; Cadwell 2015; Munro 2013; Wylie 2012). Nevertheless, these professional efforts have been somewhat limited in scope and direction and have frequently taken place in the context of large, international humanitarian organisations using a dominant lingua franca of the humanitarian sector (Fisher *et al.* 2018; Moser-Mercer, Kherbiche and Class 2014). *Ad hoc*, local and voluntary translation and interpreting efforts are valuable. Nonetheless, such efforts can lead to inefficiencies. Uncoordinated local volunteers working spontaneously may needlessly reproduce information that has already been translated elsewhere or may fail to recognise the translation and interpreting tasks that are needed most. For instance, a lack of coordinated translations in the 2018 monsoon season in Bangladesh led the Rohingya community there to feel that they lacked sufficient information in their language about flood safety, while having adequate information about other topics, such as health or security (Marzotto 2019).

In addition to the *ad hoc*, local and voluntary aspects of much disaster translation and interpreting, it is important to emphasise the significance of intercultural issues in disaster situations. Disasters are characterised by and experienced within varying contexts of cultural beliefs and world views that influence vulnerabilities, risk interpretations, preparedness and response decisions, and other forms of information processing (e.g. Cornia, Dressel and Pfeil 2016; Eiser *et al.* 2012; Harro-Loit, Vihalemm and Ugur 2012). There are many possible definitions of translation and interpreting. (For an overview of core ideas and debates, see, e.g. House 2018; Munday 2016; Pym 2014). Not all of these definitions include consideration of culture. However, definitions of disaster translation and interpreting should include culture as a key defining characteristic. For example, since 2017, the New Zealand Red Cross has been coordinating a project to involve residents of the Wellington Region from diverse linguistic and cultural backgrounds in the translation of earthquake-preparedness guides for recent migrants. Certain cultural concepts of disaster preparedness in New Zealand that were unproblematic for longer-terms residents – such as, working bees (voluntary groups set up for a charitable goal) or camping (the items and practices to lodge safely outdoors) – proved challenging for recent migrants to New Zealand to understand (Federici and Cadwell 2018; Shackleton 2018). Conduct of this project has caused coordinators to question some cultural assumptions of disaster preparedness communication in a New Zealand context (Shackleton 2018).

In sum, there is a substantial amount of evidence to suggest that studying disasters can deepen our understanding of translation and interpreting. At the same time, existing scholarship in Translation and Interpreting Studies can inform our understanding of disaster situations. Research on non-professional interpreting and translation practices (e.g. Antonini 2017; Pérez-González and Susam-Saraeva 2012), community translation and interpreting (e.g. Taibi and Ozolins 2016; Valero-Garcés and Tipton 2017), and the functioning and motivation of global communities of linguistic volunteers (e.g. McDonough Dolmaya 2012; Olohan 2014) are particularly relevant to describing and explaining communicative phenomena observed in disasters. Various directions are possible for future research. However, it is possible to indicate a number of critical issues on which future efforts could focus.

4 Critical issues and future directions

Disaster situations cause us to examine the ethics of translation and interpreting. They have much to tell us about the training of linguistic and cultural volunteers, whether these are professional or non-professional translators or interpreters. Disasters also cause us to consider appropriate modalities for the delivery of linguistically and culturally mediated information, and raise important issues about the relationship between policy and practice in translation and interpreting.

4.1 Ethics

Some scholars argue that issues arising from translation or interpreting encounters are not just practical but fundamentally ethical (e.g. Baker and Maier 2011; Goodwin 2010). Disaster situations affirm this and provide the basis for complex examinations of ethical questions for all those involved, including those who translate and interpret (O'Mathúna *et al.* 2020). Not all translation and interpreting in a disaster situation will be carried out in the immediate response phase: the shift to a proactive paradigm in Disaster Studies implies the need for consideration of longer timelines that focus on translation and interpreting in the recovery as well as mitigation and preparedness phases. Therefore, while disaster translators and interpreters will always have limited resources, time will not always be a limiting factor. Time for ethical thinking can and should be found in disaster settings. Indeed, even in situations where time is of the essence (e.g. emergency rooms in hospitals or in the immediate response phase of a disaster), those involved are trained in advance and given support afterwards in how to make and deal with complex ethical decisions quickly. Disaster translators or interpreters could benefit from such training and support to enable them to cope with complex ethical situations.

People who translate or interpret in disaster situations sometimes question what they ought to do, as well as the rightness or wrongness of their actions (Businaro 2012). Ethical questions in disaster translation and interpreting relate to issues of quality and accuracy, neutrality and bias, fairness and marginalisation, and the prudent use of limited resources in disasters (see, e.g. Hanson-Easey *et al.* 2018; McKee 2014; Moser-Mercer, Kherbiche, and Class 2014). Let us imagine some of the challenging questions that a translator or interpreter or someone who manages translation or interpreting in a disaster may be confronted with:

- Is the quality of translation or interpretation that will be produced in a high-stress, highly constrained environment good enough to be of use?
- Should translation or interpreting proceed if the translator or interpreter is not confident that they will produce accurate texts?
- Can and should a translator or interpreter be impartial if the disaster-related information affects them directly?
- Will translating or interpreting for one linguistic/cultural group put other groups who have no-one translating or interpreting for them at further disadvantage?
- Is the priority of translation or interpreting high enough to take limited resources away from another disaster preparedness or response need?

None of these questions has an obvious answer, and translators and interpreters and those who manage such activities would benefit from assistance in resolving such ethical dilemmas. One strategy – based on the principle of beneficence – is popular in healthcare settings, and especially in relation to the ethics of medical research in disasters; it involves balancing the potential benefits and likely harms of a particular action before making a decision (Beauchamp 2019). Another strategy – the deontological approach – has been to propose principles that guide ethical decision-making; codes of ethics put forward by associations of professional translators and interpreters illustrate this approach (Lambert 2018). A further strategy – developed from virtue ethics – encourages personal integrity and the development of character traits such as honesty and courage to promote ethical behaviour (O'Mathúna *et al.* 2020). While translators, interpreters and those who manage their activities might find these strategies useful, it is first important that they know about them. Some university-level courses for translators and interpreters have introduced ethical training onto their curricula (see, e.g. Baker and Maier 2011; Drugan and Megone 2011). Including disasters as cases studied in these curricula could help prepare disaster translators and interpreters of the future. However, as many disaster translators and interpreters are untrained volunteers who provide their services *ad hoc*, mechanisms for ethical support outside of traditional academic and professional settings are still required. Designing and testing mechanisms to provide *ad hoc* ethical support for translators and interpreters in disasters should be a matter of priority.

4.2 Training

Training on topics beyond ethics alone is another critical issue, especially to support those who volunteer. There is a widespread perception in the literature on volunteering of '… good-hearted, well-meaning volunteers doing important and challenging work but with little training or accountability' (Erickson 2012: 167). Systematic, scalable models of training that can be delivered at short notice in self-sustaining ways are required for disaster situations (Moser-Mercer, Kherbiche and Class 2014). Researchers at the InZone Project at the University of Geneva have carried out pioneering work to develop innovative, technology-supported training for multilingual communication in conflict and crisis settings (InZone 2019). Other initiatives to design and deliver training in the fundamentals of translation for culturally and linguistically diverse communities engaged in disaster-related translation projects have also been developed and evaluated (Federici and Cadwell 2018). Moreover, mechanisms involved not only in the training but also in the recruitment, coordination and motivation of linguistic volunteers are of critical importance for disaster translation and interpreting. Work has begun to examine existing successful models of linguistic volunteer training and management, and apply them to disaster settings (Cadwell, Bollig and Reid 2019).

4.3 Modalities

It is also of critical importance for researchers and practitioners involved in disaster-related translation and interpreting to consider appropriate modes of delivery for translated and interpreted communication. It may be reasonable to assume that a need for interpreting will be greatest at the response phase of a disaster immediately following the onset of an event when the situation is rapidly changing. In contrast, translation will make a greater contribution at the preparedness or recovery phases of disaster when timelines are longer, the situation is more stable and communication may not involve spontaneous, face-to-face interactions to the same extent. Nonetheless, a strict dichotomy between translation and interpreting activities in disaster settings might not be useful. Phenomena such as sight-translation, translation dictation, and audiovisual translation already establish fluidity between the modal boundaries of translated information (see, e.g. Kaindl 2013). Furthermore, a body of research (Fu *et al.* 2010; Nsiah-Kumi 2008; Yip *et al.* 2013) indicates that translated texts in disaster situations should be delivered not only in written formats but also orally through alternative channels such as community or faith-based centres. Doing so takes into account issues such as literacy, accessibility and cultural norms when communicating with older adults, children, those with physical or mental disabilities, or other particularly vulnerable groups. Technology also has an important function to perform here. Researchers have begun to examine how technology can assist in the generation of culturally and linguistically appropriate communication for and by diverse groups in disaster settings through, for instance, crowdsourcing, machine translation or other novel forms of information processing, distribution and translation (Lewis, Munro and Vogel 2011; Munro 2013; Ogie *et al.* 2018; Sutherlin 2013; Tanaka *et al.* 2007). More work exploring the intersection between technology, modality, translation and interpreting is required in disaster contexts.

4.4 Policies

A final issue of critical importance is that of public policy. Governments make disaster-related policies to protect the public from the impacts of disasters and to improve the public's resilience to future disasters (Birkland 2016). Policies are an expression of what the government views as problems and the actions they intend to take or not to take when confronted with these problems (Birkland 2011). Research carried out on a small sample of national governments (in Ireland, the UK, New Zealand, Japan and the United States) has indicated that several of them have yet to develop translation and interpreting significantly as tools in their disaster management policies (O'Brien *et al.* 2018). Without sufficient recognition of translation and interpreting as problems in need of solutions in disaster situations, responsibilities will remain unclear, funding will not be allocated, and detailed plans cannot be actualised. Following a disaster, a process of learning may take place leading to the formation of new policy (Birkland 2011). However, Gerber (2007) cautions that this learning may not always occur, or occur sufficiently, especially if there is a lack of political will. A critical issue for researchers and practitioners interested in translation and interpreting in disaster situations, therefore, is to advocate to key stakeholders – especially those holding political power – for the benefits of enshrining translation and interpreting in public policies on disasters.

5 Conclusion

The study of translation and interpreting in disaster situations is worthwhile, especially because the future is likely to bring more disasters involving large-scale displacements of diverse groups. It may be difficult to define a disaster clearly: any overwhelming social disruption with potential for serious, negative consequences, especially for the health and wellbeing of those affected, could probably be termed a disaster. Whatever the label used, it is widely agreed that clear, timely, accurate and reliable communication is vital in such situations. Much research up to now overlooked or downplayed the roles of language, culture, translation and interpreting in achieving this communication. Nevertheless, other research indicated that consideration of these factors in disaster communication is important to avoid misunderstanding of risks, improve decision-making, encourage participation of disaster-affected communities, access in-depth local knowledge, recognise a human right to accessible information, and achieve equity, justice and dignity. Analysis in this chapter of research about disasters in Turkey, Haiti, New Zealand, Japan, Kenya, Bangladesh and elsewhere revealed certain common characteristics of translation and interpreting in these settings. These include the *ad hoc*, local, and voluntary nature of the activities and the importance of cultural issues to the communication. In future research on translation and interpreting in disaster situations, it could be useful to examine other critical issues. In particular, ethics, training, communication modality and public policy in relation to disaster translation and interpreting are matters of interest.

Further reading

Federici, F. M. (2016) *Mediating Emergencies and Conflicts: Frontline Translating and Interpreting*. London: Palgrave Macmillan.

This book brings together fieldwork and analysis from a variety of disaster situations, health emergencies and conflicts to underline the need for adequate language mediation in these settings. It reviews a broad range of literature from relevant domains and introduces theoretical concepts for the study of disaster translation and interpreting.

Translators without Borders (2015) *Words of Relief: Ebola Crisis Learning Review*. Available at: https://translatorswithoutborders.org/wp-content/uploads/2015/10/20150529-Ebola-Learning-Review_FINAL.pdf (Accessed: 28 May 2019).

This report examines a non-profit organisation's efforts to improve communication with people affected in West Africa in the Ebola outbreak of 2014 and 2015. It focuses on practice and provides a useful overview of key issues involved in translation and interpreting when disaster strikes.

Munro, R. (2013) 'Crowdsourcing and the Crisis-Affected Community: Lessons Learned and Looking Forward from Mission 4636', *Journal of Information Retrieval*, 16(2), pp. 210–266.

This article uses the example of the 2010 earthquake in Haiti to focus on translation in disaster settings and especially on the intersection between human translation efforts – largely carried out by volunteers – and enabling technologies, such as mobile phones, social media and the Internet.

Moser-Mercer, B., Kherbiche, L. and Class, B. (2014) 'Interpreting Conflict: Training Challenges in Humanitarian Field Interpreting', *Journal of Human Rights Practice,* 6(1) pp. 140–158.

This article focuses on interpreting in conflicts and disasters and argues for the importance of sustainable and scalable training as a solution to linguistic mediation needs.

Related topics

Translating Global Epidemics, Machine Translation in Healthcare, Inter- and Intralingual Translation of Medical Information

References

Abrahams, J. and Murray, V. (2017) *Health Emergency and Disaster Risk Management: Overview.* Available at: www.who.int/hac/techguidance/preparedness/who-factsheet-overview-december2017.pdf?ua=1 (Accessed: 28 May 2019).

ActionAid (2012) *ActionAid/infoasaid Learning Review of the Pilot Communications Project in Isiolo*, Available at: http://actionaid.org/sites/default/files/isiolo_learning_review_-_final_oct_2012_0.pdf (Accessed: 28 May 2019).

Aitsi-Selmi, A. *et al.* (2016) 'Reflections on a Science and Technology Agenda for 21st Century Disaster Risk Reduction', *International Journal of Disaster Risk Science*, 7(1) pp. 1–29.

Alexander, D. (2002) *Principles of Emergency Planning and Management.* Oxford: Oxford University Press.

Alexander, D. (2005) 'Towards the Development of a Standard in Emergency Planning', *Disaster Prevention and Management*', 14(2) pp. 158–175.

Altay, N. and Labonte, M. (2014) 'Challenges in Humanitarian Information Management and Exchange: Evidence from Haiti', *Disasters*, 38(s1), pp. S50–72.

Antonini, R. (2017) *Non-Professional Interpreting and Translation: State of the Art and Future of an Emerging Field of Research.* Amsterdam and Philadelphia: John Benjamins

Athey, J. and Moody-Williams, J. (2003) *Developing Cultural Competence in Disaster Mental Health Programs: Guiding Principles and Recommendations.* Washington, DC: US Department of Health and Human Services.

Baker, M. and Maier, C. (2011) 'Ethics in Interpreter and Translator Training: Critical Perspectives', *The Interpreter and Translator Trainer,* 5(1), pp. 1–14.

Beauchamp, T. (2019) 'The Principle of Beneficence in Applied Ethics', in Zalta, E. N. (ed.) *The Stanford Encyclopedia of Philosophy* (*Spring 2019 Edition*). Available at: https://plato.stanford.edu/archives/spr2019/entries/principle-beneficence/ (Accessed: 28 May 2019).

Birkland, T. A. (2011) *An Introduction to the Policy Process: Theories, Concepts, and Models of Public Policy Making*, 3rd ed. Armonk, NY: Sharpe.

Birkland, T. A. (2016) 'Policy Process Theory and Natural Hazards', in *Oxford Research Encyclopedia of Natural Hazard Science.* Available at: https://oxfordre.com/naturalhazardscience/view/10.1093/acrefore/9780199389407.001.0001/acrefore-9780199389407-e-75 (Accessed: 28 May 2019).

Birkmann, J. (2013) *Measuring Vulnerability to Natural Hazards: Towards Disaster Resilient Societies.* Tokyo: United Nations University Press.

Bolton, P. and Weiss, W. (2001) 'Communicating across Cultures: Improving Translation to Improve Complex Emergency Program Effectiveness', *Prehospital and Disaster Medicine*, 16(4), pp. 252–256.

Bulut, A. and Kurultay, T. (2001) 'Interpreters-in-Aid at Disasters: Community Interpreting in the Process of Disaster Management', *The Translator*, 7(2), pp. 249–263.

Businaro, R. (2012) *Relief Operations across Language Barriers: The Interpreter Factor.* Master's dissertation. University College Dublin.

Cadwell, P. (2015). *Translation and Trust: A Case Study of How Translation was Experienced by Foreign Nationals Resident in Japan for the 2011 Great East Japan Earthquake.* PhD thesis. Dublin City University.

Cadwell, P., Bollig, C. and Reid, J. (2019) 'Management and Training of Linguistic Volunteers: A Case Study of Translation at Cochrane Germany', in Federici, F. M. and O'Brien, S. (eds.) *Translation in Cascading Crises*. London and New York: Routledge, pp. 152–174.

Cadwell, P. and O'Brien, S. (2016) 'Language, Culture, and Translation in Disaster ICT: An Ecosystemic Model of Understanding', *Perspectives*, 24(4), pp. 557–575.

Carroll, T. (2012) 'Multilingual or Easy Japanese? Promoting Citizenship via Local Government Websites', in Gottlieb, N. (ed.) *Language and Citizenship in Japan*. New York: Routledge, pp. 193–216.

Clerveaux, V., Spence, B. and Katada, T. (2010) 'Promoting Disaster Awareness in Multicultural Societies: The DAG Approach', *Disaster Prevention and Management*, 19(2), pp. 199–218.

Comfort, L. K. (2007) 'Crisis Management in Hindsight: Cognition, Communication, Coordination, and Control', *Public Administration Review*, 67(s1), pp. 189–197.

Coombs, W. T. (2012) 'Crisis Communication and Its Allied Fields', in Coombs, W. T and Holladay, S. J. (eds) *The Handbook of Crisis Communication*. Chichester: John Wiley & Sons, pp. 54–64.

Coppola, D. P. (2011) *Introduction to International Disaster Management,* 2nd ed., Boston: Butterworth-Heinemann.

Cornia, A., Dressel, K. and Pfeil, P. (2016) 'Risk Cultures and Dominant Approaches towards Disasters in Seven European Countries', *Journal of Risk Research,* 19(3), pp. 288–304.

Council of the European Union (2008) *Charter of Fundamental Rights of the European Union*. Paris: Éditions BIOTOP.

Coyle, D. and Meier, P. (2009) *New Technologies in Emergencies and Conflicts: The Role of Information and Social Networks*. Washington, DC and London: UN Foundation-Vodafone Foundation Partnership.

Department of Homeland Security (2019) *FEMA: About the Agency*. Available at: www.fema.gov/about-agency (Accessed: 7 August 2019).

Doğan, A. (2016) 'Anybody Down There? Emergency and Disaster Interpreting in Turkey', in Federici, F. M. (ed.) *Mediating Emergencies and Conflicts: Frontline Translating and Interpreting*. London: Palgrave Macmillan, pp. 44–53.

Doğan, A. and Kahraman, R. (2011) 'Emergency and Disaster Interpreting in Turkey: Ten Years of a Unique Endeavour', *Hacettepe University Journal of Faculty of Letters*, 28(2), pp. 61–76.

Drabek, T. E. (2003) *Strategies for Coordinating Disaster Responses*. Boulder, CO: Institute of Behavior Sciences.

Drabek, T. E. (2010) *The Human Side of Disaster*. Boca Raton, FL: CRC Press.

Drugan, J. and Megone, C. (2011) 'Bringing Ethics into Translator Training: An Integrated, Inter-disciplinary Approach', *The Interpreter and Translator Trainer*, 5(1), pp. 183–211.

Eiser, R. J. *et al.* (2012) 'Risk Interpretation and Action: A Conceptual Framework for Responses to Natural Hazards', *International Journal of Disaster Risk Reduction.* 1, pp. 5–16.

Erickson, J. (2012) 'Volunteering with Refugees: Neoliberalism, Hegemony, and (Senior) Citizenship', *Human Organization,* 71(2), pp. 167–175.

European Commission (2018) *Commission Staff Working Document: General Guidelines on Operational Priorities for Humanitarian Aid in 2019*. Available at: https://ec.europa.eu/echo/sites/echo-site/files/ggophafinal.pdf (Accessed: 28 May 2019).

Federici, F. M. (2016) *Mediating Emergencies and Conflicts: Frontline Translating and Interpreting*. London: Palgrave Macmillan.

Federici, F. M. and Cadwell, P. (2018) 'Training Citizen Translators: Design and Delivery of Bespoke Training on the Fundamentals of Translation for New Zealand Red Cross', *Translation Spaces*, 7(1), pp. 23–43.

Fischer, H. (2008) *Response to Disaster*, 3rd ed. Lanham, MD: University Press of America.

Fisher, D., Hagon, K., Lattimer, C., O'Callaghan, S., Swithern, S. and Walmsley, L. (2018), *World Disasters Report 2018: Leaving No One Behind.* Geneva: International Federation of Red Cross and Red Crescent Societies.

Fu, K., White, J., Chan, Y., Zhou, L., Zhang, Q. and Lu, Q. (2010) 'Enabling the Disabled: Media Use and Communication Needs of People with Disabilities During and After the Sichuan Earthquake in China', *International Journal of Emergency Management*, 7(1), pp. 75–87.

Geale, S. K. (2012) 'The Ethics of Disaster Management', *Disaster Prevention and Management*, 21(4), pp. 445–462.

Gerber, B. J. (2007) 'Disaster Management in the United States: Examining Key Political and Policy Challenges', *Policy Studies Journal*, 35(2), pp. 227–238.
Goodwin, P. (2010) 'Ethical Problems in Translation', *The Translator*, 16(1), pp. 19–42.
Greenstone, J. L. (2010) 'Use of Interpreters with Crisis Intervention Teams, Behavioral Health Units, and Medical Strike Teams: Responding Appropriately and Effectively', *International Journal of Emergency Mental Health*, 12(2), pp. 79–82.
Greenwood, F., Howarth, C., Escudero Poole, D., Raymond, N. A. and Scarnecchia, D. P. (2017) *The Signal Code: A Human Rights Approach to Information During Crisis*. Available at: https://hhi.harvard.edu/publications/signal-code-human-rights-approach-information-during-crisis (Accessed: 28 May 2019).
Haddow, G. D., Bullock, J. A. and Coppola, D. P. (2017) *Introduction to Emergency Management*. Amsterdam: Elsevier.
Hanson-Easey, S., Every, D., Hansen, A. and Bi, P. (2018) 'Risk Communication for New and Emerging Communities: The Contingent Role of Social Capital', *International Journal of Disaster Risk Reduction*, 28, pp. 620–628.
Harro-Loit, H., Vihalemm, T. and Ugur, K. (2012) 'Cultural Experience as a (Critical) Factor in Crisis Communication Planning,' *Journal of Contingencies and Crisis Management*, 20(1), pp. 26–38.
Harvard Humanitarian Initiative (2011) '*Disaster Relief 2.0: The Future of Information Sharing in Humanitarian Emergencies*', Washington, DC: UN Foundation & Vodafone Foundation Technology Partnership.
Henrich, N. and Holmes, B. J. (2011) 'Communicating during a Pandemic: Information the Public Wants about the Disease and New Vaccines and Drugs', *Health Promotion Practice*, 12(4), pp. 610–619.
Holmes, B. J., Henrich, N., Hancock, S. and Lestou, V. (2009) 'Communicating with the Public during Health Crises: Experts' Experiences and Opinions', *Journal of Risk Research*, 12(6), pp. 793–807.
House, J. (2018). *Translation: The Basics*. London and New York: Routledge.
ICRC (International Committee of the Red Cross) (2019) *Languages and Interpreting – Working with Us*. Available at: www.icrc.org/en/who-we-are/jobs/languages-profiles (Accessed: 28 May 2019).
IDMC (Internal Displacement Monitoring Centre) (2018) *Global Report on Internal Displacement 2018*. Available at: www.internal-displacement.org/global-report/grid2018/ (Accessed: 28 May 2019).
InZone (2019) *Who We Are*. Available at: www.unige.ch/inzone/who-we-are/ (Accessed 28 May 2019).
Kaindl, K. (2013) 'Multimodality and Translation', in Millán, C. and Bartrina, F. (eds) *The Routledge Handbook of Translation Studies*. Abingdon: Routledge, pp. 257–269.
Kapucu, N. (2006) 'Examining the National Response Plan in Response to a Catastrophic Disaster: Hurricane Katrina in 2005', *International Journal of Mass Emergencies and Disasters*, 24(2), pp. 271–299.
Kelly, M. and Footitt, H. (2012) *Languages and the Military: Alliances, Occupation and Peace Building*. Basingstoke and New York: Palgrave Macmillan.
Kendra, J. M. and Wachtendorf, T. (2003) 'Elements of Resilience after the World Trade Center Disaster: Reconstituting New York City's Emergency Operations Centre', *Disasters*, 27(1), pp. 37–53.
Kirsch, T., Sauer, L. and Guha Sapir, D. (2012) 'Analysis of the International and US Response to the Haiti Earthquake: Recommendations for Change', *Disaster Medicine and Public Health Preparedness*, 6(3), pp. 200–208.
Koenig, K. L. (2013) 'Adventures in Disaster Medicine: A United States Experience that Illustrates Key Public Health Policy Principles', *Journal of Acute Medicine*, 3(4), pp. 119–124.
Kurultay, T. and Bulut, A. (2012) 'Re-Evaluating Community Interpreting: Emergency and Disaster Interpreting', *I. U. Journal of Translation Studies*, 3(6), pp. 23–43.
Lambert, J. (2018) 'How Ethical are Codes of Ethics? Using Illusions of Neutrality to Sell Translations', *Journal of Specialised Translation*, 30, pp. 269–290.
Lewis, W. (2010) 'Haitian Creole: How to Build and Ship and MT Engine from Scratch in 4 Days, 17 Hours, and 30 Minutes', in *Proceedings of the 14th Annual Conference of the European Association for Machine Translation (EAMT 2010)*, Saint-Raphaël, France, 27–28 May.

Lewis, W., Munro, R. and Vogel, S. (2011) 'Crisis MT: Developing a Cookbook for MT in Crisis Situations', in *Proceedings of the 6th Workshop on Statistical Machine Translation*, Edinburgh, 30–31 July, pp. 501–511.

Longstaff, P. H. and Yang, S. (2008) 'Communication Management and Trust: Their Role in Building Resilience to "Surprises" such as Natural Disasters, Pandemic Flu, and Terrorism', *Ecology and Society*, 13(1): 3. Available at: www.ecologyandsociety.org/vol13/iss1/art3/ (Accessed: 28 May 2019).

Marzotto, M. (2019) *The Language Factor: Lessons for Communication and Community Engagement from Translators without Borders' Experience*. Available at: https://odihpn.org/magazine/language-factor-lessons-communication-community-engagement-translators-without-borders-experience/ (Accessed: 8 August 2019).

McDonough Dolmaya, J. (2012) 'Analyzing the Crowdsourcing Model and Its Impact on Public Perceptions of Translation', *The Translator*, 18(2), pp. 167–191.

McKee, R. (2014) 'Breaking News: Sign Language Interpreters on Television during Natural Disasters', *Interpreting*, 16(1), pp. 107–130.

Moser-Mercer, B., Kherbiche, L. and Class, B. (2014) 'Interpreting Conflict: Training Challenges in Humanitarian Field Interpreting', *Journal of Human Rights Practice*, 6(1), pp. 140–158.

Munday, J. (2016) *Introducing Translation Studies: Theories and Applications*, 4th ed. London and New York: Routledge.

Munro, R. (2013) 'Crowdsourcing and the Crisis-Affected Community: Lessons Learned and Looking Forward from Mission 4636', *Journal of Information Retrieval*, 16(2), pp. 210–266.

Naito, M. (2012) 'Community Interpreting at the Time of Great East Japan Earthquake', *Interpretation and Translation*, 14(1), pp. 97–115.

Nepal, V., Banerjee, D., Perry, M. and Scott, D. (2012). 'Disaster Preparedness of Linguistically Isolated Populations: Practical Issues for Planners', *Health Promotion Practice*, 13(2), pp. 265–271.

Nsiah-Kumi, P. A. (2008). 'Communicating Effectively with Vulnerable Populations during Water Contamination Events', *Journal of Water and Health*, 6(s1), pp. 63–75.

O'Brien, S. and Cadwell, P. (2017) 'Translation Facilitates Comprehension of Health-Related Crisis Information: Kenya as an Example', *JoSTrans: The Journal of Specialised Translation*, 28, pp. 23–51.

O'Brien, S., Federici, F. M., Cadwell, P., Marlowe, J. and Gerber, B. (2018) 'Language Translation during Disaster: A Comparative Analysis of Five National Approaches', *International Journal for Disaster Risk Reduction*, 31, pp. 627–636.

Ogie, R., Castilla Rho, J., Clarke, R. J. and Moore, A. (2018) 'Disaster Risk Communication in Culturally and Linguistically Diverse Communities: The Role of Technology', *Proceedings*, 2(19): 1256.

O'Hagan, M. (2011) 'Community Translation: Translation as a Social Activity and Its Possible Consequences in the Advent of Web 2.0 and Beyond', in O'Hagan, M. (ed.) *Translation as a Social Activity: [Community Translation 2.0]*. Brussels: University Press Antwerp, pp. 111–128.

Olohan, M. (2014) 'Why Do You Translate? Motivation to Volunteer and TED Translation', *Translation Studies*, 7(1), pp. 17–33.

O'Mathúna, D. P., Parra Escartín, C., Roche, P. and Marlowe, J. (2020). Engaging Citizen Translators in Disasters: Exploring Ethical Challenges. *Translation and Interpreting Studies*, 15(1), pp. 57–79.

Pérez-González, L. and Susam-Saraeva, Ş. (2012) 'Non-Professionals Translating and Interpreting: Participatory and Engaged Perspectives', *The Translator*, 18(2), pp. 149–165.

Perry, R. W. (2007). 'What is a Disaster?', in Rodríguez, H., Quarantelli, E. L. and Dynes, R. R. (eds.) *Handbook of Disaster Research*. New York: Springer, pp. 1–15.

Powell, C. and Pagliara-Miller, C. (2012) 'The Use of Volunteer Interpreters during the 2010 Haiti Earthquake: Lessons Learned from the USNS COMFORT Operation Unified Response Haiti', *American Journal of Disaster Medicine*, 7(1), pp. 37–47.

Purtle, J., Siddiqui, N. J. and Andrulis, D. P. (2011) 'Language Issues and Barriers', in Penuel, K. B. and Statler, M. (eds.) *Encyclopedia of Disaster Relief*. Thousand Oaks, CA: Sage Publications, pp. 379–382.

Pym, A. (2014) *Exploring Translation Theories*, 2nd ed. London and New York: Routledge.

Quarantelli, E. L. (1987) *The Social Science Study of Disasters and Mass Communications.* Newark, DE: Disaster Research Center, University of Delaware.
Quarantelli, E. L. (2000) 'Disaster Research', in Borgatta, E. and Montgomery, R. (eds) *Encyclopedia of Sociology Vol. 1*, 2nd ed. New York: Macmillan, pp. 682–688.
Rodríguez, H., Quarantelli, E. L. and Dynes, R. (2006) *Handbook of Disaster Research.* New York: Springer.
Sahana Software Foundation (2019) *People with Literacy Challenges are 'Left Behind' in Disaster Communication.* Available at: www.elrha.org/project-blog/people-with-literacy-challenges-are-left-behind-in-disaster-communication/ (Accessed: 28 May 2019).
Salama-Carr, M. (2007) *Translating and Interpreting Conflict.* Amsterdam: Rodopi.
Santos-Hernández, J. M. and Hearn Morrow, B. (2013) 'Language and Literacy', in Phillips, B. D., Thomas, D. S. K., Lovekamp, W. E. and Fothergill, A. (eds) *Social Vulnerability to Disasters*, 2nd ed. Boca Raton, London and New York: CRC Press, pp. 265–280.
Sellnow, T. L. and Seeger, M. W. (2013) *Theorizing Crisis Communication.* Chichester: Wiley-Blackwell.
Shackleton, J. (2018). 'Preparedness in Diverse Communities: Citizen Translation for Community Engagement', in Stock, K. and Bunker, D. (eds) *Proceedings of ISCRAM Asia Pacific 2018*, Auckland: Massey University, pp. 400–406.
Shiu-Thornton, S., Balabis, J., Senturia, K, Tamayo, A. and Oberle, M. (2007) 'Disaster Preparedness for Limited English Proficient Communities: Medical Interpreters as Cultural Brokers and Gatekeepers', *Public Health Reports*, 122(4), pp. 466–471.
Slade, D. (2011) *Communication for Health in Emergency Contexts: Final Report.* Strawberry Hills, NSW: Australian Learning and Teaching Council.
Smith, K. (2013) *Environmental Hazards: Assessing Risk and Reducing Disaster*, 6th ed. Abingdon: Routledge.
Snellman P. (2016) 'Constraints on and Dimensions of Military Interpreter Neutrality', *Linguistica Antverpiensia*, 15, pp. 260–281.
Sutherlin, G. (2013) 'A Voice in the Crowd: Broader Implications for Crowdsourcing Translation during Crisis', *Journal of Information Science*, 39(3), pp. 397–409.
Taibi, M. and Ozolins, U. (2016) *Community Translation.* London: Bloomsbury Academic.
Tanaka, S., Miyao, M., Okamoto, K. and Hasegawa, S. (2007) 'Template Translation for Multilingual Disaster Information System', in Kaneda, Y., Kawamura, H. and Sasai, M. (eds.) *Frontiers of Computational Science.* Berlin: Springer-Verlag, pp. 353–356.
Tanner, A., Friedman, D. B., Koskan, A. and Barr, D. (2009) 'Disaster Communication on the Internet: A Focus on Mobilizing Information', *Journal of Health Communication*, 14(8), pp. 741–755.
Tierney, K. J. and Waugh, W. L. (2007) *Emergency Management: Principles and Practice for Local Government.* Washington, DC: ICMA Press.
Translators without Borders (2019) *Crisis Response: Words of Relief.* Available at: https://translatorswithoutborders.org/our-work/crisis-response/ (Accessed: 28 May 2019).
United Nations (1948) *The Universal Declaration of Human Rights.* Available at: www.un.org/en/universal-declaration-human-rights/ (Accessed: 28 May 2019).
UNDAC (United Nations Disaster Assessment and Coordination Team) (2018) *UNDAC Field Handbook*, 7th ed. Geneva: United Nations.
UNDRR (United Nations Office for Disaster Risk Reduction) (2017) *Terminology: Disaster.* Available at: www.unisdr.org/we/inform/terminology#letter-d (Accessed: 28 May 2019).
UNHCR (United Nations High Commissioner for Refugees) (2017) *UNHCR's New Emergency Policy: How to Better Prepare for and Respond to the Needs of Displaced People.* Available at: www.refworld.org/cgi-bin/texis/vtx/rwmain?docid=59d4d5354 (Accessed: 7 August 2019).
Valero-Garcès, C. and Tipton, R. (2017) *Ideology, Ethics and Policy Development in Public Service Interpreting and Translation.* Bristol: Multilingual Matters.
World Health Organisation (2012) *Toolkit for Assessing Health-System Capacity for Crisis Management.* Copenhagen: World Health Organization, Regional Office for Europe.
Wylie, S. (2012) *Best Practice Guidelines for Engaging with Culturally and Linguistically Diverse (CALD) Communities in Times of Disaster.* Christchurch: Christchurch City Council.
Yip, M. P. *et al.* (2013). 'The Role of Self-Efficacy in Communication and Emergency Response in Chinese Limited English Proficiency LEP Populations', *Health Promotion Practice*, 14(3), pp. 400–407.

16

Translating global epidemics

The case of Ebola

Tony Joakim Sandset

1 Introduction

Global epidemics and global responses to them set into motion human networks that are meant to curb the epidemic, heal the sick and help the dying. However, there are often different ways of explaining the epidemic, 'clashing' with each other and/or competing for hegemony in order to maintain control over its spread. In such situations, the concept of 'culture' is often invoked, i.e. it is assumed that differences in culture will lead to differences in medical knowledge, and in the perspectives towards disease, illness, body and mind. As a result of the dominance of so-called 'Western medicine', minority perspectives on wellbeing and disease are often 'translated' and made intelligible through the hegemonic system of biomedicine. This foregrounds the role of language within global epidemics and the ways in which language needs to be used efficiently and appropriately in order to convey knowledge about how to prevent infections, care for the sick, and, in certain cases, how to conduct funerals for the dead. Language can thus be seen as both a potential barrier to the transference of biomedical knowledge from 'source text', i.e. clinical research, to 'target text', i.e. clinical practice, as well as a key facilitator for the transference of crucial and life-saving information and knowledge. For instance, as the non-profit organisation Translators Without Borders (TWB)[1] formulated it in relation to the 2014–2015 Ebola outbreak, the Ebola 'crisis was one of information, and especially information in the right language, as much as anything else. Information provided in languages people can understand can help save lives in a crisis'.[2]

The departure point of this contribution is that translation can serve as a useful analytical tool for understanding how medical knowledge is circulated during global epidemics, such as the Ebola outbreak in 2001 in Uganda, the 2003 outbreak in Congo (Hewlett and Hewlett 2007; Hewlett and Amola 2003) and the wider outbreak in 2014–2015 (Park and Umlauf 2014; Burci 2014; Benton 2014; Li 2014). The contribution will first offer a brief conceptual analysis of the term 'translation', discussing some fundamental aspects of the term, in particular 'translation' as a means of transferring knowledge from one culture to another and/or from one language to another. It will then look at how the Ebola epidemics have been approached within three interrelated fields: first, how it has been

DOI: 10.4324/9781003167983-21

approached 'on-the-ground' within epidemic spaces; second, how it has been tackled in anthropology as a field of analysis; and finally, how it has been mediated and 'translated' in the Global North through the mediatisation of Ebola. Following this, the contribution will offer a section on further directions.

2 Definitions

2.1 Translation

Within the lexicon of Ebola epidemics, translation occupies a space which is not only defined by its connection to the translation of language, but also linked to the concept of 'translational medicine', that is, how medical knowledge can be 'translated' from 'bench side, to bedside, and to the community side' (Cohrs *et al.* 2015). This implies that medical knowledge produced in laboratories, modelling studies and research-based interventions is 'moved', so to speak, from 'bench to bedside', to ensure that proven strategies for healthcare and disease prevention actually reach the communities that are affected by epidemics (Woolf 2008). In this frame, translation can be linked to the movement and circulation of knowledge from clinical research to clinical practice. The emphasis here is on the movement of knowledge, and thus, the notion of 'transfer' and 'fidelity' across sites wherein medical knowledge is circulated. This, of course, also involves actual translation of information and knowledge from one language to another, which brings us into the second frame wherein translation figures in Ebola epidemics.

In this second frame, translation can be seen as the process in which medical knowledge is aimed at the public in an effort to provide information meant to prevent infections as well as encourage people who suspect they are sick to seek out medical treatment. Here, translation of information is based on two interconnected premises. The first one is that knowledge is key in order to halt and stop the ongoing epidemic. By 'arming' people with knowledge about a particular disease, people will be able to protect themselves and their families, thus halting the spread of the disease. However, this premise also rests on the assumption that there is only a certain set of knowledges that should be disseminated in order to curb an epidemic. In the case of the various Ebola epidemics, this set has often been seen as biomedical information about Ebola such as its aetiology, the way it spreads, how deadly it is, and what to do if people do get sick, that is, the treatment of the disease (Southall, Deyoung and Harris 2017; Li 2014). As Li observes:

> Biomedicine, as a form of science, thus holds a privileged position in Western societies, as the arbiter of the divide between 'knowledge' and 'belief', the first denoting universal truth and the latter a mere presupposition with a connotation of error.
>
> *Li 2014: 3*

It is this biomedical information that needs to be translated, both linguistically – often from English or French to local languages – and intersemiotically, from text to images – i.e. from medical texts to flyers describing how to avoid contagion and what to do if one does fall ill.

Once again, this complicated pattern points to the importance of movement and circulation, highlighting how knowledge is perceived as being moved from one point to another, from a sender to a receiver or from a 'source text to a target text' (Engebretsen, Sandset and Ødemark 2017). In implying that knowledge about disease patterns, prevention and care is circulated and disseminated through a process of translation, we are reminded about a key feature of the process, which Michael Wintroub points out when he states that translation

> is a common word. However, its meaning cannot be reduced to common usage: to turn one language into another. Made from the combination of two other words, trans, meaning to cross over or go beyond, and fero (whose supine form is latum), meaning to bear or carry, translation signifies movement and transference, transport, and carrying over.
>
> *Wintroub 2015: 1*

When brought into the context of how translation works in global epidemics, such as those involving Ebola, we can note that the translation of (Western) biomedical knowledge is predicated upon a vast array of processes in which this knowledge is 'carried across' from one site to another. One process is the linguistic translation of information from one language to another; the other is the translation of textual messages to images used in public health information. A third process in which translation is linked to the transference and transportation of information is the vast apparatus of medical personnel who communicate on-the-ground with local communities on a daily basis and thus translate medical knowledge into a community setting (Southall, Deyoung and Harris 2017; Hewlett and Hewlett 2007; Hewlett and Amola 2003). This last point links the more conceptual aspects of translation within global epidemics to the very practical and on-the-ground work of translation. It points to the ways in which information needs to be made accessible and intelligible according to local languages and cultures, which brings us into the discussion of how the practical work of translation also intersects with the issues of so-called 'cultural grids'.

2.2 Cultural grids/conceptual grids

An important way of understanding how translation works within global epidemics is to look at the ways in which information and knowledge pass through what Lefevere and Venuti have called 'textual and conceptual grids' within translation studies (Lefevere 2002; Lefevere 1999; Venuti 2009; Venuti 2012). These grids imply a move away from a 'purely' linguistic focus on translation to how conceptual schemes and cultural framings 'around' or 'above' sentences influence translation, as well as occasionally becoming obstacles to translation. Referencing earlier work with Lefevere, Bassnett has noted that in

> formulating our notion of textual grids, we pointed out (Bassnett and Lefevere 1998: 5) that some cultures (such as French, German and English) share a common textual grid that derives from the Christian and Greco-Roman traditions. Other cultures (such as Chinese and Japanese) share less with others.
>
> *Bassnett 2007: 19*

These 'grids' reflect 'patterns of expectations that have been interiorised by members of a given culture' (Bassnett 2007: 19). Bassnett states that the notion of textual or conceptual grids is a useful one in translation studies, since it can help us understand how meaning is made through the movement between a source text to a target text, or rather from one culture to another (Bassnett 2007). Lefevere points out that by introducing the concept of textual grids as a metaphor for understanding the process of meaning making within translation, we can see that questions of translatability have more to do with cultural factors, what he refers to as 'discrepancies in the conceptual and textual grids', rather than with 'discrepancies in languages' (Lefevere 1999: 75–76). This becomes particularly acute in relation to the ways in which the West has constructed non-Western cultures by translating them into Western categories, a process that both distorts and falsifies (Bassnett 2007: 20). This important conceptual part of translation is also present in the everyday work of people within the Ebola crisis. Once again, TWB offers an example by highlighting that translation within local settings needs to take into consideration both local linguistic variants of different national languages and local cultural contexts.[3] The same idea is echoed by the World Health Organization (WHO), in a report on the 2014–2015 Ebola outbreak, which notes that it was key to 'ensure that documents [we]re translated into local languages and explained'.[4] To translate medical information in an Ebola epidemic is just as much about 'cultural translation' as it is about crossing or overcoming language barriers, by offering cultural and locally specific ways of conveying biomedical knowledge in a crisis. This brings us to the next section, which will directly link these conceptual issues of translation in global epidemics with the on-the-ground work that is being done by medical personnel and non-profit organisations, exemplified in this case by TWB.

3 Critical issues

Several critical issues and topics emerge in the novel field of translation of medical knowledge in connection to epidemics. One of the most pressing, and perhaps most obvious of these issues is to provide life-saving information as fast as possible, adapting this information to local languages as well as to local cultural contexts. This involves looking at how the ongoing information dissemination work unfolds, and how campaigns are launched as the epidemic rages on. Within this dissemination and campaign work, several questions arise in relation to translation proper: who actually translates the informational material? Are the translations outsourced to medical translators, or carried out by on-the-ground healthcare providers? Into which languages are they translated? Does the choice of language reflect the regional dynamics in terms of 'major'/ 'minor' language distribution? Through which media and outlets is the information distributed? Last but not least, does the distributed information work or is it problematic? In the following, this contribution will engage with some of these questions in the form of what we can call 'critical issues on-the-ground' in connection to translation and the Ebola epidemic.

3.1 The role of language: international, national and local variations

One of the clearest examples of translational work in the times of the Ebola epidemics is the one carried out by TWB; it offers a good starting point for looking at the critical issues of translation during and after the epidemics. The first issue belongs to the realm of an 'epistemology of epidemic translation'. Here, the question is why to translate in an epidemic and what role translation has in an Ebola epidemic. In order to address this topic, it is important to understand the role of *language* as it is understood by TWB.

TWB states that 'Ebola is a crisis of language' and that 'language was one of the main difficulties faced by humanitarian workers responding to the Ebola crisis'.[5] Translation here is seen as a way of overcoming the language barrier. TWB states that 'Words of Relief is the first crisis response translation network intended to improve communications between crisis-affected communities and humanitarian responders before, during and after a crisis, by *eliminating the language barriers that can impede vital relief efforts*' (emphasis in the original).[6] Translation in this perspective becomes crucial since the proverbial 'language barrier' is perceived to be overcome only through translation. The emergence of the field of 'crisis translation' is considered by TWB to have been spurred on by a neglect amongst humanitarian aid organisations, as well as national and international health organisations. As TWB states, 'language is usually not seen as a priority in emergency responses. As a result, misinformation, mistrust, fear and panic can spread quickly'.[7] This is due to the fact that information flow during a crisis is vital: relief workers scale up their work rapidly and they must be able to communicate with the local population to provide information on food, water, health and other life-saving issues, and to collect information from affected populations on the challenges they face.[8]

The issue of communication, language barriers and translation has also been noted by the Harvard Humanitarian Initiative, which pointed out in 2011 that 'the lack of appropriate translation' is a 'perennial hidden issue that results in delaying critical communications and disenfranchising affected populations'.[9] As TWB states, the 'Ebola crisis in West Africa was a crisis of communication and the translation of Ebola messages was critical to curbing the emergency. The affected people desperately needed information; not in any language but in the language they understood most'.[10] Here translation is connected with two interrelated issues. First is the practical issue of translating medical information, often produced in either English or French, into national and local languages. Second, there is the issue of translating often highly biomedicalised protocols and information into vernacular and culturally appropriate language. The latter has been the subject of several studies and scholarship, focusing on the ways in which biomedical information is disseminated from 'bench to trench' and from clinicians to patients in an effort to increase patient 'health literacy' (Engebretsen, Sandset and Ødemark 2017; Nutbeam 2008; Nutbeam 2000). Increasing people's health literacy has come to be seen as an important public health outcome, lowering morbidity and risk amongst the population by empowering people with the ability to understand and act upon biomedical advice and knowledge. This goal presupposes a process of translation and carries the same epistemological underpinning which we have seen in the work of TWB, WHO and the Harvard Humanitarian Initiative.

As such, the role of translation proper in the Ebola epidemics goes beyond the idea that there is a language barrier which needs to be crossed. Rather, the work of translation is not only providing life-saving information in local languages as stated by TWB, but also aiding the local population in increasing their health literacy. A standard definition of health literacy provided by the WHO reads as follows: 'The cognitive and social skills which determine the motivation and ability of individuals to gain access to, understand and use information in ways which promote and maintain good health' (Nutbeam 1998). However, as Sørensen *et al.* found in a systematic review of the term, there are 17 different definitions of it, making it a highly polysemous concept (Sørensen *et al.* 2012). For instance, health literacy may mean 'the wide range of skills, and competencies that people develop to seek out, comprehend, evaluate and use health information and concepts to make informed choices, reduce health risks and increase quality of life' (Sørensen *et al.* 2012: 4); or it may mean 'the ability to read, filter and understand health information in order to form sound judgments' (Sørensen *et al.* 2012: 4). In all these definitions, health literacy involves a process of being able to locate, access, evaluate and utilise different forms of health information which is expected to 'empower' the individual with the 'right kind' of knowledge, and that can in turn bolster health, mitigate risk, and, in emergencies such as the Ebola outbreaks, save lives.

As such, translation proper as it unfolds in medical emergencies cannot be understood without its relationship to concepts such as (il)literacy. This raises two other critical issues in connection to translation within epidemics: one is the question of multiple languages that need to be addressed in the translational work being carried out; the other is the question of literacy.

The notion that the Ebola crisis was a 'crisis of language' not only highlighted the need for health information to be translated from English or French to the local languages, but also implied the need to translate into the *right local language*. TWB states

> People at risk of contracting Ebola need information to keep themselves and their families safe. Information they don't understand will not help them. They need clear communication in plain, localized language, in a format they understand, and through channels they trust.[11]

The emphasis on localised languages is key in the TWB report. TWB notes, for instance, that

> The local form of Swahili is the most effective language for risk communication [...] Participants did not reliably understand key concepts in French and standard Swahili [...] In more rural and linguistically diverse areas, people may have greater difficulty understanding the Swahili used in Goma [centralised capital of the Northern province of Kivu in the DRC].[12]

As such, a critical issue in bolstering health literacy through correct translation is to translate medical information into a language which is as local as possible. In practical terms, this meant that TWB translated English and French information into Congolese Swahili rather than standard Swahili. However, TWB notes that 'professional translators in most West African languages do not exist, and the project had to focus on the more widely spoken languages. This meant that requests for languages like Susu, Kpelle, Bassa, Mano and Mandingo could not be met'.[13] This underscores the difficulties faced by a country rich in linguistic diversity. Translation during an emergency needs to cope with the 'language politics' wherein certain variants or languages have come to be hegemonic or dominant. Regional dynamics of 'major' and 'minor' languages are clearly an issue to be confronted with and a cause for concern for the translators.

Another critical issue connected to 'health literacy' is the issue of actual illiteracy on-the-ground. TWB states: 'Although in the right language and using graphics elements [*sic*], posters and other written materials are not effective if people can't read them'.[14] Illiteracy is an important issue in translating medical information to local people during an epidemic. Countries affected by the 2014 Ebola epidemic, e.g. Sierra Leone, Guinea and Liberia, provide an illustration of this. UNICEF reports that literacy rates in these three nations are 43.4 per cent in Sierra Leone,[15] 42.9 in Liberia[16] and 25.3 per cent in Guinea.[17] As such, translation in this case is not only concerned with the literal linguistic translation from one language into another in an effort to help people protect themselves through medical information, but also involves the 'translation' of words into images. TWB states that 'Visual content should be simple and culturally relevant',[18] alluding to the need to bridge the language barrier not only through the translation of a foreign language into a local language, but also by bridging the language gap by utilising images which also are contextually relevant and sensitive to cultural frames of reference. This type of translation locates 'crisis translation' within the domain of 'cultural translation' (Trivedi 2007; Bhabha 2000; Asad 1986; Lefevere 2002). The use of images as part of crisis translation is seen as a crucial way of addressing the issue of illiteracy, as images are expected to convey medical information on how to protect oneself from Ebola, how to respond if oneself or a family member gets sick, or how to bury those who died of Ebola. However, even here TWB warns about the risk of employing a sort of 'universal iconography' of Ebola as 'illustrations and icons do not carry universal meaning'.[19] Once again, translation seems to highlight the need for contextual and localised systems of meanings and should always be 'culturally and linguistically specific'. This last point also touches upon another key issue within crisis translation, which pertains to the role of the translator in communicating knowledge about the Ebola epidemic.

3.2 The role of the translator: insider or outsider?

Just as the multiplicity of local languages and the need to address local literacy levels have been important and highlighted in the emerging field of crisis translation, so too has the role of the translator. As mentioned earlier, crisis translation in West Africa in the midst of an Ebola epidemic was challenging not only due to the nature of the situation, but also due to the lack of access to translators. In the case of the translator's role in the Ebola epidemic, it has been defined as being the mediator of life-saving knowledge from a source text, a biomedical protocol, or a leaflet produced in either French or English, into local languages, often supplemented by visual aids. The role is clearly that of a mediator, not only of a particular language but also of a particular genre, that of medical texts meant to be clearly understood.

The practical work of recruiting translators to a region of the world which has a vast number of local languages was conducted through what TWB calls a 'spider network of translators'. These were

> virtual teams of translators trained to respond rapidly to language needs [...] They were based around the world, in the United States, Ghana, Sierra Leone, Mali, France, Switzerland, Germany and Kenya. They were recruited because they are native speakers and have strong links to the affected countries. Their languages skills [*sic*] were vetted and they underwent online training focusing on rapid translation. The training sessions addressed topics such as 'What is translation' and 'How to translate'. They also included tips for translators and best practice for terminology problems and quality assurance.[20]

However, the recruitment of translators in this manner also leads to challenges, which can tell us something about the role of the translator in relation to crisis translation. TWB notes that 'non-professional translators recruited from the diaspora via the spider networks often lack experience in translating', but that this is mitigated by basic training in translation in order 'to provide contextual and key aspect of rapid response translation'.[21] On the other hand, the training of non-professional native speakers by a set of professional translators also point to a strength of this approach which is the 'power of crowdsourcing' (Gao, Barbier and Goolsby 2011), a point that has also been highlighted in relation to relief efforts in the aftermath of the Haiti earthquake (Norheim-Hagtun and Meier 2010). However, this also has the weakness of, as TWB notes, requiring training of translators within the network, as well as running the risk of recruiting translators who might not have any medical training. Another potential pitfall is that the 'non-professional' translators must rely on the fact that the medical information they are translating is accurate and in line with 'best practice' information. If the information is not quality assured, then at best this might lead to delay in seeking help for those who are sick, or lead to confusion and contradictory information on what to do in an epidemic. Conversely, in a worst-case scenario, information of low-evidence grade might indeed exacerbate the epidemic and lead to potentially harmful outcomes for patients and communities alike.

Since translators are 'outsourced' from a diasporic network, the need for quality assurance is also key in crisis translation. TWB ensures that quality assurance was maintained through a process in which 'two people reviewed each translation. This also helped address another issue associated with the multiple dialects of a language'.[22] Since the spider network draws its translators from a diasporic and online community, the distinction between local/global spaces of locality vanishes; that is, while it is true that TWB uses people with a 'strong diasporic connection' to the areas of concern, the dichotomy between local/global or near/far is downplayed through this form of translational work.

Since TWB insists that information should be communicated in the most locally specific dialect/language possible, and that concepts should be explained 'using familiar words and clear sentence structure', avoiding 'technical jargon and words that are not commonly used',[23] a certain degree of adaptation and 'betrayal' of the language of biomedicine seem inevitable. However, this type of translation, and the accompanying role of the translator, should be seen as a form of pragmatism wherein the main concern is to provide information 'in languages people can understand' to 'help save lives in a crisis'.[24] The pragmatic approach is important, as the question of local versus professional translators must also account for the difficulty of access to personnel in an Ebola crisis. This brings us to another topic of concern in terms of the translation of knowledge in Ebola epidemics, as translators on-the-ground are not the only people who provide what we can call crisis translation. So too are anthropologists.

3.3 Cultural contexts: other 'translators' in an epidemic

Conceptualising the work of the anthropologist as that of a translator is not a very new or original approach. A vexing and peculiar problem *of* translation lies at the heart of anthropology: how to 'translate' the Other, i.e. how to avoid the many pitfalls and distortions in interpreting indigenous concepts and modes of thinking through a foreign conceptual system, then re-presenting them through the languages, categories and conceptual systems of meaning associated with the 'Western world' (Brisset 2010: 71). As for the anthropologist as translator in global epidemics – and in this case, Ebola epidemics – the function of translation and the translator can be seen through the following prism provided by Bolten and Shepler (2017). Calls for anthropological engagement and subsequent 'translation' came from 'frustrated officials who, for example, could not understand why local people persisted in "traditional" burial rituals. They also came from frustrated anthropologists concerned that officials were treating African cultures as backwards and unchanging' (Bolten and Shepler 2017: 353). Within the same call to action and to translation, Bolten and Shepler highlight the duality of the work of translation provided by anthropologists: on the one hand, anthropologists were seen as mediators who could 'tell' or 'translate' the correct biomedical information to local people, thus preventing them from continuing their 'traditional' funeral practices. On the other hand, anthropologists were afraid that public health officials would 'mistranslate' local customs and practices, thus they themselves also highlighted the *need* for translation, but one that would go beyond 'getting the biomedical message across' to local populations.

Seen as experts on both language and 'culture', the anthropologists are then regarded as translators *par excellence*, able to translate language and context in an epidemic, and benefiting from the expertise gained through social practice and long term engagement 'in the field', which in turn cultivates 'local knowledge' and causes them to *'act[...] as a kind of translator'* (Bolten and Shepler 2017: 357, my emphasis). In some cases, anthropologists have been called upon to explain, that is, to 'translate', what public health officials deemed 'nonsensical actions' such as bush meat consumption, engaging in 'traditional funeral rites' and seeking out 'traditional healers' (Goguen and Bolten 2017; Bolten and Shepler 2017; Wilkinson and Leach 2015; Spencer 2015). Importantly, as Bolten and Shepler state, these 'African others' in need of translation, have traditionally been stereotyped in the Western imaginary as acting nonsensically according to Western norms and have thus been perceived as 'ranking below' Western people in relation to various hierarchies and in particular when it comes to knowledge claims about health and illness (Bolten and Shepler 2017: 357). The call to translate here seems to cast anthropology as the handmaid of epidemiology (Li 2014: 5); what translation entails in such cases seems to be a transfer of 'Western' biomedical knowledge to local populations in such a way as to ensure fidelity between the biomedical message being sent out and the end result, which is not the *integration* of 'Western biomedical knowledge' into local health-related knowledge but rather the total *assimilation* of such knowledge within the target population.

Since Ebola epidemics have often been conceptualised as being driven by 'local, traditional burial rites', practices of bush meat consumption and the use of local indigenous knowledge and resources, such as 'traditional healers', the anthropologist as translator alludes to an underlying notion wherein a generic 'African culture' is regarded as a risk factor for the acquisition of an Ebola infection (Li 2014: 2). For the purposes of looking at the role of translation here, one can argue that 'African culture' becomes an obstacle which Western biomedical knowledge needs to overcome; in this frame of analysis, the anthropologist then becomes the translator with the means and skills to overcome these cultural barriers on the road to ensuring epidemic control. However, this also rests on the assumption that there is such an entity as 'African culture', a gross homogenisation of an entire continent. It also assumes that 'African' countries' experience with and response to the Ebola epidemics are homogeneous and that the patterns of disease spreading, as well as responses to them, are similar across vastly different geographical regions. Finally, it also stipulates that translation, here understood as the mediation of Western biomedical knowledge, is hindered by *cultural* forces, while leaving out, or at least pushing aside, systemic issues such as economy and material disparities.

Anthropology within epidemic settings, then, is predicated on translation. It is, as DiGiacomo states, 'raided for bits of information about "culture" which can then be plugged into a statistical model that generates correlations amendable to being represented as causal' (DiGiacomo 1999: 438). In this light, anthropology in epidemic settings becomes a discipline that, seen through the eyes of epidemiologists and public health administrators, promises to overcome the 'problem' of culture by way of providing translations. Here translation is conceptualised as being the work that is done by anthropologists in translating knowledge about conditions on-the-ground in Ebola settings back into the matrix of public health epidemiology and statistics in order to get a view of how culture allegedly influences the spread of the epidemic. Packard and Epstein note that this form of translational work can be envisioned when public health bureaucrats and medical researchers

> define the parameters of the social science input in line with dominant models of behavior within disease epidemiology and as such, anthropologists are presumed to have the knowledge of culture which they then can package into discrete units which can be used by public health experts in order to make epidemic control more effective.
>
> *Packard and Epstein 1991*

Conversely, the other work of translation is when anthropologists and other social scientists are called upon to re-translate biomedical information back into the local context, so that local populations take the necessary precautions in limiting their risk of infection. In both cases, culture becomes 'the obstacle' that is to be overcome, and the movement of knowledge between a 'target text' and a 'source text' can be conceptualised as the relationship between 'biomedical knowledge' (source text) to be translated into local systems of knowledge (target text). Of course, this also presupposes that local systems of knowledge are homogeneous, as well as sealed off from biomedical regimes offered by the Western global health systems.

3.4 Media translations

Global epidemics not only mobilise vast networks of political engagement, various health initiatives, military and medical personnel on-the-ground, economic funding streams, and the transportation of goods and supplies; they also mobilise international streams of media coverage. Epidemic knowledge that circulates in the media follows along the same lines of rational inquiry that circulates on-the-ground within zones of epidemics. As in the case of anthropology as a discipline which is often called upon to 'translate' the 'what, why, and how' of global epidemics, questions of aetiology – why the disease spreads, how it spreads, how deadly it is and who gets the disease – are also mediated in and across diverse media platforms.

The concept of 'translation' can be used here to investigate how various media outlets 'decode' information collected on the epidemic, as well as how they mediate the very nature of the epidemic. In this understanding of translation, the notion of conceptual grids discussed above becomes just as important a tool kit for examining the tropes used in order to mediate causality, explain patterns of disease, and distribute blame and moral responsibility, since it is through these grids the information gets filtered through.

The mediatisation of global epidemics can be exemplified by studies on the HIV/AIDS epidemic (Lovelock 2018; Miller 1998; Lyttleton 1994; Zhang and Matingwina 2016), the 'bird flu' or H1N1 pandemic (Klemm, Das and Hartmann 2016; Mccauley, Minsky and Viswanath 2013; Briggs and Hallin 2016; Hallin and Briggs 2015) and Ebola (Zhang and Matingwina 2016; Abeysinghe 2016; Joffe and Haarhoff 2002). In these studies, many scholars have produced analyses similar to the one discussed above, wherein *culture* becomes the culprit for the spread and emergence of various epidemics. As such, in a translational framework, we can state that the conceptual grid knowledge and information pass through in the mediatisation of global epidemics plays on the notion of 'other cultures' as being *the cause* for the spread of the disease in question. Case in point can be the early mediatisation of the AIDS epidemic, wherein the invocation of 'gay lifestyle' was a frequent trope utilised in order to understand the spread of the disease (Epstein 1996). Other examples of this type of conceptual grid analysis can be the continual mediatisation of Ebola epidemics with culture given as cause, in particular the focus on bush meat consumption as an 'African cultural practice' (Abeysinghe 2016: 463; Monson 2017: 13). Once again, culture becomes part of the decoding object that information is filtered through in many of the Western media outlets and as such knowledge about the epidemic is 'translated' by way of tropes such as 'African backwardness' (Dionne and Seay 2016). It is worth noting, as Morris did, that 'while anthropologists introduced "culture" into the public debate over managing the Ebola crisis to change medical practices, the mainstream media often tended to use "culture" in ways that represented those communities as the West's quintessential, abject Other' (Morris 2015: 542). In such an analysis, 'culture' becomes the conceptual filter or grid through which information about the Ebola epidemics are filtered, and with this comes an understanding of the epidemic in which the well-known patterns of homogenising the continent of Africa into the 'Africa-as-a-country' become widespread (Monson 2017:5). Furthermore, this understanding of Ebola as a disease that is 'culturally contingent' flattens differences across and within the geographical places that Ebola does emerge in, and, last but not least, it turns Ebola into an 'African disease' (Monson 2017: 11; Dionne and Seay 2016).

However, we should note that examples of more nuanced and multi-layered media representations often do circulate side by side with the more culturalist narratives of causality. While 'culture' can be said to be a dominant trope within the conceptual grid of Western translations of Ebola epidemics, other narratives have also emerged and have come to fill the conceptual grids related to Ebola. For instance, once the epidemic was brought under a tentative control, more and more analytical pieces emerged that moved the focus away from *culture* to *structure*, pointing out that the epidemic was due to 'African infrastructure' and the issue of economy. While this was an important and more nuanced approach, this tendency to point to economy and infrastructure as distal vectors that drove the epidemic risked ending up as a black box in itself. Just as culture had acted as a black box and became reified, so did economy and infrastructure. Suddenly, there was such a thing as 'an African economical problem' or 'an African health care system', once again flattening differences and homogenising heterogeneous contexts within nations and across countries.

Here is a paradox of translation, and of the analysis of conceptual grids within the Ebola epidemics as they emerge: how to account for culture without reifying it, without black-boxing it, in such a way that it does not filter out complexities or leave out complex networks of contagion; how to translate the biomedical message to a local context in a way that accounts for local particularities; and finally, how to communicate and mediate disease aetiology and causality between systems of beliefs in a way that minimises suffering and the loss of human life.

4 Future directions

While scholarship on anthropologists as translators of culture and language as well as media representations of epidemics abounds, the emerging field of 'crisis translation' is still relatively new (O'Brien *et al.* 2017; Federici and O'Brien 2019). TWB highlights this by drawing our attention to some potential avenues of future research and practice. Case in point would be to address the ways in which aid organisations utilise and access translation services in epidemic crises.[25] As TWB states,

> translation is not always considered a priority by governments and aid agencies. This challenge was reflected in the difficulty in getting content from aid organizations. While there was demonstrated interest, follow through, whereby organizations actually provide the content to be translated, has been weak.[26]

Another challenge, as well as direction for future research and innovation, lies in the need to develop digital tools that can ease and speed up the process of translating medical information from one language to another. This is highlighted by TWB in their call for more technological innovations and subsequent research into the use of machine translation.[27] The call for more research on charting, testing and evaluating different modalities of crisis communication is also important, such as SMS services and audio messages played on radio or mobile devices, as well as finding out what forms of images and icons relay the most effective message about Ebola prevention and care.[28] Yet another avenue of future research on the concept of 'crisis translation' and its connection to epidemics lies at the intersection between linguistic studies, media studies and what has been called 'a sociology of translation' (Heilbron 1999; Callon 1984). Here the future of crisis translation lies in combining perspectives on 'on-the-ground' translation, the mediation of medical knowledge and crisis information in the media, and the transfer and mediation of translated medical knowledge by various media modalities. Finally, and perhaps of more fundamental epistemological concern, is the call made by some within the medical humanities and medical anthropology for a new form of knowledge translation – one that is not just a 'soft supplement' to the 'hard sciences' such as biomedicine (Kristeva *et al.* 2018; Engebretsen, Sandset and Ødemark 2017). This direction of future research would ask how translations and translators can become agents for change both in the 'target culture' *and* in the 'source culture'. This would help uncovering how translation studies can develop methods and epistemological perspectives that not only aid in medical crises, but can also change and transform biomedical cultures by insisting on the primacy of textual and linguistic meaning making that goes beyond the biomedical. This would be one of many epistemological concerns that translation studies could contribute to in expanding on the 'knowledge translation metaphor' so often used in translating (Western) biomedical knowledge to the West's alleged Others and even within the West itself (Engebretsen, Sandset and Ødemark 2017; Wieringa *et al.* 2017; Greenhalgh and Wieringa 2011).

Notes

1 Translators Without Borders, https://translatorswithoutborders.org/ (Accessed: 3 March 2020).
2 See article at the Humanitarian Practice Network (HPN) webpage; https://odihpn.org/magazine/ebola-a-crisis-of-language/ (Accessed: 3 March 2020).
3 See Translators without Borders report on the topic of translation in the Democratic Republic of Congo; https://translatorswithoutborders.org/wp-content/uploads/2019/03/DRC_Ebola_Assessment_English.pdf (Accessed: 3 March 2020).
4 See the WHO report; www.who.int/medicines/ebola-treatment/background_briefing_on_data_results_sharing_during_phes.pdf (Accessed: 3 March 2020).
5 See the HPN webpage for more; https://odihpn.org/magazine/ebola-a-crisis-of-language/ (Accessed: 3 March 2020).
6 See TWB's own webpage for this; https://translatorswithoutborders.org/our-work/crisis-response/ (Accessed: 3 March 2020).
7 See the HPN webpage for more, https://odihpn.org/magazine/ebola-a-crisis-of-language/ (Accessed: 3 March 2020).

8 See https://translatorswithoutborders.org/wp-content/uploads/2016/05/alnap-innovation-wordsofrelief-case-study.pdf, page 7 (Accessed: 3 March 2020).
9 See the Harvard Humanitarian Initiative's 2011 report; https://hhi.harvard.edu/sites/default/files/publications/2011-humanitarian-action-summit.pdf (Accessed: 3 March 2020).
10 See TWB's blogpost on the issue of their project Words of Relief; www.elrha.org/project-blog/when-translation-saves-lives/ (Accessed: 3 March 2020).
11 See TWB 2019 report on translation under the Ebola epidemic; https://translatorswithoutborders.org/wp-content/uploads/2019/03/DRC_Ebola_Assessment_English.pdf, page 4 (Accessed: 3 March 2020).
12 See TWB 2019 report on translation under the Ebola epidemic; https://translatorswithoutborders.org/wp-content/uploads/2019/03/DRC_Ebola_Assessment_English.pdf, page 4 (Accessed: 3 March 2020).
13 See the HPN article for more information; https://odihpn.org/magazine/ebola-a-crisis-of-language/ (Accessed: 3 March 2020).
14 See the HPN article for more information; https://odihpn.org/magazine/ebola-a-crisis-of-language/ (Accessed: 3 March 2020).
15 See fact sheet from UNICEF, www.unicef.org/infobycountry/sierraleone_statistics.html (Accessed: 3 March 2020).
16 See fact sheet from UNESCO, http://uis.unesco.org/country/LR (Accessed: 3 March 2020).
17 See fact sheet from UNESCO, www.unicef.org/infobycountry/guinea_statistics.html (Accessed: 3 March 2020).
18 See TWB 2019 report on translation under the Ebola epidemic; https://translatorswithoutborders.org/wp-content/uploads/2019/03/DRC_Ebola_Assessment_English.pdf, page 15 (Accessed: 3 March 2020).
19 See TWB 2019 report on translation under the Ebola epidemic; https://translatorswithoutborders.org/wp-content/uploads/2019/03/DRC_Ebola_Assessment_English.pdf, page 16 (Accessed: 3 March 2020).
20 See more information on the spider network; https://odihpn.org/magazine/ebola-a-crisis-of-language/ (Accessed: 3 March 2020).
21 See more information on the spider network; https://odihpn.org/magazine/ebola-a-crisis-of-language/ (Accessed: 3 March 2020).
22 See more information on the spider network; https://odihpn.org/magazine/ebola-a-crisis-of-language/ (Accessed: 3 March 2020).
23 See the TWB practical guidelines on crisis translation; https://translatorswithoutborders.org/wp-content/uploads/2019/03/DRC_Ebola_Assessment_English.pdf (Accessed: 3 March 2020).
24 See https://odihpn.org/magazine/ebola-a-crisis-of-language/ (Accessed: 3 March 2020).
25 See https://odihpn.org/magazine/ebola-a-crisis-of-language/ (Accessed: 3 March 2020).
26 See https://odihpn.org/magazine/ebola-a-crisis-of-language/ (Accessed: 3 March 2020).
27 See on this topic; www.elrha.org/project-blog/when-translation-saves-lives/ (Accessed: 3 March 2020).
28 See TWB recent report of these topics, https://translatorswithoutborders.org/wp-content/uploads/2019/03/DRC_Ebola_Assessment_English.pdf (Accessed: 3 March 2020).

Further reading

Li, V. (2014) 'Ebola, Emerging: The Limitations of Culturalist Discourses in Epidemiology', *The Journal of Global Health*, 385(9975), pp. 1275–1277.

This article gives an excellent critique of the 'culturalist' paradigm of analysing Ebola epidemics as well as offering a nuanced reading of the ways in which 'culture' operates within the lexicon of global epidemics.

O'Brien, S. (2016) 'Training Translators for Crisis Communication: Translators Without Borders as an Example', in Federici, F. M. (ed.) *Mediating Emergencies and Conflicts*. Basingstoke and New York: Palgrave Macmillan, pp. 85–111.

This chapter offers one of the few scholarly efforts of engaging with Translators without Borders and how their work can be analysed as part of the field of 'crisis communication'.

DiGiacomo, S. M. (1999) 'Can There Be a "Cultural Epidemiology"?', *Medical Anthropology Quarterly,* 13, pp. 436–457.

This article offers a thought-provoking foray into the interconnectedness between medical anthropology and medical epidemiology. It addresses the role of 'culture' and its interception with epidemiology. Implicitly, this article also touches on issues of translation and health.

Engebretsen, E., Sandset, T. J., and Ødemark, J. (2017) 'Expanding the Knowledge Translation Metaphor', *Health Research Policy and Systems*, 15(1), p. 19.

This article addresses the role of knowledge translation, medical knowledge and culture as a primary locus of how knowledge is produced, how it is translated and how biomedicine and cultural contexts of care interact with each other.

Related topics

Translation and Interpreting in Disaster Situations, Healthcare Interpreting Ethics, Machine Translation in Healthcare

References

Abeysinghe, S. (2016) 'Ebola at the Borders: Newspaper Representations and the Politics of Border Control', *Third World Quarterly,* 37, pp. 452–467.

Asad, T. (1986) 'The Concept of Cultural Translation in British Social Anthropology', *Writing Culture: The Poetics and Politics of Ethnography,* 1, pp. 141–164.

Bassnett, S. (2007) 'Culture and Translation', in Kuhiwczak, P. and Littau, K. (eds) *A Companion to Translation Studies*. Clevedon, Buffalo and Toronto: Multilingual Matters, pp. 13–23.

Benton, A. (2014) 'The Epidemic Will be Militarized: Watching Outbreak as the West African Ebola Epidemic Unfolds', Hot Spots, *Fieldsights*, 7 October. Available at: https://culanth.org/fieldsights/the-epidemic-will-be-militarized-watching-outbreak-as-the-west-african-ebola-epidemic-unfolds (Accessed: 15 December 2020).

Bhabha, H. K. (2000) 'How Newness Enters the World: Postmodern Space, Postcolonial Times, and the Trials of Cultural Translation', in Procter, J. (ed.) *Writing Black Britain: An Interdisciplinary Anthology.* Manchester, Manchester University Press, pp. 300–306.

Bolten, C. and Shepler, S. (2017) 'Producing Ebola: Creating Knowledge In and About an Epidemic. *Anthropological Quarterly,* 90, pp. 349–368.

Briggs, C. L. and Hallin, D. C. (2016) *Making Health Public: How News Coverage Is Remaking Media, Medicine, and Contemporary Life*. London and New York: Routledge.

Brisset, A. (2010) 'Cultural Perspectives on Translation', *International Social Science Journal,* 61, pp. 69–81.

Burci, G. L. (2014) 'Ebola, the Security Council and the Securitization of Public Health', *Questions of International Law,* 10, pp. 27–39.

Callon, M. (1984) 'Some Elements of a Sociology of Translation: Domestication of the Scallops and the Fishermen of ST Brieuc Bay', *The Sociological Review,* 32, pp. 196–233.

Cohrs, R. J., Martin, T., Ghahramani, P., Bidaut, L., Higgins, P. J. and Shahzad, A. (2015) 'Translational Medicine Definition by the European Society for Translational Medicine', *New Horizons in Translational Medicine*, 2, pp. 86–88.

DiGiacomo, S. M. (1999) 'Can There Be a "Cultural Epidemiology"?', *Medical Anthropology Quarterly,* 13, pp. 436–457.

Dionne, K. Y. and Seay, L. (2016) 'American Perceptions of Africa During an Ebola Outbreak', in Evans, N. G., Smith, T. C. and Majumder, M. S. (eds.) *Ebola's Message: Public Health and Medicine in the Twenty-First Century*. Cambridge and London: MIT Press, pp. 95–110.

Engebretsen, E., Sandset, T. J. and Ødemark, J. (2017) 'Expanding the Knowledge Translation Metaphor', *Health Research Policy and Systems,* 15(19). Available at: https://health-policy-systems.biomedcentral.com/articles/10.1186/s12961-017-0184-x (Accessed: 6 January 2021).

Epstein, S. (1996) *Impure Science: Aids, Activism, and the Politics of Knowledge*. Berkeley: University of California Press.
Federici, F. M. and O'Brien, S. (eds) (2019) *Translation in Cascading Crises*. London and New York: Routledge.
Gao, H., Barbier, G. and Goolsby, R. (2011) 'Harnessing the Crowdsourcing Power of Social Media for Disaster Relief', *IEEE Intelligent Systems,* 26, pp. 10–14.
Goguen, A. and Bolten, C. (2017) 'Ebola Through a Glass, Darkly: Ways of Knowing the State and Each Other', *Anthropological Quarterly,* 90(2), pp. 423–449.
Greenhalgh, T. and Wieringa, S. (2011) 'Is It Time to Drop the "Knowledge Translation" Metaphor? a Critical Literature Review', *Journal of the Royal Society of Medicine,* 104(12), pp. 501–509.
Hallin, D. C. and Briggs, C. L. (2015) 'Transcending the Medical/Media Opposition in Research on News Coverage of Health and Medicine', *Media, Culture and Society,* 37(1), pp. 85–100.
Heilbron, J. (1999) 'Towards a Sociology of Translation: Book Translations as a Cultural World-System', *European Journal of Social Theory,* 2(4), pp. 429–444.
Hewlett, B. S. and Amola, R. P. (2003) 'Cultural Contexts of Ebola in Northern Uganda', *Emerging Infectious Diseases,* 9(10), pp. 1242–1248.
Hewlett, B. S. and Hewlett, B. L. (2007) *Ebola, Culture and Politics: The Anthropology of an Emerging Disease*. Boston; Cengage Learning.
Joffe, H. and Haarhoff, G. (2002) 'Representations of Far-Flung Illnesses: The Case of Ebola in Britain', *Social Science and Medicine,* 54(6), pp. 955–969.
Klemm, C., Das, E. and Hartmann, T. (2016) 'Swine Flu and Hype: A Systematic Review of Media Dramatization of the H1N1 Influenza Pandemic', *Journal of Risk Research,* 19(1), pp. 1–20.
Kristeva, J., Moro, M. R., Ødemark, J. and Engebretsen, E. (2018) 'Cultural Crossings of Care: An Appeal to the Medical Humanities', *Medical Humanities,* 44(1), pp. 55–58.
Lefevere, A. (1999) 'Composing the Other', in Basnett, S. and Trivedi, H. (eds) *Post-colonial Translation: Theory and Practice.* London: Routledge, pp. 75–94.
Lefevere, A. (2002) *Translation/History/Culture: A Sourcebook*, London and New York: Routledge.
Li, V. (2014) 'Ebola, Emerging: The Limitations of Culturalist Discourses in Epidemiology', *The Journal of Global Health*, 385(9975), pp. 1275–1277. DOI:10.1016/S0140-6736(14)62382-5.
Lovelock, M. (2018) 'Sex, Death and Austerity: Resurgent Homophobia in the British Tabloid Press', *Critical Studies in Media Communication,* 35(3), pp. 225–239.
Lyttleton, C. (1994) 'Messages of Distinction: The HIV/Aids Media Campaign in Thailand', *Medical Anthropology*, 16(4), pp. 363–389.
Mccauley, M., Minsky, S. and Viswanath, K. (2013) 'The H1N1 Pandemic: Media Frames, Stigmatization and Coping', *BMC Public Health,* 13, 1116.
Miller, D., Kitzinger, J., Williams, K. and Beharrell, P. (1998) *The Circuit of Mass Communication: Media Strategies, Representation and Audience Reception in the Aids Crisis.* London and Thousand Oaks: Sage.
Monson, S. (2017) 'Ebola as African: American Media Discourses of Panic and Otherization', *Africa Today,* 63(3), pp. 3–27.
Morris, C. D. (2015) 'Where It Hurts: 2014 Year in Review', *American Anthropologist,* 117(3), pp. 540–552.
Norheim-Hagtun, I. and Meier, P. (2010) 'Crowdsourcing for Crisis Mapping in Haiti', *Innovations: Technology, Governance, Globalization,* 5(4), pp. 81–89.
Nutbeam, D. (1998) 'Health Promotion Glossary', *Health Promotion International,* 13(4), pp. 349–364.
Nutbeam, D. (2000) 'Health Literacy as a Public Health Goal: A Challenge for Contemporary Health Education and Communication Strategies Into the 21st Century', *Health Promotion International,* 15(3), pp. 259–267.
Nutbeam, D. (2008) 'The Evolving Concept of Health Literacy', *Social Science and Medicine,* 67(12), pp. 2072–2078.
O'Brien, S. *et al.* (2017) 'The INTERACT Project and Crisis MT', *Proceedings of the MT Summit XVI*, 2017, 2, pp. 56–76.
Packard, R. M. and Epstein, P. (1991) 'Epidemiologists, Social Scientists, and the Structure of Medical Research on Aids in Africa', *Social Science and Medicine,* 33(7), pp. 771–783.

Park, S.-J. and Umlauf, R. (2014) 'Caring as Existential Insecurity: Quarantine, Care, and Human Insecurity in the Ebola Crisis', *Somatosphere*. Available at: http://somatosphere.net/2014/caring-as-existential-insecurity.html/ (Accessed: 15 December 2020).

Southall, H. G., Deyoung, S. E. and Harris, C. A. (2017) 'Lack of Cultural Competency in International Aid Responses: The Ebola Outbreak in Liberia', *Frontiers in Public Health,* 5(5). Available at: www.ncbi.nlm.nih.gov/pmc/articles/PMC5281539/ (Accessed: 6 January 2021).

Spencer, S. (2015) 'Invisible Enemy: Translating Ebola Prevention and Control Measures in Sierra Leone', *DFG Working Papers*, 13, Leipzig and Halle.

Sørensen, K., Van Den Broucke, S., Fullam, J., Doyle, G., Pelikan, J., Slonska, Z. and Brand, H. (2012) 'Health Literacy and Public Health: A Systematic Review and Integration of Definitions and Models', *BMC Public Health,* 12(80).

Trivedi, H. (2007) 'Translating Culture vs. Cultural Translation', in St-Pierre, P. and Kar, P. C. (eds) *In Translation – Reflections, Refractions, Transformations*. Amsterdam and Philadelphia: John Benjamins, pp. 277–287.

Venuti, L. (2009) 'From Translation, Community, Utopia', in Damrosch, D., Melas, N. and Mbongiseni, B. (eds.) *The Princeton Sourcebook in Comparative Literature.* Princeton, NJ: Princeton University Press, pp. 358–379.

Venuti, L. (2012) *The Translation Studies Reader*. London and New York: Routledge.

Wieringa, S., Engebretsen, E., Heggen, K. and Greenhalgh, T. (2017) 'Has Evidence-Based Medicine Ever Been Modern? A Latour-Inspired Understanding of a Changing EBM', *Journal of Evaluation in Clinical Practice,* 23(5), pp. 964–970.

Wilkinson, A. and Leach, M. (2015) 'Briefing: Ebola–Myths, Realities, and Structural Violence', *African Affairs,* 114(454), pp. 136–148.

Wintroub, M. (2015) 'Translations: Words, Things, Going Native, and Staying True', *The American Historical Review,* 120(4), pp. 1185–1217.

Woolf, S. H. (2008) 'The Meaning of Translational Research and Why It Matters', *JAMA,* 299(2), pp. 211–213.

Zhang, Y. and Matingwina, S. (2016) 'A New Representation of Africa? the Use of Constructive Journalism in the Narration of Ebola by *China Daily* and the BBC', *African Journalism Studies,* 37, pp. 19–40.

17

Interpreter-mediated communication with children in healthcare settings

Anne Birgitta Nilsen

1 Introduction

Although most of an interpreter's assignments in healthcare settings will involve interpreting between adults, interpreting for children is also a common occurrence. Therefore, it is important that both the interpreters and those who use their services know how to handle interpreter-mediated conversations with children. In this chapter, I will focus on oral interpreter-mediated communication with children in healthcare settings from the perspectives of both practice and research. First, I will provide a literature review of the research related to interpreter-mediated communication with children with a focus on methodology. Based on this review, I will attempt to answer some theoretical, as well as some practical questions. The former will look at which research methods and what types of data have been used in interpreter-mediated communication with children, and which research themes have, to date, been explored. The review findings will show that very little research has been done in interpreting for children in general and in the healthcare context in particular. Studies coming from areas unrelated to health services nevertheless can provide invaluable knowledge and information about interpreter-mediated communication with children in healthcare.

Most of the extant research on the subject is based on qualitative methods and interviews. Several of the studies considered in the review highlight the need for special training for interpreters, as well as for service users in interpreter-mediated communication with children. They also indicate that there is a need for information on how to train professional interpreters with a view to interpreting for children.

In the second part of this contribution, I will discuss some practical questions based on existing knowledge drawn from research and practice. The questions that will be posed will focus on the facilitation of interpreter-mediated communication with children, how interpreting for children differs from interpreting for adults, and what kind of skills, training and knowledge interpreters and service users need when conducting interpreter-mediated dialogues with children. The chapter will then conclude with some recommendations for future research.

DOI: 10.4324/9781003167983-22

2 Research on interpreter-mediated communication with children

Interpreting for children, and especially for young children, is a largely unexplored field within public service interpreting (for the few exceptions, see Gotaas 2007; Hitching and Nilsen 2010; Nilsen 2013; van Schoor 2013). A few researchers have conducted studies on sign-language interpreting for children in schools (e.g. Hjelmervik 2009; Schick, Williams and Kupermintz 2006; Winston 2004), but in this chapter, the focus is on interpreting in the public sector in general and in the health services in particular, therefore I will not be covering this education-focused literature.

Of the limited number of studies found for this review, very few are from the healthcare sector. In fact, the only research that I was able to find from the field of healthcare were two Swedish studies from childhood cancer care centres in Sweden (Granhagen Jungner *et al.* 2016; Granhagen Jungner *et al.* 2018). The other studies mentioned below are not located within healthcare, but nevertheless provide valuable knowledge about interpreter-mediated communication with children in general, including within healthcare settings.

The studies covered in this review (see Table 17.1 below) are based on qualitative methods (20 studies), with the exception of one survey (in Balogh and Salaets 2015) undertaken by the EU Co-Minor/INQUEST project, which investigated the questioning of minors in six different European jurisdictions. The results from the survey testify to the frequent occurrence of pre-trial interpreted interactions involving children in several European countries. It also reveals that interpreted child interviews in pre-trial settings are still unexplored territory. Another important finding from this survey is that 'the professional group of child support workers apparently knows the least about the role of

Table 17.1 Overview of data and methods used in qualitative studies of interpreter-mediated communication with children

Method and data	*Reference and country*
Interviews with interpreters (3)	Granhagen Jungner *et al.* (2018), Sweden Granhagen Jungner *et al.* (2016), Sweden Balogh and Salaets (2015), Belgium
Interviews with minors and families (3)	UNICEF (2018), Belgium Keselman *et al.* (2010), Sweden Keselman *et al.* (2008), Sweden
Interviews with service users in the public sector (4)	Powell *et al.* (2017), Australia Fontes and Tishelman (2016), USA Balogh and Salaets (2015), Belgium Matthias and Zaal (2002), South Africa
Experimental studies (3)	Kanstad and Gran (2016), Norway Balogh and Salaets (2015), Belgium Nilsen (2013), Norway
Audio recorded institutional dialogues with minor asylum seekers (2)	Kjelaas and Eide (2015), Norway Keselman, Cederborg and Linell (2010), Sweden
Literature reviews (4)	Böser and La Rooy (2018), Nilsen (2015), van Schoor (2013), Fontes (2010)

the interpreter' (Balogh and Salaets 2015: 199). This research is relevant for interpreter-mediated encounters with children in healthcare settings and may serve as an inspirational example to follow in healthcare. So far, there is no knowledge about the frequency of interpreter-mediated encounters with children in healthcare settings. We also do not know the extent of healthcare workers' knowledge about the role of the interpreter or how interpreter-mediated communication is handled in healthcare settings.

Most of the qualitative studies relating to interpreter-mediated communication with children collected their data through interviews (10 studies), and most of these studies were based on data gathered in Sweden (5 studies) and Belgium (4 studies). These studies utilised interviews to explore the experiences of the interpreters, the minors and the users of interpreting services. The studies based on interviews include:

1) Interviews with interpreters:
   a) who interpreted for healthcare staff and patients/families with limited Swedish proficiency in childhood cancer care centres in Sweden (Granhagen Jungner *et al.* 2016; Granhagen Jungner *et al.* 2018)
   b) who interpreted in the legal sector in Belgium (Balogh and Salaets 2015)
2) Interviews with minors:
   a) investigating their experiences with interpreter-mediated asylum hearings in Sweden (Keselman *et al.* 2010; Keselman *et al.* 2008)
   b) who are immigrant and refugee children in Belgium (UNICEF 2018)
   c) who were participants in an experimental study in Belgium (Balogh and Salaets 2015)
3) Interviews with service users:
   a) who are conducting investigative interviews with child complainants of sexual abuse in Australia (Powell *et al.* 2017)
   b) who are child forensic interviewers and child advocacy centre directors in the United States. The interviews in question investigated their experiences, practices and opinions regarding their daily interviews with children and families who are not native speakers of English (Fontes and Tishelman 2016)
   c) in the legal sector in Belgium (Balogh and Salaets 2015) and in South Africa (Matthias and Zaal 2002)

In addition to the studies based on interviews, two studies are based on linguistic analyses of audio recordings of institutional dialogues with minor asylum seekers, one in Sweden (Keselman, Cederborg and Linell 2010) and one in Norway (Kjelaas and Eide 2015). There are also three experimental studies with very young children: a pilot study based on linguistic analyses of video-recorded experiments (Nilsen 2013), a study based on video recordings, interviews and observations in a kindergarten in Norway (Kanstad and Gran 2016), and a study based on interviews with children who participated in interpreter-mediated experiments in Belgium (Balogh and Salaets 2015). All the experimental studies focus on how the children respond to the interpreter's translating activities and address the children's understanding of the interpreter's role.

For this review, in addition to the studies mentioned above, four theoretically-based literature reviews were examined. These focus on the challenges of interpreter-mediated interviews with minors in a criminal context (Böser and La Rooy 2018); on perspectives gained from studies on multilingualism (Nilsen 2015); on interpreter-mediated interviews with child witnesses and victims (van Schoor 2013); and, on forensic interviews with children (Fontes 2010). In the following sections, I will present the main themes arising from this literature review, including the interpreters' competence and lack of competence, as well as the competence of those using the interpreters' services concerning selecting interpreters, facilitation of interpreter-mediated communication with children, and training for both interpreters and users.

3 Critical issues

3.1 The interpreter's competence

The interpreter's competence is fundamental to successful communication in interpreter-mediated sessions with children in healthcare. Several studies in the review refer to interpreters' competence or lack thereof. In one of the studies, researchers explore the interpreters' experience of interpreting for healthcare staff and patients/families with limited Swedish proficiency in childhood cancer care (Granhagen Jungner *et al.* 2016). This study suggests that interpreters must have the understanding and ability to manage cultural differences between the staff, patients and families; to consider the general health literacy of the family, i.e. their ability to understand the information they are provided at the hospital; to acquaint themselves with the competence of the interpreters who preceded them if they are to bridge any existing gaps in knowledge and provide continuity (Granhagen Jungner *et al.* 2016: 143). The results from this study show that healthcare staff are too focused on giving information in a unidirectional way. Despite the interpreters' efforts, this affects the possibility for the family to understand the information and gain knowledge about their child's illness and treatment. In addition, the study also finds that interpreters struggle with their colleagues' lack of linguistic competence, meaning that they cannot trust that the information is consistent throughout the whole period of treatment.

Furthermore, Granhagen Jungner *et al.* (2016: 144) note that, for the interpreters in this study, the issue of neutrality becomes increasingly problematic, as they interpret for very ill children and therefore are emotionally affected. This means that they have to balance between their own compassion and professionalism, 'as one interpreter put it, "sparing them my tears"' (Granhagen Jungner *et al.* 2016: 142). In another article based on experience from the same hospital in Sweden, the authors observe:

> The fact that the study was conducted in a pediatric oncology care context gives deeper understanding of the interpreters' perspective of a complex situation and how they deal with it. This specific context means that interpreters had experiences of emotionally heavy situations, meeting children with life-threatening diseases, situations that possibly force interpreters to stretch their discretionary power to carry the bilingual conversation, and they reported doing so by using strategies clearly outside of their assignment.
>
> *Granhagen Jungner et al. 2018: 6*

The observations cited above add to the call for a better clarification of the interpreter's responsibilities, as noted by Powell *et al.* (2017: 99).

Van Schoor (2013: 65) notes that interpreters need to be particularly aware of their own potential influence on the communication during interviews with child witnesses and victims. Furthermore, the nature of the communication calls for a sensitive, child-friendly attitude from the interpreter, where friendliness is carefully balanced with neutrality (*ibid.*). These points may be of particular importance in contact with sick or otherwise vulnerable children in healthcare settings. Similarly, Wadensjö's study involving a medical examination (1998: 185) and Nilsen's experimental study (2013) show that interpreters may be able to engage in coordinating initiatives to ensure a child's continued cooperation during the interpreter-mediated communication.

3.2 The interpreter's lack of competence and its consequences

Several studies in this review refer to their observation of lack of competence on the interpreters' part. Although these studies refer to other contexts than healthcare, there is no reason to believe that interpreter competence in healthcare is any higher than the competence of interpreters in courts or elsewhere in the public sector. Furthermore, we also have no reason to believe that the consequences of this lack of competence are less serious in healthcare than for example in the courtroom. Therefore, similar concerns about the interpreter's lack of competence would be valid for interpreter-mediated communication with children in healthcare settings.

Matthias and Zaal (2002) discuss the inability of many interpreters to relate to or communicate appropriately with child witnesses in South Africa. They claim that serious difficulties are encountered in many cases where children are expected to work with interpreters in the courts (Matthias and Zaal 2002: 368). These difficulties are such that South African courts frequently fail to meet the child-participation standards set in article 12 of the UN Convention on the Rights of the Child and article 4(2) of the African Charter on the Rights and Welfare of the Child. Child witnesses are sometimes harmed by the experience, and the result is frequently a failure of justice as the courts are hearing only 'a faint echo' of what the children would have been able to communicate if translation services had been improved (Matthias and Zaal 2002: 371).

In a Swedish study of asylum interviews with minors (Keselman *et al.* 2010; Keselman *et al.* 2008), the researchers demonstrated how a child's right to be heard can be jeopardised by the use of non-professional interpreters. This occurred when the interpreters put leading questions to the children or omitted, distorted or caused doubts about things that the children had said. On the other hand, a study including professional interpreters (Nilsen 2013) suggests the opposite: that some professional interpreters pay more attention to what the child says than to what the adult says. Nilsen describes this as an instance of the child being empowered by the interpreter:

> [...] The example illustrates Birgitte Englund Dimitrova's discussion of the interpreter's responsibility in the interaction process (Englund Dimitrova, 1997). Englund Dimitrova asks what the interpreter should do when the two parties in a dialogue compete for the floor. Which party should the interpreter choose to interpret for? Amongst our informants, the answer is in favour of the weaker party, meaning the party with less power in the communicative event, the child.
>
> *Nilsen 2013: 26*

Nevertheless, the results of both studies indicate that there is a clear need to improve the competence of both the interpreters and the professionals who use their services. The studies also indicate a need for more research in this field.

In their article, Kjelaas and Eide (2015) use one case to emphasise how the interpreter's omissions and changes can hamper communication between a minor asylum seeker and a social worker, to the extent that the communication eventually collapses. Similarly, a report based on interviews in Belgium states that:

> These refugee children highlight the lack of support from guardians or lawyers. They bemoan the interventions of interpreters, which are too limited or ill-intentioned. And in the reception centers, children would like more help and to be given better information, right from the beginning, so they can better understand what game they are playing.
>
> *UNICEF 2018: 12*

Thematic analysis of semi-structured interviews with professionals about the interpreting process revealed the interpreters' insufficient understanding of 'best-practice' in the child interview process; consequently, the recommendations focus on the need for more specialised training for the interpreters (Powell *et al.* 2017).

An important distinction between interpreter-mediated communication involving children and that involving adults lies in the consequences of inadequate and non-professional interpreting. Children are less able to assert their rights due to their status as minors and their generally less advanced communicative skills. As a result, an interpreter who does not take a child seriously and whose interpreting lacks accuracy is likely to reinforce the asymmetry of the relationship. Examples of such problems appear in the Swedish research (Keselman *et al.* 2008; Keselman *et al.* 2010), which found that interpreters sometimes cast doubt on children's stories in asylum interviews. Compared to adults, children can be more easily transformed (or can transform themselves) from a person talked and listened to into an object that is talked about. The cross-cultural nature of the interaction may give legitimacy to the interpreters' expressions of their own opinion, and this may reflect or reinforce the impression caseworkers have of children as less than able interlocutors (Böser and La Rooy 2018; Keselman, Cederborg and Linell 2010).

4 Practical issues

In what follows, I will focus on some practical issues related to interpreter-mediated communication with children, including the facilitation of such communication, and what kind of skills, training and knowledge interpreters and service users need when conducting interpreter-mediated dialogues with children.

4.1 The competence of those using interpreting services

In healthcare as well as in other public services, the competence of the users of interpreting services includes knowledge about planning and conducting an interpreter-mediated meeting with children. Nilsen (2015) argues that in public sector services we need to shift from a monolingual to a multilingual perspective when planning and conducting meetings with children and their families from linguistic minorities. The argument is based on research into interpreting, mostly in Norway, and on the broader research into children's multilingual competences and multilingual practices. Once we have shifted to a multilingual perspective, it becomes clear that the planning of a meeting must include the following steps:

1. Seek information about the multilingual competences and multilingual practices of the child and the parents in order to assess whether an interpreter is required
2. If needed, book a professional interpreter, as opposed to a bilingual helper; and
3. Check that the interpreter has the necessary competence to interpret specifically for children (Nilsen 2015: 128–129)

Planning involves first establishing whether there is a need for an interpreter. There is an obvious need for interpreters in cases where children do not speak the language of the public sector worker. However, there are cases with bilingual children where it is not so easy to determine whether an interpreter is needed. Fontes and Tishelman (2016: 55) note that participants in their interviews reported difficulties in deciding whether an interpreter should be called in to work with a specific bilingual child. In their study, comments by respondents such as this one was fairly typical: 'Kids say they speak English but then you get into the room and it seems chopped up' (Fontes and Tishelman 2016: 55). When assessing children's linguistic skills and their need for an interpreter, there are many possible sources of error that may lead to a wrong assessment (Nilsen 2015). For example, it is well known that a child's language choice is not necessarily controlled by the language in which the child is addressed (Nilsen 2015: 128). A multilingual child may choose not to speak the majority language in a particular situation because they wish to create a certain distance from, or not to relate to, a majority language-speaking person – for example, a doctor. In such a situation, the child may opt for the parents' language if they are present, even when the child has greater command of the majority language than of the family's language. In such cases, there may well be a need for an interpreter.

Studies of forensic interviews with children stress the importance of interviewing children in their preferred languages (Fontes 2010; Fontes and Tishelman 2016). This may also be important in healthcare. Experience shows that both memory and presentation are affected by the language chosen for an interview. Interviewees are apt to provide more details and demonstrate the full range of their competence when they speak in their preferred language (Fontes 2010: 285).

4.2 The 'right' interpreter

The necessary competence for those who use interpreting services includes knowledge about choosing the 'right' interpreter. An evaluation by the Norwegian Directorate of Immigration indicates that experience and formal education in interpreting in general are not in themselves indicators of success in interpreting for children (Hitching and Nilsen 2010: 41). The main concern expressed by asylum interviewers is that some interpreters are too dominant; on the other hand, there were also issues with interpreters whose manner was too passive and distant. Factors such as personality and body language emerged as important. For instance, some children were reported to be afraid of certain interpreters who interpret in the Norwegian public sector services. The Directorate's findings suggest that not all interpreters are suitable for assignments involving children. As Matthias and Zaal observe:

> It is thus necessary to move away from the idea that interpreters are interchangeable if they have the same language familiarity. As a starting point in developing improved selection procedures, court administrators should identify which of their interpreters actually want to work with children.
>
> *2002: 364*

These observations are consistent with the views of Jareg and Pettersen (2006: 45) who write that some interpreters are better suited than others to work in what they call sensitive situations, and interviews with children may well come into this category. Importantly, Jareg and Pettersen do not consider that the personal qualities that may render someone suitable or unsuitable for interpreting in sensitive situations are immutable. A person may be made aware of the need of, and then cultivate, the necessary qualities.

4.3 The facilitation of interpreter-mediated communication with children

Van Schoor (2013) concludes from her literature review that interpreters should be involved in the interview preparation process, as is prescribed by the UK Ministry of Justice[1] (van Schoor 2013: 63). However, in the field of interpreting for children, very few articles or reports exist on how to facilitate oral interpreter-mediated communication. Such studies are often based on research into children's cognitive development and the use of sign language (e.g. Rainò 2012; Schick 2001) or on personal experience (Bjørnås 2006; Phoenix Children's Hospital 2008; Veritas Language Solutions 2012; Wilson and Powell 2001). According to Bjørnås (2006), who works as a consultant in Trondheim's municipal interpreting services in Norway, there is little distinction between an interpreted meeting with children and one with adults, provided that both the interpreter and the user of the interpreting services follow the basic rules for conversing through an interpreter. In Norway, these rules are explained in an online document published by the Norwegian Health Directorate with the title 'Guidance for interpreter-mediated communication'.[2] In this document, the healthcare workers are, for example, instructed to talk directly to the patient, keep eye contact with the patient and not with the interpreter, and not to involve the interpreter in the dialogue. Nilsen (2013) supports Bjørnås' views on children's abilities to participate in interpreter-mediated communication and notes that a child's participation is dependent on their understanding and acceptance of the system of turn-taking that is fundamental to consecutive interpreting. An important condition, however, is that the adult participants know how to handle such communication and can act as a role model for the child on how to communicate through an interpreter.

As noted by van Schoor (2013: 65), it is crucial to delineate the roles of the participants accurately at the start – particularly the difference between the roles of the interpreter and the interviewer. This should be done through a clear introduction and by strictly sticking to these roles during the interaction. Thus, health personnel should explain to the children who the interpreter is and what their function and role are. Children are very different depending on their age and level of cognitive development; furthermore, in many countries, 'children' as a group may include individuals from infancy to 18 years of age. Hence, this introductory information needs to be adapted to the child's age and cognitive development. The following could, for instance, serve as an example adapted for a five-year-old:

> This is the interpreter. Her name is Jamila. Jamila is here to help us so that you and I can talk together. Jamila speaks both Arabic and Norwegian. Jamila will never tell anybody what you have told us.

Böser and La Rooy (2018) highlight the importance of building rapport and draw attention to the necessity of establishing some ground rules in order to set the desired framework for participation. An example of such a rule could be that it is the person in charge of the communication who introduces the interpreter to the child, and not the interpreter themselves.

The complexities of rapport building in interpreter-mediated communication with children is also highlighted in experimental studies (Nilsen 2013; Kanstad and Gran 2016). Based on their experimental study in the Norwegian kindergarten context, Kanstad and Gran (2016) emphasise the importance of the child having full confidence in the interpreter; to achieve this, interpreters have to stretch their professional guidelines in a flexible manner. The interpreters interviewed by Kanstad and Gran (2016: 73) say that to gain the children's trust they talk to the children or play with them before they interpret for them. Nilsen also finds that interpreters must maintain rapport during the interpreting process in order to connect with a child. Non-verbal language such as eye contact seems to play an important role in maintaining a desirable framework for participation. This confirms the findings of Böser and La Rooy, reported in their review article (2018: 214), about the importance of gaze patterns on the establishment of participant status in children's interaction with adult interpreters.

Böser and La Rooy (2018: 214) also state that studies of face-to-face interpreting with adults in diverse institutional settings have highlighted varying degrees of asymmetry in the distribution of institutional and interactional power between participants. They acknowledge that this asymmetry may be further exacerbated in situations involving particular groups of participants, such as children. Böser and La Rooy (2018: 220) quote an interpreter from Catherine King's research (2015: 72), working with children, who argues that '[i]f it is not possible to build up trust or rapport, then it may be more productive to arrange for another interpreter in order to carry out the interview', a view that is supported by Balogh and Salaets (2015: 72). This may also be a solution in healthcare settings when there is a problem of building trust.

4.4 Training

Several studies recommend special training for interpreters to build competence in handling interpreter-mediated communication with children. I believe these recommendations also apply for healthcare. Matthias and Zaal (2002: 368) conclude that there is an urgent need to introduce new measures to improve the interpreting services available for children required to testify in South African courts. Furthermore, they recommend that a course should be designed that will lead to official certification of interpreters as 'qualified to interpret for children'. Powell *et al.* (2017: 98) state that

> interpreter training in the area of child abuse investigation needs to extend its focus beyond simply translating questions and responses in order to maintain their structure and meaning. Training should also build interpreters' competency in maintaining

> a non-verbal demeanour that facilitates accurate disclosure and maintains a context where children feel heard, understood and not judged.
>
> *Powell et al. 2017: 98*

Balogh and Salaets (2015) suggest that training for interpreters who will be handling child interviews could include some background knowledge of the developmental stages of childhood and adolescence, possible disorders, the functioning of memory in children and language acquisition. They note that some knowledge about trauma and victimisation and the corresponding behaviours (e.g. panic, distrust, reluctance) are essential for all professionals working with child victims and witnesses. This is confirmed by the United Nations Office on Drugs and Crime (UNODC) *Handbook for Professionals and Policymakers on Justice Matters Involving Child Victims and Witnesses of Crime* (2009). Such skills would enable interpreters to anticipate certain behaviours and deal with them in the best possible way when working in a challenging environment (van Schoor, Balogh and Salaets 2015: 22). According to Matthias and Zaal (2002: 365), a study-participant who was a criminal court magistrate with considerable experience of working with court interpreters stated that a future course of child-competence training for interpreters should include the following outcomes:

- the ability to understand the stages of child development
- the ability to assess a child's level of comprehension
- the ability to appreciate the more common effects of trauma on a child, especially the effects of rape; and
- knowledge about the way in which young, mentally-challenged or traumatised children tend to give evidence – for example, that it will not necessarily be in a logical sequence

This magistrate also emphasised that there is frequently a need for tremendous patience and gentleness when interviewing a child. Properly trained interpreters must, for example, be able to deal appropriately with the child breaking down and crying whilst giving evidence. Similar concerns arise when children suffer from chronic illnesses, may be recovering from highly stressful events, such as accidents, or are traumatised as a result of physical and/or sexual abuse. When these children are offered healthcare, their interpreters in healthcare settings will have to undergo similar training in dealing with sensitive situations.

4.5 Joint training

Already in 2002, Matthias and Zaal had highlighted an important point that emerged from their study, namely that interpreters (no matter how well-trained) will not be able to work effectively with children if other persons in positions of authority expect them to convey inappropriately complex language to children (2002: 368). It may therefore be suggested that a basic course of certification for working with children, as recommended above for interpreters, could very usefully be extended to other staff involved in interpreter-mediated communication within health care. Granhagen Jungner *et al.* (2016: 144) note that healthcare staff need training in the use of interpreters and that integrated systems need to be created for the booking and evaluation of interpreters.

Many studies have found that communication through an interpreter is a skill that must be learnt, as it differs significantly from other types of communication (e.g. Radanović

Felberg 2016). Of particular importance is an understanding of the intersection between the interpreter's and the public servant's areas of expertise. Successful communication in interpreter-mediated institutional dialogues requires specific skills from the interpreters and matching skills from the public service employees about how to communicate through an interpreter. It is imperative that training for interpreters and users is synchronised in order to avoid contradictory modes of operation (Radanović Felberg 2016: 154).

Several studies in this review recommend specialised training, not only for interpreters but also for other professionals who deal with interpreted communication with children (e.g. within the legal context, see Balogh and Salaets 2015; van Schoor 2013). Van Schoor (2013: 64) writes that 'the key for guaranteeing high-quality interpreter-mediated interviews with child witnesses and victims lies in close collaboration between all involved professionals. Not only during the interviews, but also in the training phase, through the development of a joint training programme'. Van Schoor (2013: 64) comments that the main advantage of multidisciplinary training is that professionals from several fields can exchange their expertise on central topics. In healthcare settings, the benefits of bringing together the expertise of paediatricians, nurses, child psychologists and the interpreters could shed significant light on supporting children with health issues, communication techniques when the patients are children, as well as child development and psychology. This type of training would also provide an ideal opportunity to set up role plays where participants could practise interacting with children and learn how to work together to guarantee a smooth sequence of events. During such courses, audiovisual recordings of interactions with child patients could be analysed to provide learners with further understanding, provided that necessary ethical hurdles could be overcome and permissions obtained. Such training for interpreters would ideally be complemented by a continuous evaluation mechanism, including debriefings after a session and regular feedback by experts (i.e. interpreters as well as professionals from related fields).

An interdisciplinary approach to training is also supported by van Schoor, Balogh and Salaets (2015: 22). Training in interpreter-mediated communication with children is not only the concern of interpreters, but also of other professionals. Doctors, nurses and psychologists should also have competence related to the particular characteristics of interpreter-mediated communication with children and be taught the basic principles of working with an interpreter. Van Schoor, Balogh and Salaets (2015: 22) suggest that these principles can be practised in joint role plays, imitating a real interpreted child interview. Similarly, these principles can be practised in role plays including doctors, nurses and psychologists.

These are, of course, important suggestions, but I would rather argue for specialised training for interpreters and for users of their services who work with children in the public sector in general. The components of working with children are the same across all public sectors; what differs is the context. It is no less important in healthcare that the interpreters and users of their services know, for example, how to ask developmentally appropriate questions of children, than it is in the court rooms or in investigative interviews. It is important across all sectors to have knowledge about the specifics of children's language use and the most constructive way in which to relate to children.

5 Recommendations for future research

There is a need for more research-based knowledge on interpreting in public service meetings with children from linguistic minorities, and in particular, research that relates to healthcare. Themes that emerged as important from this review highlight some of the differences between interpreting for children and for adults. One theme is trust, and several researchers refer to the importance of establishing rapport and connection through non-verbal communication. Another theme is the need for cooperation between healthcare workers and interpreters, and the clear separation of their roles. We need to know more about the types of situations in which there is a need to interpret for children in healthcare, and how to facilitate interpreter-mediated communication with children in healthcare settings. We also need to know more about good practice and about the multilingual practices currently taking place in encounters with children and their families in public sector services (Nilsen 2015: 129).

Kanstad and Gran (2016) show that interpreting may be important to safeguard children's rights to express themselves, to participate in interactions, and to prevent social exclusion resulting from a lack of shared language with others in the kindergarten. These aspects of interpreting are important in healthcare, for example so that the children can contribute to the dialogues about their own health and express their pain and/or concerns. In their study on paediatric healthcare, where the participants had interpreted in multi-party bilingual consultations that included children, Granhagen Jungner *et al.* (2018) observe:

> Participants described experiences of interpreting between healthcare personnel and the family (parents). However, the participants did not mention experiences of including the child in the multi-party consultation. Thus, further research is needed exploring the complexity of multi-party consultations that includes children, especially from the child's perspective.
>
> *Granhagen Jungner et al. 2018: 661*

Balogh and Salaets (2015) note that interpreter-mediated communication with children is, intrinsically, an interdisciplinary research topic; thus, the research methods or perspectives employed should also be interdisciplinary. Balogh and Salaets' project CO-Minor-IN/QUEST survey could serve as a good example of such an interdisciplinary approach.

Research into interpreter-mediated communication with children inevitably presents particular challenges relating to ethical issues, due to the vulnerability that goes with young age and the considerable imbalance of power between adults and children. At different ages, children have varying cognitive capacities to make decisions about their own involvement in research, to express meaningful assent or to refuse to participate. However, only one of the studies mentioned above (Nilsen 2013) discusses ethical issues, and then only cursorily. In that study, the experiments conducted with very young children were, for example, set up in such a way that they would cause as little stress as possible to the children (Nilsen 2013: 17). The author notes that one of the children may not have fully understood the differences between the primary speaker and the interpreter, and also that he or she may not have had a clear understanding of the interpreter's role. The child's lack of understanding of the interpreter's role as a translator did not, however, seem to hinder the communication, although the situation may raise certain ethical concerns (Nilsen 2013: 20–21).

6 Conclusion

In this chapter, I have presented a literature review of interpreter-mediated communication with children. The review shows that communication through an interpreter is a skill that must be learnt. Of particular importance is an understanding of the intersection between the interpreter's and the public servant's areas of expertise, which means that training for interpreters and users must be synchronised in order to avoid contradictory modes of operation.

The review shows that extant research generally relates both to the (lack of) competence of interpreters and to those who use their services, and to the training of these two professional groups. There is a need to train interpreters and interpreter users in how to handle interpreter-mediated communication with children of different ages, and there is a need for more knowledge about what to teach the interpreters and users. In turn, this knowledge will help to improve meetings in the public sector services with children who have not mastered the language spoken or who have limited linguistic skills. Most of all, there is a demand for more knowledge about the best practices related to interpreter-mediated communication with children of all ages in healthcare, as well as in other public service areas. In that respect, it is important to note the asymmetry of the relationship in interpreter-mediated communication involving children – children are less able to assert their rights due to their status as minors and their generally less advanced communicative skills.

Based on the literature review this chapter has also provided some recommendations for future research. In particular, I would like to highlight the fact that interpreter-mediated communication with children is an interdisciplinary research topic. Hence, the research methods or perspectives employed should also be interdisciplinary.

Notes

1 www.cps.gov.uk/sites/default/files/documents/legal_guidance/best_evidence_in_criminal_proceedings.pdf (Accessed: 9 March 2020).

2 www.helsedirektoratet.no/veiledere/kommunikasjon-via-tolk-for-ledere-og-personell-i-helse-og-omsorgstjenestene/God%20kommunikasjon%20via%20tolk%20–%20Veileder%20for%20ledere%20og%20personell%20i%20helse-%20og%20omsorgstjenestene%20(fullversjon).pdf/_/attachment/inline/90658993-97c6-44db-a9c0-6ea6e2d2f4e7:eb7dc3bc5ab2de93f379fbb9f0313ef3182f2007/God%20kommunikasjon%20via%20tolk%20–%20Veileder%20for%20ledere%20og%20personell%20i%20helse-%20og%20omsorgstjenestene%20(fullversjon).pdf (Accessed: 9 March 2020).

Further reading

Balogh, K. and Salaets, H. (eds) (2015) *Children and Justice: Overcoming Language Barriers*. Cambridge: Intersentia.

The book addresses the challenges in interpreting for minors during an interview as part of (pre-trial) criminal proceedings.

Granhagen Jungner, J., Tiselius, E., Blomgren, K., Lützén, K. and Pergert, P. (2018) 'The Interpreter's Voice: Carrying the Bilingual Conversation in Interpreter-Mediated Consultations in Pediatric Oncology Care', *Patient Education and Counseling*, 102(4), pp. 656–662. DOI:10.1016/j.pec.2018.10.029.

Granhagen Jungner, J., Tiselius, E., Lützén, K., Blomgren, K., and Pergert, P. (2016) 'Creating a Meeting Point of Understanding: Interpreters' Experiences in Swedish Childhood Cancer Care', *Journal of Pediatric Oncology Nursing*, 33(2), pp. 137–145. DOI:10.1177/1043454215600148.

These two articles focus on interpreting in Swedish childhood cancer care.

Nilsen, A. B. (2015) 'Interpreted Communication With Children in Public-Sector Services', *The International Journal for Translation and Interpreting Research*, 7(3), pp. 121–131. DOI:10.12807/ti.107203.2015.a09.

This article discusses interpreter-mediated communication with children based on knowledge from research on multilingualism.

UNICEF (2018) The Voice of Migrant and Refugee Children Living in Belgium. What Do You Think? Available at: https://emnbelgium.be/publication/what-do-you-think-voice-migrant-and-refugee-children-living-belgium-unicef (Accessed: 7 May 2019).

The report is based on testimonies of 170 migrant and refugee children from 36 nationalities in reception centres and schools. The children talk about their experiences in their country of origin and their new environment, the disaster they fled from, the trials they endured on the way, their joys and sorrows.

Related topics

Healthcare Interpreting Ethics, Remote (Telephone) Interpreting in Healthcare Settings, Community/Liaison Interpreting in Healthcare Settings

References

Balogh, K. and Salaets, H. (eds) (2015) *Children and Justice: Overcoming Language Barriers*. Cambridge: Intersentia.

Bjørnås, B. M. (2006) 'Arbeid med tolk', in Nasjonalt kunnskapssenter om vold og traumatisk stress (ed.) *Psykososialt arbeid med flyktningbarn – Introduksjon og fagveiledning*. Psykososialt senter Midt-Norge og Nord-Norge. Available at: www.nkvts.no/biblioteket/Publikasjoner/PsykososialtArbeidFlyktningbarnVeileder.pdf (Accessed: 15 December 2020).

Böser, U. and La Rooy, D. (2018) 'Interpreter-Mediated Investigative Interviews With Minors', *Translation and Interpreting Studies*, 13(2), pp. 208–229.

Englund-Dimitrova, B. (1997) 'Degree of Interpreter Responsibility in the Interaction Process', in Carr, S. E., Roberts, R. Dufour, A. and Steyn D. (eds) *The Critical Link: Interpreters in the Community*. Amsterdam: Benjamins, pp. 147–164.

Fontes, L. A. (2010) 'Interviewing Immigrant Children for Suspected Child Maltreatment', *The Journal of Psychiatry and Law*, 38(3), pp. 283–305. DOI:10.1177/009318531003800304.

Fontes, L. A. and Tishelman, A. C. (2016) 'Language Competence in Forensic Interviews for Suspected Child Sexual Abuse', *Child Abuse and Neglect*, 58, pp. 51–62. DOI:10.1016/j.chiabu.2016.06.014.

Gotaas, N. (2007) 'Bruk av tolk i barnevernet', in Holm-Hansen, J., Haaland, T. and Myrvold, T.M. (eds.) *Flerkulturelt barnevern. En kunnskapsoversikt*. NIBR-rapport 10. NIBR: Oslo, pp. 93–132.

Granhagen Jungner, J., Tiselius, E., Lützén, K., Blomgren, K., and Pergert, P. (2016) 'Creating a Meeting Point of Understanding: Interpreters' Experiences in Swedish Childhood Cancer Care', *Journal of Pediatric Oncology Nursing*, 33(2), pp. 137–145. DOI:10.1177/1043454215600148.

Granhagen Jungner, J., Tiselius, E., Blomgren, K., Lützén, K. and Pergert, P. (2018) 'The Interpreter's Voice: Carrying the Bilingual Conversation in Interpreter-mediated Consultations in Pediatric Oncology Care', *Patient Education and Counseling*, 102(4), pp. 656–662. DOI:10.1016/j.pec.2018.10.029.

Hitching, T. R. and Nilsen, A. B. (eds) (2010) *Tolking for barn – en statusrapport*. HiO-rapport 2010 nr. 20. Høgskolen i Oslo. Avdeling for Lærerutdanning og internasjonale studier.

Hjelmervik, E. (2009) 'Tolking for barn i skolen', in Hansen, A. L., Garm, N. and Hjelmervik, E. (eds) *Hørsel – språk og kommunikasjon: en artikkelsamling*. Levanger: Kompetansesenteret, pp. 91–98.

Jareg, K. and Pettersen, Z. (2006) *Tolk og tolkebruker – to sider av samme sak*. Bergen: Fagbokforlaget.

Kanstad, M. and Gran, J. (2016) *Kommunikasjon med barn via tolk*. Fagrapport. Trondheim: Dronnig Mauds minne, Høgskole for barnehagelærerutdanning.

Keselman, O., Cederborg, A.-C., Lamb, M. E. and Dahlström, Ö. (2008) 'Mediated Communication with Minors in Asylum-Seeking Hearings', *Journal of Refugee Studies*, 21(1), pp. 103–116.

Keselman, O., Cederborg, A.-C., Lamb, M. E. and Dahlström, Ö. (2010) 'Asylum Seeking Minors in Interpreter-Mediated Interviews: What Do They Say and What Happens to Their Responses?', *Journal of Child and Family Social Work*, 21(1), pp. 103–116.

Keselman, O., Cederborg, A.-C. and Linell, P. (2010). '"That Is Not Necessary for You to Know!" Negotiation of Participation Status of Unaccompanied Children in Interpretermediated Asylum Hearings', *Interpreting,* 12(1), pp. 83–104.

King, C. (2015) 'Highly Vulnerable Child Suspects. Signed Language Interpreter', in Balogh, K. and Salaets, H. (eds) *Children and Justice: Overcoming Language Barriers.* Cambridge: Intersentia, pp. 158–165.

Kjelaas, I. and Eide, K. (2015). 'Barnets stemme i tolkemedierte samtaler', *Tidsskriftet Norges Barnevern,* 02(92), pp. 109–122.

Matthias, C. and Zaal, N. (2002) 'Hearing Only a Faint Echo? Interpreters and Children in Court', *South African Journal on Human Rights,* 18(3), pp. 350–371. DOI:10.1080/02587203.2002.11827650.

Nilsen, A. B. (2013) 'Exploring Interpreting for Young Children', *The International Journal for Translation and Interpreting Research,* 5(2), pp. 14–29. DOI:http://dx.doi.orgti.105202.2013.a02.

Nilsen, A. B. (2015) 'Interpreted Communication with Children in Public-Sector Services', *The International Journal for Translation and Interpreting Research,* 7(3), pp. 121–131. DOI:10.12807/ti.107203.2015.a09.

Phoenix Children's Hospital (2008) *Spanish Bilingual Assistant. Introduction to Medical Interpreting.* Section 8 Interpreting for Children. Phoenix: Phoenix Children's Hospital.

Powell, M. B., Manger, B., Dion, J. and Sharman, S. J. (2017) 'Professionals' Perspectives About the Challenges of Using Interpreters in Child Sexual Abuse Interviews', *Psychiatry, Psychology and Law,* 24(1), pp. 90–101. DOI:10.1080/13218719.2016.1197815.

Radanović, F. T. (2016) 'Towards a Unified Model for Interpreter User Training', in Munyangeyo, T., Webb, G. and Rabadán-Gómez, M. (eds) *Challenges and Opportunities in Public Service Interpreting.* London: Palgrave Macmillan.

Rainò, P. (2012) *Language Choices and the Need for Interpreting Services for Deaf Children and Young People With Cochlear Implants.* Series F, HUMAK publication. Helsinki: HUMAK University of Applied Sciences.

Schick, B. (2001) 'Interpreting for Children – How it's different', *Odyssey: New Directions in Deaf Education,* Winter/Spring.

Schick, B., Williams, K. and Kupermintz, H. (2006) 'Look Who's Left Behind: Educational Interpreters and Access to Education for Deaf and Hard-Of-Hearing Students', *Journal of Deaf Studies and Deaf Education,* 11(1), pp. 3–20.

United Nations Children's Fund (UNICEF) (2018) *The Voice of Migrant and Refugee Children Living in Belgium. What Do You Think?* Available at: https://emnbelgium.be/publication/what-do-you-think-voice-migrant-and-refugee-children-living-belgium-unicef (Accessed: 7 May 2019).

United Nations Office on Drugs and *Crime* (UNODC) (2009). *Handbook for Professionals and Policymakers on Justice Matters Involving Child Victims and Witnesses of Crime.* Available at: www.un.org/ruleoflaw/files/Handbook%20for%20Professionals%20and%20Policymakers%20on%20Justice%20in%20Matters%20involving%20Child%20Victims%20and%20Witnesses%20of%20Crime.pdf (Accessed: 15 December 2020).

Van Schoor, D. (2013) *Interpreter-Mediated Interviews of Child Witnesses and Victims: Status Quaestionis.* MA Thesis. University of Leuven:

Van Schoor, D., Salaets, H. and Balogh, K. (2015) 'Introduction', In Balogh, K. and Salaets, H. (eds) *Children and Justice: Overcoming Language Barriers.* Cambridge: Intersentia, pp. 1–46.

Veritas Language Solutions (2012) *Interpreting for Children – Points to Consider.* Swansea: Veritas Language Solutions. Available at: www.veritaslanguagesolutions.com/ interpreting-for-children-points-to-consider/ (Accessed: 15 December 2020).

Wadensjö, C. (1998) *Interpreting as Interaction.* London: Longman.

Wilson, J. C. and Powell, M. B. (2001) *A Guide to Interviewing Children: Essential Skills for Counsellors, Police, Lawyers and Social Workers.* Canberra: Allen and Unwin.

Winston, E. A. (2004) *Educational Interpreting: How It Can Succeed.* Washington, DC: Gallaudet University Press.

18
Disability in translation

Eva Spišiaková

1 Introduction[1, 2]

The *World Report on Disability*, issued in 2011 by the World Health Organisation (WHO), estimated that more than 1 billion people worldwide – about 15 per cent of global population – are living with some kind of disability (WHO 2011: xi). While various disabilities were historically seen as separate issues and their study was the domain of the medical profession, recent waves of activism and a widespread shift towards the so-called social model of disability have supported a view of disabled people[3] as a distinct minority group united by a fight for equal rights with the non-disabled population. These changes were also accompanied by the birth of disability studies in the 1990s (see Davis 1999, for a detailed history), an academic discipline whose aim is to 'weave disabled people back into the fabric of society, thread by thread, theory by theory' (Linton 2005: 518).

As this new conceptualisation of disability spreads across the world, it is increasingly tied to the questions of interlingual transfer. New words associated with disability activism (such as 'ableism') are adopted, modified or rejected in different linguistic environments, while formerly widespread terms (such as those used as counterparts for 'handicapped' or 'invalid' in English) are now considered offensive in some languages but remain in regular use in others. Legal documents, such as the Convention on the Rights of Persons with Disabilities (CRPD, United Nations 2006) are ratified and signed by hundreds of nations and subsequently require translations into their respective languages. Increased migration leads to the transfer of medical records between different healthcare systems with different conceptualisations of disability. The question of accessibility for people with sensory impairments is also frequently tied to translation, such as interpreting into sign language, or the use of subtitles or audio descriptions in audiovisual material for the benefit of Deaf and Hard of Hearing (DHH) or blind/visually impaired people. Disability is also increasingly seen as part of a person's identity, in the same way as race or sexuality, and this leads to questions about how we translate stories from and about disabled people in various textual and audiovisual forms.

However, despite these and many more areas in which disability and translation intersect, research that would bring together the fields of disability and translation studies has

DOI: 10.4324/9781003167983-23

thus far been scattered and limited. This chapter will first provide basic definitions of disability underpinned by the change from the individual towards the social model, and then explore some of the issues in the translation of terminology related to disability, which is currently undergoing rapid changes with the rise and spread of disability activism. The chapter will then survey the existing works in the field of translation studies that relate to disability, and then briefly highlight the issues that accompany the translation of legal documents such as the UN's CRPD. The chapter will conclude by identifying some possible future directions for research on disability in translation studies.

2 Defining disability

The Convention on the Rights of Persons with Disabilities, adopted by the United Nations in 2006, aims 'to promote, protect and ensure the full and equal enjoyment of all human rights and fundamental freedoms by all persons with disabilities' (United Nations 2006: 4). The term 'persons with disability' is, for the purposes of this convention, defined in Article 1 and is formulated as follows:

> [p]ersons with *disabilities* include those who have long-term physical, mental, intellectual or sensory *impairments* which in interaction with various *barriers* may hinder their full and effective participation in society on an equal basis with others.
>
> *United Nations 2006: 4, my emphases*

The CRPD's emphasis on social inequalities created by the interaction of *impairments* with various *barriers* is significant here, as it places the UN's concept of disability in line with the social model of disability. The term 'social model of disability' was first coined by Mike Oliver in 1983 (Shakespeare 2006: 197; see also Oliver 1996), who was building on ideas proposed by UK's Union of the Physically Impaired Against Segregation (UPIS) in their *Fundamental Principles of Disability* (1976) document. The social model was developed in direct opposition to the individual (also known as biomedical) model of disability. The differences between these two models are crucial in understanding how the concept of disability changed over the past few decades, and as such, requires a brief explanation. In necessarily simplified terms, the individual model sees disability as a consequence of a person's impairment (e.g. a missing limb, visual impairment, chronic illness), and therefore, as a problem that requires medical care and treatment, whereas the social model sees disability as a consequence of socially constructed barriers and lack of accessibility, and therefore, as a societal issue. A simple example of this difference is a wheelchair user facing a flight of stairs. While the individual model sees the person's inability to walk as an issue, the social model sees the problem in the absence of a lift.

The language used is of particular significance here, as the social model makes a clear distinction between the terms *disability* and *impairment*: disability is a societal issue manifested through barriers and other forms of discrimination against people with various impairments. The concept also relies on the idea that disabled people are a distinct social minority; while disabled people have different impairments that affect their daily lives in different ways, they are all collectively oppressed by societal structures, as well as by non-disabled people and the institutions led by them (Shakespeare 2006: 199). Other models of disability have been conceptualised alongside this main distinction, including the charity model, which sees disabled people as victims deserving pity, or moral/religious models which see disability as a punitive mechanism imposed by a higher power. In recent years, the human rights model, which builds on the social model in acknowledging the societal factors contributing to disability, but focuses on 'the inherent dignity of the human being and subsequently, but only if necessary, on the person's medical characteristics' (Quinn and Degener 2002: 14) has become prominent. The aforementioned UN CRPD can also be seen as a representative of this human rights model.[4]

The social model has become particularly influential in the UK where it was first developed (Shakespeare 2006: 198), as can be seen from the emphasis on impairments as the sole cause of inequalities in the official definition of disability in the UK Equality Act of 2010: 'A person has a disability [...] if he or she has a physical or mental impairment and the impairment has a substantial and long-term adverse effect on his or her ability to carry out normal day-to-day activities' (Office for Disability Issues 2010: 7).[5] The model's simplicity, memorability and easy applicability to various forms of social activism, as well as its suitability as a heuristic device within the field of disability studies, have caused it to become one of the most popular and widespread ideas of present-day disability discourse. However, it is also necessary to acknowledge some of the weak points of the premise. Amongst the most prominent issues is the possible erasure of the very real difficulties impairments present to many people's lives (such as chronic pain), and which are unrelated to wider societal structures. Another frequently mentioned problem is the impracticability of any 'barrier-free utopia' (Shakespeare 2006: 201). While it is tempting to envision a world so accessible that disability would cease to exist, it is necessary to acknowledge that different impairments need different provisions; visually impaired people prefer pavements with defined kerbs, but these become a barrier for wheelchair users (Shakespeare 2006: 201). Owens (2015: 41–43) provides a comprehensive list of other criticisms of the model, including the tendency to ignore the embodied experiences of disabled people, as well as theoretical issues, such as difficulties in defining 'oppression', or the creation of false dichotomies between disability and impairment.[6]

In light of these issues, other institutions such as the WHO prefer definitions of disability which blend together both models into a so-called 'bio-psycho-social model' (WHO 2011: 4), rather than seeing them as polar opposites. The International Classification of Functioning, Disability and Health (ICF), which is the basis for the World Report on Disability, defines it as:

> the umbrella term for impairments, activity limitations and participation restrictions, referring to the negative aspects of the interaction between an individual (with a health condition) and that individual's contextual factors (environmental and personal factors)
>
> *WHO 2011: 4*

This definition makes a distinction between impairments (e.g. paralysis), activity limitations (e.g. difficulties in walking), and participation restrictions (e.g. workplace discrimination), and understands all of them as being part of disability, rather than perceiving disability as exclusively the result of societal barriers. As all other models however, the bio-psycho-social model likewise has its critics. Its focus on the interaction between the individual and their contextual factors can be easily interpreted as a claim that some disabled people take responsibility for the barriers they experience. In more practical terms, the model is easily (mis)used by social institutions to limit the number of people receiving disability benefits by redefining the concept of 'work readiness', as was the case in the UK Government's Work Capability Assessment (Shakespeare, Watson and Alghaib 2017).

Although the stereotypical image of a person with a disability is usually limited to the idea of someone with paraplegia using a wheelchair (further strengthened by the internationally recognised symbol for accessible spaces), it is necessary to stress that all of the aforementioned definitions encompass a broad spectrum of different experiences of disability. The WHO report provides the following examples as an insight into the breadth as well as fluidity of the category:

> Disability encompasses the child born with a congenital condition such as cerebral palsy or the young soldier who loses his leg to a land-mine, or the middle-aged woman with severe arthritis, or the older person with dementia, among many others. Health conditions can be visible or invisible; temporary or long term; static, episodic, or degenerating; painful or inconsequential.
>
> *WHO 2011: 7–8*

The social model in particular encourages an identity-based understanding of the term where each individual can decide whether they consider their impairment(s) to be disabling in their daily lives and whether they want to identify themselves as being disabled. The Deaf and Hard of Hearing (DHH) communities are an important example of the relativity and individuality of the label 'disabled'. As Harlan Lane explains, 'nowadays, two constructions of deafness in particular are dominant and compete for shaping deaf peoples' destinies. The one construes deaf as a category of disability; the other construes deaf as designating a member of a linguistic minority' (Lane 2006: 80). As he further elaborates, the difference is frequently tied to the circumstances of how a person becomes deaf; an adult losing their hearing due to an accident is likely to see themselves as living with a disability, whereas a Deaf child of Deaf parents is likely to perceive themselves as part of a distinct linguistic and cultural heritage (Lane 2006: 81).

The question of which impairments to include under the disability label becomes even more complicated once it enters the domains of law and healthcare. Governmental decisions on whether an impairment is disabling 'enough' to warrant disability benefits or provision of a carer are usually taken according to a spectrum, rather than a simple disabled/non-disabled dichotomy. These decisions also frequently involve a requirement to 'prove' that one is 'disabled enough' to receive support. Moreover, the delineations of which impairments are considered disabling may vary between countries and legal systems; coeliac disease, a chronic auto-immune disorder of the small intestine, is at the time of writing considered a disability in Slovakia (meaning that the diagnosis warrants a disability ID card and it is possible to claim some degree of financial support), but it is not considered a disability in the UK. These differences also reflect the ways in which disability is understood across different geographical regions, cultures and linguistic systems. Ingstad and Whyte (1995: 5) describe the conceptual problems associated with the attempts to find a universal definition of disability, and highlight the fact that the very notion of disability is rooted in Western tradition (Ingstad and Whyte 1995: 7). Their volume *Disability and Culture* (1995) provides an insight into different lived experiences of disabled populations around the world. Although primarily an anthropological survey, the volume highlights the need for a global study of disability that would pay attention to the nuanced culture- and language-specific definitions of the term, and the importance of interdisciplinary research with fields such as translation studies. The following section will highlight how some of these differences are embodied in the variations of the vocabulary associated with disability.

3 Translating the language of disability

Apart from campaigning for large-scale social, political and legislative changes (see Berghs *et al.* 2019 for a detailed examination of these efforts), one of the key challenges posed by the disability movement is to change the way disability is spoken about in media and amongst wider public, similar to the changing discourse surrounding sexuality, gender or race. As the WHO stresses in their *World Report on Disability*, '[n]egative imagery and language, stereotypes, and stigma – with deep historic roots – persist for people with disabilities around the world' (WHO 2011: 6). The aim of these linguistic changes is to question and ultimately abolish common phrases that vilify or victimise people with various disabilities, contribute to the deep-seated stigmatisation of non-normative bodies, and associate disability with negative stereotypes. These changes spread together with disability activism across the world, and their local linguistic variations present some interesting translation challenges.

The most obvious, as well as the most widely observed change related to these shifts, is the gradual removal of words associated with disabilities that were widely used as expletives. Words such as 'cripple',[7] 'freak' and 'retarded' are now considered highly offensive and have largely disappeared from public discourse and most forms of polite conversation in English. This is widely mirrored in languages that use terms with the same etymological base; the German variation of cripple, *Krüppel*, is flagged as 'diskriminierend' [discriminatory] in the newest online version of the *Duden* dictionary,[8] whereas the Slovak version *kripel* is labelled as pejorative in the *Dictionary of Present-day Slovak Language* from 2015 (*Slovník súčasného slovenského jazyka*).[9] The situation becomes more complicated in the case of terms which are not used as expletives per se, but that are nonetheless considered outdated and unsuitable for (Anglophone) public discourse. Perhaps the most prominent example of this category is the term 'invalid'. The UK government's *Guidance for Inclusive Language Related to Disability* recommends that the term is replaced with 'disabled person', and the accompanying table detailing the use of correct and incorrect terms suggests that it is synonymous with 'cripple'.[10] On the other hand, both the Slovak and Czech languages use the term 'invalid' in its adjectival form as the legal and official term for disability benefits (*invalidný dôchodok/invalidní důchod*, lit. invalid pension). This fact is not lost on local disability activists; a recent guide on *How to Speak and Write about and to Persons with Disabilities* published by the Czech Ombudsperson (*Jak mluvit a psát o lidech a s lidmi s postižením, Ombudsman veřejný ochrance práv* 2020: 8) advises: '[w]e do not recommend using the expression "invalid", although we are aware that the term is still in use within the legal parlance', citing the term's association with illness and inability to do things as their reasons for this recommendation.[11] A similar case is the term 'handicapped', which is now considered inappropriate in Anglophone disability discourse but remains in regular use in many other languages. As an example, the French translation of the aforementioned CRPD definition of disability translates 'persons with disabilities' as 'personnes handicapées' ('handicapped persons', Nations Unies 2006: 4).

Another interesting example is the term 'ableism', defined by the Oxford English Dictionary as '[d]iscrimination in favour of able-bodied people; prejudice against or disregard of the needs of disabled people', and first recorded in the English language in 1981.[12] The noun was created on the same principle as 'sexism' or 'racism', using the 'able' part of 'disabled' at its core.[13] However, 'disability' is not a widely used term outside of the Anglophone realm, and most languages will have a local expression which typically does not allow for the same linguistic cut-and-paste operation as in English.

The German language recognises the term *Behindertenfeindlichkeit* [lit. hostility against the disabled] which follows the same pattern as *Islamfeindlichkeit* (Islamophobia, lit. hostility against Islam) and *Fremdenfeindlichkeit* (Xenophobia, lit. hostility against the foreign). However, the expression does not fully cover the semantic range of the English term; *phobia/Feindlichkeit* suggests an irrational or excessive fear of a group, as opposed to 'ism' in racism or sexism, which implies active and often institutionalised discrimination against said group. Some voices within disability activism in Germany have already noted this discrepancy (Maskos 2010), and the term ableism is gradually becoming more widespread (sometimes spelt as 'Ableismus' or 'Able-ismus', see *Interessenvertretung Selbstbestimmt Leben in Deutschland* 2016). Neither the Slovak nor the Czech language have a local word for ableism, which further emphasises the fact that the issue of discrimination against disabled people has been systemically overlooked throughout the history of these countries. Both the Czech transliteration ('ableismus') and the Slovak one ('ableizmus') have recently entered these countries' disability discourse, but for now they can only be found in activist blogs and webpages (such as articles from the Czech portal *Mujautismus*[14] or Slovak *Transfúzia*[15]).

While the examples above might suggest that global disability discourse relies solely on changes adapted from Anglophone models, this is decidedly not the case. For example, the aforementioned Czech guidance on language related to disability considers the term 'čtení ze rtů' (lit. reading from lips; lipreading) as inappropriate, as it wrongly suggests that the practice is as precise and easy as the 'reading' of the alphabet, and places an overly strong emphasis on lips only, as opposed to a whole range of gestures accompanying the practice (Ombudsman veřejný ochrance práv 2020: 11). The guidance instead recommends 'odezírání' (lit. closest 'looking/staring from') as the correct term, whereas most Anglophone DHH communities use the term 'lipreading' without objection.

Apart from opposing harmful or offensive expressions, disability activism also places an emphasis on what is referred to as 'people-first' language, which promotes a view of disabled people as whole beings, not defined by their disability alone. For this reason, 'people with epilepsy' is the preferred term to 'epileptics' (which suggests epilepsy is the only trait of these people) or 'victims of epilepsy' (which promotes the victim-centric, pity-inducing view of disability). Similarly, 'wheelchair user' is a preferred term to 'wheelchair-bound' or 'confined to a wheelchair', as the term foregrounds the image of the mobility aid and a supposedly helpless, immobile person 'bound' to it. At the same time, it overlooks the fact that many people use wheelchairs on an ambulatory basis, meaning that they are able to walk under certain circumstances and use wheelchairs to conserve energy, prevent vertigo and many other reasons. These changes are likewise mirrored in the aforementioned Czech guidelines, which recommend the omission of terms such as *vozíčkář* (compound noun from 'wheelchair user') and to replace it with *'Člověk pohybující se na vozíku/člověk s omezením hybnosti'* [Person moving in a wheelchair/person with limited mobility] (Ombudsman veřejný ochrance práv 2020: 8).

It is also important to note that not all variations of English use people-first language when it comes to the term 'people with disabilities'. While this is the expression preferred in the United States and most Anglophone disability discourse, the UK community largely chooses to refer to themselves as 'disabled people'. The UK nomenclature shows a strong influence of the social model whose proponents suggest that 'persons with disabilities' implies that disabled people have ownership or responsibility over their experience of disability, rather than disability being an intrinsic part of who they are.

These discrepancies even within the English language itself highlight the importance of a nuanced and informed approach to the various languages of disability, which would account for the individual voices within the disabled communities and actively encourage the de-stigmatisation of its members.

4 Disability in translation studies

Although an academic area that would combine disability and translation has as of yet not been established, the discipline of translation studies has over the past few decades generated a number of works that are related to disabled people and issues of accessibility. Given the fluidity of the term disability and its changing conceptualisation in recent decades, it is difficult to decide which works within translation studies to include in this category; furthermore, there is naturally a large degree of overlap between different subfields, including those explored elsewhere in this volume, such as interpreting for the DHH people.

One of the first studies explicitly mentioning disability in a translated context is an article titled 'Disability Issues in Translation/Interpretation' by Smart and Smart (1997). Although primarily focusing on translation and interpreting in rehabilitation services, it is one of the first texts directly mentioning the specific requirements of disabled people within the context of healthcare interpreting and under the direct influence of the anti-discriminatory legislation based on the Americans with Disabilities Act (United States Department of Justice 1990). The article also acknowledges the cultural differences in the conceptualisation of disability, mentioning for example that most Native American languages have no equivalent expression for 'learning disability' (Smart and Smart 1995: 16, cited in Smart and Smart 1997: 124), or that it is difficult to find expressions related to disability in Chinese that would not perpetuate stereotypes of weakness or helplessness (Ong 1993; cited in Smart and Smart 1997: 124).

After Smart and Smart's article, studies pertaining to disabled people have largely been scattered in various subfields of translation studies, typically without an explicit reference to disability. The largest number of these studies can be found in the field of audiovisual translation (AVT), which surveys both subtitling for the deaf and the hard of hearing (SDH, also known as close captioning in US English) and audio description for the blind and the partially sighted (AD). Both areas are of growing interest within AVT and there is an increasing number of studies on these topics in several of the most recent works in the field (e.g. Díaz-Cintas and Remael 2014; Baños Piñero and Díaz-Cintas 2015). The *Routledge Handbook of Audiovisual Translation* (Pérez-González 2019) has dedicated entries that detail the history and current issues in both subfields (see Neves 2019 for SDH; and Perego 2019 for AD). Although SDH and AD are perhaps the most obvious connection between AVT and disabilities, it is important to stress that audiences with sensory impairments are not the only group benefiting from subtitles or audio descriptions. For instance, Franco, Medina Silveira and dos Santos Carneiro (2015) explore whether AD aimed at the blind and visually impaired can also ensure better understanding for people with learning disabilities.

Although, as explained in the previous section, some DHH people prefer to see themselves as part of a linguistic minority instead of the disabled community, it is necessary to mention sign language interpreting as another substantial area of research related to disability within translation studies. *The Sign Language Interpreting Studies Reader* (Roy and Napier 2017) provides a detailed overview of the field's history and addresses the sometimes problematic connection with disability studies (p. 368). Volumes by Janzen (2005),

Napier (2009) and Roberson and Shaw (2018) provide further insights into this academic area, and the contribution by Moreland and Swabey in this volume discusses the specific issues associated with sign language interpreting in healthcare settings and the related disparities faced by DHH patients.

Other works that link disability with translation are more diffused and isolated. Studies within the field of interpreting, such as the one from Salaets and Balogh (2015), focus on the specific requirements of interpreter-mediated questioning of disabled and vulnerable children. In relation to blind and visually impaired communities, machine translation technology is used for the transcription of texts into Braille in languages that are not using the Latin alphabet (Sugano *et al.* 2010; Wang *et al.* 2017). Inga Wagner's research considers terminological standardisation of the Spanish version of the aforementioned International Classification of Functioning (ICF) published by the WHO in 2010, with a brief reference to German and Italian translations (Wagner 2004). Many other areas, such as intralingual translation (e.g. into Simple English) which could benefit people with learning disabilities (Brøgger and Zethsen, this volume), interpreting in mental health settings (Bot, this volume) and child language brokering (Nilsen, this volume) could provide further insights into how various disabilities overlap with translation or interpreting within healthcare settings, despite not mentioning disability studies explicitly. While this is by no means a complete list, it attempts to emphasise both the scarcity of works at the intersection of translation and disability, and the broad possibilities for future research, which will be further stressed in the final section.

One last category whose absence is particularly striking comprises studies that would consider disability as an identity category that provides its own unique lens for the study of translation. This category is already well established in literary studies (see e.g. Hall 2016, 2020; Barker and Murray 2017). Thus far, the only work within the field of translation studies that uses disability as a theoretical framework to consider how stories written by and about disabled people are translated is a volume edited by Someshwar Sati and G. J. V. Prasad titled *Disability in Translation: The Indian Experience* (2019). The entries in this collection are centred around the translations of 18 short stories with motifs of disability from various Indian languages into English. Each translator details their experiences in the de- and reconstruction of the various themes, metaphors and images of disability in the process of translation. The volume remains the sole example of such an undertaking and foregrounds the need for further attention to be given to the use of disability as a critical framework for the exploration of literature, language and translation.

5 Translating the CRPD

The last part of this contribution will offer a small comparative case study focusing on the translation of international disability legislation published by the UN. All official UN documents are translated into the six official languages of the organisation; Arabic, Chinese, English, French, Russian, and Spanish (United Nations DGACM, no date); however, some documents, such as the CRPD, are adopted into the legal systems of its signatory countries and are therefore translated directly into their respective languages. The CRPD has so far been signed by 163 countries (UN Department of Economic and Social Affairs, no date). As this document sets out some of the most important anti-discriminatory regulations for disabled people, the wording in these translations has far-reaching consequences and a direct effect on the lives of disabled people in these signatory countries. Here I would like to offer a brief insight into the possible issues associated with these translations, using the Slovak, Czech and German definitions of disability from Article 1 of the CRPD, already cited in the section above discussing the social model of disability.

The Slovak version of the CRPD (Organizácia Spojených Národov 2010) was ratified in May 2010 and signed in September of the same year. The definition of 'persons with disabilities' reads as follows:

> Dohovor OSN o právach ľudí so **zdravotným postihnutím** definuje osoby so **zdravotným postihnutím** ako osoby s dlhodobými telesnými, mentálnymi, intelektuálnymi alebo zmyslovými **postihnutiami**, ktoré v súčinnosti s rôznymi **prekážkami** môžu brániť ich plnému a účinnému zapojeniu do spoločnosti na rovnakom základe s ostatnými.
>
> *Organizácia Spojených Národov 2010*

> [The UN convention on the rights of people with **health impairments** defines persons with **health impairments** as persons with long-term physical, mental, intellectual or sensory **impairments**, which in concurrence with various **barriers** can hinder their full and effective integration into the society on the same basis as others.]

As is visible from the back translation, the Slovak version uses the same term *postihnutie* for both disability and impairment, and the Slovak language currently does not have separate terms for the two concepts. The noun *postihnutie* (lit. closest to 'affliction') serves as a generic description of various impairments, usually preceded by a classification (*telesné postihnutie*/physical impairment etc.). The term 'disabled person' translates in both the medical and legal sense into *osoba s [ťažkým] zdravotným postihnutím* [person with a [severe] health impairment]. In everyday parlance, this is shortened into the acronym ZŤP (from the adjective *zdravotne ťažko postihnutý/á*), and functions in the same way as the English disability status; a person can indicate they 'have' a ZŤP when claiming a disability discount, e.g. when using public transport.

A similar situation is present in the translation of the CRPD into Czech, a language closely related to Slovak, which likewise shows the absence of a differentiation between a disability (*osoby se zdravotním postižením [persons with health impairments]) and impairment (postižení* [impairment]) (Organizace Spojených Národů 2007: 98, signed in March 2007). Interestingly, the aforementioned guide published by the Czech Ombudsperson (Ombudsman veřejný ochrance práv 2020: 8) recommends to omit the 'health' [zdravotní] part in 'person with health impairments', as it is seen as related to the outdated, individual model of disability.

While it would be erroneous to claim that this lack of linguistic differentiation between disability and impairment makes the explanation or adaptation of a social model of disability impossible, the fact remains that the easy and memorable definition of disability as a social inequality caused by impairments in interaction with barriers is much more difficult to convey in both Slovak and Czech. These linguistic discrepancies indicate one of the most significant areas for future research into disability and translation, represented by the differences in the very conceptualisation of the most basic terms, such as disability or impairment.

Let us now return to the CRPD definition of disability and compare the Slovak and Czech versions with the German translation. The German version was signed in March 2007 (Vereinte Nationen 2009a: 2), ratified in March 2009, and serves as the official and joint translation for Germany, Austria, Switzerland and Liechtenstein. The definition of disability is as follows:

> Zu den Menschen mit **Behinderungen** zählen Menschen, die langfristige körperliche, seelische, geistige oder Sinnes**beeinträchtigungen** haben, welche sie in Wechselwirkung mit verschiedenen **Barrieren** an der vollen, wirksamen und gleichberechtigten Teilhabe an der Gesellschaft hindern können.
>
> *Vereinte Nationen 2009a: 4*
>
> [Amongst people with **disabilities** count people who have long-term physical, mental, cognitive or sensory[-] **impairments**, which can, in interaction with various **barriers**, hinder their full, effective and equal participation in the society.]

The German version makes a clear distinction between *Behinderung* (lit. disability; the Germanic root of the noun is the same as the English *to hinder*), and *Beeinträchtigung* (lit. impairment; the verb *zu beeinträchtigen* can be translated as *to affect* or *to interfere with*), and as such follows the distinction between disability and impairment rooted in the social model of disability. This difference not only helps to easily convey the idea of the social model of disability, but the clear distinction between disability and impairment is much easier to integrate into the local legislations based on the CRPD in all four signatory countries.

Interestingly however, the official German version of the CRPD evoked some criticism from German-speaking disability activists, who felt that the translation did not mirror the meaning of the original English text sufficiently, and resulted in the publication of a 'shadow translation' ('Schattenübersetzung', Vereinte Nationen 2009b; translation prepared by the German Association for Human Rights and Equality for Disabled People Netzwerk Article 3). The primary reason for this dissatisfaction was the fact that the official version did not pay sufficient attention to 'awareness raising through the **right** translation' (UN-Behindertenrechtskonvention, no date, emphasis in original), and used too many loanwords from English (such as 'disability mainstreaming' 'peer support' and 'capacity-building', among others). The use of these Anglicisms, it was felt, 'do not sharpen the consciousness of the society about the concerns of people with disabilities' (*ibid.*). The need for this unofficial German shadow translation highlights the (over)use of English in non-Anglophone disability discourse discussed above, but also the crucial need for nuanced and informed translations done by experts who are trained not only in the translation of legal documents, but also understand the role of language in disability activism. It also highlights the question of agency; the shadow translation emphasises the direct involvement of the disabled community in the preparation of the document as the main defining feature of this alternative translation (Vereinte Nationen 2009b: 3), and as such underscores the importance of the inclusion of disabled people not only in the process of drafting, but also in the translation and editing of official documents.

6 Conclusion and future directions

With disability activism becoming a prominent international issue joining the fight against racism, sexism, ageism and other inequalities, the study of disability from the perspective of translation studies becomes increasingly relevant. The examples in this chapter sketch out some of the possible areas for future research at the intersection of disability studies and translation studies, such as the fast-changing language of disability activism and how its vocabulary travels across linguistic borders; the predominance of English in international disability discourse; the conceptual problems of translating models of disability into different languages and cultures; and, the question of agency in the translation of legal documents related to disability. Alongside these, the overlap between the two disciplines provides a broad range of further research directions. A better understanding of the different cultural and linguistic perceptions of disability could be used to improve translation standards in healthcare and help to represent disabled people in different linguistic environments. Questions of how disabilities affect the work of translators and interpreters could also become a subject of future study, including surveys about what could make translation and interpreting a more accessible occupation for disabled people. Training of interpreters and translators could be built with an awareness of the specific needs of disabled groups in mind, and the training itself could be more inclusive towards disabled interpreters and translator. Ensuring accessibility through translation could likewise expand beyond the present-day issues of sign language interpreting and SDH/AD in AVT, and could encompass intralingual translation, tactile writing and specific provisions for people with learning disabilities.

Another large and hitherto unexplored area is literary translation, where disability can be used as a critical tool similar to a queer perspective; future works could map the historical developments of disabled characters in translation, explore the work of disabled authors in translation and attempt retranslations of literary works through the lens of disability. Lastly, the presence of disability discourse within the field of translation studies could also raise awareness about the practical needs of disabled communities when teaching in academia or organising conferences and other events in the field of translation studies, and contribute to the creation of a truly inclusive and diverse academic field.

Notes

1 This project was completed with the support of the University of Vienna and has received funding from the European Union's Horizon 2020 research and innovation programme under the Marie Skłodowska-Curie grant agreement No 847693.
2 The author would like to thank Miro Griffiths for his generous comments and detailed feedback on an earlier draft of this chapter.
3 This chapter uses the term 'disabled people' as opposed to 'people with disabilities', given that this term is prevalent in the UK where the author wrote most of this chapter. A detailed discussion of the difference between these two expressions is included in Section 3.
4 See Lawson and Beckett (2020) for a comparison of the social and human rights models.
5 Compare also with the definition in the Americans with Disabilities Act (ADA) of 1990: '[t]he term "disability" means, with respect to an individual (A) a physical or mental impairment that substantially limits one or more major life activities of such individual; (B) a record of such an impairment; or (C) being regarded as having such an impairment' (United States Department of Justice 1990).
6 See also Barnes and Mercer (2004) for a discussion of the social model as an oppositional device.
7 Interestingly, parts of the (primarily Anglophone) disabled community are now reclaiming the term 'cripple' (and particularly the shortened form 'crip') as a way to take back the agency over their own identity, similar to how the term 'queer' was re-appropriated by many members of the LGBTQ+ community (see McRuer 2006, particularly Chapter 1 'Coming out crip: Malibu is burning').

8 www.duden.de/suchen/dudenonline/Kr%C3%BCppel.
9 https://slovnik.juls.savba.sk/?w=kripel&s=exact&c=Jae3&cs=&d=kssj4&d=psp&d=sssj&d=orter&d=scs&d=sss&d=peciar&d=hssjV&d=bernolak&d=noundb&d=orient&d=locutio&d=obce&d=priezviska&d=un&d=pskcs&d=psken#.
10 www.gov.uk/government/publications/inclusive-communication/inclusive-language-words-to-use-and-avoid-when-writing-about-disability.
11 All back translations are the author's, unless otherwise specified.
12 www.oed.com/view/Entry/240190?redirectedFrom=ableism#eid.
13 See also e.g. Wolbring (2008) and Campbell (2009) for further discussions of the concept of ableism and the associated issues.
14 https://mujautismus.cz/2018/02/nelitujte-me-nelitujte-me-deti/.
15 www.transfuzia.org/kniznica-archiv/clanky/ableizmus-dostupnost-a-transsexualizmus_49.

Further reading

Sati, S. and Prasad, G. J. V. (2019) *Disability in Translation: The Indian Experience*. London: Routledge.

The volume brings together essays from 18 translators who were invited to share their experiences in translating short stories with themes of disabilities from various Indian languages into English.

Smart, J. F. and Smart, D. W. (1997) 'Disability Issues in Translation / Interpretation', in Babirecki-Labrum, M. (ed.) *The Changing Scene in World Languages*. Amsterdam and Philadelphia: John Benjamins.

One of the first texts connecting disability and translation studies. Published as a response to the Americans with Disabilities Act of 1990, the article provides a succinct list of issues in translation and interpreting pertaining specifically to disability.

Ingstad, B. and Whyte, S. R. (1995b) *Disability and Culture*. Berkeley and Los Angeles: University of California Press.

Ingstad and Whyte's anthropological survey compares different cultural perceptions of disability in a range of countries, including Southern Somalia, Borneo, Uganda, Nicaragua and Botswana.

Davis, L. J. (2006) *The Disability Studies Reader*, 2nd ed. New York and London: Routledge.

The Reader brings together key texts from the field of disability studies, and as such presents a good starting point for those interested in the history and development of the field.

Related topics

The Impact of Interpreters and the Rise of Deaf Healthcare Professionals, Medical Humanities and Translation, Queer Feminisms and the Translation of Sexual Health

References

Baños Piñero, R. and Díaz Cintas, J. (2015) *Audiovisual Translation in a Global Context: Mapping an Ever-changing Landscape*. Basingstoke and New York: Palgrave Macmillan. DOI:10.1017/CBO9781107415324.004.

Barker, C. and Murray, S. (eds) (2017) *The Cambridge Companion to Literature and Disability*. Cambridge: Cambridge University Press.

Barnes, C. and Mercer, G. (2004) *Implementing the Social Model of Disability: Theory and Research*. Leeds: The Disability Press.

Berghs, M. *et al.* (2019) *The Routledge Handbook of Disability Activism*. London and New York: Routledge. DOI:10.4324/9781351165082.

Campbell, F. K. (2009) *Contours of Ableism: The Production of Disability and Ableness*. Houndmills Basingstoke and New York: Palgrave Macmillan. DOI:10.1177/0094306111425016h.

Davis, L. J. (1999) 'Crips Strike Back: The Rise of Disability Studies', *American Literary History*, 11(3), pp. 500–512. DOI:10.1093/alh/11.3.500.

Díaz-Cintas, J. and Remael, A. (2014) *Audiovisual Translation: Subtitling*. London and New York: Routledge. DOI:10.4324/9781315759678.
Franco, E. P. C., Medina Silveira, D. M. and dos Santos Carneiro, B. C. (2015) 'Audio Describing for an Audience with Learning Disabilities in Brazil: A Pilot Study', in Baños Piñero, R. and Díaz Cintas, J. (eds) *Audiovisual Translation in a Global Context: Mapping an Ever-changing Landscape*. Basingstoke and New York: Palgrave Macmillan, pp. 99–109.
Hall, A. (2016) *Literature and Disability*. London and New York: Routledge.
Hall, A. (2020) *The Routledge Companion to Literature and Disability*. London and New York: Routledge.
Ingstad, B. and Whyte, S. R. (1995) *Disability and Culture*. Berkeley and Los Angeles: University of California Press.
Interessenvertretung Selbstbestimmt Leben in Deutschland (2016) *Ableismus erkennen und begegnen: Strategien zur Stärkung von Selbsthilfepotenzialen*. ISL e. V.
Janzen, T. (2005) *Topics in Signed Language Interpreting: Theory and Practice*. Amsterdam and Philadelphia: John Benjamins. DOI:10.1075/intp.9.2.09pet.
Lane, H. (2006) 'Construction of Deafness', in Davis, L. J. (ed.) *The Disability Studies Reader*. New York and London: Routledge, pp. 79–92.
Lawson, A. and Beckett, A. E. (2020) 'The Social and Human Rights Models of Disability: Towards a Complementarity Thesis', *International Journal of Human Rights*, pp. 1–32. DOI:10.1080/13642987.2020.1783533.
Linton, S. (2005) 'What Is Disability Studies ?', *PMLA*, 120(2), pp. 518–522.
Maskos, R. (2010) 'Was heißt Ableism? Überlegungen zu Behinderung und bürgerlicher Gesellschaft [What does Ableism mean? Thoughts on disability and civil society]', *arranca!*, 43(December).
McRuer, R. (2006) *Crip Theory: Cultural Signs of Queerness and Disability*. New York and London: New York University Press.
Napier, J. (2009) *International Perspectives on Sign Language Interpreter Education*. Washington, DC: Gallaudet University Press.
Nations Unies (2006) *Convention relative aux droits des personnes handicapées*. Available at: www.un.org/disabilities/documents/convention/convoptprot-f.pdf (Accessed: 15 December 2020).
Neves, J. (2019) 'Subtitling for Deaf and Hard of Hearing Audiences: Moving Forward', in Pérez-González, L. (ed.) *Routledge Handbook of Audiovisual Translation*. London and New York: Routledge, pp. 82–95.
Office for Disability Issues (2010) *Equality Act 2010*. Available at: www.equalityadvisoryservice.com/ci/fattach/get/586/1354033333/redirect/1/session/L2F2LzEvdGltZS8xNTg2NTI2MjA3L3NpZC8xWlYqVTJHbw==/filename/disability-definition.pdf (Accessed: 15 December 2020).
Oliver, M. (1996) *Understanding Disability: From Theory to Practice*. New York: Macmillan Education. DOI:10.1017/CBO9781107415324.004.
Ombudsman veřejný ochrance práv (2020) *Jak mluvit a psát o lidech a s lidmi s postižením [How to speak and write about and to persons with disabilities]*. Available at: www.ochrance.cz/fileadmin/user_upload/CRPD/Doporuceni/6-2020_doporuceni_media.pdf (Accessed: 28 June 2020).
Ong, W. M. A. (1993) *Asian American Cultural Dimensions in Rehabilitation Counseling*. San Diego: San Diego State University Rehabilitation Cultural Diversity Initiative.
Organizace Spojených Národů (2007) *Úmluva o právech osob se zdravotním postižením, Ministerstvo zahraničních věcí České Republiky, sbírka mezinárodních smluv*.
Organizácia Spojených Národov (2010) *Dohovor o právach osôb so zdravotným postihnutím, Ministerstvo zahraničných vecí Slovenskej Republiky, zbierka zákonov*.
Owens, J. (2015) 'Exploring the Critiques of the Social Model of Disability: The Transformative Possibility of Arendt's Notion of Power', *Sociology of Health and Illness*, 37(3), pp. 385–403. DOI:10.1111/1467-9566.12199.
Perego, E. (2019) 'Audio Description: Evolving Recommendations for Usable, Effective and Enjoyable Practices', in Pérez-González, L. (ed.) *Routledge Handbook of Audiovisual Translation*. London and New York: Routledge, pp. 114–129.
Pérez-González, L. (2019) *Routledge Handbook of Audiovisual Translation*. London and New York: Routledge. DOI:10.4324/9781315717166-3.

Quinn, G. and Degener, T. (2002) *Human Rights and Disability: The Current Use and Future Potential of United Nations Human Rights Instruments in the Context of Disability*. New York and Geneva: United Nations.

Roberson, L. and Shaw, S. (2018) *Signed Language Interpreting in the 21st Century: An Overview of the Profession*. Washington, DC: Gallaudet University Press.

Roy, C. B. and Napier, J. (2017) *The Sign Language Interpreting Studies Reader*. Amsterdam and Philadelphia: John Benjamins.

Salaets, H. and Balogh, K. (2015) *Children and Justice: Overcoming Language Barriers*. Cambridge, Antwerp and Portland: Intersentia Ltd. DOI:10.1017/9781780685144.

Sati, S. and Prasad, G. J. V. (2019) *Disability in Translation: The Indian Experience*. London: Routledge.

Shakespeare, T. (2006) 'The Social Model of Disability', in Davis, L. J. (ed.) *The Disability Studies Reader*. London and New York: Routledge.

Shakespeare, T., Watson, N. and Alghaib, O. A. (2017) 'Blaming the Victim, All Over Again: Waddell and Aylward's Biopsychosocial (BPS) Model of Disability', *Critical Social Policy*, 37(1), pp. 22–41. DOI:10.1017/CBO9781107415324.004.

Smart, J. F. and Smart, D. W. (1995) 'The Use of Translators/Interpreters in Rehabilitation', *Journal of Rehabilitation*, 61(2), pp. 14–20.

Smart, J. F. and Smart, D. W. (1997) 'Disability Issues in Translation / Interpretation', in Babirecki-Labrum, M. (ed.) *The Changing Scene in World Languages*. Amsterdam and Philadelphia: John Benjamins.

Sugano, A. *et al.* (2010) 'eBraille: A Web-Based Translation Program for Japanese Text to Braille', *Internet Research*, 20(5), pp. 582–592. DOI:0.1108/10662241011084121.

The Union of the Physically Impaired Against Segregation (1976) 'Fundamental Principles of Disability'. DOI:10.1787/9789264218789-5-en.

UN-Behindertenrechtskonvention (no date) *Schattenübersetzung*, www.behindertenrechtskonvention.info. Available at: www.behindertenrechtskonvention.info/schattenuebersetzung-3678 (Accessed: 25 June 2020).

UN Department of Economic and Social Affairs (n.d.) *Convention on the Rights of Persons with Disabilities (CRPD)*. Available at: www.un.org/development/desa/disabilities/convention-on-the-rights-of-persons-with-disabilities.html (Accessed: 28 June 2020).

United Nations (2006) *Convention on the Rights of Persons with Disabilities (CRPD)*. DOI: 10.1057/palgrave.development.1100310.

United Nations DGACM (n.d.) *Translation*. Available at: www.un.org/Depts/DGACM/Translation.shtml (Accessed: 25 June 2020).

United States Department of Justice (1990) *Americans with Disabilities Act of 1990, as amended with ADA Amendments Act of 2008*. Available at: www.ada.gov/pubs/adastatute08.htm#12102 (Accessed: 10 April 2020).

Vereinte Nationen (2009a) *Übereinkommen der Vereinten Nationen über die Rechte von Menschen mit Behinderung*. Die amtliche, gemeinsame Übersetzung von Deutschland, Österreich, Schweiz und Lichtenstein. DOI:10.5771/0042-384x-2010-2-57.

Vereinte Nationen (2009b) *Übereinkommen der Vereinten Nationen über die Rechte von Menschen mit Behinderung (Schattenübersetzung)*. Die Schattenübersetzung des Netzwerks Artikel 3. DOI:10.5771/0042-384x-2010-2-57.

Wagner, I. (2004) 'Aspetti terminologici e traduttivi dell'ICF', *Rivista internazionale di tecnica della traduzione*, 8, pp. 129–145.

Wang, X. *et al.* (2017) 'Chinese to Braille Translation Based on Braille Word Segmentation Using Statistical Model', *Journal of Shanghai Jiaotong University (Science)*, 22(1), pp. 82–86. DOI:10.1007/s12204-017-1804-x.

WHO (2011) *World Report on Disability*. Geneva. Available at: www.who.int/disabilities/world_report/2011/report/en/ (Accessed: 15 December 2020).

Wolbring, G. (2008) 'The Politics of Ableism', *Development*, 51(2), pp. 252–258. DOI:10.1057/dev.2008.17.

19

Queer feminisms and the translation of sexual health

Michela Baldo

1 Introduction

This chapter focuses on the notion of health, which will be discussed through the lenses of translation on the one hand, and gender and sexuality studies on the other. It will make references to the way health has been theorised by a range of contemporary queer feminists in the United States, Europe, Latin America and China, who were inspired mainly by the feminist initiatives in the 1970s, like self-help clinics and self-awareness groups in the United States. For queer feminisms, health becomes synonymous with freedom of choice on matters such as one's own body, affective and sexual relationships, and reproduction. Many queer feminist groups are actively engaged in the production of counter-knowledge on health, i.e. new and peripheral knowledge that opposes the official mainstream one, for two main reasons: first, to subvert the asymmetrical relationship between expert mainstream knowledge and the needs expressed by women and LGBTQ* subjects on these topics; second, to challenge institutional medical narratives, which have marginalised or censored this counter-knowledge. Pivotal in the production of an understanding of health in feminist terms is translation, given that it can make up for the lack of specific knowledge in a given cultural context. In this chapter I will discuss a number of translation scenarios, touching on health concerns that were raised by feminists in the 1970s and are still of interest to queer feminisms in the present day, namely the questions of female sexual health and reproductive choices, which appear to be the main topics that the translations focus on.

2 Definitions and historical perspectives

This section will provide a brief historical outline of the concept of sexual health in feminist terms. The 1970s can be considered a crucial moment in the feminist history of sexuality in Italy, the United States, the UK, France and Spain, among other countries. The feminist movements in these countries had felt the urge to revolutionise the patriarchal medical system that was silencing women's needs and desires in relation to health and sexuality. This urge was part of the general feminist revolution that fought against patriarchal control on women's bodies, which the healthcare system was especially contributing

DOI: 10.4324/9781003167983-24

to perpetuate, given its focus on bodily health. Such a patriarchal medical system was operating by making use of the binarism 'normal/pathological' (Busi and Fiorilli 2014: 5), which constrained any form of women's rebellion through a control of their sexuality, and by silencing those needs that exceeded the sphere of reproduction. Feminists thus elaborated on, and at the same time contested, the notion of 'medicalisation' (Busi and Fiorilli 2014), understood not only as the violence perpetrated by the medical institutions on women's bodies, but also as 'the performative effects of medical/scientific categories in the organisation of the possibilities of expression'[1] (Busi and Fiorilli 2014: 6) in relation to women's bodies. The effects of medicalisation are as familiar to the feminist movements as they are to the LGBTQ* movements. For instance, during the HIV epidemic of the 1990s, the latter campaigned for life and health rights against a medical system that considered 'non-reproductive and non-heteronormative bodies, sexuality and pleasures to be "sick"' (Busi and Fiorilli 2014: 6). Moreover, the concept of medicalisation has been fundamental to more recent reflections by the international transgender movement on the de-pathologisation of trans people; this movement has reclaimed self-determination of bodies beyond the constraints of the medical/institutionalised sex/gender transitioning practices (Busi and Fiorilli 2014). The idea of de-pathologisation has also been central to the intersex movement, which – starting in the 1990s – has opposed the surgical treatments used to 'normalise' ambiguous genitals; these treatments have been, and still are, guided by a perception of intersex bodies as pathological.

Through their conceptualisation of the notion of medicalisation, feminists in the 1970s thus tried to find new ways of understanding and experiencing their bodies and sexualities. In order to do so, they started a series of practices ranging from self-help interventions via the publication of informative material (e.g. leaflets, booklets, books) to the creation of self-awareness groups and self-managed health clinics and centres. In the United States, for example, the Feminist Women's Health Centre was founded in Los Angeles between 1971 and 1972. This initiative would be replicated in Italy in the following two years (Percovich 2005: 11),[2] alongside the birth of self-managed women's health clinics. Some of these Italian clinics also practised illegal abortions.[3]

The birth of these health centres and clinics, and especially of the self-help groups (Voli 2007: 109), was partly influenced by the important and popular book, *Our Bodies, Ourselves* (hereafter *OBOS*),[4] published in 1971 by a group of women in Boston. These women wanted to share knowledge about their bodies among themselves and with other women. *OBOS* became pivotal for international women's movements and was translated into several languages,[5] including Italian in 1974, under the title *Noi e il Nostro Corpo* (We and our Body). The book touched on topics such as contraception, abortion, menopause, venereal diseases and medication (Percovich 2005). What was striking about this project was that personal experience was transformed into collective political experience and knowledge of women's bodies was no longer relegated to male experts but to the women themselves (Percovich 2005: 38–39). In Italy, the book was used within the consciousness-raising feminist groups along with another book, *Donne è Bello* (Women is Beautiful),[6] a translation of three texts written mainly by the New York radical feminists (NYRF).[7]

Given this historical background, this chapter will build on the importance of a notion of health as conceptualised by feminisms in the 1970s, taking also into account the prominence transgender issues have gained in the last 20 years.[8] The chapter will also examine the resurgence of feminist practices within certain contemporary queer feminisms, such as the health clinics inspired by the feminist practices of the 1970s. Finally, it will take into account the rise of transnational feminist movements engaged in the struggle to stop 'male' violence against women, inspired by the feminist movement *Ni Una Menos* (Not One Woman Less),[9] born in Argentina in 2015 to combat violence against women, which led to the creation of other feminist movements with the same name in many Latin American countries and in Europe (i.e. Spain, Italy, the UK, the United States, Germany, Switzerland).[10] These transnational feminist movements' agenda touches on many of the concerns raised by *OBOS* and by the feminist movements of the 1970s, such as women's sexual health, violence against women and reproductive choices. In doing so, the chapter will also examine the fundamental role of translation in the development of ideas around health understood in feminist terms.

3 Critical issues and current research

3.1 *Transfeminism and health*

In the previous section we have seen that the notion of health and sexuality has been an important object of investigation, and a field of intervention, for feminist movements. In this section I will make particular reference to the way health has been theorised within queer feminisms. However, I will refer also, and more specifically, to a strand of queer feminism called transfeminism, which is a type of feminism more in line with my understanding of, and involvement in, feminist activism.

Transfeminism can be considered a form of feminism that is informed by transgender politics. Transfeminism has developed mainly in countries such as the United States, Spain, Italy and France, and also in some Latin American countries. In the United States, the term transfeminism was used for the first time by Emi Koyama, in her *Transfeminist Manifesto* of 2001, where it is defined as a feminism by and for trans women, also open to queer and intersex people, trans men, non-trans women, and non-trans men who are sympathetic toward the needs of trans women. In Spain, on the other hand, the term transfeminism first appeared during an annual conference entitled *Jornadas Feministas Estatales* (Feminist National Days) held in Córdoba in 2000. By 2009, the term had become 'a familiar and persistent expression for reclaiming space for feminist trans people excluded from feminist circles' (Espineira and Bourcier 2016: 87). As Italian transfeminist scholar Rachele Borghi (2018) writes, when discussing Spanish and Italian transfeminisms, the prefix trans does not only refer to the inclusion of the trans subject within feminism – which is more the case for US transfeminism – but to a total shift of paradigm. The prefix trans challenges (Borghi 2018) the epistemology of dominant feminisms centred on a feminine identity conceived as a natural essence or biological fact and moves beyond that. Spanish transfeminism, for example, is based on non-hierarchical alliances; it is a feminism that crosses various social spheres, touching mainly on questions of social justice. As clearly expressed in the *Manifiesto para la insurrección transfeminista* (Manifesto for a Transfeminist Revolution), written in Córdoba in 2009 by a group of collectives and feminist activists, transfeminism puts emphasis on building a feminism based on a coalition of subjects living at the margins, such as 'squatters, lesbians, anticapitalists, fags and transgender people' (Solà 2013: 19).

Because of its intersectional nature, Spanish transfeminism can be defined as queer feminism. Since the first inception of the term at a conference in 1990 delivered by Teresa de Lauretis (1991), the adjective 'queer' was used to highlight the differences between gay and lesbian subjects, despite their shared non-heteronormative sexuality. The adjective 'queer', as used by de Lauretis and others who followed her, was meant to stress, among other things, the importance of taking into account the intersection between the notions of gender and sexuality, and race, class, ability, age, migration, etc. However, according to Karine Espineira and Marie-Hélène/Sam Bourcier (2016), Spanish transfeminism prefers to use the prefix trans instead of the term 'queer', which is associated with 'Anglo white queer theory and English as an imperialistic language' (2016: 88), especially considering 'the theoretical excesses' (2016: 88)[11] of the first wave of white queer theory. Transfeminism instead places the questions of the body and of embodiment at the centre of its theorisations and practices.

The Spanish transfeminist movement has had significant influence on the Italian and French ones. In Italy, the term transfeminism has been circulating at least since the translation of the above-mentioned *Manifiesto para la insurrección transfeminista* into Italian in 2010 by the Italian diasporic art collective *ideadestroyingmuros*, which is based in Spain. Like Spanish transfeminism, the Italian one is centred on the critique of binarisms, cisnormativity[12] and essentialism, and is a form of feminism from the margins, based on alliances of micro-groups and identities, with strong anti-capitalist, postcolonial, antiracist, transnational and sex-positive connotations. As for France, the transfeminist movement started through the queer group *Le Zoo* and its seminars, organised by Marie Helène/Sam Bourcier between 1996 and 2003. It formally went public when the trans collective *OUTrans* published a statement in 2009 (and in a revised form, again in 2012) entitled *Transfeminismes*. French transfeminism, like the Spanish one, can be considered a form of third-wave feminism, a queer feminism that stresses the importance of building a politics of resistance and alliances, and places emphasis on anti-capitalist struggles.

Spanish, Italian and French transfeminisms, which share similarities with Latin American transfeminisms (Bettcher and Stryker 2016: 12), are the main coordinates within which this chapter develops its analysis, as these feminisms are closer to my experience as an Italian. This chapter, however, will also make reference to other geographical contexts when possible. Transfeminisms constitute the ideal background against which to place an analysis of feminist health issues, given that the theme of health is a 'natural object of transfeminist politics', as Beatrice Busi and Olivia Fiorilli put it (2014: 9). The reason for this is that transfeminism has placed a great deal of emphasis on the body, as mentioned above. Spanish transfeminism, for instance, is closely linked to the post-porn movement (Egaña and Solà 2016: 77), which in Spain emerged in the 1990s, in the wake of the post-porn movement that originated in the United States in the 1980s. The movement[13] represents practices that are not represented by the mainstream porn scene. Such practices, according to Egaña and Solà (2016: 77), 'problematise the male/female binary and compulsory heterosexuality', and use the body 'as a support for making visible abject, antinormative, and pathologised sexualities'. Moreover, the post-porn movement emphasises the political value of sexuality by bringing it into the public sphere, thus breaking not only the public/private binary, but also the divide between theory and practice, by considering practitioners of post-porn as authoritative voices on sexuality (Borghi 2014: 170).

The body as theorised within transfeminism therefore differs from the body as theorised by feminists of difference, as it is based on an anti-essentialist and anti-binary epistemology, which is centred on a transgender epistemology and on the idea of transformation, or better still, of an 'ongoing transformation', to quote Espineira and Bourcier (2016: 88).

Moving from these premises, Busi and Fiorilli (2014) perceive the transfeminist movement's fight against medicalisation as one that is especially centred not on a complete dismissal of technologies, seen as representatives of a sort of techno-patriarchy, but rather, on their re-appropriation. This re-appropriation follows in the footsteps of the self-help practices of the 1970s (e.g. tools for self-abortion, menstrual aspiration practices and so forth). Yet, it places a stronger emphasis on the desires that such practices pay attention to, which mainly stem from transgender people's refusal to accept the pathologisation of themselves as the only way to gain access to medical technologies. Moreover, the transfeminist post-porn movement also fights against the pathologisation of non-mainstream sexual practices and androgynous bodies, by making them visible through performances and creative practices, where the body serves as a tool to expose and fight against such pathologisation. The term used to describe this is to 'hack' (Kinki 2013: 305). For transfeminists, technologies are thus desirable because in post-porn transfeminist practices, the body is closely connected to the concept of technology and can be itself conceived as technology (Kinki 2013) – a sort of open software, a machine that can be hacked and deprogrammed from the influence of the hegemonic medical system. For transfeminism, the body can thus become a tool of resistance against heteropatriarchal power, as it makes us imagine ways in which we can manipulate and transform our bodies outside of the framework of compulsory heterosexuality and gender binarism.

The next subsections will refer to the themes that have emerged from my introduction to transfeminism in relation to translation and health: transgender issues and, specifically, the medicalisation of sex reassignment; female sexuality, in particular female genitalia and sexual pleasure; and technology and reproductive choices. In terms of the translation scenarios, I will start by illustrating examples of translations from Italy, Spain and France, and I will then make references to other countries, including the United States, Poland, Turkey, Morocco, Brazil and China, taking into account similarities and differences between the diverse contexts. The translations analysed here are mainly located within the political/activist strand of translation studies (Baker 2013; Tymoczko 2010) and, more specifically, within the feminist strand (Castro and Ergun 2017b); the latter focuses on the feminist/activist role of translation as a tool for social transformation. Although there are several studies on feminist translation, which have gained prominence since the 1990s, very little has been written on the translation of transfeminism, apart from some sporadic articles (see for example Gramling and Dutta 2016; Baldo 2019). This chapter, then, also aims to fill this gap.

3.2 Translating trans issues

Taking inspiration from the feminist self-help practices of the 1970s, several transfeminist initiatives originated in Spain in the 21st century. One example is GynePunk,[14] a Catalan collective who developed first-aid DIY (do it yourself) – and DIT (do it together) – gynaecological tools for disadvantaged women, sex workers and refugees (but also for themselves). Italy saw the birth, from 2013 onward, of *Consultorie Transfemministe Queer* (queer transfeminist self-help clinics),[15] borrowing their name from the self-help clinics of the 1970s, which were called *consultori*, though using the feminine grammatical gender instead of the masculine one. These are political spaces of personal and collective awareness, which use the practice of self-enquiry, that is the practice by which needs and desires are collectively shared starting from a reflection on one own's life experiences and political positioning. These spaces are based on the re-appropriation of discourses on, and practices of, sexual health from a queer transfeminist perspective, in view of the possibility of experimenting with new relationships.

Particularly interesting for our discussion is the case of the 2015 translation of *Testo Yonqui* (Preciado 2008) into Italian, under the title *Testo Tossico* (Junkie Text) (Preciado 2015). This is a book by Spanish queer transfeminist scholar Paul B. Preciado, who is considered a major theoretical inspiration for transfeminism.[16] Preciado's text is a memoir about the self-injection of testosterone outside of the medico-juridical protocol for sex change, as in the vast majority of cases this hormone is not prescribed for women outside the protocol. By taking small doses of testosterone, which are not aimed at making the transition to a male body, Preciado, an assigned woman at birth, wanted to sabotage the norm that is based on a strict gender binarism, which contemplates the existence of strictly male (testosterone being one) and female hormones.[17] The story of this voluntary intoxication is interspersed with a theoretical and political critique of what Preciado (2008) calls the 'pharmaco-pornographic regime' in which we live, referring to the processes of production of masculinity and femininity that are mediated by the pharmaceutical and pornographic industries. In this text, Preciado understands the body as a site of investigation, a training lab, in line with transfeminist understandings.

Prior to the publication of the Italian translation, parts of the text were translated by the activists of the *Consultoria Transfemminista Queer Bologna*, to be read within a seminar focusing on testosterone, as part of a cycle of seminars centred on 'endogenous and synthetic hormones' and on issues such as 'transitioning, pharmacological contraception and medicalisation of the menopause' (*Consultoria Transfemminista Queer Bologna* 2014: 17). The chosen extracts were read and commented on by interspersing them with personal narratives shared within the group.

The political value of the translations used by the *Consultoria Transfemminista Queer Bologna* within the seminars is reflected in the topics of the extracts chosen for the translation. Some of these include passages that revolve around the idea of 'techno-gender' (Preciado 2008: 99), similar to the idea of techno-patriarchy mentioned above, that is, the mechanisms of the production of subjectivity, affects, desires and identity by the heteropatiarchal pharmaceutical and capitalist regime in which we live.[18] Other extracts were selected to confirm the practical and instrumental aspects of these translations. These extracts contain information (like that contained in information leaflets) on the composition of testogel (testosterone in form of gel), on its use and practical effects (e.g. increased energy, increased sexual desire, better concentration, etc.), and on the fact that testosterone is not a masculine hormone per se, or a property of biological men (since also biological women produce it), and that masculinisation[19] is only one of the outcomes of testosterone, since the physical effects of the hormone need to be understood as not separated from the mediation of our gendered subjectivities.

The translations are thus used in discussions that insist on the importance of giving visibility to an alternative imaginary, one based not on gender binarism, but on the importance of legitimising fluid embodiments of masculinity and femininity. Although such alternative imaginary cannot be built merely on disruptions of ideas linked to a hormone like testosterone, the discussions conveyed by these translations help to legitimise the desires of re-appropriating, collectively, body practices and technologies, which are otherwise conventionally reserved to assigned males at birth. Like the practices they put forth, the translations here can be considered a DIY/DIT activity, for they are carried out by non-professional translators who are activists. Moreover, the DIY ethics is centred on grassroots politics and autonomous cultural production (Kempson 2015). It relies on personal bodily experience, which in the post-porn movement is valued as more important than an expert's knowledge of sexuality (Preciado 2013), and it aims at eventually creating 'alternative spaces of social production' (Cuffman 2015: 6). Such alternative spaces, whose construction is enabled by translation, strive to produce new narratives on health, gender and sexuality, and to fulfil desires not even contemplated by the mainstream heteropatriarchal medical system. Therefore, the fight against medicalisation in this case is a fight against the medical system's failure to recognise and cater for the health and desires of women and LGBTQ* subjects.

A similar scenario is described in the study by Álvaro Jarrín (2016). Jarrín explains how the medical system in Brazil, despite having covered the cost of sex reassignment surgeries in some hospitals since 2008, does not consider 'travestis' as patients. Travestis are individuals who are assigned male at birth, identify as female, have no desire for sex reassignment surgery, but might require 'other forms of medical treatment such as hormone therapy or breast implants' (Jarrín 2016: 358). Since they wish to retain their sexual/genital organs, and their identity therefore does not fit within the normative medical definition of transsexuality, travestis are barred from medical care in relation to gender identity and their manifestations. This scenario bears some similarities to the Italian case discussed above, where individuals assigned women at birth may resort to taking testosterone outside the medical protocol for sex change. Jarrín (2016) argues that this has to do with the way medical categories like 'transsexuality' are translated from one context to another. In this case the reference is to an Anglophone (specifically an American) medical discourse that frames 'transsexuality as a psychiatric disturbance that entails a complete transition from maleness to femaleness' (Jarrín 2016: 359). Thus, the medicalised concept of transsexuality translates well into the Brazilian context, as it colludes with the political aim of excluding subjects who do not fall neatly into the gender binarism of 'female/male'.

3.3 Translating female sexuality

Another interesting case of silence, distortion of information and pathologisation of sexuality is that concerning the anatomy of the vulva. This is the subject of a book written by transfeminist Spanish writer and post-porn performer Diana Torres, titled *Coño potens* (Powerful Cunt, Torres 2015a) and translated into Italian with the title *Fica potens* in 2015 (Torres 2015b) by two transfeminist activists, Valentine and Luciana Licitra. The text is a manual about female sexuality and is centred on female ejaculation, a topic censored and pathologised by institutional medicine for centuries. In the book, Torres narrates her own episodes of squirting, which were dismissed by the gynaecologists who examined her as incontinence. This text is therefore the outcome of her personal research and investigation into female ejaculation, and of the theoretical and practical workshops she organised on the topic, which later became the inspiration for her book. Her thesis once again challenges gender binarism, since for Torres every woman should have the capacity to ejaculate; women, like men, have a prostate,[20] which traditional medicine has instead given the name of 'skene glands'.[21]

As I have written elsewhere (Baldo and Inghilleri 2018; Baldo 2019), it is interesting to look at the Italian translation of *Coño potens,* which was published by Golena edizioni, a small publisher in Rome. One of the translators of this text, Valentine, had participated and acted as an interpreter in Torres's workshops on female ejaculation. Subsequently, she started running workshops herself,[22] including presentations of the Italian translation, under the stage name *Fluida Wolf*. Translation thus becomes another DIY/DIT tool that facilitates self-experimentation with the body and self-learning. Moreover, along with the source text, translation becomes a way to fight the censorship and lack of research within a traditionally misogynist and sexist medical establishment on topics revolving around expressions of female pleasure and sexuality, which fall outside the field of reproduction; it also allows fighting against the shame and stigma associated with this phenomenon. The stigma is accurately described in Torres's book, and has to do with feelings of being dirty or perceived as 'a slut'. This is not the only translation from Torres. Challenging the prospect of censorship, Golena edizioni has published other translations of texts by the performer, such as *Pornoterrorismo* (Torres 2011/2014) and *Vomitorium* (Torres 2017a, 2017b), which contributed a great deal to the growth of transfeminist activism in Italy.

The prejudices and silences surrounding vulvas and vaginas are also described by American transgender writer Julia Serano, whose essays have been translated into Italian, Spanish, French and Turkish, and whose popular book *Whipping Girl* (Serano 2007), on misogyny and transphobia against transsexual women, was translated into French by Naomi Grunenwald (2018). In a chapter of this book Serano argues that women are not even told the name of their own sexual organs, that some are unaware of the existence of the clitoris, and that vaginas are understood to be 'simply the hole where the penis is supposed to go' (Serano 2007: 230).

Another important work addressing these issues is Eve Ensler's (1998) *The Vagina Monologues*, whose translations have been examined within translation studies, such as in Chinese (Yu 2015; 2016) and Turkish (Bircan and Koçak 2016). *The Vagina Monologues* is a feminist play that made its debut in 1996 in New York. It is a series of monologues based on a number of interviews Ensler conducted with several women of different ages, sexualities and races, and which revolve around consensual and non-consensual sexual experiences, descriptions of the vulva (a word that some feminists claim should be used instead of or alongside the word vagina),[23] genital mutilation, rape, reproduction, sex work, and lesbian relationships. Ensler also created the V-day movement, a global activist movement whose aim is to stop violence against women and which has been funded through the ticket sales of performances of the play *The Vagina Monologues*. In 2004 Ensler, in conjunction with Jane Fonda and Deep Stealth Productions, produced and directed the first all-transgender performance of *The Vagina Monologues*.

The monologues, as Ensler states, are intended to celebrate the vulva/vagina, a word still considered taboo in many societies. As Zhongli Yu (2015; 2016) demonstrates, this is certainly the case in China. Yu analyses three translations of *The Vagina Monologues* in Chinese, two carried out by two male translators – respectively a Chinese playwright, Rongjun Yu, and a Taiwanese professor of English, Cangduo Chen – and a third translation carried out by a female translator, Xiaoming Ai, who is a feminist activist and a former professor of gender studies. Zhongli Yu reaches the conclusion that the female translator's strategies reveal her feminist positioning, while the strategies adopted by the male translators disclose a heteropatriarchal perspective, for example in their negative views toward lesbianism and their toning down of the descriptions of female pleasure. Yu's study should not, however, make us jump to the conclusion that the gender of the translator is the most important indicator of the outcome of a translation. José Santaemilia (2015), who analysed the translations of terms related to female sexuality from English or French into Spanish and vice versa, states that what is more important is the explicit or implicit feminist stance of the translator.

This partial manipulation of *Vagina Monologues* in China not only stemmed from the translators' self-censorship, but also from the censorship imposed by Chinese authorities. However, ever since the publication of the translation by the above-mentioned feminist professor Xiaoming Ai, the play has become an empowering tool for feminist and women's groups all over China, as documented in the *VaChina Monologues* by queer activist Fan Popo (2013); this documentary chronicles 10 years of the play's performances throughout the country. Some of these performances were organised by LGBTQ activists, like the one staged in 2012 by members of the Zhehe Club in Fudan, who rewrote parts of the play to include LGBTQ topics (such as the wives of gay men for example) in order to fight discrimination against LGBTQ subjects.[24]

In a study of the Turkish translation of *The Vagina Monologues*,[25] Bircan and Koçak (2016) similarly stress the determination of the feminist translator and stage director Amula Merter, who managed to fight the strict censorship that topics related to female sexuality and pleasure usually provoke within Turkish institutions. The play was translated into Turkish in 2002. The district governor of Kadıköy in Istanbul banned it from being performed in public on the pretext of the 'indecent title', that he himself was allegedly ashamed to pronounce, let alone shout in a theatre. Despite this, Merter and her actresses were invited to perform the play in many conservative cities around the country and the media were generally supportive of the play (*ibid.*). Merter's translation also inspired the publication in 2008 of a Turkish book titled *İşte Böyle Güzelim* (There You Go, My Dear) (Düzel *et al.* 2012), hailed as the Turkish *Vagina Monologues*[26] and written by four academics.

The way *Vagina Monologues* often requires the audience to repeat the word 'cunt' after the actresses, as a way to reclaim the slang word, mirrors what happens in relation to Torres's *Conõ potens*. The book – translated into Italian using the equivalent of the obscene slang term for cunt, *fica* – not only exposed a topic, namely female ejaculation, which is completely dismissed by the medical heteropatriarchal system, but also reclaimed the use of taboo words in relation to female sexuality, bringing what is considered private into the public sphere, following the post-porn attempts of bridging the divide between private and public. Indeed, Diana Torres reclaims the use of obscenity – which she calls 'pornoterorismo' (porn terrorism) – in her performances, in order to destabilise the audience, to make them feel the violence being perpetrated on women and LGBTQ* subjects by the society we live in. Another Spanish transfeminist and post-porn writer of Basque origin, whose work has been translated into Italian and gained popularity within Italian transfeminism, is Itziar Ziga. Her 2009 book *Devenir perra* (Becoming a Bitch/Slut) was translated into Italian in 2014, by a group of five activist translators,[27] with the title *Diventar Cagna* (Ziga 2014), a title which uses the same derogatory words in Italian. The translation thus echoed the attempt to reclaim, in a positive way, the word 'bitch' or 'slut' (*perra* in Spanish and *cagna* in Italian) in order to fight misogyny and slut-shaming, challenging the use of these words as a rhetorical device to control women (see Baldo and Inghilleri 2018; Baldo 2019). 'Slut' has also been used more recently in the compound *SlutWalk*, a protest march that first appeared in Canada in 2011 against rape culture and the shaming of its victims (Robinson 2017). The SlutWalk campaign was translated into many different languages and cultural contexts. In Italy the first slut walk was organised in 2013, by a transfeminist collective called *Le Ribellule*, and expressed the same messages contained in the translation of Ziga's book *Devenir perra*. The term 'slut walk' was borrowed from English and was not translated into Italian. This is not the case for all the contexts in which the campaign was translated. As Rebecca Robinson (2017) states in her study of the translation of the *SlutWalk* in Morocco, the feminist activists decided to change the name because the term slut was too offensive for Moroccan sensibilities. They eventually chose one that focused on sexual harassment in the street, rather than on slut-shaming and rape, calling the movement 'Woman Choufouch'. The combination of terms is a wordplay on the Moroccan Arabic term 'Manchoufouch', which means 'What's up?', a phrase used by men to catcall women on the street (Robinson 2017: 214).

3.4 Translating reproductive issues

One of the pivotal feminist issues of the 1970s was the question of reproductive rights and technologies, and, more specifically, the topic of abortion. As I mentioned at the beginning of this chapter, as part of the Italian feminist movement, self-help feminist clinics in Italy in the 1970s practised abortions before abortion was legalised in 1978. However, despite the legalisation of abortion, nowadays in Italy this practice is still not guaranteed due to the high number of doctors and pharmacists refusing to perform abortions or to provide abortion pills, invoking a 'conscience clause' (Salvatori 2018: 75).

Many Italian feminist movements – including the transfeminist one – have placed the topic of abortion at the top of their political agenda, like many other feminisms around the world. This happened especially after the mass women's strike in Poland in October 2016, called Black Monday,[28] against the proposal for a total ban on abortion in the country. This strike took inspiration from the first massive demonstrations held in 2015 and 2016 by the above-mentioned movement *Ni Una Menos*. It also inspired a series of protests organised by the movement for the legalisation of abortion in Argentina[29] and in other Latin American countries.

Availability and legalisation of abortion is only one of the topics that feature in the agenda of *Ni Una Menos* (others include femicide, domestic violence, rape, sexual harassment, gender roles, sexual objectification, and the gender pay gap) but is certainly a major concern of the movement. Translation has played – and continues to play – a pivotal role in the internationalisation of this movement. Documents, including articles, assembly reports, public announcements and calls for demonstrations and strikes,[30] which circulate on the movements' web pages and social media accounts or through internal newsletters, are constantly and collectively translated by teams of volunteer translators into e.g. Spanish, Italian, German and English. Moreover, volunteers also act as interpreters during assemblies or at demonstrations.

The international demonstration and assembly organised in Italy by the Italian branch of the movement, *Non Una di Meno*, which took place in 2019 in Verona, defined itself as characterised by a strong transfeminist agenda; the event was called 'Verona città transfemminista' (Verona transfeminist city),[31] and was meant to oppose the 13th International Conference of the World Congress of Families, an American Christian coalition that promotes the value of the 'natural family' and opposes abortion and LGBTQ* rights. The Verona branch of this conference was funded by local authorities and had the support of the far-right League party and other neo-fascist groups. The call for demonstration by *Non Una di Meno*,[32] which was translated into English and Spanish, stressed its opposition to these 'lords of patriarchy', and the fact that behind the 'natural family' lie patriarchal violence and the reproduction of gender hierarchies. The Verona Congress of Families is indeed described as the imposition of compulsory heterosexuality against the freedom of women and LGBTQ* subjects, who refuse to conform to established and prescribed identities and social roles, such as those that see maternity as a destiny and try to subordinate women to a caring role within the family. As part of this control toward non-confirming bodies, we can also include the issue of forced sterilisation imposed on transgender people for years in many European countries, as a condition for legal gender change. In light of this, we can state that reproductive issues (used either to impose reproductive work or deny reproduction rights) have been and still are a weapon used to subjugate certain bodies to the heteronormative dominant system.

This is a scenario that is certainly worth analysing further from a translation studies point of view. A strong emphasis on collective translation (that is, signed simply by the name of the movement) characterises *Non Una di Meno* and other similar movements. This is confirmed in a recent and interesting study by Sergi Mainer (2017) on German anarcho-feminist texts by the collective *Rote Zora*, on reproductive technology and abortion, which were translated into Spanish in 2012. The Spanish translation of the texts by *Rote Zora* refuses to make the names of the translators visible, due to their anarchist critique of private property and authority, and of capitalism in general, stating that this is a collective enterprise. Rote Zora's anarchist translation gives emphasis to egalitarian collaboration between various agents involved in the translation and reception process, validating all their voices and putting them in dialogic relation to each other. It does so in the belief that this de-authorisation can make translation a more efficient instrument of contestation and transformation.

The transfeminist interest in reproductive issues is also confirmed by the references Italian, and especially Spanish, transfeminism makes to the thought of the scholar Donna Haraway, who has been translated into Italian by Claudia Durastanti and Claudia Ciccioni (Haraway 2019b) and by Angela Balzano (Haraway 2019c), as well as into Spanish by transfeminist translator Helen Torres (Haraway 2016c; 2019a).[33] Donna Haraway's 'Chthuchulene Manifesto' in *Manifestly Haraway* (2016b) and her book *Staying with the Trouble. Making Kin in the Chthulucene* (2016a) focus on the importance of making kin both with and among other humans and non-humans. Making kin among humans involves getting connected to persons not bounded by ancestry or genealogy, outside of normative familial (or species-bound) structures. These texts do not discourage giving birth to children but stresses the need to conceive natality more as a collective choice. In her translation of these texts Helen Torres (Haraway 2016c; 2019a)[34] has paid attention to the question of invoking, in a performative way, the idea of making alliances by producing, based on the translation, collective performances, collective writings and games inspired by collective readings. This understanding of translation is indeed in line with the DIY/DIT and the collective and performative uses of translations by transfeminist collectives, mentioned throughout the chapter. Haraway's idea of reproduction that generates kinship instead of children has been also influential for Italian transfeminism, as anticipated above. For Italian transfeminist groups, Haraway's suggestion, which can also be understood as a remedy against the environmental crisis, is meant to encourage us to pay attention to all living species on earth and make alliances especially with migrants, in order to create better conditions of living for all.

4 Conclusion

This chapter has discussed the role of activist translation (see Tymoczko 2010; Baker 2013) in the construction of queer feminist understandings of health: a construction that refuses pathologisation and places emphasis on the concept of self-determination and subjectivity, fighting trans exclusionary, 'essentialist, whoraphobic and technophobic' (Bourcier 2015: 125) views on health and sexuality. It has done so by analysing the translation of trans issues, and of taboo topics in relation of female sexuality and genitalia, and reproductive choices (in particular, abortion), as these are some of the most prominent topics discussed within queer transfeminisms in relation to the concept of health. The translation genres discussed here range from volunteer draft/unpublished translations circulated among collectives and used within workshops, to translations published either by small publishing houses or online (e.g. on websites, Facebook pages, Twitter, Instagram) and to volunteer interpreting. Two main topics have emerged: first, to challenge pathologising heteropatriarchal notions of health requires translation of knowledge and language that have traditionally been censored; second, these translations, generally done collectively, are political tools for the co-creation of new feminist knowledge on health, which involve much experiential knowledge and bodily self-experimentation.

As for the question of censorship, the chapter has shown that terms considered obscene or taboo in relation to female sexuality can be reclaimed in activist translation scenarios, when these act in solidarity with the (trans)feminist cause, as a means to fight against a mainstream heteropatriarchal medical and social system that has silenced these terms. It has also shown that this act of reclaiming is not a smooth one, as it might entail a series of negotiations and self-censorship depending on the specific cultural context in which translation occurs.[35]

In relation to the second topic mentioned above, this chapter has discussed the political importance of translation in the fight against pathologising and heteropatriarchal notions of health by resorting to the idea of DIY (do it yourself) and DIT (do it together) translations. Given the centrality of the notion of self-help in feminism, which I discussed in reference to the recent birth of self-help clinics and practices inspired by those of the 1970s, translation can likewise be understood as a DIY/DIT political practice. On the one hand, this is so because it is used in bodily self-experimentations, and its transformative role thus stems from the profound impact that self-knowledge on body and sexuality can have for political struggles (starting from the feminist idea that the personal is political). On the other hand, volunteer activist translation performed by non-professional translators who are activists can be understood, according to the ethics of the DIY/DIT, as a radical practice that relies on the participants doing as much as possible themselves, given the lack of help and understanding from the institutions. I have written on this DIY/DIT aspect of translation elsewhere (Baldo 2019; Baldo and Inghilleri 2018); I have also analysed the performative aspect of these translations, as they produce new translations, discourses, networks and even performers (as in the case of translator Valentine, aka Fluida Wolf).

Finally, in relation to the DIT aspect of translation, this chapter has focused on the collective dimension of the translation of health issues, performed by groups of volunteer translators/activists. The collective aspect of translation reflects the political importance queer feminisms – especially transfeminisms – have placed on transforming female and LGBTQ* private issues into politically widespread issues, taking them out from the private and invisible space to which they have been relegated by, in this case, a heteropatriarchal medical system aimed at controlling them.

Future research is needed in order to investigate further translational contexts in relation to the topics discussed in this chapter, especially with reference to the translations produced as part of the growing transnational feminist movements which took inspiration from *Ni Una Menos*. These movements are communicating with each other more and more and using translation as part of such communication.

Notes

1 All the back translations of quotes from Italian and other languages into English are mine.
2 See for example the *Centro di Salute per le Donne di Padova* (Women's Health Centre of Padua) founded in 1974. www.femminismo-ruggente.it/femminismo/pdf/salute/salute_1.pdf (Accessed: 30 July 2019).
3 For more information see https://historyitalianfeminism.co.uk/the-fight-for-abortion/the-birth-of-the-self-help-clinics-in-rome/ (Accessed: 30 July 2019).
4 See www.ourbodiesourselves.org/our-story/history/ (Accessed: 28 July 2019).
5 As of April 2019 the book has been translated into 31 different languages. See www.ourbodiesourselves.org/global-projects/ (Accessed: 28 July 2019).
6 *Donne è bello* places much emphasis, like *OBOS*, on sexuality, which was one of the most prominent topics to be discussed within the feminist consciousness-raising groups: a theme that had become important also thanks to the translations into Italian of these and other texts by American radical feminism, to which Italian feminism was looking up to as a source of inspiration (Basilio 2017).
7 New York Radical Women (NYRW) was a feminist group founded in New York city by Shulamith Firestone. The group was active between 1967–1969. For more information see www.thoughtco.com/new-york-radical-women-group-3528974 (Accessed: 30 January 2020).
8 It is interesting to note that in 2014 a book called *Trans Bodies, Trans Selves* (Erickson-Schroth 2014) was published, which was inspired by *OBOS*, and which contained an afterword written by one of the founders of *OBOS*.
9 Although the Italian branch of the movement, called *Non Una di Meno*, states that patriarchy is not only a system of oppression perpetrated by men, the use of male here reproduces the slogan used by the movement, which focuses on the fact that violence against cis and trans women, such as rape and femicides, is almost exclusively a problem related to the heteropatriarchal construction of masculinity.
10 In the UK the movement is called 'Women Strike Assembly' (I am a member of the Leicester branch of this movement). *Ni una Menos* inspired the birth of Women's Marches in the United States. See further info at https://womensmarch.com (Accessed: 31 July 2019).
11 By 'theoretical excesses' Espineira and Bourcier (2016: 88) refer to the fact that the first-wave white Anglophone queer theory relied heavily on poststructuralism, with the consequence of promoting an abstract concept of political subjectivity and dismissing the importance of the embodiment of the political subject.
12 Cisnormativity is the assumption that all human beings are 'cisgender' or 'cissexual', i.e. their gender identity matches the sex assigned to them at birth.
13 I will be discussing the post-porn movement more in depth further in this chapter.
14 See www.makery.info/en/2015/06/30/gynepunk-les-sorcieres-cyborg-de-la-gynecologie-diy/ (Accessed: 31 July 2019).
15 These *consultorie* (self-help clinics) were born in Bologna, Padua and Rome. For the *Consultoria Transfemminista Queer* in Bologna see www.facebook.com/consultoriatfqbologna/ (Accessed 31 July 2019); for the *Consultoria Transfemminista Queer* in Padua, called 'queersultoria' and is now closed, see the description at www.dwf.it/queersultoria-esperimenti-di-welfare-dal-basso-per-un-nuovo-diritto-alla-salute-e-alla-vivibilita/; for a talk on the project of the *Consultoria Transfemminista Queer* in Rome, see www.ondarossa.info/redazionali/2018/02/consultoria-transfemmista-e-riflessioni (Accessed: 31 July 2019).
16 Paul B. Preciado worked for a long period in France as he was Professor of Political History of the Body, Gender Theory, and History of Performance at Université Paris VIII. *Testo yonqui* was also translated into French and English.
17 This is confirmed also by the lack of availability of testosterone for post-menopausal women in the UK to treat hypoactive sexual desire dysfunction (HSDD). Testosterone for women is not licensed by the UK's regulatory authorities and is only available privately. This is in stark contrast to the fact that men are allowed to get testosterone and Viagra prescribed on the National Health Service for their sexual needs. See e.g. the following article www.theguardian.com/society/2019/sep/11/testosterone-postmenopausal-women-uk-hormone (Accessed: 30 January 2020).

18 The concept of techno-gender as formulated by Preciado refers to the idea that bodies are produced and controlled by technology, and more specifically, by the pharmaco-pornographic industrial technology, which regulates and reduces the messy nodes of both sex and gender to a binary form. Technology per se, however, is not considered negative by transfeminism, which instead conceives bodies as tools or technologies through which we can experiment with ways to resist and subvert this techno-patriarchal system.
19 Here I do not want to emphasise a biological masculinity separated from the cultural construction of masculinity. The argument put forward by the assigned women who experimented with testosterone is that the symptoms it produces vary according to our gender expectations and specific bodily configurations. Therefore, the outcome is a mediation between biochemical physical processes and gendered subjectivity and culture.
20 Diana Torres prefers to use the term 'female ejaculation' instead of squirting to challenge gender binarism. This term is also used in the Italian translation.
21 Skene glands were named after the Scottish gynaecologist Alexander Skene, who wrote about it in Western medical literature in 1880.
22 Valentine named her workshops 'ejaculation for cunts'.
23 Some feminist claims that in *The Vagina Monologues* the word 'vulva' should have been used instead. Vagina and vulva are both medical terms, but whereas vulva refers to the external part of the female sexual organ, which is devoted to pleasure due to the presence of the clitoris, vagina is a term preferred by mainstream heteropatriarchal medicine, as it refers to the reproductive part of the female sexual organ.
24 For further information on this aspect, see www.gaystarnews.com/article/china-vagina-monologues170412/ (Accessed: 5 March 2020).
25 For an analysis of other translations of the *Vagina Monologues* see Castro and Ergun (2017a. 2017b).
26 'Türkiye'nin "Vajina Monologları"' (18 May 2008). Available at: www.milliyet.com.tr/pazar/turkiye-nin-vajina-monologlari-545547 (Accessed: 6 March 2020).
27 The translators were Valentine, feminoska, Serbilla Serpente, Elena Zucchini and lafra.
28 See further information at www.bbc.co.uk/news/world-europe-37540139 (Accessed: 31 July 2019).
29 Argentina legalised abortion on 24 January 2021, after the corresponding bill was passed by the National Congress in December 2020. This law was possible thanks to the battles for legal abortion by the aforementioned feminist movement, *Ni Una Menos*.
30 *Non Una di Meno* in Italy produced a document called 'Piano Antiviolenza' (Anti-violence programme) which is currently being translated into English and German.
31 See https://nonunadimeno.wordpress.com/2019/03/29/verona-trans-feminist-city/ (Accessed: 31 July 2019).
32 The text of the call is available at https://nonunadimeno.wordpress.com/2019/03/29/verona-trans-feminist-city/ (Accessed: 31 July 2019).
33 Haraway's thought has greatly influenced transfeminism and the post-porn movement. Her emphasis on the fact that the body becomes an experimentation site, which can be modified and altered by technology, resonates with post-porn ideas about the body as a machine that can be altered.
34 Interview with the author of this chapter, October 2018.
35 For further reading and a list of bibliographic entries on the notion of censorship of taboo/sensitive words in written and audiovisual translations, see the works of José Santaemilia (2014, 2015), who has looked into the nuances of censorship, and the chapter by Martín Ruano (2018), as part of the *Routledge Handbook of Translation and Culture* (Harding and Carbonnell Cortés 2018).

Further reading

Gramling, D. and Dutta, A. (eds) (2016) *Translating Transgender*. Special issue of *TSQ Transgender Studies Quarterly*, 3(3–4).

This special issue focuses on the translation of transgender issues in a variety of cultural contexts and includes many references to health and medicine which can be useful to further clarify concepts discussed in this chapter.

Castro, O. and Ergun, E. (eds) (2017a) *Feminist Translation Studies. Local and Transnational Perspectives*. London and New York: Routledge.

This book is a collection of chapters that analyses feminist translation from a transnational perspective, touching on some of the topics mentioned in this chapter.

Bettcher, T. and Stryker, S. (eds) (2016) *Trans/Feminisms*. Special issue of *TSQ Transgender Studies Quarterly*, 3(1–2).

This edited collection of articles introduces the question of transfeminisms and contains some of the articles mentioned in this chapter along with many others touching on different geographical areas and periods. A very useful resource for examining transfeminism more in depth.

Baldo, M. (2019) 'Translating Spanish Transfeminist Activism into Italian. Performativity, DIY, and Affective Contaminations', *g/s/I*, special issue 'Italian Queer cultures', 6, pp. 66–84.

This chapter gives more background information on the concept of DIY in relation to translation and to the concept of performativity associated with it.

Santaemilia, J. (ed.) (2014) *Gender, Sex, and Translation: The Manipulation of Identities*. New York and London: Routledge.

This book is a useful resource that examines the translation of gender and sexuality and the question of censorship which have been mentioned in this chapter.

Related topics

Translation and Women's Health, Translation in Maternal and Neonatal Health, Disability in Translation

References

Baker, M. (2013) 'Translation as an Alternative Space for Political Action', *Social Movement Studies*, 12(1), pp. 23–47.

Baldo, M. (2019) 'Translating Spanish Transfeminist Activism into Italian. Performativity, DIY, and Affective Contaminations', *g/s/I*, special issue 'Italian Queer cultures' , 6, pp. 66–84.

Baldo M. (2020) 'Queer Translation as Performative and Affective Un-Doing. Translating Butler's *Undoing Gender* into Italian', in Baer, B. J. and Kaindl, K. (eds) *Queering Translation/Translating the Queer*. London and New York: Routledge, pp. 188–205.

Baldo, M. and Inghilleri, M. (2018) 'Cultural Resistance, Female Voices. Translating Subversive and Contested Sexualities', in Harding S-A. and Cortes, O. C. (eds) *The Routledge Handbook of Translation and Culture*. London and New York: Routledge, pp. 296–313.

Basilio E. (2017) '*Donne è bello* and the Role of Translation in the Migration of "Consciousness Raising" from the US to Italy', in Castro, O. and Ergun, E. (eds) *Feminist Translation Studies. Local and Transnational Perspectives*. London and New York: Routledge, pp. 167–180.

Bettcher, T. and Stryker, S. (eds) (2016) *Trans/Feminisms*. Special issue of *TSQ Transgender Studies Quarterly*, 3(1–2).

Bircan, G. A. and Koçak, M. I. (2016) 'Translating Women's Sexuality as Resistance', *Studia filologiczne uniwersytetu Jana Kochanowskiego*, 29(2), pp. 19–31.

Borghi, R. (2014) 'Post-porn. Or: Alice's Adventures in Sexland', in Biasin, E., Maina, G. and Zecca, F. (eds) *Porn after Porn. Contemporary Alternative Pornographies*. Gorizia: Mimesis International, pp. 165–188.

Borghi, R. (2018). *Tran(s)femminismo*. Unpublished paper.

Bourcier, M-H/S. (2015) 'Conclusion. TransRévolution', in Maud-Yeuse, T., Grüsig, N. B. and Espineira, K. (eds) *TransFéminismes*. Paris: L'Harmattan, pp. 125–129.

Busi, B. and Fiorilli, O. (2014) 'Introduzione. Per una prospettiva (trans)femminista sulla salute ai tempi del neoliberismo', *DWF*, 103–104, pp. 5–14.

Castro, O. and Ergun, E. (eds) (2017a) *Feminist Translation Studies. Local and Transnational Perspectives*. London and New York: Routledge.

Castro, O. and Ergun, E. (2017b) 'Pedagogies of Feminist Translation: Rethinking Difference and Commonality across Borders', in Castro, O. and Ergun, E (eds) *Feminist Translation Studies: Local and Transnational Perspectives*. London and New York: Routledge, pp. 93–108.
Consultoria Transfemminista Queer Bologna (2014) 'Ormonautica. Le favolose avventure della consultoria queer nel mondo degli ormoni "sessuali"', *DWF*, 103–104, pp. 17–26.
Cuffman, T. (2015) 'Idle Musical Community: Dischord Records and Anarchic DIY Practice', *Contemporary Justice Review*, 18(1), pp. 4–21.
De Lauretis, T. (1991) 'Queer Theory: Lesbian and Gay Sexualities: An Introduction', *differences*, 3(2), pp. iii–xviii.
Düzel, E., Gül Altınay, A., Adak, H. and Bayraktar, N. (2012) *İşte Böyle Güzelim*. Istanbul: Kitapsepeti.
Egaña Rojas, L. and Solà, M. (2016) 'Hacking the Body. A Transfeminist War Machine', *TSQ: Transgender Studies Quarterly*, 3(1–2), pp. 74–80.
Ensler, E. (1998) *The Vagina Monologues*. New York: Villard.
Erickson-Schroth, L. (ed.) (2014) *Trans Bodies, Trans Selves. A Resource for the Transgender Community*. Oxford: Oxford University Press.
Espineira, K. and Bourcier, M-H/S. (2016) 'Transfeminism. Something Else. Somewhere Else,' *TSQ: Transgender Studies Quarterly*, special issue on Trans/feminisms, 3 (1–2), pp. 84–94.
Grunenwald, N. (2018) 'Non mots, nous-même: aventures de la traduction e de l'édition militantes', unpublished paper presented at the CIRFF conference in Nanterre, 30 August 2018.
Haraway, D. (2016a). *Staying with the Trouble. Making Kin in the Chthulucene*. Durham, NC and London: Duke University Press.
Haraway, D. (2016b) *Manifestly Haraway*. Minneapolis, MN: University of Minnesota Press.
Haraway, D. (2016c) *Manifiesto chthuluceno*. [*Manifestly Haraway*]. Translated by Helen Torres. Laboratory Planet. Available at: https://laboratoryplanet.org/es/manifeste-chthulucene-de-santa-cruz/ (Accessed: 15 December 2020).
Haraway, D. (2019a) *Seguir con el problema: generar parentesco en el chthuluceno* [*Staying with the Trouble. Making Kin in the Chthulucene*]. Translated by Helen Torres. Bilbao: Consonni.
Haraway, D. (2019b) *Chthulucene. Sopravvivere su un pianeta infetto*. [*Staying with the Trouble. Making Kin in the Chthulucene*]. Translated by Claudia Durastanti and Claudia Ciccioni. Milan: Nero edizioni.
Haraway, D. (2019c) *Le promesse dei mostri*. Translated by Angela Balzano. Rome: DeriveApprodi.
Harding, S-A., and Carbonnell Cortés, O. (eds) (2018). *The Routledge Handbook of Translation and Culture*. London and New York: Routledge.
Jarrín, A. (2016) 'Untranslatable Subjects: Travesti Access to Public Health Care in Brazil', *TSQ*, special issue 'Translating Transgender', 3(3–4), pp. 357–375.
Kempson, M. (2015) 'My Version of Feminism: Subjectivity, DIY and the Feminist Zine', *Social Movement Studies*, 14(4), pp. 459–472.
Kinki, K. (2013) 'Ofensiva Transhackfeminista: Your Machine is a Battleground', in Solà, M. and Urko, E. (eds) *Transfeminismos. Epistemes, fricciones y flujos*. Tafalla: Txalaparta, pp. 305–312.
Koyama, E. (2001) *Transfeminist Manifesto*. Available at: http://eminism.org/readings/pdf-rdg/tfmanifesto.pdf (Accessed: 27 July 2019).
Mainer, S. (2017) 'Rote Zora in Spanish. Anarcha-Feminist Activism in Translation', in Castro, O. and Ergun, E. (eds) *Feminist Translation Studies: Local and Transnational Perspectives*. New York and London: Routledge, pp. 181–194.
Martín Ruano, R. (2018) 'Issues in Cultural Translation. Sensitivity, Politeness, Taboo, Censorship', in Harding, S-A. and Carbonell Cortes, O. (eds) *The Routledge Handbook of Translation and Culture*. New York and London: Routledge, pp. 258–278.
Percovich, L. (2005) *La coscienza nel corpo: donne, salute e medicina negli anni settanta*. Milan: Franco Angeli Editore.
Popo, F. (2013) *VaChina Monologues*. Documentary. Available at: https://queerasia.com/vachina-monologues/ (Accessed: 31 August 2020).
Preciado, P. (2008) *Testo Yonqi*. Barcelona: Espasa libros.
Preciado, P. (2015) *Testo tossico. Sesso, droghe e biopolitiche nell'era farmacopornografica*. Translated by Elena Rafanelli. Milan: Fandango.

Robinson, R. (2017) '"Slut" in Translation. The *SlutWalk* Movement from Canada to Morocco', in Castro, O. and Ergun, E. (eds) *Feminist Translation Studies: Local and Transnational Perspectives*. New York and London: Routledge, pp. 208–221.
Salvatori, L. (2018) '"Lost Between the Waves" or Riding a New Tide? Drawing Connections Between Italian and Polish Digitally Mediated Feminism', *Studies in Russian, Eurasian and Central European New Media*, 19, pp. 73–91.
Santaemilia, J. (2009) 'La vie sexuelle de Catherine M: A Journey Through "Woman", Sexual Language and Translation', *Sendebar* 20, pp. 123–141.
Santaemilia, J. (ed.) (2014) *Gender, Sex, and Translation: The Manipulation of Identities*. London and New York: Routledge.
Santaemilia, J. (2015) 'Translating Sex(uality) from English into Spanish and Vice-versa: A Cultural and Ideological Challenge', *ATLANTIS. Journal of the Spanish Association of Anglo-American Studies*, 37(1), pp. 139–156.
Serano, J. (2007) *Whipping Girl, A Transsexual Woman on Sexism and the Scapegoating of Femininity*. Seattle, WA: Seal Press.
Solà, M. (2013) 'Pre-textos, con-textos y textos', in Solà, M. and Urko, E. (eds) *Transfeminismos, epistemes, fricciones y flujos*. Tafalla: Txalaparta, pp. 15–30.
The Boston Women's Health Collective (1971) *Our Bodies, Ourselves*. New York: Simon and Schuster.
The Boston Women's Health Collective (1974) *Noi e il nostro corpo*. Translated by Angela Miglietti. Milan: Feltrinelli.
Torres, D. (2011) *Porno terrorismo*. Tafalla: Txalaparta.
Torres, D. (2014) *Pornoterorismo*. Rome: Golena edizioni.
Torres, D. (2015a) *Coño potens: manual sobre su poder, su prostata y sus fluidos*. Tafalla: Txalaparta.
Torres, D. (2015b) *Fica potens. Un manuale sul suo potere, la sua prostata e i suoi fluidi*. Translated by Luciana Licitra and Valentine Braconcini. Rome: Golena.
Torres, D. (2017a) *Vomitorioum*. Mexico: Self-publication thanks to the project Verkami.
Torres, D. (2017b) *Vomitorium*. Translated by Luciana Licitra. Rome: Golena Edizioni.
Tymoczko, M. (ed.) (2010) *Translation, Resistance, Activism*. Amherst and Boston: University of Massachusetts Press.
Voli, S. (2007) 'Angela Miglietti. Noi e il nostro corpo: Storia di una traduzione', *Zapruder*, 13, pp. 108–115.
Yu, Z. (2015) *Translating Feminism in China: Gender, Sexuality and Censorship*. New York and London: Routledge.
Yu, Z. (2016) 'Translation as Adaptation and Selection: A Feminist Case', *Perspectives*, 25(1), pp. 49–65.
Ziga, I. (2009) *Devenir perra*. Barcelona: Melusina.
Ziga, I. (2014) *Diventar cagna*. Rome: Golena Edizioni

20

Translation and women's health

Nesrine Bessaïh

1 Introduction

This chapter focuses on the translation of women's[1] health texts. It starts by defining the notion of women's health and distinguishing it from the way international organisations and national public health institutions comprehend the health and wellbeing of women. It will therefore present two interpretations of the notion of 'women's health': the one that is used by international organisations (UN, WHO, UNIFEM, etc.) and the one that has emerged from within the women's health movement; in this chapter I will adhere to the latter interpretation. The chapter will present a brief historical overview of the women's health movement and elaborate on its main tenets with regard to health and illness. Particular attention will be given to the notions of 'agency' and 'empowerment', which lie at the root of the criticism women's health movement directs at Western biomedicine and its understanding of health and body.

The second part of this chapter will address in more detail the discourse surrounding health and body. Given the scarcity of studies devoted to women's health texts within translation studies, critical issues will be drawn from research undertaken in related fields. I will present three studies tackling semiotics, grammar and terminology used in medical texts that address women. The perspectives offered in these studies can be usefully applied in translation processes, since they deal with the importance of word choices and connotations, as well as grammatical choices and their implications.

The third part of the chapter will present a multiple-case study (see Susam-Sarajeva 2009) on translation of texts focusing on women's health. It will discuss two of the most translated women's health texts: *Our Bodies, Ourselves* (BWHBC [1971] 2011), and *The Vagina Monologues* (Ensler 1998). A brief introduction to each text will be provided and the work of researchers (mainly translation studies scholars and anthropologists) who studied their dissemination will be outlined. Both of these texts are internationally well-known, as they have been translated into more than 20 languages and widely circulated. The studies will give the occasion to discuss the importance and relevance of adaptation in the area of women's health. Adaptation here will refer to the fact of supplementing or manipulating the text in order to enhance its cultural relevance in its new linguistic and

DOI: 10.4324/9781003167983-25

cultural environment. I will particularly focus on the link between the adaptation process and translator's agency, as well as the ability of the target text to support women's agency and their empowerment around health issues.

2 Definitions

While much literature on health addresses health professionals, this chapter focuses on women's health texts that directly target lay audiences. These texts are often produced with the objective of encouraging reflection or behaviours that favour the improvement of women's health and wellbeing. The World Health Organization (WHO) defines health promotion as follows:

> Health promotion is the process of enabling people to increase control over, and to improve, their health. To reach a state of complete physical, mental and social well-being, an individual or group must be able to identify and to realize aspirations, to satisfy needs, and to change or cope with the environment. [...] Therefore, health promotion is not just the responsibility of the health sector, but goes beyond healthy life-styles to well-being.
>
> *WHO 1986: 426*

Texts stemming from the women's health movement deal with the perception of health, body and intimate relationships, relationships between patients and providers, and physical and mental health. They aim to improve the overall well-being of the people who read them by encouraging them to become active agents in achieving their own health. From this angle, they are texts on health promotion, according to the criteria described by the WHO. However, they are also critical of the way biomedicine, international organisations and national public health organisations tackle the issue of health and wellbeing.

Indeed, when it comes to the concept of 'women's health', there seem to be at least two ways of approaching and defining it: the one used by international health organisations and public health agencies, and the one developed by women's health movement. I will now briefly explain the reasons why this chapter will adhere to the latter perspective.

Texts produced by international organisations (UN, WHO, UNIFEM, etc.) and national public health agencies on the health of women and their wellbeing are mainly concerned with issues like childbirth, nutrition, HIV/AIDS, violence against women and genital mutilation. International organisations usually gather these health topics under the umbrella term 'maternal and infant health' (EWEC 2015). By doing so, they continue to address women's health primarily through the lens of their role as mothers. Moreover, they adopt a perspective where people are objects of knowledge. They consider that there exists one precise way to be healthy and that the health experts are the ones able to define it. The health texts produced by international organisations and national public health institutions aim at circulating this knowledge created by experts and transmitting it to lay people.

In contrast, the women's health movement was built upon issues that affect sexual and reproductive health such as menstruation, abortion, pregnancy and birth, menopause, intimate relationships, violence against women, and sexuality, but from the perspective of the women who experience these processes and situations. The historical development of the movement is rooted in the pursuit of social justice; consequently, it highlights social, legal and institutional parameters that condition women's health and wellbeing.

Moreover, this movement is critical of the way international organisations frame women's health and confine women to an identity of motherhood (Ehrenreich and English 1978; Kuhlmann and Babitsch 2002; Löwy 2005; Vuille *et al.* 2006; Salle and Vidal 2017, Bessaïh and Bogic 2020). More recently, the women's health movement has expanded its focus to include health and safety at work, so as to examine working conditions that are specific to occupations mainly held by women (i.e. domestic workers, cashiers, administrative assistants, teachers, nurses, waitresses, etc.).

In order to better understand the fundamental differences between the two approaches to women's health, it is important to provide a brief overview of the historical development of the links between women and health. Before the 17th century, in Western Europe and North America, healthcare and healing practices were largely undertaken by women. Women were taking care of their families and communities as midwives, herbalists and healers. However, between the 17th and the 19th centuries, the emerging medical profession built its legitimacy upon creating an image of women's bodies as fundamentally dysfunctional and unstable (Ehrenreich and English 1973, 1978; Dorlin 2006). During the same period, the medical profession systematically disqualified women healers and their practices based on the use of herbal remedies and observation of lived experiences (Ehrenreich and English 1973). Already, since the 16th century, a ruthless witch hunt had been raging against independent women, especially those who took care of pregnancies and births, as well as abortions. They were literally burned at the stake (Ehrenreich and English 1973; Barstow 1994; Karlsen 1998; Federici 2004; Chollet 2018). Numbers vary enormously; some texts mention 100,000 victims, while others go up to a million (Chollet 2018: 22).

During the 19th century, medical institutions disqualified most healers apart from medically trained doctors, who continued to gain a clientele both through political pressure and by manipulating the perception of illness (Kohler 1998). During the start of the industrialisation, in upper classes of the society, women were paraded as objects of luxury and having an idle wife was considered a sign of wealth.[2] A condition labelled as 'female invalidism' spread like a fashion; in 1873, Edward H. Clarke, an American physician, claimed that all women would undergo an atrophy of the uterus, especially during puberty. According to his theory, called 'the limited energy theory', the uterus and the brain could not develop simultaneously (Weitz 1998; Oreskes 2019). Female invalidism gave rise to a variety of 'diagnoses', such as neurasthenia (great general weakness), hysteria (nervous breakdown or apathy), and nymphomania (uncontrollable or excessive sexual desire in a woman; consequently, propensity for masturbation or auto-eroticism) – 'conditions' which could easily have been linked to the extended home confinement mentioned above. Women with 'mild disorders' were prescribed bed or mental rest, isolation or diets. For others, doctors prescribed purges, bleeds and mercury-based drugs. If the symptoms were severe, doctors would resort to hysterectomy (removing the uterus) or clitoridectomy (removing the clitoris).[3] Doctors' professional interest in considering rich women as 'sick' was in line with their financial interests and with an ideology that wanted to keep upper-class women out of the labour market. The 'limited energy theory' supports the general political ideology at the time regarding the role assigned to women: reproduction. During the 19th and early 20th centuries, some researchers and physicians did criticise this approach, but it was only during the second half of the 20th century that a fully critical perspective emerged, enabling women to deconstruct this medico-patriarchal vision of their bodies and giving rise to a movement.

During the 1960s, through consciousness-raising groups in the United States, lay women began sharing their experiences around health and their interactions with the medical system and health professionals. The process of putting together these experiences, their critical thinking and the results of the research they undertook, led to the development of self-help groups in health and formed the basis of a highly critical analysis of Western biomedicine. In the following decades, research undertaken from this critical perspective has upheld the centrality accorded to lived experiences and the importance given to social and cultural factors. As Kuhlman and Babitsch observe:

> Women's health research confronts the interpretive power of biomedical discourse and biomedical structures with a complex understanding of health and experience-based competence in dealing with health and illness. Researchers in this field [...] emphasize the significance of the conditions of social life and clearly reject biomedicine's fixation on individual risk and behavior as the main factors influencing health and illness. This perspective is based on an empirical, praxis-oriented concept which questions the naturalization of health and illness and instead highlights social and cultural factors.
>
> *2002: 92*

Throughout the 1970s and 1980s, the women's health movement developed and spread this vision, mainly in North America and Western Europe. It has approached biomedicine with a pragmatic stand: reclaiming some of the progress and solutions (i.e. analgesics used during labour and birth, birth control) while maintaining their critical perspective. While it could be argued that the movement gradually has lost its strength – as more and more books, magazines and public policies took an interest in the subject of women's health, but not always from a critical perspective (Davis 2007) – today it continues to critique Western biomedicine and the way international organisations and national public health institutions approach health and wellbeing.

This critique and challenge can be grouped into three main areas. First, the women's health movement is critical of the paternalistic approach that relies solely on the experts' production of a supposedly objective knowledge. In accordance with the consciousness-raising groups at the source of its creation, the movement values 'subjective knowledge produced by individuals and shared as situated knowledges about their health and well-being', stemming from collectivised individual experiences (Bessaïh and Bogic 2020: 519). For example, biomedicine had promoted the practice of episiotomy – surgical cut of the perineum and the vaginal wall at the end of labour in order to 'facilitate' the passage of the baby (objective knowledge). It is thanks to the reports made by a multitude of women about the unjustified and across-the-board use of this intervention, and the fact that reconstitution was difficult and sometimes so poor that women had to live with incontinence for the rest of their lives (subjective/experiential knowledge), that this intervention has been gradually losing popularity.

The women's health movement is also critical of the biomedical perspective that health problems arise as a result of individuals' behaviours. Instead it proposes a global approach to health and an analysis based on social determinants of health and well-being. Moreover, the movement holds a role of surveillance and vigilance with regard to medical and pharmaceutical devices that may have fatal consequences for women users. For example, hormone replacement therapy (HRT) has been systematically prescribed during the 1980–1990s to perimenopausal women. However, during the 2000s, research has demonstrated that certain types of HRT increase the risk of breast cancer and stroke (Health Canada 2006).

Furthermore, the very concept of 'women's health' did not exist before the development of a movement around these issues. Indeed, it is only during the 1960s, when women started gathering around the project which led to the publication of *Our Bodies, Ourselves* (hereafter, *OBOS*) in the United States, that they proposed this term. According to Davis, the book is at the origin of the notion of women's health as a field of action and study. 'The concept of women's health – unknown prior to the publication of the first edition of *OBOS* – has since become a reputable field' (Davis 2007: 47). Following the first publication of *OBOS* (1971) and the rise of this movement, scientific research and public policies in this field began to appear in the United States. As Davis observes, '[*OBOS*] has not only enjoyed a widespread popularity, unique for a feminist book, but has also transformed the provision of healthcare, helped shape healthcare policies and stimulated research on women's health in the United States' (2007: 2). For all the reasons discussed above, this chapter addresses women's health according to the perspective of the movement that has developed the very concept.

3 Historical and critical perspectives

Translations of texts on women's health is a relatively new area within translation studies and so far, very few works have tackled the issue. An overview of research published between 2007–2019 in the main translation studies journals[4] reveals that only three articles have been published on this theme during this period:[5] one by Şebnem Susam-Sarajeva (2010), one by Anna Bogic and myself (2016) and one by Mwamba Chibamba (2019). I will present the content of my article with Anna Bogic in the next section on *OBOS*. The article by Chibamba displays a perspective frequently taken in relation to the translation of health texts in general: the importance of adaptation. The article by Susam-Sarajeva touches on an important and recent current in translation studies: the contribution of translation to the circulation of ideas and social changes. In this section, I will first briefly present the arguments of Chibamba and Susam-Sarajeva, then I will turn to disciplines such as linguistic anthropology and terminology to highlight a number of issues related to women's health texts.

3.1 Adaptation

Mwamba Chibamba's article is rooted in the theoretical approach of Hans Vermeer's skopos theory (2000) and analyses how cultural context shapes translational choices. The author focuses on a mother and child nutrition campaign in Zambia. The material she examines is more affiliated with the approaches of international organisations to health than to the women's health movement discussed earlier. Based on this case study, Chibamba illustrates the need for adaptation or, in other words, taking the culture into account and transforming the source text and its message, process or communication medium when necessary. Translation here is supplemented by adaptation and translators adopt the role of mediators who transfer the message interlinguistically as well as intersemiotically. According to Chibamba, 'the most important consideration in the communicative process is not how much the target text adheres to the source text but rather how the message is designed and packaged for a specific audience and how it is received' (2019: 13). This article is therefore in line with other research on translation of health texts intended for a lay audience, insofar as it stresses the importance of adaptation (see Colantonio *et al.* 2016, Taibi and Ozolins 2016, Rey 2007, Yoda 2007, Gilley 2006, Bernhardt 2004).

3.2 *Circulation of ideas*

In her article, Şebnem Susam-Sarajeva (2010) focuses on the contribution of translation to the circulation of ideas and schools of thought within the field of maternal and infant health. She analyses texts uploaded on the net by a non-professional translator, an obstetrician involved in the natural birth movement in Turkey. Her work reveals the various forms translation can take within cyberactivism. Direct translation, reported speech, interpretation of source text as well as 'autochtonous writings' (2010: 232) coexist within the obstetrician's web-publications, without being clearly distinguished from one another. She highlights '[...] that the electronic medium strongly influences the way translations are carried out, integrated into other textual productions and disseminated to audiences [...]' (2010: 242). Susam-Sarajeva also shows that the ideology of the natural birth movement and the personal beliefs of the obstetrician influence his translational choices, including omissions and additions. Translating thus constitutes one of the tools that the Turkish natural birth movement uses to influence and transform local maternity services and to challenge the way modernity is defined by dominant meta-narratives in Turkish society in regard to childbirth and parenthood.

3.3 *Linguistic and terminological issues in women's health texts*

Critical analyses of texts concerning women's health have identified three issues that contribute to the image of the female body as 'flawed' and 'passive': the use of the passive voice, metaphors and terminology. Here I will focus on two such analyses: first by Emily Martin (1991, [1987] 1992), a feminist anthropologist who described these linguistic and paradigmatic issues, and Lynn Bowker (2001), a terminologist and translation scholar, who studied the terminology of infertility.

Martin is interested in the way biomedicine presents women's physiological processes. She shows that in biomedicine, women are considered to be passive and lacking any control over their bodies while these processes take place:

> For example, if a woman's labor slows down because her contractions are not sufficiently strong [...] most obstetrics texts suggest these causes: the pelvis is too small; the foetus is not positioned properly; or the uterus is too distended [objective knowledge]. Nowhere it is suggested that the woman's general state of mind (fear, anxiety) [subjective knowledge] might have led her to stop her labor.
>
> *Martin 1992: 62*

Women themselves have internalised this way of seeing and understanding their own processes and this has an impact on the way they talk about the experiences they go through. For instance, they will describe their pregnancy or the birth of their babies referring to measurable and external parameters, instead of referring to their emotions, sensations or lived experiences. Martin suggests that the use of the passive voice is symptomatic of this particular conception of women's body and health.

Lisa Campo-Engelstein, a feminist bioethicist, and Nadia Johnson, a semantic scholar, have applied Martin's analysis to textbooks published in the United States between 2005 and 2010 for middle-school science classes and for medical schools. They found out that women's physiological processes were still associated with passivity. For example, while the sperm is presented as active, the ovum is seen as passive:

> In almost all textbooks, we encountered the passive language 'the egg is fertilized' [...] whereas the egg is merely the object in which this action takes place. While it is true that fertilization takes place within the egg, the egg also plays an active role in the process of fertilization [...]. This passive language could easily be substituted by more active language that includes both the egg and the sperm, such as [...] 'the sperm and egg fuse together' [or] 'combine'.
>
> *Campo-Engelstein and Johnson 2014: 206*

According to Martin, active voice contributes to restoring women's agency toward their health and promotes a perspective that favours the production of subjective knowledge on health.

On a paradigmatic level, Martin shows that metaphors used to describe reproduction are indicative of the unequal and patriarchal ways medicine approaches men and women. For instance, the ovum and the sperm are represented according to sexist stereotypes pertaining to men and women:

> [Scientists] liken the egg's role to that of sleeping beauty: 'a dormant bride awaiting her mate's magic kiss, which instils the spirits that brings her to life'. Sperm by contrast have a 'mission' which is to 'move through the female genital tract in quest of the ovum'. One popular account has it that the sperm carry out a 'perilous journey' into the 'warm darkness' where some fall 'exhausted'. 'Survivors' 'assault' the egg, the successful candidates 'surrounding the prize'.
>
> *Martin 1991: 104*

In light of these observations, while translating women's health texts, arguably more so than any other text type, one must pay a great deal of attention to metaphors and their implications. As Martin puts it, 'one clear feminist challenge is to wake up sleeping metaphors in science, particularly those involved in the description of the egg and the sperm' (1991: 112).

Lynne Bowker studied the terminology of infertility used in scientific and lay health texts (2001). She discusses the terms and their collocations in order to characterise the ways gender, body and sexuality are conceptualised in medical texts. Bowker underscores that biomedicine tends to define the woman's body as 'faulty' and this perception is reflected in the terminology. She gives the example of the 'incompetent cervix', which is the term given to 'a situation in which a woman's cervix does not remain closed during pregnancy and which can therefore result in an extremely premature birth' (Bowker 2001: 598). Through an analysis of a general corpus (language for general purposes in texts that target lay audiences), she identifies that 'incompetent' is associated with words like 'idiots', 'fool' or 'morons'. These collocations indicate that 'incompetent' has a negative connotation and is generally used to devalue something or someone. In contrast, medical texts on infertility choose to qualify a male 'ejaculation' as being 'retrograde', rather than 'incompetent' – a term generally associated with other terms like 'flow', 'motion' and 'rotation', which are more neutral (2001: 598).

Similarly, when infertility is due to a malfunction in the immune system, it is referred to as 'hostility' for the female body – a particularly negative term – while much more neutral terms are used when this malfunction is found in male bodies, such as 'antibodies' or 'auto-immunity' (2001: 595). Bowker gives numerous examples such as 'insufficiency', 'faulty', 'inadequate' on the feminine side and 'low', 'too few', 'reduced' on the masculine side. The terms used to talk about women's bodies are systematically more negative than the ones used for men's bodies. In Bowker's words,

> In the semi-specialized literature, men are clearly perceived to be suffering from a serious medical condition with a seriously technical name; women in contrast, are not perceived to be suffering from a medical condition but are simply at fault – they HAVE problems, ARE abnormal or FAIL in their task [...].
>
> *2001: 597*

To sum up this section, research undertaken in translation studies on the translation of health texts addressing lay people stresses the importance of adaptation and the contribution of translation to the circulation of ideas and schools of thought. Research in related fields highlights the impact of grammatical choices (active versus passive voice), terminological choices (collocations and connotations), and metaphors in health texts on women's positive perception of themselves and on their empowerment as agents for their own health and wellbeing.

4 Current contributions and research

In this section, I will turn to research that has analysed translation of texts stemming from the women's health movement and focus on literature which studies two of the most translated texts in this area: *The Vagina Monologues* (Ensler 1998; hereafter *TVM*), and *OBOS* (BWHBC 2011), both originating from the United States. They are thus characteristic of the prevalent international translation flows: the majority of source texts in general are in English or French and are translated into other languages, while information flow in the opposite direction is significantly less frequent (Benmessaoud and Buzelin 2018; UNESCO 2019). This flow is indicative of the cultural and geopolitical domination of the United States and former colonial states (United-Kingdom and France) over other cultures in the world (Robinson 1997).

The circulation of *TVM* and of *OBOS* have been framed differently from each other and allowed varying degrees of freedom to the translators in the adaptation of these texts. While translators of *OBOS* are actively encouraged to reappropriate the text and adapt it to their own cultures, *TVM* circulates mostly under a fixed format determined by its author and the institution she built around the book. These translational conditions determine whether or not the target texts will be culturally relevant and therefore will support readers' agency, a notion of great importance to the women's health movement.

4.1 The Vagina Monologues

TVM was created between 1996 and 1998 by the American feminist playwright Eve Ensler. Ensler interviewed about 200 women, mostly living in the United States, from different ethnic and racial groups and sexual orientations, and with a range of life experiences.

Their narratives were based on their experience of sexuality, sexual health and violence against women (sexual abuse, rape, genital mutilation, domestic violence) and were then turned into monologues gathered together in a theatrical play. It is difficult to establish exactly how many monologues formed the 'original' play as it was staged at different events and did not always comprise the same number of monologues. Moreover, in 2001, Ensler launched an annual campaign called the V-Day,[6] for which she continues to write new monologues every year, based on new interviews she conducts with women in and outside the United States. The V-day campaign aims at raising funds for grassroots organisations which fight to end violence against women, girls and gender non-conforming[7] people. No fees are charged to use the rights of the play staged around the V-Day (14 February) each year; in return, all proceeds must go to organisations working to stop gender-based violence. In 2019, for the 20th anniversary of the play, the V-day campaign offered the monologues in 45 different languages and noted that the play would be performed in 140 countries. The map of the campaign website reveals that these locations are mostly in North America and Western Europe but also, to a lesser extent, in Eastern Europe, Asia, South America and Africa.[8] There are however, two more stipulations:[9] If the local groups are to link their performances to the V-day campaign and benefit from the rights exemption, the performance has to take place between 1 February and 8 March each year, and, most importantly for the purpose of this chapter, the scripts should be those translated by V-day campaign coordinators based in the United States and thus cannot be adapted locally. Hereafter, I present three studies documenting the translation projects of TVM, some of which have a dimension of adaptation.

Jelena Djordjevic is a Serbian activist working against the trafficking of women and girls; she is one of the founders of the Anti-Trafficking Center, a local NGO dedicated to the issue. In 2006, she coordinated the organisation of a local performance of *TVM* that involved several of the region's languages. Djordjevic observes that 'the performance of *Vagina Monologues* in different Slavic languages enabled women across regional borders to understand each other through the universal language of their bodies' (2006: 1). She describes her work in the context of a recently established Serbian state and underscores that the collaboration of activists from various Serbian, Bosnian and Croatian organisations, together with actresses from different ethnic backgrounds, allowed the (re)construction of solidarities beyond the ethnic divide:

> Having all those activists present, including KOLO [Women's Cross-Cultural Collaboration] from Bosnia and Herzegovina, and an actress from Croatia, showed that the lines of ethnic divide that fuelled [*sic*] the war in former Yugoslavia can be crossed with such a small step.
>
> *Djordjevic 2006: 5*

Thus, she asserts that the circulation of the play served local interests in terms of cohesion building.

Sea Ling Cheng, an anthropology professor at the Chinese University of Hong Kong, has been part of the project of translating and adapting *TVM*, and organising venues for its stage production in Hong Kong. As her work was not staged during the prescribed period around the V-day, and, most importantly, as she undertook a process of adaptation of the monologues, she did not benefit from the rights' exemption. In her article (2009), Cheng addresses the fact that the conditions of circulation established by the V-day campaign (using only the original text or the translation produced by the campaign itself, and not being allowed to add, modify or omit any parts or passages) form an obstacle to the localisation of *TVM*. Cheng notes:

> I attempted to negotiate for an adaptation of the play. But I never received a response to my inquiries from the V-day agent and these attempts consequently failed. Therefore, I finally decided to devise a production that could speak more directly to a local audience rather than through 'borrowed voices'.
>
> *2009: 23*

Cheng raises important questions about the ways an American text, which necessarily entails a culturally specific understanding of body, sexuality and violence, can be transferred to another geopolitical and cultural environment that has its own social, historical and political contexts, and still manages to respect local women's struggles. She points out that 'concerned feminists may develop more effective coalitions with local women by recognizing and identifying locally derived creative efforts to respond to issues that are pertinent to their lives' (Cheng 2009: 32).

Through the adaptation process, Cheng managed to address local terminological issues linked to passivity and agency, as raised by the women's health movement discussed above. The term 'vagina' itself entails notions of passivity in Chinese (Cantonese) as it is composed from the root 'yin' (陰) that designates a feminine principle associated with passivity:

> The literal translation of 'vagina' in Chinese is 'the yin channel/road (陰道)'– as opposed to 'the yang instrument (陽具)', the penis. The terms directly reflect the gender distinction in the yin/ yang concept within Chinese cosmology. The passive/ active dichotomy is also obvious in the distinction between 'channel/road' and 'instrument'.
>
> *Cheng 2009: 24*

The title of the play was translated as *Stories of Our Little Sisters*; Cheng explains that 'little sisters' is a label that young Chinese women use to designate their vaginas, in a gesture of re-appropriating male language (labelling penises as 'little brothers') and gaining power over their own bodies: 'Through this discursive appropriation of a predominantly male linguistic practice, these women are able to invest the muted part of the female body as a site of desire with a certain subjectivity' (Cheng 2009: 24).

Beyond Cheng's adaptation/translation into Cantonese, there are two translations of *TVM* in Mainland China into Mandarin that were not undertaken by the V-day campaign. Zhongli Yu (2017) compares the trajectories of these two different translations: one conducted by Rongjun Yu, the manager of the Shanghai Dramatic Arts Center, and the other one carried out by Xiaoming Ai, a professor of Chinese at the University of Sun Yat-sen in Guangzhou, who is also known for her feminist engagement. Whereas Rongjun Yu maintained most of the content of the play and even kept American slang words in English to designate the vagina, Xiaoming Ai omitted parts of the text and used several translation and adaptation strategies. For example, Ai presented the American monologues in her classes and used them to trigger new local narratives that she then added to the play.

Zhongli Yu draws a correlation between the degree of adaptation and the positive reception of the text within the target culture. The version by Rongjun Yu was quickly censored while Xiaoming Ai's version continues to circulate online and at universities. Yu demonstrates that adaptation, or what she frames as 'the three-dimensional transformations (i.e. linguistic, cultural and communicative dimensions)' (2017: 50), are essential to the survival of the text in its host culture. Ai had much more agency when translating the text. She took the freedom to transform it by bringing in local and significant experiences. Her agency enhanced the target text and made it more relevant to the target culture. It has thus more chances to support women's agency and empowerment within local contexts. By creating their own versions of a source text, translators develop new local knowledges that can be viewed as more relevant and that can also contribute to the strengthening of women's activism locally.

4.2 Our Bodies, Ourselves

As mentioned earlier, *OBOS* is a major book in women's health; its first publication in 1971 has been associated with the rise of the women's health movement in the United States (Morgen 2002; Davis 2007). *OBOS* is characterised by three key features that set it apart from other women's health texts: it comprises women's personal narratives that echo the sharing of experiences in consciousness-raising groups; medical information researched by the women themselves that has allowed them to better understand their health, body and sexuality; and, critical social and political analyses that reflect the awareness raised by the women's liberation movement. The combination of these features has contributed to the success and transformative power of *OBOS*. It has been able to reach women readers, challenge them and afford them a position of agency with regard to their own health (Morgen 2002; Löwy 2005; Davis 2007). As Davis observes, 'from the beginning, the authors of *OBOS* [...] believed that by providing experientially based, critical knowledge they were opening up individual and collective avenues of empowerment to all women' (2007: 48).

OBOS touches on numerous subjects: anatomy, sexual orientation, masturbation, contraception, abortion, pregnancy, birth, menopause and aging, as well as violence against women. The book has been a tremendous success and the American version has sold over four million copies since 1971 in the United States and abroad. It has been revised and edited eight times (1973, 1976, 1979, 1984, 1992, 1998, 2005 and 2011). As Morgen argues, it 'would be difficult to exaggerate the impact of *Our Bodies, Ourselves* [...]. Erupting into the void (there were few popular books about women's health before it), *Our Bodies, Ourselves* created its own niche' (2002: 19). Immediately after the first edition, translations followed in the 1970s and 1980s, and continue to be undertaken today by different women's groups.[10] To date, there are more than 30 translations around the world.

Kathy Davis offers the most extensive study of *OBOS* translations. She identifies three waves of translation activity: from 1970 to 1982 in Western Europe and Japan, from 1982 to 1996 in Asia, Africa and the Middle East, and from 1996 to 2006 in Eastern Europe (2007: 52–53). Davis raises the issue of the conditions of translation, adaptation and dissemination of a book stemming directly from American culture. She suggests that *OBOS* is a transnational phenomenon, one that does not impose itself through cultural imperialism. She argues that *OBOS* is locally adapted by women who are the most concerned in terms of its content. In fact, with the first translations in the 1970s, the authors (The Boston Women's Health Book Collective) found out that the success of the book made it attractive for publishers who simply wanted to make a profit. In order to preserve the potential of the book in supporting women's empowerment, they decided to award publication and translation rights only to feminist publishers or to women's groups dedicated to the defence of women's rights. They thus established the conditions according to which the book could be adapted; this could only be done by those intimately familiar with the cultural and social realities affecting women readers locally.

Following Davis, several scholars have studied the translations of *OBOS*. Here I will discuss three of them: Boya Li's study of the Chinese version (2018), Ester Shapiro's of the Latin-American version (2013) and our study with Anna Bogic on the translations into French (2016).

Boya Li (2018) examines the Chinese translation published in 1998. Based on interviews with the translators and on comparisons between the source text and the target text, Li traces the social and historical conditions underlying the Chinese translation. In 1995, when China welcomes the 4th United Nations conference on women, the country was gradually opening up to the market economy. At the political level, this positioning was reflected in the introduction of new texts into China, including feminist ones such as *OBOS*, which was first presented at a course on the history of Western feminism at Tianjin University in 1993. Li's work demonstrates the importance of adaptation as well as the way it is negotiated through various actors involved in the translation process. The translation team consisted of medical doctors, scholars in social sciences and literary translators. Some translation negotiations took place within this team. For example, physicians routinely used the term 'patients', while feminist team members insisted that the term 'women' should be used instead. Another example is when the translation team chose to use the term 'self-consolation' when talking about masturbation, and not the more commonly used term 'hand lewdness'. Through their negotiations and by using their critical lens, the translation team sought to deconstruct the prevalent negative perspective on sexuality and replace it with a more positive one. Publishers also had an impact on translation and adaptation choices. For example, it was at the level of the publishing house that the decision was made to remove the chapter on homosexuality. Some members of the translation team circumvented this censorship by circulating a version of the target text that maintained the chapter through underground channels of gay rights NGOs and Chinese universities. Through their negotiations, their strategies and their agency throughout all stages of the project, the more feminist translators in the team sought to support women's empowerment locally.

Shapiro, an American of Cuban origin, is a professor at the University of Massachusetts in Boston. From 1994 to 2000, she was the coordinator of the second translation and adaptation of *OBOS* into Spanish, *Nuestros cuerpos, nuestras vidas* (2000). In her study, she adopts an empirical approach and takes an activist stance to explore the context underlying the translation, as well as the cultural and political aspects that frame the process. She asks: 'What makes it possible to translate a feminist women's health text so both health education knowledge and messages activating women's empowered connections to local/global social movements successfully cross cultural borders in new sociopolitical contexts and evolving historical times?' (2013: 22). She describes the background to her decision to coordinate the translational and editorial choices made during the process. She presents the political orientations of the translators involved and their anchoring in the Latin-American tradition of social action. For her, the elaboration of a Spanish version of *OBOS* supports social change, as long as the process implies the participation of several people and organisations involved in critical thinking and knowledge construction. Shapiro notes that the 'overview of *NCNV* [*Nuestros cuerpos nuestras vidas*] translation/

adaptation decisions illuminates guiding frameworks and pedagogical practices that can help community-engaged health educators convey specific knowledge while also inspiring shared processes leading to societal change' (2013: 23). Thus, Shapiro demonstrates the importance of grounding the translation in local culture and of the fact that a translation and adaptation works best if undertaken by individuals who have at heart the rights and wellbeing of the people primarily addressed by the content. She illustrates how the specific parameters of the circulation of *OBOS* allow for the creation of knowledge and support local actions that aim to improve women's living conditions.

Anna Bogic and I studied the translations of *OBOS* into French published over a period of 40 years: the French version of 1977 in France, the Senegalese version of 2004 and the French-language version for Quebec published in 2019. Our study (Bessaïh and Bogic 2016) is based on interviews with the translators, textual analysis, ethnography (including participant observation)[11] and genetic criticism.[12] Through these three versions, we examined the use of the phrase 'nous les femmes [us, the women]'. Historically, and in the source text, this sentence has played the role of a slogan that has the power to unite women and call them to action: 'The pronoun "we" as a discursive element hails women reading the book and invites them to join the feminist movement. It constitutes a perlocutionary act [...], that is, a speech act that calls women readers to action'[13] (Bessaïh and Bogic 2016: 45). However, this particular role is less obvious in the French-language versions. These translations shed light on the shifting meaning of 'nous [we]' and the obstacles to a universalising conception of the term. In the French version of the 1970s, the 'we' sometimes stands for the French team undertaking the translation; sometimes it echoes the 'we' of the American team of authors; and, at other times, it represents the universalising 'we, the women'. Just as in the source text, the call to action uses the perlocutionary power of the expression to trigger action; however, the shifting meanings of 'we' in this translation cause confusion. In the West African version of 2004, the 'we' designates West Africans. The collective identity the translators refer to has more to do with ethnicity and race rather than with sex and gender. In the Quebecois version, the 'we' designates the translation and adaptation team. This is mainly because, in the feminist movement in Quebec in the 2010s, the use of a universalising 'we' is perceived as a negation of the diversity of experiences and identities of women and gender non-conforming people.

In all the French-language versions discussed above, the differential usage of the 'nous [we]' opens a window on to the translators' agency in the translation and adaptation process. Their ideology, as well as the social, cultural and political environments they work in, cause them to invest the definition of a collective identity with different meanings. In doing so, they construct a significant text for their local movements; and, they also develop knowledges that empower women collectively in accordance with their cultural and socio-historical realities.

To conclude this section, it is important to note that the most recent research on translation and women's health texts focuses primarily on agents and processes. This research is in accordance with the reflections of the women's health movement on women's agency and it looks at terminology and grammar with a view to supporting this agency locally. In addition, similar to research on the translation of health texts in general, research on translation and women's health underscores the importance of adaptation for the benefit of lay people, and illustrates that, when translators seek to promote women's agency, their own agency allows them to support the local production of subjective knowledge on women's health and wellbeing.

5 Conclusion

The notion of women's agency is at the heart of the issues surrounding women's health. It constitutes a key element in the rise of this movement as well as in the critique that this movement has articulated about Western biomedicine. In the same way, analysis of women's health texts has insisted on the importance of agency whether it be through the deconstruction of established patriarchal metaphors or the attention accorded to terminology and use of passive/active voices. Thanks to translation, these women's health texts travel across linguistic and cultural borders and seek to support local women's agency and empowerment worldwide.

However, as we have seen in the discussion on *TVM* and *OBOS* translations, these travels may come with their own significant issues. The circulation of *TVM* is framed in a rigid way: the author and the American institution she has built around the book maintain control over the translation process and limit any possibility of adaptation. This is despite the fact that, according to the studies quoted above, the adapted versions of *TVM* – the ones that do not benefit from the rights' exemption – seem to have a longer lifespan and are more meaningful locally. In the case of *OBOS*, the translators are encouraged to adapt the text and integrate elements that stem from local women's life conditions, as well as socio-economic and historical contexts. As Kathy Davis argues,

> The translators adopted this process of collective knowledge making, using their translations to generate similar discussions among women in their own context. It is this feature of *OBOS* – more than its informational content, its format, or its specific feminist politics of health – that ultimately proved to be universally translatable.
> *(Davis 2007: 195)*

Most importantly, the examples analysed in this chapter illustrate the crucial link between translators' agency and women's agency, revealing the far-reaching impact of text circulation not only on individual readers but also on the entire women's health movement.

Notes

1 It is important to note that the use of the term 'woman' in this chapter is non-essentialist. 'Woman' here refers to a social category that is still socially, economically, politically, symbolically and representationally minoritised at local and international levels. It can therefore include any person who identifies as a woman: trans and cis women, as well as non-binary people who identify themselves somewhere on the spectrum of femininity. It can even include, in certain aspects, individuals who have been assigned female at birth but who do not identify with this label, although they do share certain organs and physiological experiences with cis women.

2 In working classes, women had to work, and often had to work hard, to support their families. However, when a man was rich enough, it was a sign of wealth that his wife stayed at home, using a cook, gardener, nanny and servants to fulfil the domestic tasks. The 'lady of the house' was not supposed to do anything – neither work for money outside the house nor do much inside the house. This 'idleness', and the consequent dedication of all her time to being 'a beautiful object', could thus bear witness to her husband's wealth.

3 In the United States, the last clitoridectomy prescribed to 'cure' disorders related to an alleged 'womanly condition' was performed in the mid-20th century (Rodríguez 2014).

4 *Meta*, *Target*, *The Translator*, *Traduction Terminologie et Rédaction (TTR)*, *Translation and Interpreting Studies*, and *Translation Studies*.

5 There is also one article by Rebecca Tipton (2017) on interpretation in a context related to violence against women; however, this article is out of the scope of the present chapter.

6 www.vday.org/homepage.html (Accessed: 11 July 19).

7 www.vday.org/organize-event.html (Accessed: 2 April 2020).
8 See the V-Day campaign map at https://vspot.vday.org/vday/events (Accessed: 29 May 2019).
9 See the 'Organize an event' section of the V-Day website: www.vday.org/organize-event.html (Accessed: 20 February 2020).
10 See the 'Global initiative' section on OBOS website: www.ourbodiesourselves.org/global-project (Accessed: 20 February 2020).
11 I had been involved in the collective project of translating *Our Bodies, Ourselves* into Quebec French and adapting it to the Quebec context. I had thus access to the process and could observe through participation even before the publication of the target text.
12 Genetic criticism is an emerging methodology in translation studies that consists of studying the various drafts that preceded the final text (Fenoglio and Chanquoy 2007; Lavieri 2015).
13 My translation from the French original: 'Le "nous", en tant qu'élément discursif, interpelle ainsi les lectrices et les invite à joindre les mouvements féministes. Il constitue un acte perlocutoire, c'est-à-dire un acte de parole qui provoque l'action en incitant les lectrices à agir' (Bessaïh and Bogic 2016: 45).

Further reading

Davis, K. (2007) *The Making of* Our Bodies, Ourselves. *How Feminism Travels Across Borders.* Durham, NC and London: Duke University Press.

This study offers a global, critical and transnational vision of the dissemination and impact of translations of a women's health text.

Ehrenreich, B. and English, D. (1973) *Witches, Midwives and Nurses: A History of Women Healers.* New York: The Feminist Press.

Ehrenreich, B. and English, D. (1978) *For Her Own Good: 150 Years of the Experts' Advice to Women.* Garden City, NY: Anchor Press/Doubleday.

Ehrenreich and English's work constitutes a milestone in the development of feminist knowledge and research about women's historical relation to health in the Western world. These are key books in understanding the women's health movement's criticism of Western biomedicine.

Cheng, S. L. (2009) 'Questioning Global Vaginahood: Reflections from Adapting the *Vagina Monologues* in Hong Kong', *Feminist review*, 92(1), pp. 19–35.

This article illustrates the importance of translators' agency in the process of translating and circulating a text on women's health. It also gives an occasion to read about the circulation of women's health texts in China.

Related topics

Translation in Maternal and Neonatal Health, Queer Feminisms and the Translation of Sexual Health, Quality, Accessibility and Readability in Medical Translation

References

Barstow, A. L. (1994) *Witchcraze. A New History of the European Witch Hunt.* New York: Harper Collins.

Benmessaoud, S. and Buzelin, H. (2018) 'Publishing Houses and Translation Projects', in Harding, S. A. and Carbonnell Cortés, O. (eds) *The Routledge Handbook of Translation and Culture.* London and New York: Routledge, pp. 154–176.

Bernhardt, J. M. (2004) 'Communication at the Core of Effective Public Health', *American Journal of Public Health*, 94(12), pp. 2051–2053.

Bessaïh, N. and Bogic, A. (2016). '"Nous les femmes" de 1970 à 2017 à travers les traductions et adaptations de Our Bodies Ourselves en français', *TTR: Traduction, Terminologie et Rédaction*, 29(2), pp. 43–71.

Bessaïh, N. and Bogic, A. (2020) 'Translating Texts on Women's Sexual and Reproductive Health', in von Flotow, L. and Kamal, H. (eds) *Handbook on Translation and Feminism*. London and New York: Routledge, pp. 518–527.

Bowker, L. (2001) 'Terminology and Gender Sensitivity: A Corpus-Based Study of the LSP of Infertility', *Language in Society*, 30(4), pp. 589–610.

BWHBC, Boston Women's Health Book Collective ([1971, 1973, 1976, 1979, 1984, 1992, 1998, 2005] 2011) *Our Bodies, Ourselves*. New York: Simon & Schuster.

BWHBC, Boston Women's Health Book Collective (2000) *Nuestros cuerpos, nuestras vidas*. New York: Seven Stories Press.

Campo-Engelstein, L. and Johnson, N. (2014) 'Revisiting "the Fertilization Fairytale": An Analysis of Gendered Language Used to Describe Fertilization in Science Textbooks from Middle School to Medical School', *Cultural Studies of Science Education*, 9, pp. 201–220.

Cheng, S. L. (2009) 'Questioning Global Vaginahood: Reflections from Adapting the *Vagina Monologues* in Hong Kong', *Feminist Review*, 92(1), pp. 19–35.

Chibamba, M. (2019) 'Translation and Communication for Development: The Case of a Health Campaign in Zambia', *The Translator*, 24(4), pp. 1–17.

Chollet, M. (2018) *Sorcières, la puissance invaincue des femmes*. Paris: La Découverte.

Colantonio, L., Pena, L., Whittaker, R. and Mejia, R. (2016) 'Cross-Cultural Adaptation of a Text Message-Based Program for Smoking Cessation in Buenos Aires, Argentina', *Nicotine & Tobacco Research*, 18(3), pp. 314–320.

Djordjevic, J. (2006) 'Vagina Sisters, Crying Men, Soap Opera Stars and Sushi: The Story of the *Vagina Monologues* in Belgrade', *Institute of Development Studies Bulletin*, 37(5), pp. 127–133.

Dorlin, E. (2006). *La matrice de la race. Généalogie sexuelle et coloniale de la nation française*. Paris: La Découverte.

Ehrenreich, B. and English, D. (1973) *Witches, Midwives and Nurses: A History of Women Healers*. New York: The Feminist Press.

Ehrenreich, B. and English, D. (1978) *For Her Own Good: 150 Years of the Experts' Advice to Women*. Garden City, NY: Doubleday Anchor Books.

Ensler, E. (1998) *The Vagina Monologues*. New York: Villard.

EWEC, Every Woman Every Child (2015) *Saving Lives, Protecting Futures, Progress Report on The Global Strategy for Women's and Children's Health 2010–2015*, New York: United Nations.

Federici, S. (2004) *Caliban and the Witch: Women, the Body and Primitive Accumulation*. New York: Autonomedia.

Fenoglio, I. and Chanquoy, L. (2007) 'Avant-propos. La notion d'avant texte: point de rencontre pour une compréhension de l'écriture en acte', *Langue Française*, 3(155), pp. 3–7.

Gilley, B. (2006) '"Snag Bags": Adapting Condoms to Community Values in Native American Communities', *Culture, Health and Sexuality*, 8(6), pp. 559–570.

Health Canada (2006) *Benefits and Risks of Hormone Replacement Therapy*. Government of Canada. Available at: www.canada.ca/en/health-canada/services/healthy-living/your-health/medical-information/benefits-risks-hormone-replacement-therapy-estrogen-without-progestin.html (Accessed: 21 February 2020).

Karlsen, C. (1998) *The Devil in the Shape of a Woman. Witchcraft in Colonial New England*. New York: W. W. Norton.

Kohler, C. (1998) 'Women and Medicalization: A New Perspective', in Weitz, R. (ed.) *Politics of Women Bodies*. Oxford: Oxford University Press.

Kuhlmann, E. and Babitsch, B. (2002) 'Bodies, Health, Gender? Bridging Feminist Theories and Women's Health', *Women's Studies International Forum*, 25(4), pp. 433–442.

Lavieri, A. (2015) 'L'archivio come dispositivo. dalle pratiche discorsive alle comunità del tradurre', *Transalpina*, 18, pp.19–32.

Li, B. (2018) *Translating Feminism in 'Systems': The Representation of Women's Sexual and Reproductive Health and Rights in the Chinese Translation of Our Bodies, Ourselves.* Master's thesis. University of Ottawa.

Löwy, I. (2005) 'Le Féminisme a-t-il changé la recherche biomédicale? Le women's health movement et les transformations de la médecine aux États-Unis', *Travail, Genre et Société*, 2(14), pp. 89–108.

Martin, E. (1991). 'The egg and the sperm. How science has constructed a romance based on stereotypical male-female roles', in Hunt, K. and Annandale, E. (eds) *Gender and Health, Major Themes in Health and Social Welfare*. London and New York: Routledge, pp. 101–116.
Martin, E. ([1987] 1992). *The Woman in the Body, A Cultural Analysis of Reproduction*. Boston: Beacon Press.
Morgen, S. (2002) *Into Our Own Hands: The Women's Health Movement in the United States, 1969–1990*. New Brunswick, NJ: Rutgers University Press.
Oreskes, N. (2019) *Why Trust Science*? Princeton, NJ: Princeton University Press.
Rey, J. (2007) 'Traduction et adaptation des éléments culturels dans les textes scientifiques', *Babel*, 53(2), pp. 132–146.
Robinson, D. (1997) *Translation and Empire: Postcolonial Theories Explained*. London and New York: Routledge.
Rodríguez, S. B. (2014) *Female Circumcision and Clitoridectomy in the United States: A History of a Medical Treatment*. Rochester, NY: University of Rochester Press.
Salle, M. and Vidal, C. (2017) *Femmes et santé, encore une affaire d'hommes?* Paris: Éditions Belin/Humensis.
Shapiro, E. (2013) 'Translating Latin American/US Latina Frameworks and Methods in Gender and Health Equity: Linking Women's Health Education and Participatory Social Change', *International Quarterly of Community Health Education*, 34(1), pp. 19–36.
Susam-Sarajeva, Ş. (2009) 'The Case Study Research Method in Translation Studies', *The Interpreter and Translator Trainer*, 3(1), pp. 37–56.
Susam-Sarajeva, Ş. (2010) 'Whose "Modernity" is it Anyway? Translation in the Web-based Natural-birth Movement in Turkey', in Daldeniz, E. (ed.) *Translation Studies*, special issue 'Contemporary Perspectives on Translation in Turkey', 3(2), pp. 231–245.
Taibi, M. and Ozolins, U. (2016) *Community Translation*. London and New York: Bloomsbury.
Tipton, R. (2017) 'Contracts and Capabilities: Public Service Interpreting and Third Sector Domestic Violence Services', *The Translator*, 23(2), pp. 237–254.
UNESCO, United Nations Educational, Scientific and Cultural Organization (2019) 'Top 50 original languages', *Index Translationum*. Available at: www.unesco.org/xtrans/bsstatexp.aspx?crit1L=3&nTyp=min&topN=50 (Accessed: 15 May 2019)
Vermeer, H. (2000) 'Skopos and Commission in Translational Action', in Venuti, L. (ed.) *The Translations Studies Reader*. London and New York: Routledge.
Vuille, M., Rey, S., Fussinger, C. and Cresson, G. (2006) 'La santé est politique', *Nouvelles questions féministes*, 2(25), pp. 4–15.
Weitz, R. (1998) 'A History of Women's Bodies', in Weitz, R. (ed.) *Politics of Women Bodies*. Oxford: Oxford University Press.
WHO, World Health Organization (1986) 'Milestones in Health Promotion: Statements From Global Conferences', *Canadian Journal of Public Health/Revue Canadienne de Santé Publique*, 77(6), pp. 425–430.
Yoda, L. A. (2007). 'Traduction et messages de santé au Burkina Faso: Le cas du français vers le mooré', *La Revue*, 3(49), pp. 89–98.
Yu, Z. (2017) 'Translation as Adaptation and Selection: A Feminist Case', *Perspectives*, 25(1), pp. 49–65.

21

Translation in maternal and neonatal health

Şebnem Susam-Saraeva and Luciana Carvalho Fonseca

1 Introduction

Conception, pregnancy, birth, labour and postpartum periods are crucial life events which have a bearing on the future health of individuals, as well as the collective health of families and societies. How one begins life or becomes a parent can have a lasting impact on their physical, mental and emotional health for the rest of their lives. Strictly speaking, pregnancy, labour, birth and postnatal period are not 'medical' events or processes per se. They are normal physiological processes with deep-rooted social, cultural, psychological, emotional, historical, spiritual and familial dimensions.

Practices surrounding childbirth vary from one culture to another. 'Although the common aim is to maintain the wellbeing and safety of mother and child,' there are great variations between the 'notions of human reproduction, care of the expectant mother and the unborn child, methods of giving birth and postnatal care [...] according to cultural beliefs and traditional practices' (Hoang, Le and Kilpatrick 2009: 2). Regardless of these variations, there has been a gradual and global shift from a midwifery-led and woman-centred approach focused on normality in pregnancy and birth, to obstetric dominance, led by physicians and focused on the foetus. The latter perspective is mostly on the lookout for problems in birth and treating women's bodies as factories/containers and mothers as patients/consumers.[1] This shift took place in tandem with the move of births from home to hospital, transforming birth from a social event shared within female circles to a medical event overseen by (male) physicians (for a succinct summary, see Colton 2004: 697–699; see also Arms 1975; Davis-Floyd 1992; Hensley Owens 2015; Wolf 2001; for a history of the development of obstetrics vis-à-vis midwifery, see Rich 1976: 128–155; for the control of reproduction, see Federici 2004). Especially in countries where healthcare systems are financially and technologically driven, birth has become 'a complexly negotiated minefield of litigation, politics, vested interests, money, and beliefs about who holds the power over the delivery room' (Wolf 2001: 18).[2]

We, the authors of this chapter, come from countries with high intervention rates. Caesarean section rates, for instance, are 53.1/100 live births in Turkey (first in the world among OECD countries in 2017)[3] and 52/100 in Brazil (Oswaldo Cruz Foundation 2014).

DOI: 10.4324/9781003167983-26

A life-saving operation has become the 'normal' way of giving birth in both countries.[4] We have both worked as translators, interpreters, editors and translation scholars in maternal and neonatal health (Fonseca is also a publisher in this field; Susam-Saraeva works as a doula)[5] and we both self-identify as birth activists. We believe that empowerment of mothers is crucial not only for the physical, but also emotional and social wellbeing of the whole family. Our main theoretical perspective in this contribution is therefore a feminist approach to women's health and to translation, and the next section will provide an overview of what such an approach entails.

2 A feminist approach to women's health and to translation

This chapter approaches women's health from the perspective of women's health movements, which are part of the feminist struggle against patriarchal domination and capitalist exploitation. Although we are addressing translation in pregnancy and childbirth, we acknowledge that these are but two of the many areas in women's health (e.g. reproductive rights, menstruation, abortion, menopause, domestic violence, birth control, genital mutilation, etc.). Translating women's health, therefore, involves a translator's agency that is aware of the various oppressions of women. The foci of the interpreting contexts and translated materials discussed in this chapter are: promoting wellbeing and women-centeredness during childbirth, strengthening the role of professionals who ensure the former (such as interpreters, doulas and midwives), and challenging the factors and infrastructures which account for the high intervention rates worldwide.

In the case of Brazil, for instance, c-section rates have increased by 400 per cent in 40 years. The rates for women in the highest income bracket is 88 per cent and there are high-income maternity hospitals in São Paulo with rates of over 90 per cent (Fonseca 2015: 84). This could imply that educated women with financial means are 'choosing' c-section: According to a study of medical narratives, Brazilian doctors[6] claim that women 'pressure' them into performing c-sections (Hopkins 2000). However, the *Nascer no Brazil* (Born in Brazil)[7] survey (Oswaldo Cruz Foundation 2014) tells a different story, revealing that when women start their antenatal care, 84.6 per cent of them in public healthcare and 63.9 per cent in private healthcare prefer a vaginal birth. During antenatal care – which in Brazil is carried out by obstetricians/ gynaecologists (OBGYNs) – the c-section preference rate for women in the public healthcare remains unaltered; however, the rate for women who access the private healthcare goes up, indicating that they 'change their mind'. This group's c-section 'preference' rate rises from 36.1 per cent before the start of antenatal care to 63 per cent during the antenatal care. It is worth noting that this rate is still lower than the group's actual c-section rate of 88 per cent mentioned above.[8] This mismatch between what pregnant women desire and what they actually experience is not exclusive to Brazil; birth movements worldwide have been fighting for women's rights to experience birth as they choose, on their own terms, and based on informed decisions.

Because a feminist approach to women's health means placing women at the centre and in control of their own decisions, a feminist approach to translation in relation to pregnancy and childbirth entails choosing and translating texts that circulate within global women's health movements and introducing these texts into target systems where they challenge hegemonic discourses and practices of exploitation; build collective memories of women's embodied experiences; empower expecting women to achieve a more satisfying and liberating birth experience; and, contribute to transforming the contexts of reception.

In feminist studies, culture is seen as a field of conflict between oppressors and oppressed, and language as a domination tool (Ballestrin 2017: 1037). This conflict can take place on/in/over women's bodies, which are both a source of identity and a 'prison' (Federici 2004: 15) and a 'territory' to be conquered (Ballestrin 2017: 1038). Women's bodies are not only vulnerable in prototypical situations of violence and conflict which threaten them from the outside, such as urban violence and war. Because the driving force of capitalist exploitation and patriarchal domination have waged 'a war against our body, making it a signifier for all that is limited, material, and opposed to reason' (Federici 2019: 190), many women believe their bodies are dysfunctional and need to be fixed. This signification of women's bodies becomes most apparent in pregnancy and childbirth.

In this context, translation can be a powerful discursive, ideological and cultural tool to foster feminist causes through numerous genres. In this chapter, we first address linguistic and cultural issues in interpreting for immigrant women during perinatal care. Then, we move on to the translation of childbirth narratives, which lie between oral and written genres. Finally, we focus on written genres, such as books for expecting families and midwifery textbooks.

3 Interpreting in maternal and neonatal health: linguistic and cultural issues

Research on linguistic and cultural issues in maternal and neonatal health has so far been conducted in disciplines such as midwifery, nursing, and perinatal healthcare improvement, and not in translation and interpreting studies. This is surprising given the high proportion of women giving birth in countries which are 'foreign' to them and the linguistic support they need throughout their pregnancies, births and postnatal recoveries. Within the last three to four decades, as a result of the increasing pressures of migration and globalisation, the number of foreign nationals giving birth abroad has steadily increased. Today it is estimated that between 15–30 per cent of women giving birth in a given country were born elsewhere and more often than not, come from a different linguistic and cultural background from that of their host country (e.g. Akhavan and Lundgren 2012; Fredsted Villadsen, Ims and Nybo Andersen 2019: 2; Yelland *et al.* 2016: 2; Yelland *et al.* 2017: 500).

Migrant mothers in high-income countries are reported to experience considerable inequalities in healthcare provision (Hughson *et al.* 2018: 11) and more perinatal complications (Sami *et al.* 2019: 2). Multiple factors underlie this situation: a lack of social support in the host country, of cultural competence and health literacy, and, of course, language barriers (Sami *et al.* 2019: 2; Yelland *et al.* 2016:7). To complicate matters further, many of these women come from cultures where 'the doctor knows best'; therefore, they do not necessarily ask questions or enquire about their options (Binder *et al.* 2012: 1178). They are often 'reticent "in speaking out" as a result of ingrained unassertiveness and inhibition, cultivated from childhood in many cultures for all genders but especially for women' and therefore, they may 'have less access to resources and may not be able to receive the services they are entitled to' (Hoang, Le and Kilpatrick 2009: 7). If parents do not know that interpreting services are available, for instance, they do not request them. They may not 'feel that they had the right to ask for a professional interpreter or to request a different interpreter [...]' (Yelland *et al.* 2016: 6).[9] Different solutions have been suggested to address this issue. For example, in a Melbourne hospital in Australia, notices reminding staff about engaging interpreters were placed where midwives would regularly see them: on the doors of staff toilets. The notice said: 'Offer interpreter early in labour; Gently insist if declined; Offer again' (Yelland *et al.* 2017: 501).

There seems to be a strong correlation between being a foreigner and rating one's intrapartum care experience as poor (Yelland *et al.* 2017: 500). Parents who experience communication difficulties tend to seek medical care rather late during their pregnancies; some are known to seek medical help only when labour begins (Igarashi, Horiuchi and Porter 2013: 782). They may have a poor understanding of treatment plans and may feel unable to participate in medical decision-making processes (Yelland *et al.* 2016: 1). This inability to seek help when needed reportedly contributes to maternal or neonatal deaths as a result of e.g. ectopic pregnancies or eclampsia (Yelland *et al.* 2017: 500). In the case of refugees, motherhood in a new country may take place against a complex backdrop of hardship, a history of torture and subsequent PTSD, loss of loved ones, ethnic and religious persecution, inadequate accommodation, lack of transport, poverty, racism, malnutrition, sexual slavery and female genital mutilation (Correa-Velez and Ryan 2012; 14; Fredsted Villadsen, Ims and Nybo Andersen 2019: 2; Hoang, Le and Kilpatrick 2009: 2; Sami *et al.* 2019: 6; Tobin, Murphy-Lawless and Tatano Beck 2014: 832–833). Healthcare providers, social workers and interpreters working with refugees in maternity settings need to be educated on the impact of this background on new parents.

Even in cases where women move to a foreign country as a result of a new job, relationship or other factors based on personal choice, the lack of a support network and familial role models may increase the new mothers' sense of isolation (Sami *et al.* 2019: 4; Taniguchi and Baruffi 2007: 90), which is only exacerbated by linguistic barriers. In a study focusing on Japanese women living in Hawaii, 'language barrier, the distance from family and friends, and different culture and healthcare attitudes' emerged as key factors impacting on the mental and physical health of new mothers (Taniguchi and Baruffi 2007: 92). Childbirth in a foreign country thus emerges as a particularly stressful event, especially for those giving birth for the first time, in some cases multiplying postpartum depression rates six-fold (e.g. 31 per cent for Japanese women in the United States, compared to the Japan average of 5 per cent; Taniguchi and Baruffi 2007: 94). Furthermore, even if the women have high proficiency in the language of their new country, it is well-documented that people 'tend to revert to their first language during times of stress, such as medical encounters' (Maher, Crawford and Neidigh 2012–2013: 474), and especially during labour and birth, which necessitate the activation of ancient limbic parts of one's brain.

While in translation and interpreting studies communication issues per se tend to dominate the discussion, in midwifery and healthcare 'lack of connection, communication and cultural understanding' are seen as interrelated issues, which exacerbate women's experiences of alienation, loneliness, exhaustion, fear and vulnerability, 'increasing their risk of mental health issues' (Tobin, Murphy-Lawless and Tatano Beck 2014: 831, 837). Culturally appropriate and competent care, on the other hand, ensures that women will be treated with more respect and dignity (Tobin, Murphy-Lawless and Tatano Beck 2014: 837). However, it is also important to remember that healthcare providers belong to a culture of its own, i.e. the biomedical one (Fredsted Villadsen, Ims and Nybo Andersen 2019: 2), and this particular culture may need to be clearly explained to new parents. More often than not, 'women have reported feeling that their intergenerational cultural knowledge was devalued or disregarded in the western maternity culture' (Hughson *et al.* 2018: 11).

Interpreters have traditionally been the main link in the communication between healthcare providers and expectant women and their partners. The importance of using interpreters is widely recognised in maternity services and in research which focuses on remedying linguistic and cultural incongruence. However, a common pattern across countries is that interpreters are accessed less frequently during labour and birth (due to their unpredictability and protracted timeframe) compared to antenatal and postnatal care, which includes appointments with midwives, scans and tests at hospitals, ward stays or home visits (Yelland *et al.* 2017: 500). Even for routine antenatal appointments, it is common that interpreters are booked for the first appointment, but not for the subsequent ones (Yelland *et al.* 2016: 1, 4). There seems to be a general perception that appointments with an interpreter take twice or three times longer than appointments without (Binder *et al.* 2012: 1176; Hughson *et al.* 2018: 13), and this seems to hinder the booking of interpreters more widely. There are some common misconceptions amongst healthcare staff, such as 'the perception that using interpreters for women in early labour would have unacceptable cost implications for the unit's interpreting budget and that accessing an interpreter for a woman more than once in labour was not acceptable practice' (Yelland *et al.* 2017: 502).

In labour and birth, there seems to be a tendency to ask for interpreting services only when consent for a procedure is sought or when there is an urgent need, such as in an emergency (Yelland *et al.* 2017: 503). However, enlisting an interpreter early on in labour is found to reassure the mothers and give them better support (Yelland *et al.* 2017: 502–503). In order to ensure this, language requirements could be noted on to the triage admissions or women could be informed about how to access the telephone interpreting service themselves (Yelland *et al.* 2017: 502). Targeted care for immigrant women can afford more flexibility for healthcare providers in, for instance, arranging the length of meetings and booking times. However, it also risks stigmatising immigrants by e.g. assigning interpreters based on the women's names and surnames, rather than their actual need for interpreting services or assuming parents from a certain culture will have certain expectations, values, and belief systems, and thus homogenising a potentially heterogeneous group (Fredsted Villadsen, Ims and Nybo Andersen 2019: 1, 5). Furthermore, 'emphasizing too much the culture behind a health issue might ultimately hand the problem over to the patient as a private matter' (Binder *et al.* 2012: 1183).[10]

In the surveys conducted, women who had interpreters were overall fairly positive about their experience, as they found it easier to ask questions, express themselves and share their concerns (Binder *et al.* 2012: 1176–1177; Yelland *et al.* 2017: 502). Some appreciated the distance, privacy and anonymity afforded by the use of remote interpreting (Yelland *et al.* 2016: 4), while others indicated a preference for face-to-face interpreters (Yelland *et al.* 2017: 502). Studies from Australia show that remote interpreting can be challenging for the midwives as well, due to issues such as delays in telephone connections, getting access on weekends and overnight, questionable quality of the ensuing communication and no provision for the languages required (Yelland *et al.* 2016: 4; Yelland *et al.* 2017: 503; Hughson *et al.* 2018: 13). In addition, amongst the maternity healthcare staff, skills and professionality of interpreters appear to be a recurrent concern (Binder *et al.* 2012: 1180; Hughson *et al.* 2018: 14; Tobin, Murphy-Lawless and Tatano Beck 2014: 833). Many, for instance, are unsure about the interpreters' grasp of medical terminology and professional training, which indicates that there are issues regarding accreditation and cooperation.

Reproductive health has its own characteristics when it comes to the use of interpreters. Given the intimate nature of labour and birth, women may decline offers of interpreting services. The presence of interpreters may be perceived as disruptive to the birth process, causing embarrassment (Yelland *et al.* 2017: 502). Therefore, women may choose to rely on their partners or female members of their family, such as sisters, cousins, etc. (Yelland *et al.* 2017: 501). In other cases, it may be the partners who insist on interpreting; occasionally, they are known to request certain information not to be passed on to the mothers, presumably trying to protect them from worry and anxiety, acting as 'gatekeepers' (Yelland *et al.* 2016: 5). In fact, although bilingual or multilingual healthcare providers and hospital staff are occasionally called upon (Hughson *et al.* 2018: 13), it is often the partners and other family members interpreting for pregnant women, with varying degrees of success (Sami *et al.* 2019: 7; Yelland *et al.* 2016: 1, 5; Yelland *et al.* 2017: 500).

Some health professionals may also express a preference for the partners interpreting: 'It's not impartial or whatever but it's superior (to telephone interpreting) in many ways' says one midwife, especially when she has to show something to the women physically (Yelland *et al.* 2016: 5). However, the use of partners as non-professional interpreters within the context of maternal health inevitably discourages healthcare professionals from asking questions on domestic violence and may inhibit women from giving full and frank answers (Yelland *et al.* 2016: 6); it also endangers confidentiality (Sami *et al.* 2019: 7).

When professional interpreting services are available and called for, female interpreters are preferred overall (e.g. Binder *et al.* 2012: 1180; Yelland *et al.* 2017: 502), encouraging women to disclose 'health or family concerns, asking questions and seeking clarification at pregnancy visits. [...] Several women noted that they were embarrassed to ask health professionals about "feminine issues" via a male interpreter' (Yelland *et al.* 2016: 4). In the words of one mother: 'I was unhappy when a male interpreter was called when I had a miscarriage [...] I didn't like it and it took me a while to forget what happened' (Correa-Velez and Ryan 2012: 16). A further complication arises when the mothers know that some accredited interpreters are members of the local and relatively small ethnic community. In such cases they are more reluctant to talk about sensitive issues, concerned that their personal information 'could become "community gossip"' (Yelland *et al.* 2016: 4).

In studies ranging from Australia to Sweden, Japan to Switzerland, researchers agree on similar solutions for ensuring optimum care for immigrant mothers (Binder *et al.* 2012: 1172, 1180; Hoang, Le and Kilpatrick 2009: 9; Hughson *et al.* 2018: 14; Sami *et al.* 2019: 7; Tobin, Murphy-Lawless and Tatano Beck 2014: 831):

- Dedicated community-based services
- Mandatory training for healthcare providers in cultural awareness and competence
- 24/7 access to professional interpreters during labour and birth (making sure that both the parents and healthcare providers are aware of the availability of interpreting services)
- Social assistance providers to guide parents through the local healthcare system and administrative procedures
- Use of technology, such as carefully screened or locally-developed eHealth resources (e.g. smartphone pregnancy apps in multiple languages)
- Training bi- or multilingual hospital staff so that they can interpret to a more professional standard
- Diversifying the healthcare workforce so that it is representative of the population it serves
- Information leaflets, videos or audio recordings in multiple languages

It is clear that in these research findings, interpreting is seen as only one, albeit a crucial and often underused, tool.

In the area of maternal health, it is well-known that continuity of carer, i.e. the consistency in healthcare providers who support a woman and her baby throughout pregnancy, labour and the postnatal period,[11] increases women's satisfaction, trust and confidence, 'improves communication, and enhances women's sense of control and ability to make informed decisions' (Correa-Velez and Ryan 2012: 14). In the research surveyed, continuity of interpreters is highlighted for the same reason (Correa-Velez and Ryan 2012: 21), making sure that the same interpreter accompanies the mother in all antenatal appointments, as well as during labour and birth. In a project in Sweden, a further step was taken to train doula-interpreters who could provide such continuity of care. These were 'foreign-born women (mainly non-European immigrants) who were interested in this project, had given birth, had their own child/children, could speak Swedish and could attend a birth at any time'; they were then 'trained by midwives to become doulas and support their peers before, during and after childbirth' (Akhavan and Lundgren 2012: 81). A similar project in the United States opted to work with trained medical interpreters and offered them additional doula training, with similarly successful results, increasing trust and cooperation between them and the healthcare providers (Maher, Crawford and Neidigh 2012–2013: 477, 479).[12] Needless to say, an additional doulaing role blurs the professional boundaries of interpreters and can make any transition between these two roles rather tricky. It becomes vital for the doula-interpreter 'to ensure that all involved understand exactly when she is interpreting and when she is speaking on her own behalf' (Maher, Crawford and Neidigh 2012–2013: 478).

Despite this caveat, the midwives in the Swedish project note that they regard the doula-interpreters as 'assets', 'facilitators' and 'part of the team' (Akhavan and Lundgren 2012: 81). They appreciate the continuous physical presence and involvement of the doula-interpreters (as opposed to e.g. remote interpreters or interpreters sent from agencies), the support and assistance they offer to the midwives (e.g. in explaining cultural differences), the interaction and affinity between mothers and doulas (who had a chance to get to know each other throughout pregnancy), as well as doulas' interest in and knowledge of childbirth and related terminology and procedures (Akhavan and Lundgren 2012: 82). According to the findings of this project, a doula-interpreter coming from the same linguistic and cultural background as the mother can also 'create a sense of community' (Akhavan and Lundgren 2012: 83), precisely what is demonstrated to be missing from the experience of women giving birth in foreign lands.

4 Translation of childbirth narratives

Regardless of any cultural or linguistic differences, what women most want during childbirth is respect, warmth, support, a sense of security and affirmation (Igarashi, Horiuchi and Porter 2013: 782). Within the medicalised model of birth, however, this is often rather difficult to achieve. As mothers have felt compelled to tell their birth stories, the term 'obstetric violence'[13] has slowly gained ground.[14] In the absence of stable and strong female communities and wisdom worldwide, and of familiarity with life transitions such as birth and death, women have turned to listen to each other's birth stories, shared orally, in print, and online. 'The shared birth story provides a vicariously learned experience' for expectant mothers (Staton Savage 2001: 4). It partially fills the gap created by the lack of 'significant observational and participatory experience with the process and with different women's ways of handling different births', compensating for 'individual bodily experience and [...]

collective observational experience to draw on' (Hensley Owens 2015: 95). Therefore, birth stories by women outside one's own immediate circle can become a source of information and support.

Birth stories help the mothers to relive the events, incorporate them into their memory and sense of self (Nelson 2004: 803). Writing them down, sharing them publicly and reaching out to other women preparing for birth or grappling with their own birth-related emotions and memories help women avoid victimhood, censorship and silence (Hensley Owens 2010: 353). Especially in the case of traumatic events and their subsequent narration, birth stories may help turn disappointment into acceptance and reconciliation, which are crucial for mental health.[15] This rewriting/rewiring of past events (Hensley Owens 2015: 137–138) enables women to gain more control over what has happened to them and to heal themselves, at least partially.

Second-wave feminism's slogan 'the personal is political' resonates deeply in the writing and sharing of birth stories (Hensley Owens 2010: 356). While these stories are replete with emotional, physical, spiritual and psychological detail, and seem to solely focus on personal experiences and memories, they set off concrete social and political ramifications by presenting different choices in childbirth, critiquing societal and medical expectations, and advocating certain stances. They inspire resistance against standard practices and rigid social norms about where, how and with whom to give birth. As a social practice, birth stories are a way of being, because they express identities; a way of acting in the world, because they have the power to enact change in society; and, a way of representing birth, because they shape discourses and ideologies revolving around childbirth (Fonseca 2015: 29–32).

There is growing recognition within medical humanities that subjective experience can be a legitimate source of knowledge and that experiential information can complement, enhance, as well as challenge, the conventional wisdom disseminated by institutions and authorities. Medical humanities 'attempts to bridge the gap between biologically based medical theory and reality-based human/patient experience' (Hashish 2020: 165). Birth stories are noteworthy examples of such experiential, visceral and feminist experience and knowledge passed on from one person to another, one generation to the next, and, in the case of translation, one language and culture to another.

The significance of translating childbirth narratives is multi-fold. Infrastructures supporting maternity services vary considerably from country to country – and even within one and the same country – depending on socio-economic profiles, demographics and approaches to maternal healthcare. It is therefore important for parents to hear what is possible and available elsewhere. For instance, home-birth stories shared across languages and cultures have increased the interest in the possibility of giving birth at home, especially during the COVID-19 pandemic.[16] Translating these stories also gives voice to parents who have taken unconventional decisions depending on their personal circumstances, education, research, convictions, etc. Being exposed to these decisions helps other parents question their own stance vis-à-vis the birthing choices presented to them by the medical establishment.

Despite the growing interest in childbirth narratives within diverse academic disciplines, such as rhetoric and discourse studies, comparative literature, motherhood/mothering studies, women studies, and midwifery (e.g. Akrich and Pasveer 2004; Colton 2004; Cosslett 1994; Fonseca 2014; Hensley Owens 2015; Nelson 2009; Podnieks and O'Reilly 2010), there has been almost no research on the circulation of these narratives beyond their languages and cultures of origin from a translation studies point of view. To date, the only research in this area is by Susam-Saraeva (2020), focusing on *Ina May's Guide to Childbirth* (Gaskin 2003) and its Turkish translation (2015), which both include 44 birth stories. Her article compares and contrasts the US-American and Turkish maternity systems and cultural attitudes towards childbirth outside hospital settings by using the lens of translation. Adopting the framework of narrative theory, the article demonstrates that even though translational agents (translators, editors, revisers) may be open to new ideas and possibilities, they may still be unable to harness the full transformative power of personal narratives in translation. The public and meta-narratives about childbirth circulating in society exert their dominance in translational and editorial decisions both on macro- and micro-levels.

Stories of natural/positive births[17] are part of a worldwide social movement enabling such births. Translating stories from countries with respectful, women-centred birthing practices can inspire expecting parents in target cultures and help transform interventionist medical institutions. Translated birth stories can also influence birth professionals who are open to challenging the status-quo in their countries. Although stories, as well as personal observations, are considered 'low-level' evidence in medicine (as opposed to e.g. randomised controlled trials), the power of these stories should be acknowledged and taken into account.

5 Translation of (text)books on pregnancy and childbirth

This section explores translated books and textbooks aimed at birth professionals and expectant families within the natural/positive birth movement. The examples are taken from the work of Fonseca, as a translator and publisher. These books, translated from American English – and in one case, Mexican Spanish – into Brazilian Portuguese, are mostly written by birth professionals and relate to each other in terms of their common goal, i.e. reducing c-section rates in Brazil through materials that support informed decision making and reconnect women with their bodies and traditional knowledge on birthing.

The target audience of these translations are women in the upper-middle class bracket. Although this group is statistically the best-read and has full access to relevant information, it also has the highest c-section rate in Brazil, due to the association of c-sections with economic status and of medicalisation with 'risk avoidance' and 'state-of-the-art technology'. Other demographic groups in the society, in turn, try to imitate the choices of the upper-middle class whenever they can.

Among the discourses operated to encourage c-sections for the women in this group is the claim that their body cannot cope with a vaginal birth. This is part of a global discourse observed in diverse areas of medicine which represents women's bodies as dysfunctional (Martin 2001). In the case of Brazil, however, it is further boosted by structural racism rooted in coloniality. White European women have historically been represented as fragile in contrast to non-white women, who, in turn, have been considered strong enough to cope with any kind of work (Lugones 2008: 95). As a result, the present-day upper-middle class woman in Brazil, who defines herself as white, perceives her inability to give birth due to her allegedly frail constitution as a means to come closer to the idealised notion of whiteness. Moreover, many women in the targeted group think they have control over their body and sexuality, and that oppression is reserved for poor black women (Martin 2001: 202).

To reach this group, a feminist translation approach should necessarily use a variety of genres. Women in this group are surrounded by birth professionals, their social peers and family. When a woman considers swimming against the c-section current, she has to be able to find materials not only to educate herself and make informed decisions, but also to educate those around her. In her study of birth stories, Fonseca found that Brazilian VBAC (Vaginal Birth after Caesarean) stories represent partners as key allies in achieving a vaginal birth; without their support it was more difficult, if not impossible, to have a VBAC (2015: 123–125). Moreover, birth professionals who challenge the dominant c-section culture also require resources to educate themselves and their clients, and to show that their profession is 'written about', and therefore, 'exists'. The birth professionals targeted by these translations are first, Brazilian doulas and midwives, and second, OBGYNs and nurse-midwives.

What the translated books have in common is their focus on the normalcy of childbirth, the celebration of women's bodies, their power and ability to give birth, and women controlling time-space. Thus, although many of the books are targeted at professionals, they depict them in a supporting role in the pregnancy and birthing process. From a feminist translation perspective, the woman-centred birthing ideology these books convey deliberately antagonises the Brazilian c-section culture; and, from a marketing perspective, it targets an audience too small to attract mainstream publishers. As a result, only feminist translators and independent publishers take on this work, largely supported by the community of birth activists.

The work and encouragement of leading birth activists have been crucial to these feminist translation projects.[18] Brazilian movement's leadership is very active in São Paulo,[19] and among other activities, holds the main annual humanised birth conference in Brazil (Simpósio Internacional de Assistência ao Parto, SIAPARTO) and promotes international exchange of birth professionals and activists. Three of the authors of the translations discussed in this section have been regular speakers at SIAPARTO. The birth movement's role in promoting the authors is essential to the circulation of their books in translation. Because the authors, local birth professionals and activists frequently work together, their books circulate through word-of-mouth. As for the production of these translations, the movement's role is equally crucial. Translations of all the books in this section have been carried out by birth activists who are professional or non-professional translators. Revision is also supported by birth professionals (doulas, midwives, nurses, doctors, and birth photographers), activists and/or graduate students and academics in Public Health at the University of São Paulo and other public universities. The networked and collective effort that goes into activist translation and publishing, especially of non-hegemonic women's health texts, is a phenomenon widely researched (see, Davis 2009; Rosas *et al.* 2020; Sánchez 2020; Shapiro 2013; Susam-Saraeva 2020; Tymoczko 2007).

Having touched upon the complex networked endeavour of translating in the field of pregnancy and childbirth, we will now discuss specific feminist goals and rationale of each translation, and explicate translational strategies.

5.1 Heart and hands: a midwife's guide to pregnancy and birth – new front cover and neologisms

Heart and Hands is a textbook by the American midwife, educator and consultant Elizabeth Davis (2012). The title was translated as *Com as mãos e o coração: manual de parteria* (With the Hands and the Heart: Midwifery Manual, Davis forthcoming). This 320-page textbook is targeted mainly at midwives, but also at doulas and expectant families. It was translated by a team of three translators, with different specialisms.[20] The revision of each chapter was carried out by activists who are also professionals and/or researchers in the topic of the relevant chapter.[21]

Studies show that gender bias is rife in textbooks across all levels of education and disciplines (Baldwin and Baldwin 1992; Blumberg 2007). In medicine, it has been found that gender bias not only affects how women are represented (Martin 2001) but also the diagnosis and treatment of common ailments (Blumberg 2007; Dijkstra, Verdonk and Lagro-Janssen 2008). This is also the case in translated textbooks. Leonardi (2017) studied gender and ideology in original and translated anatomy textbooks in English and Italian to assess whether sexism is maintained or omitted linguistically and semiotically. She found that the 'textbooks analysed show a disproportionate use of male-centred anatomy' and that 'sexism in both language and imagery helps reinforce the sexist social structure', concluding that 'it is important to rethink language used in *all* medical publications, including textbooks, and rethink visual language, even in translation' (Leonardi 2017: 27; emphasis added). Accordingly, it is important to look at the packaging of and illustrations in translations, as well as any bias in the language used.

A midwifery textbook such as *Heart and Hands*, which focuses on the normalcy of childbirth, is inherently feminist and woman-centred. Yet, the front covers of the five editions in English to date have become increasingly baby-centred.[22] Up until and including the 3rd edition, the front cover had a coloured photo of a dark-skinned baby's head being born vaginally into the waiting hands of a midwife. In the 4th edition, the same photo was used for the cover, but this time in close-up and black and white, therefore not as clear as in the former editions. In the 5th edition, a different photo was chosen, showing a rosy-pink baby asleep on its white mother's chest on top of a white blanket. The mother is out of focus, only the contours of her shoulder and chin are identifiable, and the baby is wearing a white bonnet hat.

Judging by the covers of the later editions, in addition to the characters having been whitened, the midwife has progressively left the scene. On the cover of the 5th edition, a tranquil baby, well past the moment of birth, was brought to the foreground and the mother was placed in fuzzy background in a much more conventional, restful position. The latest edition of this textbook on midwifery has thus completed the phasing out of the midwife from the front cover, as well as blurring the mother and her bodily powers. This is in accordance with the worldwide marginalisation of the midwife that started the process in which

> [...] Women lost the control they had exercised over procreation, and were reduced to a passive role in child delivery, while male doctors came to be seen as the true 'givers of life' (as in the alchemical dreams of the Renaissance magicians). With this shift, a new medical practice also prevailed, one that in the case of a medical emergency prioritized the life of the fetus over that of the mother. This was in contrast to the customary birthing process which women had controlled; and indeed, for it to happen, the community of women that had gathered around the bed of the future mother had to be first expelled from the delivery room, and midwives had to be placed under the surveillance of the doctor, or had to be recruited to police women.
>
> *Federici 2004: 89*

The feminist translation project of this book revolves around birthing in Brazil, and the challenges of having a vaginal birth in this context. Therefore, a very different photo[23] (by award-winning birth photographer Lela Beltrão) was chosen: a birthing woman and her partner in an upright position. The woman's right hand is on her pregnant belly, and her left hand is partially on top of her partner's hand whose fingers are crossed over her breasts, at the height of their hearts, as he holds her. The choice of the photo was motivated by the lack of powerful imagery showing vaginal births in (text)books in Brazil, and due to the key role partners play in helping women achieve a respectful and midwife-assisted birth in the target culture. The semiotically translated cover photo is intended to enable couples to see themselves birthing and to build their individual representations and collective memory pool, in addition to subtly warn women that they seldom achieve a natural birth in Brazil unsupported.

The translation of the term *midwifery* throughout the book has been another issue. It is known that students learn 5,000 new words in the first year of medical school (Bordelois 2016: 14), but what is the dominant ideology behind the words they learn? If most textbooks are linguistically and semiotically gender biased, their vocabulary – or the lack thereof – would mirror this bias. In Brazilian Portuguese, there is no word for 'midwifery' – neither in medicine nor in nursing. There is, however, a term for midwife, *parteira*, but it is ideologically charged and stigmatised. *Parteiras* correspond to 'self-taught or traditional midwives' who attend births in rural areas. Trained midwives in Brazil are called *obstetrizes*, their field of knowledge being *obstetrícia* (obstetrics), and 'nurse-midwives' are called *enfermeiras-obstetras* (nurse-obstetricians). Activist and trained birth professionals, on the other hand, make a point of being called *parteiras* and even *parteiras urbanas* (urban midwives).

Because our feminist translation approach aimed at raising the status of midwifery as a profession in order to challenge the interventionist birth culture, we wanted to create a counterpart for the word 'midwifery'. After a number of exchanges with the reviewers, our attention was called to the fact that Spanish has the term *partería* (midwifery). This term is transparent to Brazilian readers. Therefore, it was decided that the translation would introduce the term *parteria* (without the accent) into the Brazilian birth culture. The need to use a Spanish neologism in a translation from English was clarified in the paratext, and the term was presented as a dictionary entry at the beginning of the book, as well as being used in the title.

Creating new words has always been part of a feminist agenda. Since language is a social phenomenon, new words that expurgate sexism in society must be created (Saffioti 2015: 51). In the discourse surrounding childbirth in Brazil, women have been masterfully excluded from the lexicon. There is no grammatical equivalent for 'I give birth' or 'she gives birth'; the verb *parir* (to give birth) cannot be conjugated with first- or third-person singular. OBGYNs, on the other hand, systematically use the phrase *fazer o parto*, which literally means 'to perform a (vaginal) birth', rather than 'to assist a birth'; and, maternity hospitals identify their operating rooms as *sala de parto* (vaginal birth room). The lexicon attached to those supporting the mothers can also be vague and misleading. Feminist translation can raise awareness about the biases reflected in such terms and phrases, as well as about the urgent need to create new ones.

5.2 The Belly Mapping Workbook – *enlarging readership*

The Belly Mapping Workbook: How Kicks and Wiggles Reveal Your Baby's Position was written by the American midwife Gail Tully, who is also the author of the well-known book and website *Spinning Babies* (2010).[24] The original was a 45-page-long A4 spiral-brochure targeted mainly at 'pregnant women', according to the title, but also at 'maternity care providers' (Tully 2010: 1). The workbook was translated as *Guia prático de Belly Mapping: descobrindo a posição do bebê na barriga pelo tato* (Practical Guide to Belly Mapping: Finding the Baby's Position Through Touch; Tully 2015).[25] The translation, in square back binding, 21 × 21cm, has 126 pages. This expansion is due to the objective of the translation project, which was to appeal to a wider audience in the target language. This was achieved by enlarging all the photos; rewording the title to address midwives as well as mothers; changing the front cover;[26] adding an entire chapter on belly painting; and, whenever possible, replacing the photographs in the original with those of Brazilian women and birth professionals – not only doulas and midwives, but also physicians – so that they could see themselves represented in the book and thus perceive woman-centred pregnancy and birth as tangible and possible in their own culture.

As a result, the book has become popular among doulas and young or in-training nurses and doctors. Doulas use it to teach their clients how to feel their baby in the womb, and by doing this, they encourage expecting women to touch, feel and know their body. Mothers who use the Belly Mapping techniques become less alienated from their pregnancy, gain confidence in their ability to give birth, and begin to value women's knowledge about their own bodies. Enabling women to (re)gain this knowledge about themselves is subversive because 'science' and the medicalisation of birth have undermined women's knowledge for centuries (Federici 2004; Schiebinger 1999).

This translation project holds 'translating and editing as a mutually implicated process whose points of divergence are also points of contact' (Emmerich 2017: 13). The 'original' workbook was translated into an expanded version to fulfil the feminist agenda of both the original author and the editor in the target culture. By enlarging readership, the editor instrumentalised a wider range of birth professionals and activists, who can then attend to expecting women and empower them. At the same time, these professionals gain visibility in the process, through belly painting and birth photographing – two activities which celebrate women's bodies.

Finally, in terms of the discourse of translation, which 'has consistently served to express the difference in value between the original and its "reproduction"' (von Flotow 1991: 81), this feminist approach to editing subverts traditional hierarchies and power relations by making the work of 'reproduction' fruitful and valuable. Feminist translation in women's health challenges the static notion of the 'original'; every interpretation is guided by the present context and its current struggles and challenges.

5.3 Un bebé nace naturalmente / Nasce um bebé… naturalmente/ A baby is born… naturally – memory in the making

The first edition of this multilingual book was written in Spanish and illustrated by the Mexican midwife Naolí Vínaver, translated into English and Brazilian Portuguese,[27] and published in 2005 (retranslated in 2015). The book has also been published in another trilingual edition since then (Italian, German and French; Vínaver 2009).[28]

A Baby is Born… Naturally is a birth story told by Alelí, the older sister of a soon-to-be-born baby. Although the book is primarily for older siblings in families planning a home birth and conveys Vínaver's experience as a midwife, it is a book Brazilian doulas and midwives carry with them to show to pregnant women, due to the lack of available home-birth imagery. It is lavishly illustrated by the author in bright colours and in marked Latin American aesthetics. The drawings depict scenes which may be considered taboo in children's books, such as the baby crowning, Alelí kneeling facing her mother's open legs, and the naked mother catching her baby. In the story, Alelí learns to wait, helps the midwife prepare the house for the birth, watches her mother labour, witnesses the intimacy and cooperation between her parents, and more: 'she looks in wonder as her mother's vagina opens, widens, and slowly makes room for the baby's head' (Vínaver 2015: 14).

As stated in the section on birth stories, this story in the form of a children's book aims at building and strengthening individual and collective memory pools, for both children and adults. These memories will be accessed by older siblings, partners and birthing women when the time comes. The book goes against the countless images inflicted by the mainstream media, which feed into the interventionist and medicalised birth culture. By making the imagery in Vínaver's book available to its target readers, the feminist translation aims at compensating for the lack of observational experience related to childbirth.

In the book and its translation, the term 'naturally' takes on two meanings: the natural birth of Alelí's brother is not only free from intervention, but is also experienced as a natural part of life, with ease and without fear. 'Just as birth should be: a remarkable event, but at the same time common and constant in any growing family. Some may think it is a miracle, but it is simply life as it is' (Vínaver 2015: 15).

This book, seemingly addressing children, is intertextually connected to the previously discussed translations. As in *Heart and Hands*, it depicts the work and role of midwives, the bodily expressions of women during birth, and the process of childbirth. It is linked to the *Belly Mapping* book, as the midwife feels the baby to determine the foetal position and draws the baby on the mother's belly. The three translations discussed in this section so far reinforce each other, value the birth attendants, and encourage the mother so that she can find material support to educate those in her social and family circles, who, in turn, will be key supporters for her to birth on her own terms.

5.4 A Bun in the Oven: *how the food and birth movements resist industrialization – connecting the dots*

Unlike the authors above – all midwives – Barbara Katz Rothman is Professor of Sociology at the City University of New York. Having penned a number of other books about birth (Katz Rothman 1986, 1991, 2000), in *A Bun in the Oven* (2016) Katz Rothman takes the leap and provides women with the opportunity to connect the dots, encouraging them to identify – and fight – patriarchal domination and capitalist exploitation beyond birth:

> [...] Birth and food are a lot alike: they became institutionalized, industrialized. As did pretty much everything else in America. Prisons, schools, childcare, disease, dinner (and maybe especially breakfast), transportation, housing, clothing production – you name it. It all came under the rational, systematic gaze of science. [...] Things that used to be in the realm of the lay world become subject to medical definition [...] in a world that recognizes only medical knowledge about the body as legitimate knowledge.
>
> *Katz Rothman 2016: 75*

Because Katz Rothman writes about the United States in particular, to achieve the same eye-opening effect in the target culture, the myriad of both evidence-based and anecdotal examples of scientification and medicalisation of both food and birth were adapted whenever possible, with the agreement of the author. Adaptation took place first in the title. Translated as *Comer, parir e pensar: como os movimentos do parto humanizado e da alimentação saudável resistem à industrialização* (Eat, Birth and Think: How the Humanised Birth and Healthy Food Movements Resist Industrialization),[29] the title replaces the culturally-marked idiom of the source language – 'a bun in the oven' – with the trinomial 'Eat, Birth and Think', which intertextually resonates with Elizabeth Gilbert's bestseller *Eat Pray Love* (2006) and its Brazilian Portuguese translation. Further adaptations were introduced, for instance, when food brands unknown to the target audience were referred to (brands were replaced with local examples) or scientific studies by government agencies were mentioned (similar Brazilian studies were included). Adaptation is a common – and necessary – practice in feminist translation, especially in women's health (Davis 2009; Sánchez 2020; see also Bessaïh in this volume), which is a culturally marked area affected by local laws and policies. In the case of *A Bun in the Oven*, adaptation provides a continuum with the previously discussed translations and attempts to create a sinuous path towards emancipation. It offers readers quality information so that they can establish connections, identify implications, deconstruct the ideologies behind both modern food and birth processes, and subsequently, transfer this knowledge to other aspects of their lives.

6 Future research

As is hopefully demonstrated in this chapter, translation and interpreting within maternal and neonatal health is a complex and dynamic field. It comprises a range of outputs and situations: from oral to written genres; from offering support to the most marginalised groups in society to those who are better educated and well-off; and, from a close rendition of the words of an asylum-seeking mother in labour to extended adaptations of (text)books aiming at birth professionals. Translations can introduce a more favourable approach to disparaged practices (e.g. in *parteria*/midwifery), improve women's lives in the countries they immigrate to (e.g. integrated interpreting services), and help parents-to-be gain their own voices and challenge ingrained attitudes and existing customs (e.g. birth stories).

More research in this area is definitely called for, particularly from within translation and interpreting studies, complementing, and possibly contrasting and challenging, the existing body of research produced in other disciplines. Especially in the case of interpreting, the existing research regards interpreters as 'outsiders' – a profession deemed necessary but only partially understood and accepted by healthcare professionals. Another fruitful area of research is non-professional interpreting within this context, teasing out its advantages and disadvantages, as well as comparing it to the more recent trials with multilingual doulas.

Translation in the area of women's health in general, and maternal and neonatal health in particular, is a highly networked, feminist, collective and intersectional endeavour. Future research could examine these endeavours from the perspective of sociological approaches to translation, highlighting the embeddedness of translational activities in the transformation of societies and the infrastructures that sustain them. Furthermore, such research could focus not only on the North to South flows, as we have done so far in our own research, but also on South to North, as well as South to South ones.

Given that translations carried out within maternal health form a continuum of activist endeavours, studies focusing on a body of work, rather than individual translations, would shed light on wider translational and editorial patterns. Such research could also feed into actual practices of feminist translation which resist coercive systems of oppression, and not only in the field of maternal and neonatal health.

Notes

1 Although this chapter generally uses the term 'women' to refer to those who go through pregnancy and childbirth as a reflection of our experiences as well as of the available literature on the topic, the authors would also like to recognise that not all pregnant people identify as women.

2 For some concrete examples of how financial considerations dictate the care offered, see e.g. Wolf (2001: 169, 178).

3 https://data.oecd.org/healthcare/caesarean-sections.htm (Accessed: 27 May 2020).

4 For risks associated with unnecessary c-sections, see WHO Recommendations (2018). For financial and health costs, see Gibbons *et al.* (2010).

5 A doula is a trained companion who offers physical, emotional, informational and advocacy support to women during their pregnancy, labour and birth, as well as postnatally.

6 Given their position of power in relation to patients, it is easy to villainise doctors. However, the current birth culture turns doctors into employees of hospitals and health insurance companies, working on the basis of maximum profit and control.

7 All glosses from Spanish and Portuguese are by Fonseca.

8 This strong push for c-sections in Brazil is a structural issue, which can, for instance, be observed in advertisements of private maternity hospitals showing blow-dried celebrities after 'painless' c-sections due to 'large babies' and high-tech ICU units for 'small babies'. It results from the prevailing set up of an OBGYN practice. OBGYNs in Brazil usually have a private practice and any time away from consultations at the practice due to spontaneous labour and birth in the hospital means less income. Therefore, scheduling elective c-sections is the 'most efficient' way to run a one-person business.

9 Whereas in rich countries there is usually lack of information on the availability of interpreting services, in poor countries interpreters may simply not be available in the public healthcare system, even when there are laws in place ensuring the right to their services. There may also be differences in availability between public and private healthcare. In the city of São Paulo, the situation of immigrants is radically different from the situation of 'expats' and wealthy tourists serviced by upscale hospitals, which may have International Patient Centres where staff are bilingual and interpreters are a phone call away (e.g. www.einstein.br/en/international-patients-center. Accessed: 31 October 2020).

10 Having said that, cultural differences do have a profound impact on the parents' expectations about pregnancy and childbirth. For instance, migrant Brazilian women in the UK have difficulty understanding why they cannot 'simply' have their c-section scheduled before they go into labour as they do in Brazil (Fonseca 2014: 106), and find it odd that the UK's National Health System (NHS) 'insists' they have a vaginal birth. This is demonstrated in the numerous comments made by Brazilian women on the British birth culture in groups such as *Brasileiras Poderosas na Europa* (Powerful Women of Brazil in Europe) www.facebook.com/groups/256025137909432 and *Mães Brasileiras na Inglaterra* (Brazilian Mothers in the UK) www.facebook.com/groups/526163771057598.

11 www.england.nhs.uk/ltphimenu/maternity/targeted-and-enhanced-midwifery-led-continuity-of-carer/ (Accessed: 19 October 2020).

12 It is important to note that 'Unlike the traditional doula role, in which the doula is not affiliated with the hospital and is working solely for the birthing mother and her support persons, interpreter/doulas are hospital employees' (Maher, Crawford and Neidigh 2012 2013: 477). This shifting allegiance can erode the doula's advocacy role on behalf of the parents, defending the mothers' rights in medical settings.

13 www.may28.org/obstetric-violence/; www.who.int/reproductivehealth/topics/maternal_perinatal/statement-childbirth-govnts-support/en/ (Accessed: 11 June 2020).

14 In Brazil, the term 'obstetric violence' has been defined and criminalised by statute in some states (*Lei Estadual nº 17.097* 2017). In 2019, the Federal Health Ministry attempted to ban the use of

the term due to pressure from medical associations. The attempt was unsuccessful; the Federal Prosecutor's Office sued the Ministry, arguing that the term has been firmly established in scientific literature and is widely used by specialists and non-specialists alike. https://g1.globo.com/ciencia-e-saude/noticia/2019/05/07/ministerio-diz-que-termo-violencia-obstetrica-tem-conotacao-inadequada-e-deixara-de-ser-usado-pelo-governo.ghtml (Accessed: 21 October 2020).

15 For the transformative power of birth stories in healing birth trauma, see Colton (2004).

16 www.theguardian.com/world/video/2020/jun/10/giving-birth-at-home-during-COVID-19-black-mothers-were-already-scared-video, www.nationalgeographic.com/history/2020/05/inside-a-home-birth-in-the-time-of-coronavirus/ (Accessed: 26 June 2020).

17 It is difficult to give a single name to the movement that questions the dominance of the patriarchal/medical model of obstetrics. While 'natural' denotes that the births in question are mostly free from medical interventions and end with vaginal births, 'positive' implies that it is how supported and good parents feel during and after a birth that is crucial regardless of the type of birth they had.

18 Two of these translations have not yet been published due to the challenges faced by independent publishing, but they are forthcoming (Davis 2012; Katz Rothman 2016).

19 Ana Cristina Duarte, a Brazilian midwife based in São Paulo, not only organises marches and demonstrations, but also speaks at public legislative hearings.

20 Carla Finger, Eliana Herrman and Fonseca are all professional translators. Finger is a physician by training and Herrman a medical translator; both have almost 20 years of experience in translating medical texts but not in birth activism. Fonseca, on the other hand, is a birth activist but does not specialise in women's health.

21 Reviewers were University of São Paulo graduate students in Public Health and members of the GEMAS group (Gender, Maternity and Health).

22 Third edition front cover: www.amazon.com.br/Heart-Hands-Revised-Eli-Davis/dp/0890878382; 4th edition front cover: www.goodreads.com/book/show/15598.Heart_Hands; 5th edition front cover: elizabethdavis.com/books/heart-hands-a-midwifes-guide-to-pregnancy-and-birth/.

23 www.lelabeltrao.com/gael (Accessed: 21 October 2020).

24 www.spinningbabies.com/ (Accessed: 31 October 2020). Gail Tully's *Spinning Babies* (Tully 2016) and *Spinning Babies: Breech Birth* (Tully 2018) have also been translated into Brazilian Portuguese.

25 The translation was carried out by doula and physiotherapist Lúcia Desideri and Fonseca. Revision was undertaken by a certified Spinning Babies professional, Tania de Filippis.

26 www.emalivros.com.br/produtos/guia-pratico-de-belly-mapping/ (Accessed: 22 October 2020).

27 The English version is the work of professional translator Amanda Morris and Fonseca; the Brazilian Portuguese version is by co-editor Luciana Benatti and Fonseca.

28 Translation of the European edition was carried out by birth professionals and activists. The book was published by the School of Midwives in Florence, Italy.

29 The book was translated by anthropologist, doula and professional translator Clarissa Oliveira, social scientist and professional translator Maria Teresa Mhereb, and Fonseca.

Further reading

Fair, F., Raben, L., Watson, H., Vivilaki, V. van den Muijsenbergh, M. and Soltani, H. (2020) 'Migrant Women's Experiences of Pregnancy, Childbirth and Maternity Care in European Countries: A Systematic Review', *PLOS ONE* 15(2), e0228378. DOI:10.1371/journal.pone.02283.

This is a systematic review of articles on migrant women's experiences of pregnancy and maternity care in the European Union. According to the findings, migrant women report poor understanding of medical terminology and inadequate use of interpreters within the healthcare system, affecting their ability to choose care options, provide informed consent and establish relationships with providers.

Hensley Owens, K. (2015) *Writing Childbirth: Women's Rhetorical Agency in Labor and Online*. Carbondale, IL: Southern Illinois University Press.

The book focuses on the rhetorical analysis of birth plans and stories circulating online as part of blogs, opening up a personal space for mothers in the medicalised birthing culture of the United States.

Susam-Saraeva, Ş. (2019) 'Diversity of Translational Data in Contemporary Social Knowledge Making', in Schögler, R. Y. (ed.) *Circulation of Academic Thought. Rethinking Translation in the Academic Field.* Oxford and Bern: Peter Lang, pp. 77–91.

This contribution examines the role of translation in the spread of natural birth movement in Turkey, particularly focusing on the diverse data that support the movement (e.g. translational data available online, official and amateur subtitles of audiovisual material, and translated key publications).

World Health Organization (2018) *Improving the Health care of Pregnant Refugee and Migrant Women and Newborn Children. Technical Guidance.* Copenhagen: WHO Regional Office for Europe. Available at: www.euro.who.int/__data/assets/pdf_file/0003/388362/tc-mother-eng.pdf?ua=1.

This technical guidance addresses interpretation services and provides recommendations, such as those for the use of remote and face-to-face professional interpreters and cultural mediators rather than family members.

Yelland, J. *et al.* (2017) 'Bridging the Language Gap: A Co-Designed Quality Improvement Project to Engage Professional Interpreters for Women During Labour', *Australian Health Review*, 41, pp. 499–504. DOI:10.1071/AH16066.

The article reports on a project designed to improve the engagement of professional interpreters in maternity units in Australia, and provides a model for enhancing effective communication between healthcare providers and parents-to-be.

Related topics

Translation and Women's Health, Community/Liaison Interpreting in Healthcare Settings, Medical Humanities and Translation

References

Akhavan, S. and Lundgren, I. (2012) 'Midwives' Experiences of Doula Support for Immigrant Women in Sweden – a Qualitative Study', *Midwifery*, 28, pp. 80–85.

Akrich, M. and Pasveer, B. (2004) 'Embodiment and Disembodiment in Childbirth Narratives', *Body and Society*, 10(2–3), pp. 63–84. DOI:10.1177/1357034X04042935.

Arms, S. (1975) *Immaculate Deception: A New Look at Women and Childbirth in America.* Boston: Houghton.

Baldwin, P. and Baldwin, D. (1992) 'The Portrayal of Women in Classroom Textbooks', *Canadian Social Studies*, 26, pp. 110–114.

Ballestrin, L. M. de A. (2017) 'Feminismos subalternos (Subaltern Feminisms)', *Revista Estudos Feministas*, 25, pp. 1035–1054. DOI:10.1590/1806–9584.2017v25n3p1035.

Binder, P., Borné, Y., Johnsdotter, S. and Essén, B. (2012) 'Shared Language Is Essential: Communication in a Multiethnic Obstetric Care Setting', *Journal of Health Communication*, 17(10), pp. 1171–1186. DOI:10.1080/10810730.2012.665421.

Blumberg, R. L. (2007) *Gender Bias in Textbooks: A Hidden Obstacle on the Road to Gender Equality in Education.* Paris: UNESCO.

Bordelois, I. (2016) *A la escucha del cuerpo* (Listening to the Body). Buenos Aires: Zorzal.

Colton, A. B. (2004) 'From Trauma to (Re)Birth: The Birth Story as a Site of Transformation', *Journal of Advanced Composition*, 24(3), pp. 679–704.

Correa-Velez, I. and Ryan, J. (2012) 'Developing a Best Practice Model of Refugee Maternity Care', *Women and Birth*, 25, pp. 13–22.

Cosslett, T. (1994) *Women Writing Childbirth: Modern Discourses of Motherhood.* Manchester: Manchester University Press.

Davis, E. (2012) *Heart and Hands: A Midwife's Guide to Pregnancy and Birth*, 5th ed. Berkeley, CA: Ten Speed Press.
Davis, E. (forthcoming) *Com as mãos e o coração: manual prático de parteria* (With the Hands and the Heart: A Practical Midwifery Guide). Translated by L. Carvalho, C. Finger and E. Herrman.
Davis, K. (2009) *The Making of* Our Bodies, Ourselves*: How Feminism Travels Across Borders*. Durham, NC and London: Duke University Press.
Davis-Floyd, R. (1992) *Birth as an American Rite of Passage*. Berkeley, CA: University of California Press.
Dijkstra, A. F., Verdonk, P. and Lagro-Janssen, A. L. M. (2008) 'Gender Bias in Medical Textbooks: Examples From Coronary Heart Disease, Depression, Alcohol Abuse and Pharmacology', *PubMed* 42: 1021–1028. https://doi.org/10.1111/j.1365-2923.2008.03150.x
Emmerich, K. (2017) *Literary Translation and the Making of Originals*. New York: Bloomsbury.
Federici, S. (2004) *Caliban and the Witch*. Brooklyn, NY: Autonomedia.
Federici, S. (2019) *Re-Enchanting the World – Feminisms and the Politics of the Commons*. Oakland, CA: PM and Autonomedia.
Fonseca, L. C. (2014) '"Eu quero cesárea!" ou "Just cut it out!": análise crítica do discurso de relatos de parto normal após cesárea de mulheres brasileiras e estadunidenses à luz da linguística de corpus' (Eu quero cesárea! or Just Cut It Out! *A Corpus-Based Critical Discourse Analysis of Vaginal-Birth-After-C-Section Stories by Brazilian and American Women*). São Paulo: Universidade de São Paulo. DOI:10.11606/T.8.2014.tde-21052015-112432.
Fonseca, L. C. (2015) 'Eu não quero outra cesárea: ideologia, relações de poder e empoderamento feminino nos relatos de parto após cesarea' (I Don't Want Another C-Section: Ideology, Power Relations and Women's Empowerment in Accounts of Birth After Caesarean). São Paulo: Ema Livros.
Fredsted Villadsen, S., Ims, H. J. and Nybo Andersen, A.-M. (2019) 'Universal or Targeted Antenatal Care for Immigrant Women? Mapping and Qualitative Analysis of Practices in Denmark', *International Journal of Environmental Research and Public Health*, 16, pp. 3396. DOI:10.3390/ijerph16183396.
Gaskin, I. M. (2003) *Ina May's Guide to Childbirth*. London: Bantam.
Gaskin, I. M. (2015) *İna May'ın Doğuma Hazırlık Rehberi* (Ina May's Guide to Childbirth), Z. Birinci Güler and Ö. Altınkaya Erkök (trans.). Istanbul: Sinek Sekiz.
Gibbons, L., Belizán, J. M. Lauer, J. A., Betrán, A. P., Merialdi, M. and Althabe, F. (2010) 'The Global Numbers and Costs of Additionally Needed and Unnecessary Caesarean Sections Performed per Year: Overuse as a Barrier to Universal Coverage', *World Health Report No. Background Paper, 30*, World Health Organization.
Gilbert, E. (2006). *Eat Pray Love*. London: Bloomsbury.
Hashish, N. (2020) Towards Holistic Medical Humanities. *Alif: Journal of Comparative Poetics*, 40, pp. 164–185.
Hensley Owens, K. (2010) 'Revelations and Representations: Birth Stories and Motherhood on the Internet', in Podnieks, E. and O'Reilly, A. (eds) *Textual Mothers/Maternal Texts: Motherhood in Contemporary Women's Literatures*. Waterloo, ON: Wilfred Laurier University Press, pp. 351–366.
Hensley Owens, K. (2015) *Writing Childbirth: Women's Rhetorical Agency in Labor and Online*. Carbondale, IL: Southern Illinois University Press.
Hoang, H. T., Le, Q and Kilpatrick, S. (2009) 'Having a Baby in the New Land: A Qualitative Exploration of the Experiences of Asian Migrants in Rural Tasmania, Australia', *Rural and Remote Health*, 9, pp. 1084.
Hopkins, K. (2000) 'Are Brazilian Women Really Choosing to Deliver by Cesarean?', *Social Science and Medicine*, 51(5), pp. 725–740. DOI:10.1016/S0277-9536(99)00480-3
Hughson, A. E., Marshall, F. B., Daly, J. O. B, Woodward-Kron, R. C., Hajek, J. A. and Story, D. (2018) 'Health Professionals' Views on Health Literacy Issues for Culturally and Linguistically Diverse Women in Maternity Care: Barriers, Enablers and the Need for an Integrated Approach', *Australian Health Review*, 42, pp. 10–20. DOI:10.1071/AH17067.
Igarashi, Y., Horiuchi, S. and Porter, S. E. (2013) 'Immigrants' Experiences of Maternity Care in Japan', *Journal of Community Health*, 38, pp. 781–790. DOI:10.1007/s10900-013-9679-8.
Katz Rothman, B. (1986) *The Tentative Pregnancy: Prenatal Diagnosis and the Future of Motherhood*. New York: W. W. Norton.

Katz Rothman, B. (1991) *In Labor: Women and Power in the Birthplace*. New York: W. W. Norton.
Katz Rothman, B. (2000) *Recreating Motherhood*, 2nd ed. New Brunswick, NJ: Rutgers University Press.
Katz Rothman, B. (2016) *A Bun in the Oven: How the Food and Birth Movements Resist Industrialization*. New York and London: New York University Press.
Lei Estadual no 17.097 (2017) Available at: http://leis.alesc.sc.gov.br/html/2017/17097_2017_lei.html#:~:text=1%C2%BA%20A%20presente%20Lei%20tem,de%20Aten%C3%A7%C3%A3o%20Obst%C3%A9trica%20e%20Neonatal (Accessed: 16 December 2020).
Leonardi, V. (2017) 'Gender, Language and Translation in the Health Sciences: Gender Biases in Medical Textbooks', in Camus, C. C., Castro, C. G. and Camus, J. T. W. (eds) *Translation, Ideology and Gender*. Newcastle upon Tyne: Cambridge Scholars Publishing, pp. 8–31.
Lugones, M. (2008) '*Colonialidad y género* (Coloniality and Gender)', *Tabula Rasa*, 9, pp. 73–101.
Maher, S., Crawford, A. and Neidigh, K. (2012–2013) 'The Role of the Interpreter/Doula in the Maternity Setting', *Nursing for Women's Health*, 16(6), pp. 472–481. DOI:10.1111 / j.1751-486X.2012.01775.x.
Martin, E. (2001) *The Woman in the Body: A Cultural Analysis of Reproduction*. Boston: Beacon Press.
Nelson, F. (2004) 'Birth Stories and the Narrative Construction of Maternal Identities', in Randall, B., Furlong, D. and Poitras, T. (eds) *Narrative Matters 2004 Conference Proceedings*. Fredericton, New Brunswick: Narrative Matters Planning Committee, pp. 797–811.
Nelson, F. (2009) *In the Other Room: Entering the Culture of Motherhood*. Black Point, NS: Fernwood Publishing.
Oswaldo Cruz Foundation (2014) *Pesquisa nascer no Brasil* (Research on Birth in Brazil). Rio de Janeiro: Fiocruz.
Podnieks, E. and O'Reilly, A. (eds) (2010) *Textual Mothers/Maternal Texts: Motherhood in Contemporary Women's Literatures*. Waterloo, ON: Wilfrid Laurier University Press.
Rich, A. C. (1976) *Of Woman Born: Motherhood as Experience and Institution*. New York: Norton.
Rosas, C., Bittencourt, J., Izidoro, L. G. and Macedo, S. de O. M. (2020) 'Conjurar traducciones: la traducción colectiva de Caliban and the Witch al portugués brasileño como estrategia feminista transnacional (Conjuring Translations: The Collective Translation of *Caliban and the Witch* to Brasilian Portuguese as a Transnational Feminist Strategy)', *Mutatis Mutandis*, 13, pp. 117–138. DOI:10.17533/udea.mut.v13n1a06.
Saffioti, H. (2015) *Gênero patriarcado violência (Gender Patriarchy Violence)*, 2nd ed. São Paulo: Fundação Perseu Abramo e Expressão Popular.
Sami, J. *et al.* (2019) 'Giving Birth in Switzerland: A Qualitative Study Exploring Migrant Women's Experiences During Pregnancy and Childbirth in Geneva and Zurich Using Focus Groups', *Reproductive Health*, 16, p. 112. DOI:10.1186/s12978-019-0771-0.
Sánchez, L. (2020) 'En torno a la traducción de *Our Bodies, Ourselves* para España y la construcción de un nuevo sujeto político del feminismo en la Transición española (About the Translation of *Our Bodies, Ourselves* Into Spanish and the Construction of a New Feminist Political Subject During the Spanish Transition)', *Mutatis Mutandis*, 13, pp. 93–116. DOI:10.17533/udea.mut.v13n1a05.
Schiebinger, L. (1999) *Has Feminism Changed Science?* Cambridge, MA: Harvard University Press.
Shapiro, E. R. (2013) 'Translating Latin American/US Latina Frameworks and Methods in Gender and Health Equity: Linking Women's Health Education and Participatory Social Change', *International Quarterly of Community Health Education*, 34, pp. 19–36. DOI:10.2190/IQ.34.1.c.
Staton Savage, J. (2001) 'Birth Stories: A Way of Knowing in Childbirth Education', *The Journal of Perinatal Education*, 10(2), pp. 3–7.
Susam-Saraeva, Ş. (2020) 'Translating Birth Stories as Counter-Narratives', *Mutatis Mutandis*, 13(1), pp. 45–63. DOI:10.27533/udea.mut.v13n1a02.
Taniguchi, H. and Baruffi, G. (2007) 'Childbirth Overseas: The Experience of Japanese Women in Hawaii', *Nursing and Health Sciences*, 9, pp. 90–95.
Tobin, C., Murphy-Lawless, J. and Tatano Beck, C. (2014) 'Childbirth in Exile: Asylum Seeking Women's Experience of Childbirth in Ireland', *Midwifery*, 30, pp. 831–838.
Tully, G. (2010) *The Belly Mapping Workbook*, 2nd ed. Bloomington, MN: Maternity House Publishing.

Tully, G. (2015) *Guia prático de Belly Mapping: descobrindo a posição do bebê na barriga pelo tato* (Practical Guide to Belly Mapping: Finding the Baby's Position Through Touch), 2nd ed, Translated by L. Carvalho and L. Desideri. São Paulo: Ema Livros.

Tully, G. (2016) *Spinning babies: guia de consulta rápida para profissionais* (Spinning Babies: Guide for Birth Professionals), 2nd ed. São Paulo: Ema Livros.

Tully, G. (2018) *Spinning babies pélvico: guia de consulta rápida para profissionais* (Spinning Babies for Breech Births: Guide for Birth Professionals), Translated by L. Carvalho. São Paulo: Ema Livros.

Tymoczko, M. (2007) *Enlarging Translation, Empowering Translators*. Manchester: St. Jerome.

Vínaver, N. (2005/2015) *Un bebé nace naturalmente/Nasce um bebê naturalmente/A Baby is Born Naturally*. São Paulo: Ema Livros.

Vínaver, N. (2009) *Nasce un bambino naturalmente / Ein Kind kommt zur Welt Natürlich / Un bebé est né… Naturellement*, Translated by V. Schmid (Italian); V. Schmid and R. Byland (German); L. Uplinger, L. de Schyter, M. A. Zaldùa, B. Bureau, and V. Collin (French). Florence: Scuola Elementale di Arte Ostetrica (SEAO).

Von Flotow, L. (1991) 'Feminist Translation: Contexts, Practices and Theories', *TTR: traduction, terminologie, rédaction*, 4(2), pp, 69–94. DOI:0.7202/037094ar.

World Health Organisation (2018) Who Recommendations: Non-Clinical Interventions to Reduce Unnecessary Caesarean Sections. Available at: www.who.int/reproductivehealth/infographic-unnecessary-caesarean-section.pdf?ua=1 (Accessed: 16 December 2020).

Wolf, N. (2001) *Misconceptions: Truth, Lies, and the Unexpected on the Journey to Motherhood*. New York: Doubleday.

Yelland, J., Riggs E., Szwarc J., *et al.* (2016) 'Compromised Communication: A Qualitative Study Exploring Afghan Families and Health Professionals' Experience of Interpreting Support in Australian Maternity Care', *BMJ Qual Saf*, 25, e1. DOI:10.1136/bmjqs-2014–003837.

Yelland, J. *et al.* (2017) 'Bridging the Language Gap: A Co-Designed Quality Improvement Project to Engage Professional Interpreters for Women During Labour', *Australian Health Review*, 41, pp. 499–504. DOI:10.1071/AH16066.

22

Dialogue interpreting in mental healthcare

Supportive interference

Hanneke Bot

1 Introduction

According to Article 25 of the Universal Declaration of Human Rights by the United Nations,[1] 'everyone has the right to a standard of living adequate for the health and well-being of himself and of his family', including medical care. Article 2 stipulates that 'everyone is entitled to all the rights and freedoms set forth in this Declaration, without distinction of any kind, such as race, colour, sex, *language*, religion, political or other opinion, national or social origin, property, birth or other status'[2] (my emphasis). In reality though, language often becomes a stumbling block to accessing healthcare. If the care provider and patient do not share a common language, diagnosis and treatment become difficult, if not impossible. This is particularly so in mental healthcare, which relies heavily on the spoken word. An older but still relevant piece of research by Hertog and Van Gucht (2003) showed that 50 per cent of foreign nationals seeking help in Belgian healthcare did need language assistance, suggesting that the numbers are not insignificant. Although the European Union ensures the legal right to be assisted by a professional interpreter in judicial procedures, no such assurance is given in the case of healthcare. In most European countries, easy access to professional interpreters in healthcare is non-existent. In practice, this means that patients who do not speak the same language as the medical professional and require (mental) healthcare are either not treated at all, or receive inferior care with the help of non-professional language assistance (family members, nonmedical staff, etc.). Only few patients receive proper treatment, either by a care provider speaking the language of the patient, or through the assistance of professional interpreters. ENPSIT (European Network for Public Service Interpreting and Translation)[3] campaigns for European regulations to ensure proper language services in the entire social sector, comparable with those of the judicial sector, but there is still plenty of work to do.

Mental healthcare in particular is not a suitable setting for working with a nonprofessional interpreter. Mental health issues are usually associated with feelings and behaviour that people may be ashamed of, or with which they do not want to burden others, especially their family members. Despite these issues, the Dutch government, for instance, decided in 2011 to withdraw its central funding for interpreter services in the health sector.

DOI: 10.4324/9781003167983-27

The Minister of Health's reasoning was that it is the responsibility of each individual to make sure they either understand their care provider or bring their own language help.[4] In practice, it is frequently people with low incomes who require language assistance, which makes acquiring the services of a professional interpreter even more unattainable. As a result, the burden of supplying an interpreter is either left to individual healthcare providers and/or to the institutions they work for, creating extra costs. Alternatively, the patient has no option but to rely on their family members or similar non-professional interpreters. Mental health is the sector within healthcare that makes the most frequent use of interpreters, and, for economic reasons, 85 per cent of these services are done over-the-phone in the Netherlands.[5] Despite this, the use of professional interpreters in healthcare in the Netherlands dropped by more than 75 per cent since this governmental decision.[6]

This contribution deals with the ins and outs of professional interpreting in mental healthcare. It is based on the premise that the primary task of the interpreter is to give a faithful rendition of the words which the therapist[7] and their patient utter; should be neutral and independent; and should refrain from having an input of their own. This is the stance taken by most Codes of Conduct for interpreters, stemming from their work in the judicial realm. Although I personally would support this restricted position of the interpreter, in practice it is impossible to realise. It can even be 'dangerous' to believe that an interpreter can ever be of so little influence. Moreover, sometimes a deliberate independent input of the interpreter may enhance the therapeutic process. This means that 'drawing the line' is the critical issue here: how much of an independent input is helpful, and when does it go too far, obfuscating the conversation between the primary parties? As in all forms of communication, the key role of the interpreter is to help the healthcare provider and the patient to understand one another. However, it is equally important that they are given the opportunity to find out that they are misunderstanding one another.

This chapter begins with an outline of the main characteristics of therapeutic talk and the interpreting required in this type of conversation, and then discusses the questions of faithfulness, equivalence, and divergence in these settings. The following section provides an overview of the most common critical issues found in mental health interpreting, such as questions, small talk and communicative devices like hedging and modalisation, and uses practical examples to illustrate possible solutions to these problems. The third section introduces the concept of interactive interpreting as a general model for interpreting in mental health settings and discusses situations in which an independent input of an interpreter might become necessary. The chapter briefly touches on the benefits of special training for both therapists and interpreters and ends with a summary of the key characteristics of professional interpreting in mental health.

2 Interpreting therapeutic talk

Throughout this chapter, I use the term therapeutic talk to refer to interactions that take place between a variety of mental health workers (psychiatrists, psychologists, psychotherapists, social workers, etc.) and their patients. Generally speaking, therapeutic talk is about careful listening and understanding in a non-judgemental and open atmosphere. It is also emphatically about interacting and relating, which is conveyed through words *and* through non-verbal and paraverbal behaviour. Evidence shows that the success of therapeutic work is mostly dependent on the therapeutic relationship between the therapist and the patient, as well as on the therapists' attitude and whether they can convincingly explain and implement their treatment methods (see e.g. Wampold and Imel 2015). The key characteristics of a therapists' attitude in this relationship are described as empathic, accepting, non-judgemental and authentic, based on humanistic-existential approaches to therapy (see for example Feltham and Horton 2006, specifically part V).

The presence of an interpreter, whether in person or via telephone or video conferencing, inevitably has an impact on the therapeutic talk. This presence changes a dialogue between two people, i.e. the therapist and the patient, into a conversation between more than two parties. By the act of rendering the words of both the therapist and the patient, the interpreter influences the content of the talk as well as their mutual interaction, inevitably becoming part of the therapeutic relationship. However, in some cases, a neutral and independent stance is not enough for creating the open and empathic environment necessary for a therapeutic session. Some intentional input might become necessary, such as when interpreters have to meta-communicate in order to do justice to the words of the patient or the therapist. As the interpreter should not disturb the formation of a therapeutic relationship, it might also be necessary that the interpreter's attitude diverges from the neutral stance in order to reflect the attitude of the therapist (empathic, non-judgemental, accepting and authentic) and so to create an atmosphere in which a therapeutic relationship can prosper.

2.1 The importance of understanding 'faithfulness'

It is difficult to separate spoken words from all the other elements involved in human interaction; gaze, gesture, posture, intonation, facial expression, the process of turn-taking, overlapping speech, etc. are all important in a conversation. Nonetheless, the semantic aspects of an interpreted conversation need to be addressed first, for two main reasons.

First, therapists – and other professionals – decide to involve an interpreter because of the meaning of their words. They can observe their patients, they can see what they look like and see how they behave, but they cannot understand the language in which they speak. Those who commission the services of an interpreter therefore expect them to render the utterances spoken in the unknown language as closely as possible. Healthcare providers without training or experience with interpreting services might even expect the interpreter to give a wholly equivalent rendition. This, however, might be a dangerous expectation, as the following example with a Dutch-speaking therapist and a Farsi speaking patient will show.

Example 1[8]

Therapist: en wat is uw probleem hiermee [.. stilte] wat betekent het voor u dat u dat nog niet heeft?

Gloss: *and what is your problem with this [... silence] what does it mean for you that you still do not have it?*

Interpreter: Mîgûyand kch khob moshkcl chîst hâlâ kch masalân kârtctûn tamdîd nashodeh ya nadârîd cheh moshkelî barâtûn pîsh âmadeh?

Gloss: *he says, that it is OK, what is the problem now that for example your permit has not been prolonged, or you do not have it, what problem does it cause you?*

In this session, the patient has been talking about the fact that his residence permit has not been prolonged in time. He is worried that he will miss out on social benefits and lose everything he has built up in his new country. The therapist has already asked several questions about the matter and came to the conclusion that the patient has no reason to worry at this moment (a lawyer had already taken the necessary steps for an extension). While rendering the sentence into Farsi, the therapist starts with the word 'problem', but, after a brief silence, switches to 'what does it mean', seemingly correcting himself. The interpreter, apart from adding a lot more words, some of which have a coordinating function ('that your permit has not been prolonged' instead of 'it'), repeats the word 'problem' twice, and does not ask about 'meaning' at all. The therapist is looking for a deeper fear but does not arrive there; the patient starts repeating his worries about losing everything. A therapist assuming that the interpreter rendered his question with complete accuracy would ascribe all the answers solely to the patient. He could potentially stop going deeper into the matter with further enquiries, concluding that the patient does not want to, or is not able to do so. This would do injustice to the patient, who had in fact heard a question that was different from the one posed by the therapist, and gave an answer in line with what he heard. This example highlights some of the problems in the concept of an 'equal' rendition of the interpreted text, which often disregards the complicated nature of interpreter-mediated communication. It ascribes everything the interpreter says to the original speaker and may thus misrepresent the person for whom they are interpreting.

What happened in reality during this particular session was this: after the episode described above, the therapist returned to the residence permit, acknowledged that he knows about the issue being overseen by a lawyer, and asked whether the patient had trust in these proceedings. This time, the therapist's utterances, and especially the issue surrounding the lack of trust, were rendered accurately by the interpreter and thus opened a different area of therapeutic talk. The same therapist, when interviewed before the recorded session, offered an insight into his understanding of interpreting. He said he was aware of the fact that a rendition can differ from the original words, and that sometimes you just have to return to a topic to find out if the patient really responded to the question asked or whether any interpreting problem played a role in the interaction. In other words, he had expressed what I refer to as an interactive view of interpreting (Bot 2005a), i.e. the acceptance that the interpreter is more than an invisible go-between and that they interact with the primary parties, thus influencing both the content of the talk and the overall interaction. I call the technique this therapist uses 'recycled questioning' (Bot 2005a), which is a strategy that can be used by primary speakers to prevent some of the communicative problems in an interpreted setting.

The second reason for the importance of accurate renditions of the therapist's and patient's utterances is the need of the primary parties to get a reliable impression of each other's talk; content, style, register and specific words that are used in a conversation all give information to the listener. Interpreters who adjust the words of a primary speaker to what (they think) the other party wants to know can compromise the mutual understanding of both parties. Primary speakers have to be able to hear that their collocutors use a different register than themselves, that they give answers that do not fit the question which was posed, that they repeat or contradict themselves, etc. The ground rule here is 'let them (i.e. the primary speakers) sort out their own problems'.[9]

The problem here is of course that interpreting can never produce a completely accurate renditions of the source text. The idea of an interpreter, producing completely equal renditions and nothing else, is as attractive as it is unrealistic. One of the reasons for its attractiveness is that people want to believe in a perfect world,[10] where things are easy and manageable: one hires an interpreter and all communication problems are solved. The idea of a professional interpreter whose techniques allow for perfect renditions and the metaphor of translator-as-machine are still strong among healthcare professionals.

2.2 Rendering therapeutic talk: general issues in equivalency and divergence

Research conducted in the past two decades which compared primary speakers' utterances with their interpreted renditions in naturally occurring mental health related conversations has yielded interesting results. Bot (2005a), using a bespoke equivalency concept,[11] arrived at an average of 74 per cent equivalent renditions per session (ranging from 56–94 per cent over six sessions) and with marked differences between three interpreters (61–87 per cent, taking into account two sessions per interpreter). Annys (2013), with an equivalence concept derived from Bot's, found a percentage of 86.3 per cent, and Khawkokgraud (2015), analysing a telephone-interpreted administering of a diagnostic questionnaire and likewise using Bot's equivalence concept, arrived at 73 per cent equivalent renditions. Wang and Fang (2019) found equivalent renditions ranging from 74–78 per cent in three interpreted encounters in a simulated social service environment. Judging by these results, roughly one-fifth to one-quarter of all renditions in these studies were somehow divergent from their original turn.

Divergence does not necessarily lead to misunderstandings. Just as in a monolingual setting, speech in multilingual conversations is frequently redundant and listeners miss pieces of information, but may also correct obvious mistakes. Systematic divergence however can lead to problems, as it leaves no room for corrective action. The following example from a therapeutic session with a Dutch-speaking therapist and a Dari-speaking patient provides an example of such a situation.

Example 2

> In this session the interpreter systematically changes religious references (if God permits/gives; God forbid) into secular terms, making the patient secular and also changing the perspective from a patient relying on help and rules from god into a self-conscious acting person.
>
> *Bot 2005a: 214–223*

The interpreter, with whom the transcripts were discussed later, said he had made these adjustments as he considered the religiously inspired utterances to be idiomatic. He thought that if he had rendered them literally, the therapist would have interpreted these words as an expression of extreme religiousness, and he felt that that would not be correct. However, as became clear when analysing the two subsequent sessions in detail, the changes caused the therapist to miss the crucial nature of the patient's religiousness, and that in turn made him formulate an intervention which offended the patient a great deal. This interpreter opted for a target-oriented rendition, which did not prove to be appropriate.

In my research, I found several issues that led to information loss in interpreted renditions. Many of these were associated with overlapping speech, due to, for instance, not adhering to appropriate turn-taking measures and the therapist not assuming the role of the chair of the session. Bot (2005a) shows that long and grammatically complicated turns of the therapist and the patient were associated with divergent renditions and could frequently lead to information loss. Some argue that it is important to let the patients produce their narratives undisturbed, especially when the case concerns a traumatised patient at the beginning of their treatment (see e.g. Zimányi 2013). My stance is that it is generally unproductive to let the patient produce a narrative if the therapist is unable to understand it (see Bot 2005a). The therapist, as the 'chair' of the session, can nudge the patient into pauses in their speech. They can do this in cooperation with the interpreter, who knows best at what point to pause the narrative. This avoidance of overlapping speech and the use of short turns requires some discipline during the session, and it is helpful for the therapists to be aware of the needs of the interpreter. We see here that there is a strong connection between the faithfulness of renditions, the coordinating of the communication, and the organisation of the sessions.

The frequent use of 'he/she/they said' and similar reporting verbs, and the change in perspective (from the first into third person or third into second) usually does not affect understanding, but can lead to a certain degree of alienation (Bot 2005b) with unknown effects on the quality of the therapeutic session. An effort (Bot and Aarts, unpublished) to analyse the nature of the divergence in the material of Khawkokgraud which concerned the administering of a diagnostic questionnaire with the help of an interpreter via the telephone and its influence on the outcome of the questionnaire (i.e. the diagnosis), did not lead to a clear outcome because of extremely low interrater reliability.[12] Wang and Fang (2019) conclude to a very low percentage of unjustifiable omission and distortions, ranging from 3 to 7 per cent; other divergence that they found has either a strategic function or is minimal.

3 Rendering therapeutic talk: critical issues

As stated in the previous section, the relationship between a therapist and their patient, and the way in which this relationship develops, is a very important aspect of the treatment process. This is reflected in the therapeutic language and leads to some specific issues that frequently pose difficulties in interpreting the therapists' words. Amongst these are hedges and phatic communication (Albl-Mikasa *et al*, 2015; Bot 2005a; Iglesias-Fernández 2010), modalisations (Bührig and Meyer 2004), questions and brief introductory phrases (Bot 2005a), but also small talk, cultural issues and problems pertaining to patients with severe mental health problems that affect their speech. The following section will look at each of these subjects in an interpreted setting and provide practical suggestions on how to avoid some of the reoccurring problems.

3.1 Hedges, phatic communication and modalisations

Omitting hedges (typically adjectives, adverbs or tags used to signal caution and probability) and phatic communication (social or polite phrases) can leave out important information; while hedges play a role in showing empathy, phatic communication is crucial to relationship building. Modalisations (linguistic options used to express levels of certainty) are important in searching for hidden feelings, dealing with ambivalence, etc., in phrases such as 'is it possible that…?' At the beginning of an intervention, therapists often use phrases like, 'as you have said previously', 'do I understand correctly that you mean….' or 'I might be wrong, but didn't you just …'. These phrases involve mutuality. They emphasise that the therapist and patient are working together, and that the therapist is building on the words of the patient. If these phrases are considered phatic (or 'fringe', as an interpreter once said to me) and are omitted during the interpreting process, the therapist can come across as someone who 'already knows' and who 'is the expert', instead of someone who is looking for answers together with the patient. The same applies to false starts or other unorthodox parts of the conversation, including 'Freudian slips' and other unintentional utterances from both the therapist and the patient. Leaving these out, as some interpreters tend to do, may mean that important information is omitted. Therapists sometimes ask the interpreter not to interpret these utterances, such as when they feel that they made a mistake or said something rude or reflective of themselves, as I know from training sessions with interpreters. I do not think this is correct behaviour. It poses a dilemma for the interpreter (follow the request of the therapist or the official Code of Conduct) and places the therapist into a 'superior' position. Therapists and patients should be aware that everything they say will have to be rendered.

3.2 Questions

In many cases, therapeutic talk necessitates letting the patient talk in a scenario where the therapist assumes a 'not-knowing' position. For this reason, therapists will often ask questions, leading the patient to reflect upon what they have said or delve deeper into their emotions. However, when these questions are rendered as statements, the therapist is moved from a not-knowing position into a knowing one. The question 'So, you were angry?' is completely different from the statement 'So, you were angry.' and the difference should ideally be replicated in the rendition. Bot (2005a) found that questions are often changed into statements or their content is altered in the process of interpreting.

3.3 Small talk and self-disclosure

Small talk and self-disclosure, usually present at the beginning and the end of a session, are an important part of the therapeutic relationship. Self-disclosure usually involves the therapist sharing personal information with the patient (such as marital status or questions about their family) and is nowadays seen as an acceptable part of a therapy session, provided it contributes to the wellbeing of the patient (van Meekeren, 2017). Not disclosing such information and not indulging in small talk can lead to an alienation between the therapist and the patient; the same applies, to an extent, to the interpreters. For example, a therapist mentioning something along the lines of 'educating adolescents is not easy' suggests that they are speaking from experience; a nod by the interpreter could be a welcome supporting gesture in such a situation. However, both small talk and self-disclosure have their boundaries. Therapists receive training about what is appropriate to disclose in which circumstances, and interpreters should follow their example.

Example 3[13]

The patient in this example is very mistrustful of people from his country of origin and asks the interpreter where he comes from. The interpreter renders the question to the therapist. The therapist, knowing that the interpreter is of Dutch origin, agrees that the interpreter can disclose this to the patient. However, the information is immediately followed by a lively exchange (about food, as it turns out later) between the interpreter and the patient.

While the interpreter, as part of their professional conduct, consults the therapist about the patient's initial request for information, the following discussion about food goes beyond the bounds of an acceptable interpreter intervention. Therapists are trained to 'never volunteer information', i.e. to answer requests for personal information briefly without adding anything that has not been asked for. Here the interpreter and the patient have overtaken the conversation by sharing more information than necessary, as well as taking the lead in the conversation, which is not part of the interpreter's role.

3.4 Cultural issues

Another aspect that is often mentioned in research about interpreting in general is the question of cultural differences. The Dutch Code of Conduct for certified interpreters notes that interpreters should make sure there is 'complete and effective communication between the two parties [...] and if necessary to intervene actively to correct (culturally defined) misunderstanding'.[14] However, what is meant by 'culturally defined' is not further elaborated upon. This can take the form of the interpreter intervening in a session to give information about some specific practice or expression, but it can also lead the interpreter to adjust their renditions to how they think the receiver of their rendition will understand the other person's words (target-text orientation). These changes can again lead to various issues in the interpreting process.

> **Example 4**
>
> A therapist reported that during a session with a patient, the interpreter intervened by commenting 'you should know that there are arranged marriages in his (i.e. the patient's) country'. The therapist was surprised – it distracted him from the topic of the session, and, more importantly, he felt offended by the interpreter; 'how stupid does he think I am; does he really think I do not know this?' The experience took him completely off the course, he said.

Here we have a situation in which an interpreter, possibly with good intentions, purposefully and openly adds information he feels will contribute to the session, but ends up affecting the interaction negatively. The cultural adjustments from Example 2, with the interpreter systematically changing religiously inspired terms into secular ones, changed the overall impression of the patient. The interpreter in Example 2 made a cultural adjustment, adapting what he considered to be a culturally-impacted statement from the patient so as to be appropriate for the therapist. Such an intervention of the interpreter is very difficult to detect as neither the therapist nor the patient know that these changes are being made and subsequently cannot interfere. The responsibility for this kind of problem lies with the interpreter and it is imperative that they are aware of this danger and keep as close to the source text as possible.

'Culture' is a concept that appears frequently in discussions about treating migrant patients; interpreting agencies advertise that 'we solve language and cultural barriers'[15] or 'we connect cultures'.[16] However, 'culture' i.e. a meaningful combination of norms and values, is a group concept. Especially when it concerns groups that one has not chosen deliberately (such as national or ethnic groups), its members relate very differently to these norm and values (Bot 2020). There is no such thing as 'certified cultural information' on which the interpreter can rely. Interpreters connect people, not cultures, by interpreting faithfully and thus allowing the primary speakers to find differences, cultural or otherwise.

3.5 Psychotic patients

The utterances of severely psychotic patients can sometimes diverge from regular speech patterns or grammatical norms. They may repeat themselves, use words that do not exist, talk without pausing, speak in a sequence of seemingly unrelated words, etc. An interpreter cannot be expected to give a faithful rendition of such speech patterns. Here the interpreter has to take an active role, initiating meta-communication and explaining to the therapist how the patients is communicating, such as their use of grammar and general speech patterns, the topic of their talk, or their use of non-existent words. In these cases, it is helpful for the interpreter to know what kind of language issues the therapist is looking for (see the section on training below).

3.6 Other factors influencing therapeutic work

Therapists influence the therapeutic process just by being there for the patient. The same goes for interpreters and their very presence may have an impact on the process, even if they work remotely, e.g. via telephone. The interpreters' prosody, idiolect, fluency, pitch, and – in face-to-face interpreting – their appearance, can have a decisive impact on the atmosphere and even the success of the session. These factors can determine whether the patient feels reassured and safe enough to speak openly, whether the patient or the therapist feel criticised in any way, and whether they perceive the interpreter as interested in what is being said during the interaction. Therapists report on the importance of factors such as minor facial movements, gaze, posture, and changes in intonation or pitch. When they perceive that the interpreter does not agree with what they are doing, they feel inhibited in doing their job (Bot 2005a). The interpreter cannot prevent having an influence, but they can make sure they use this influence in a way that benefits the session (see also Iglesias-Fernández 2013). Ideally, the therapist and interpreter are working together towards a common goal, i.e. understanding what the patient wants to convey, while supporting each other's roles (Bot 2005a). Patients too report on the influence of the interpreters' attitude on their feelings of safety during the sessions (Bot 2005a).

> **Example 5**
>
> In my own clinical work as a therapist, I once worked with an interpreter who frequently laughed when hearing the patient's words before rendering them to me. Not only did I feel left out ('Apparently there is something to laugh about, do you care to enlighten me?') but I also did not think there was anything to laugh about after receiving the rendition.

Here we see a situation where the interpreter sets the tone for the upcoming statement (indicating 'this is something to laugh about') and taking charge of the session, which should be the role of the therapist. Although the interpreter's laughter annoyed the therapist and the situation might have created negative feelings that could potentially disturb the session, the therapist in this case was able to intervene and make the situation more constructive. In similar situations, the therapist could also follow up on the issue and discuss whether the patients' statements are indeed something to laugh about or not, and why. Although this may not be what the therapist wanted to talk about, at least they can thus avoid negative emotions and may arrive at a meaningful conversation. On the other hand, an interpreter choosing not to laugh while both the patient and the therapist do may cause them both to feel as if they are being looked down upon or snubbed. That is, there are times when the interpreter can come across as 'too neutral', but, on the other hand, their openly shared opinions on the matter at hand may harm – or support – the sessions.

The issue of turn transfer also impacts the quality of a session. Although the therapist should be in charge of the session, they often cannot manage the turn transfer adequately without the help of the interpreter, who knows what is being said and whether a turn transition point has been reached. The turn transfer not only influences the quality of the translation, but also the feelings of the participants. It has an impact on, for instance, whether the patient has enough time to express themselves, whether they feel hurt when they are interrupted, and whether the therapist feels their turn comes at the right time and they are still in control of the session. A successful turn transfer combines the practical needs of the interpreter and takes into account the feelings of the primary participants, making sure their statements are acknowledged and taken seriously.

4 Interactive interpreting

As the examples above have shown, a successfully interpreted therapy session usually requires the interpreter giving accurate renditions of the utterances while paying attention to coordinating turns, as well as being mindful of their own personal presence at the session. I have called this the stance of the 'interactive interpreter' (Bot 2005a) and it implies a close cooperation between the therapist, the interpreter and the patient. The following section outlines what this stance looks like.

4.1 Rendering faithfully

As in all interpreted settings, the language competency of the interpreter, including their use of relevant medical vocabulary, plays a crucial role in ensuring the success of a therapy session. However, the other participants also carry a responsibility for the smooth running of a session. The use of clear and grammatical sentences and the avoidance of jargon and long turns can help the interpreter immensely in providing proper renditions of what has been said. Preferably, the therapist assumes the role of the chairperson for the session (Bot 2005a). They are in charge of the turn transfer, although they may need some help from the interpreter. It is the therapist's role to intervene when there are problems in the communication. The therapist intervenes when the patient takes very long turns and/or produces overlapping speech. When the chairperson of the session is performing their duties correctly, the interpreter can focus on giving accurate renditions.

Even with these precautions, we know that interpreters' renditions are a form of reported speech; the interpreter constructs a dialogue which is based on the words of the primary speakers, but is biased by their translation choices and influenced by their worldview, i.e. in this case, ideas and opinions about 'what mental health talk is about' and about proper behaviour in general terms (Bot 2005a and 2005b). For example, the interpreter might think that it is best not to talk about traumatic experiences ('do not stir it up') and resist when the therapist emphasises that talking about these issues is at the core of any trauma treatment. In these cases, it is important that the therapist, and preferably also the patient, make use of the technique of 'recycled questioning', i.e. rephrasing questions or formulating new ones when there seems to be a misunderstanding. By keeping short turns, both the patient and the therapist receive feedback from one another, thus promoting mutual understanding. Furthermore, interpreters have to be fair in acknowledging possible mistakes on their part and use meta-communication as an 'emergency-buoy' for detecting these issues.

4.2 Independent input

Depending on the setting, the interpreter might deviate from a neutral stance and choose to offer an independent input in order to fit into the overall atmosphere of the session. Neutrality does not mean being aloof or distant. Empathy is essential in mental health sessions and interpreters may have more success if they are in tune with the feelings expressed in the sessions. In fact, in order to create a good working relationship, interpreters should ideally shadow the expressions of the therapist to some extent, e.g. if the therapist laughs, the interpreter smiles (Bot 2005a). The same applies to the expressions of the patient; when the patient shouts, the interpreter may also raise their voice, but to a lower level. As far as the treatment strategy is concerned, the interpreter should follow the therapist as the chair of the session. An interpreter siding with the patient as in the example below may seem like a supportive gesture but is in fact anti-therapeutic. If a patient asks the interpreter for help, for example when they disagree with the therapist or dislike them, the interpreter should encourage the patient to discuss this directly with the therapist.

Example 6

The therapist encouraged the patient to become more independent and helped her prepare for important conversations with the social services, which she was later supposed to manage on her own. Afterwards, the therapist discovered that, on the patient's request, the interpreter had accompanied the patient to the social service encounters, as the interpreter felt that the therapist expected too much from the patient.

In this example, the interpreter is going against the therapist's strategy. The action undermines the relationship of trust between the therapist and the patient, as the interpreter and the patient are effectively acting behind the therapist's back. This is a case where the interpreter acts as an independent participant. However, this problem could have been avoided. When the patient asked the interpreter for help, the interpreter could have said something along the lines of 'I understand your feelings. If you do not feel ready to do this on your own, you should speak to your therapist and see what can be done about it.' In this way, the interpreter validates the feelings of the patient but also refers the patient back to the therapist. If the interpreter really thinks the therapist is not helping the patient, they could discuss the matter with the therapist first, in order to understand their reasons for this decision. If this is not sufficient and the interpreter remains feeling bad about the sessions, it would be best for them to stop interpreting in these sessions. The basis of an effective cooperation is the mutual trust between the therapist and the interpreter, including their trust in each other's professionalism. The following example shows the complexity of this relationship.

Example 7

Therapist and patient have been working with the same face-to-face interpreter for a long time, and the patient emphasises in an interview that the interpreter is very important to her: it is *her* interpreter. The interpreter encourages her, saying supportive things like 'you're doing very well' and 'you'll get over all this, I'm sure'. Then there is a change in therapist. The new therapist does not like the way the interpreter behaves towards the patient and, moreover, she feels that the patient's Dutch is quite good. She decides to continue the therapy without an interpreter. The patient is very angry and upset about this but continues with her treatment. In an interview conducted in Dutch some years after the therapy was successfully concluded, the patient acknowledges that it had been a good decision to stop the involvement of the interpreter. She liked having the support of the interpreter, but she would not have become as independent as she is now, had she continued to rely on the interpreter's help.

In this example, we see the complex nature of the matter. The first therapist was aware of the interpreter's personal involvement but showed no objection to them going beyond their designated role. The second therapist did not approve of this relationship and, being aware of the increasing language proficiency of the patient, stopped using the interpreter during therapy sessions. The outcome was ultimately evaluated positively by the patient; we can only guess at how the therapy would have ended if the interpreter had continued to accompany the patient. We also do not know how the therapy would have proceeded had there been a less overtly supportive interpreter at the beginning of the sessions. We only know the outcome after the change: the patient learnt to speak Dutch, overcoming her shyness and worries about making mistakes, and ultimately became much more independent. It shows the importance of a careful deliberation on the part of the therapist in regard to the interpreter's involvement, as well as of the flexibility of the interpreter, who has to adjust to different therapists' methods within the limits of their professional involvement.

5 Training

In this chapter, I mentioned several times that coordination and cooperation between therapist and interpreter is important for the proper course of a session. Personally, I think it would be best if therapists and interpreters had some training in each other's trade. Some of the problems that I have discussed above might be prevented with such training. Interpreters should not become (co-)therapists, but some background knowledge about what mental health talk stands for in general will help them to interpret faithfully. The topics that should be included concern the differences between the various kinds of therapists and the overall way mental healthcare is organised; the major categories of mental illness and the specific problems these represent in the way patients talk and relate; some of the major treatment techniques and their specific ways of wording interventions; and managing severe stress and emotions. Training of skills in dealing with these problems (meta-communicating; dealing with questions directed at the interpreter or with inappropriate requests, intense emotions, etc.) should be an important part of such training.

Therapists are usually very ill-informed about what interpreting entails and often foster the naive notion of the interpreter as a translation machine. In training sessions, I often get disappointed reactions when I tell therapists that they have to adjust their conversation techniques in order to make the complicated communication work. In general, therapists should know what the role and task of the interpreters entails and be familiar with their training and Code of Conduct; have some insight into the difficulties of interpreting and what 'faithful' interpreting means; make sure they construct their interventions carefully and in a grammatically correct way; allow time for the interpreter's work; and take into account that the interpreter's words are not the patient's words. They also need to be aware of the dynamics in this three-party talk and use it to the benefit of the treatment, understand that, although they are 'the chair' of the sessions, they have to delegate the coordination of turns to the interpreters, and also accept that the attention of the patient will be shared with the interpreter.

I have conducted this type of training for both interpreters and therapists. Although the feedback I receive indicates that participants find it useful and that it brings benefits to both interpreters and therapists, it should be noted that these findings are as of yet not confirmed by any large-scale data, and much more research is needed both into the question of training and into interpreting in mental health settings in general.

6 Conclusion

Interpreting in mental health settings is a complex issue that includes not only interlingual exchange, but also verbal, non-verbal and paraverbal aspects that require careful coordination of the sessions. Its success also relies on building a solid relationship between the interpreter and the therapist, who have to coordinate their actions based on mutual trust in each other's professional abilities. Although any list of rules for mental health interpreting will be necessarily incomplete, the following hopes to give some guidance on successful interpreter-mediated (psycho)therapeutic sessions.

Accurate renditions are important: they are the *raison d'être* of interpreters, allow the primary speakers to understand (or misunderstand) one another and ultimately to solve their own communication problems. In order to help the interpreter in successfully executing their work, the primary speakers could:

- Organise the conversation, keep turns relatively short (while allowing for feedback) and avoid overlapping speech
- Talk in properly phrased sentences that are grammatically correct, avoiding complicated constructions or jargon

In practice of course, not all primary speakers will be able to follow these guidelines. Interpreters should focus on accurate renditions, but both interpreters and the users of their services should be aware that a fully accurate translation is not possible, even when the above-mentioned guidelines are followed. As a result, the following should also be observed:

- Acknowledging that renditions may not have been what the primary speaker intended to convey; the willingness to provide alternatives is important

- Using recycled questioning by primary speakers
- Source speech orientation by the interpreter
- Meta-communication, both by the interpreter and by the primary speakers when they are not able to hear or understand the message

Particularly in mental health settings, the interpreter also needs to pay attention to the overall atmosphere of the conversation and be attuned to the emotions expressed in the session. This sometimes means leaving behind the professionally 'neutral' stance (which could come across as 'too neutral' and thus inhibiting to the free flow of the conversation) while being aware of the interpreter's own influence on the outcomes of the session ('interactive interpreting'). Some points to keep in mind in this regard are:

- Following and remaining a little behind the emotions expressed in the session – 'shadowing' the therapist who determines the flow of the conversation
- Steering away from giving opinions and information that go beyond language-related issues, even when asked, and referring those questions back to the primary speakers
- Meta-communication by the interpreter to explain words or concepts that are difficult to translate, preferably in interaction with the primary speaker who used the word
- Including some small talk and self-disclosure, in close cooperation with the therapist

It is clear that both the interpreter and the therapist have their individual responsibilities during a session. Their mutual respect, as well as some knowledge of each other's fields, can greatly contribute to a successful outcome. This means that the interpreter should have some basic knowledge of the field of mental healthcare (how it is organised; what the various disciplines stand for; general knowledge of therapeutic aims; strategies and wording of therapeutic interventions) and that the therapist should know what interpreting entails and what they can do to facilitate the work of the interpreter. The patient usually does not receive any training in interpreted conversations and should, of course, be allowed to speak freely. The therapist, however, can inform the patient about the rules of the organisation of the talk via the interpreter by pointing out the importance of keeping short turns and the avoidance of overlapping speech. In interpreter-mediated mental healthcare, coming to an understanding is always a three-party responsibility.

Notes

1 www.un.org/en/universal–declaration–human–rights/.
2 *Ibid.*
3 www.enpsit.org.
4 https://zoek.officielebekendmakingen.nl/kst–32500–XVI–143.html; Kamerstuk Tweede kamer der Staten Generaal, 01–06–2011; dossiernr. 32500–XVI nr. 143.
5 Oral communication, TVcN (Dutch Interpreter and Translation Service) 2018.
6 Oral communication, TVcN (Dutch Interpreter and Translation Service) 2013.
7 The term 'therapist' is used throughout this chapter as a generic term including psychiatrists, psychologists, psychotherapists, social workers and the like.
8 Unless stated otherwise, all examples of interpreted dialogue in this chapter were collected as part of a PhD thesis (Bot 2005a) but not all of them were published or published in this format. All therapists are speaking in Dutch, interpreters in Farsi or Dari (transliterated into Latin alphabet), and the English glosses were translated by the author.
9 Thanks to Marina Sleptsova for this clear and precise wording offered at a symposium in Lausanne, 11–12 November 2009.

10 Hermans related this to 'the longing for the security of the womb, before the rupture of translating appeared' (Hermans 2004: 40, translation by the author).
11 In order to compare the original turns of the therapists with their renditions, I designed an equivalency concept which consisted of three parts: conservation of information, conservation of the perspective of person and conservation of the therapeutic perspective (Bot 2005a: 145–149). For the analysis of the therapeutic perspective, I used the Hill Counsellor Verbal Response Category System, revised for the Dutch language (Lietaer *et al.* 1995). The Hill system focuses on the 'syntactic or grammatical structure of language which implies a relationship between communicator and recipient, e.g. a question' (Hill 1986: 132). If the therapist's utterance and its rendition were scored in the same category, they were seen as equivalent.
12 The original research consisted of an assessment of the quality of renditions in a telephone interpreted administration of a diagnostic questionnaire with a French-speaking patient and a Dutch speaking therapist. In order to assess the effect of the rendition on the outcome of the questionnaire, a Dutch translation was made of the interpreted original, which was scored by two certified psychologists. Of the 20 diagnostic questions, 16 were scored differently by the two psychologists; one psychologist gave ten items the same score as the psychologist with the interpreter, the other one only four. The exercise seems to say more about the reliability of the administration of the diagnostic instrument than of the work of the interpreter.
13 This example stems from the clinical practice of the author.
14 www.bureauwbtv.nl/binaries/content/assets/wbtv/wetgeving/gedragscode–tolken–en–vertalers.pdf, page 3 (translation by the author).
15 www.tvcn.nl (Accessed: 14 February 2020).
16 www.livewords.nl (Accessed: 14 February 2020).

Further reading

Wadensjö, C. (1998) *Interpreting as Interaction*. London and New York: Longman.

Wadensjö's publication is a classic where he analyses the intricate structures of interpreter-mediated talk and shows the subtle ways in which the cooperation between the interacting persons develops.

Albl-Mikasa, M., Glatz, E., Hofer, G. and Sleptsova, M. (2015) 'Caution and Compliance in Medical Encounters. Non-Interpretation of Hedges and Phatic Tokens', *Translation and Interpreting*, 7(2), pp. 76–89.

The rendering of hedges and phatic tokens is important in interpreter-mediated psychotherapeutic sessions as these linguistic features help to build rapport and emphasise the cooperative nature of the session. The article shows that interpreters have difficulties in interpreting these phenomena.

Iglesias-Fernández, E. (2010) 'Verbal and Nonverbal Concomitants of Rapport in Healthcare Encounters: Implications for Interpreters', *JosTRAns, The Journal of Specialised Translation*, 14, pp. 216–228.

This article shows how rapport in healthcare encounters is shaped and how interpreters can render these characteristics.

Pöchhacker, F. and Schlesinger, M. (eds) (2007) *Healthcare Interpreting*. Amsterdam and Philadelphia: John Benjamins.

This publication consists of five articles on discourse-based research on healthcare interpreting, as well as a number of book reviews. The research studies show what happens in real interpreter-mediated healthcare sessions and are food for thought for practising interpreters.

Bot, H. (2005) 'Dialogue Interpreting as a Specific Case of Reported Speech', *Interpreting*, 7(2), pp. 237–261 (also included in the above-mentioned publication by Pöchhacker and Schlesinger).

In this article I focus on what is usually referred to as the rule of 'interpreting in the first person'. Based on naturalistic data, I conclude that interpreters very often neglect that rule, but this decision does not seem to compromise the quality of the understanding of the primary parties. Specifically, the use of a reporting verb (such as 'he says' before a rendition) as a 'mental space builder' seems to enhance the understanding by the primary parties about 'who is talking'.

Related topics

Healthcare Interpreting Ethics, Community/Liaison Interpreting in Healthcare Settings, Remote (Telephone) Interpreting in Healthcare Settings

References

Albl-Mikasa, M., Glatz, E., Hofer, G. and Sleptsova, M. (2015) 'Caution and Compliance in Medical Encounters. Non-Interpretation of Hedges and Phatic Tokens', *Translation and Interpreting*, 7(2), pp. 76–89.
Annys, V. (2013) *Tolken Bij Psychologisch Onderzoek*. Unpublished Master's Thesis. KU Leuven.
Bot, H. (2005a) *Dialogue Interpreting in Mental Health*. Leiden: Brill.
Bot, H. (2005b) 'Dialogue Interpreting as a Specific Case of Reported Speech', *Interpreting*, 7(2), pp. 237–261.
Bot, H. (2020). 'De Ontvreemding', *Tijdschrift voor Psychotherapie*, 46(1), pp. 50–55.
Bot, H. and Aarts, R. (n.d.) *Kwaliteit van het tolken bij de afname van een psychologische vragenlijst bij asielzoekers in Nederland: een gevalsbeschrijving.* Unpublished case study.
Bührig, K. and Meyer, B. (2004) 'Ad-Hoc Interpreting and the Achievement of Communicative Purposes in Specific Kinds of Doctor-Patient Discourse', *Arbeiten zur Mehrsprachigkeit* Folge B, Series 57. Hamburg: Universität Hamburg.
Feltham, C. and Horton, I. (eds) (2006) *The Sage Handbook of Counselling and Psychotherapy,* 2nd ed. Thousand Oaks, CA: Sage Publications.
Hermans, T. (2004) 'Huydecoper verkoopt zijn huid: over vertaalhistorie en vertaalironie', *Filter, Tijdschrift over Vertalen*, 11(3), pp. 33–50.
Hertog, E. and van Gucht, J. (2003) *Onderzoeksopdracht: Taalbijstandsbehoeften In De Belgische Algemene Ziekenhuizen*. Antwerpen: Lessius Hogeschool.
Hill, C. E. (1986) 'An Overview of the Hill Counsellor and Client Verbal Response Modes Category System', in Greenberg, L. S. and Pinsof, W. M. (eds) *The Psychotherapeutic Process: A Research Handbook*. New York: Guilford Press, pp. 131–160.
Iglesias-Fernández, E. (2010) 'Verbal and Nonverbal Concomitants of Rapport in Healthcare Encounters: Implications for Interpreters', *The Journal of Specialised Translation*, 14, pp. 216–228.
Iglesias-Fernández, E. (2013) 'Understanding Variability in Interpreting Quality Assessment: User's Sex and Judgments for Pleasant Voice', in Way, C., Vandepitte, S., Meylaerts, R. and Bartłomiejczyk, M. (eds) *Tracks and Treks in Translation Studies*. Amsterdam: John Benjamins, pp. 103–125.
Khawkokgraud, S. (2015) *Tolken In De Geestelijke Gezondheidszorg: De Kwaliteit Van Het Tolken Bij De Afname Van De CAPS-5 Vragenlijst Bij Uitgeprocedeerde Asielzoekers In Nederland.* Unpublished Master's Thesis. KU Leuven.
Lietaer, G., Leijssen, M., Vanaerschot, G. and Gundrum, M. (1995) 'Handleiding Bij een Categorieënsysteem Voor Therapeutinterventies, Nederlandstalige Bewerking Van de Hill Counsellor Verbal Response Category System', *Psychotherapeutische Bijdrage*, 8. KU Leuven.
Price, J. (1975) 'Foreign Language Interpreting in Psychiatric Practice', *Australian And New Zealand Journal of Psychiatry*, 19, pp. 263–267.
Van Meekeren, E. (ed.) (2017) *Zelf Onthulling, Openheid Van Professionals In de Ggz*. Amsterdam: Boom.
Wadensjö, C. (1998) *Interpreting as Interaction*. London and New York: Longman.
Wampold, B. E. and Imel, Z. E. (2015) *The Great Psychotherapy Debate: The Evidence for What Makes Psychotherapy Work*. London and New York: Routledge.
Wang, J. and Fang. J. (2019) 'Accuracy in Telephone Interpreting and On-Site Interpreting', *Interpreting*, 21(1), pp. 36–61.
Zimányi, K. (2013) 'Somebody Has to Be in Charge of a Session: On the Control of Communication in Interpreter-Mediated Mental Health Encounters', *Translation and Interpreting Studies*, 8(1), pp. 94–111.

23
Nutrition and translation

Renée Desjardins

1 Introduction

The *Oxford Dictionary of Food and Nutrition* (Bender 2014) defines 'nutrition' as 'the branch of science that studies the process by which living organisms take in and use food for the maintenance of life, growth, reproduction, the functioning of organs and tissues, and the production of energy'. Nutrition science differs from food anthropology, which typically focuses on food as an anthropological object or on the broader concept of foodscape. Foodscapes are 'the global flows of food and cuisines as they are produced, distributed and exchanged, and as imagined and experienced within everyone's daily lives' (Ferrero 2002 cited in Crowther 2018: xxvi). Nutrition can intersect with 'global flows of food'; for instance, as nutritional guidelines change over time, so too do the needs and behaviours of consumers. As a result, some foods might be more popular than others or they may be promoted differently in public health nutritional guidelines. For example, a century ago, Hass avocados were not part of the typical North American diet. In Mexico and Central America there is evidence that humans did cultivate *āhuacatl* around 500 BCE, but no such evidence exists for North America. Today, thanks to discourses that have extolled the nutritional value of avocados, the popularity (and, arguably, notoriety)[1] of the fruit has soared worldwide (Handwerk 2017). This example illustrates how discourses on the nutritional value of specific foods/ingredients can influence dietary and consumer behaviour in specific foodscapes. The study of nutrition, as it intersects with food anthropology and sociology, allows us to understand foodscapes more holistically.

This chapter focuses more specifically on human nutrition and translation, meaning that the perspective is inevitably more anthropocentric (i.e. what *humans* eat). Since this handbook addresses human health, primarily, it makes sense to focus on human nutrition, though this is not to discount the valuable insights that come from studying the nutrition of other living organisms or the links that can be made with non-anthropocentric perspectives (an area that is gaining ground, for instance, in fields such as Critical Animal Studies).

Public and individual health are intrinsically linked to nutrition: illnesses in the population can be related to poor nutrition or poor diet. Food contamination or food-borne

DOI: 10.4324/9781003167983-28

diseases are also a matter of public health as these relate to what we eat, where and how (e.g. the rise in food allergies and sensitivities; changes in auto-immune diseases; the growing emphasis on proper handling of food in public spaces). Although nutrition science differs epistemologically from how we understand and study food behaviours, as in food anthropology, the two disciplines can overlap: because humans generally want to perform optimally and feel *well* (maintaining optimal health), they will turn to nutrition science or dietary advice to inform their eating behaviours (which include food choices, diet, number and frequency of meals). Specific food behaviours are typically associated with cultural and social norms, and are usually forged within a food community or other community (e.g. eating locally as part of the Slow Food movement; eating plant-based foods as part of the vegan movement). As Crowther (2018: xx) states: 'what we eat is culturally and socially patterned'.

Nutritional guidance typically falls within the purview of public health. Public health issues or problems tend to be multifaceted, which means that different expertise and disciplinary lenses can examine different aspects of the same issue (cf. Tolley 2016). If we consider that language is a *foundation* of effective public health communication, it follows that we can examine nutrition using the lens of translation studies.

2 Current research on translation and nutrition

In translation studies (TS), it is well-established that translation contributes to the circulation of knowledge, and this would naturally include knowledge related to food and nutrition. Yet, little research exists in TS, food studies (using humanistic epistemology), food science (using epistemologies from chemistry, biology, nutrition, microbiology and engineering) and public health examining these various points of convergence. To complicate matters, when the term 'translation' is used in public health or nutrition science contexts, it often refers to 'knowledge translation' (KT) or 'knowledge management' (KM). Although these terms are not always used interchangeably, they are understood as generally synonymous in this chapter. According to Risku (2013: 92), '[k]nowledge management (KM) is an interdisciplinary area of management research and practice that deals with the systematic, planned coordination and development of knowledge in organisations and individuals'. The Canadian Institutes of Health Research (2010) states that, 'knowledge translation is a dynamic and iterative process that includes synthesis, dissemination, exchange and ethically sound application of knowledge to improve the health of [citizens], provide more effective health services and products and strengthen the health care system'. Thus, when public health, nutrition or dietetics researchers refer to or use the concept of translation, this may not always mean *interlingual* translation; rather, translation in these areas would mean the development, transfer, uptake, and dissemination of discipline-specific knowledge (health, nutrition, dietetics, public health). Yet, as Risku notes, KM/KT and interlingual translation relate to one another:

> In KM, the different ideas, experiences, and perspectives of people with different cultural backgrounds are considered valuable intellectual capital [...]. Translation and cross-cultural communication are thus increasingly seen as a form of KM – preserving and supporting the diversity that is essential for sustainable development.
>
> *2013: 93*

Despite the relation between these terms, literature on interlingual translation in public health and nutrition research remains rather scant and difficult to find in English due to this conceptual overlap.

For instance, in the second edition of the *Oxford Handbook of Nutrition and Dietetics* (Webster-Gandy, Madden and Holdsworth 2012) the subject of global nutrition is addressed in a stand-alone chapter. This chapter addresses a list of causes that lead to global undernutrition, and while 'low national expenditure on health and education' is listed as a risk factor, the lack of nutritional information provided in one's language (i.e. a lack of 'knowledge translation') is not mentioned, though one could hypothesise a connection. Further, the *Handbook* does not explicitly mention the role of interlingual translation in disseminating nutritional literacy (KM/KT). Nutritional literacy and food education, as part of a holistic public health strategy, cannot be adequately imparted if this knowledge is not available in the languages of a given community (see Dragan 2009, n.p.). Similarly, in the *Multicultural Handbook of Food, Nutrition and Dietetics* (Thaker and Barton 2012), one might expect to see the index include the terms 'translation' (interlingual and KM/KT) or 'language', yet neither are indexed. Translation/multilingual communication plays a role in how food knowledge circulates, but none of the chapters, which are divided by region (South Asian Sub-continent, West Indies, East Asia, Israel, Eastern Mediterranean Region, West Africa, East and South-East Europe), explicitly addresses this role, nor do the last two chapters on public health discourse on maternal and child nutrition and on nutritional management of disease (Thaker and Barton 2012). These two examples serve to illustrate the relative absence of translation in nutrition and dietetics literature, despite the fact that translation is recognised as an important part of effective public health communication. However, in recent years, some public health campaigns have been more sensitive to the needs of multicultural and multilingual societies, as we shall see further on. Moreover, as food systems have increasingly become interconnected on a global scale, the need for multilingual approaches to production, labelling, packaging, and distribution has also become more pressing. As Chiaro and Rossato state:

> [...] due to the globalisation of food production and distribution, the circulation of food items originating from the most remote parts of the planet has also increased enormously, boosting the need for documents and labels that accompany foods and the need to translate them.
>
> *2015: 237*

The subject of (interlingual) translation may be taking some time to gain visible traction within nutrition research, but it is worth noting that interest in food and translation is on the increase in TS.[2] For instance, in 2015, *The Translator* published a special thematic issue titled 'Food and Translation, Translation and Food' (Chiaro and Rossato, 2015), which generated notable engagement within the field and beyond: the issue's introduction received over 16,100 online views since 2015, while the combined views for individual contributions amount to nearly 5,000. The co-editors of the special issue remark that part of this growing interest also reflects a broader interest in food as a cultural phenomenon: '[g]enerally speaking it would appear that a sort of food mania has pervaded the post-modern world' (Chiaro and Rossato 2015: 239). It is worth noting that the publication of the special issue occurred between two editions of the FaCT (Food and Culture in Translation) conference, in 2014 (Bertinoro, Italy) and 2016 (Catania, Italy) respectively. Another conference titled *Traduire le culinaire/Culinary Translation* was originally scheduled for spring 2020 (but later rescheduled due to the COVID-19 pandemic) with subjects ranging from cookbook translation to food in translated films, culinary terminology and food ecology.

In reviewing extant literature in TS and in related fields (such as media studies, semiotics, etc.), research linking food and translation can generally be divided into the following categories:

- Food in translated literature (e.g. Wiedenmayer 2016)
- Food, tourism and translation (e.g. De Marco 2015)
- Food terminology and phraseology (comparative analyses) (e.g. Gaspari 2015)
- Translation of food-related texts (non-institutional; e.g. cookery books; menus; recipes) (e.g. Chiaro 2008; Desjardins 2011; Ghafarian, Kafipour and Soori 2016; Fuentes-Luque 2017)
- Translation of food-related texts (institutional) (e.g. public health guidelines; nutritional guides; food labels; food packaging) (e.g. Chiaro 2004; Desjardins, Cooke and Charron 2015)
- Food and 'translation' of the Other/Otherness (e.g. Chiaro 2004; Elliott 2008; Stano 2016)
- Audiovisual translation (subtitling; dubbing; closed-captioning) and food (e.g. González-Vera 2015; Baños 2019)
- Non-anthropocentric/decolonised understandings of food ecology (e.g. Cronin 2016)

For the most past, research in all these categories tends to fall under the umbrella of the social sciences and humanities: the food/translation nexus has been examined from a more humanistic perspective than a nutritional science perspective or public health perspective. In this chapter, I draw from these arenas, but also seek to shift the focus to nutrition, public health and app development, and to the question of how these fields have mobilised translation to disseminate nutritional and dietetic knowledge.

There is a need for a closer examination of the roles translation plays in discourses on nutrition where it is curiously absent. Likewise, there is a need for examining how nutritional knowledge is translated or presented multilingually in institutional contexts, such as national public health campaigns or national food regulation policies. Countries with more than one official language or multilingual policies (e.g. Canada, South Africa, Singapore, Switzerland) must ensure the availability of public health information in each of their official languages, so examining translation in these national settings may provide data to determine best practice related to equitable public health communication and nutritional guidelines. Closer study of translation's role in nutritional discourses is also relevant in spaces where geography does not determine polyglossia (the coexistence of multiple languages), but where it is undeniably present, for instance in online spaces, such as social media platforms and websites, which are transnational by definition. Finally, this chapter seeks to fill a gap noted within TS: comprehensive handbooks such as *The Routledge Encyclopedia of Translation Studies* (Baker and Saldanha 2020) and *The Handbook of Translation Studies* (van Doorslaer and Gambier 2010) do not have entries under 'food' (at the time of writing this chapter), despite the evident interest in the topic. In this chapter, the three main topics that will be considered are the translation of nutritional guidelines with a focus on Canada's *Food Guide*; health apps, translation and localisation; and the growing importance and relevance of translation in the agro-food and food-processing industry.

3 Translation of public health discourses and nutritional guidelines: the case of *Canada's Food Guide*

Dietary recommendations are part of the foundation of many public health guidelines. In North America, proper nutrition and a healthy diet are deemed integral to preventative healthcare models. Public health authorities and agencies are usually involved in developing policy and action plans on food safety, food packaging and in promoting nutritious and balanced food habits for the general population. According to the Food and Agriculture Organisation of the United Nations (FAO):

> Food-based dietary guidelines (also known as dietary guidelines) are intended to establish a basis for public food and nutrition, health and agricultural policies and nutrition education programmes to foster healthy eating habits and lifestyles. They provide advice on foods, food groups and dietary patterns to provide the required nutrients to the general public to promote overall health and prevent chronic diseases. *2020*

For instance, the United States' Office of Disease Prevention and Health Promotion, which is the body that communicates national food and nutrition guidelines in the United States, includes dietary guidelines and nutritional intake references. Similarly, Health Canada, the federal government agency that communicates health and food policy and guidelines, has produced the well-known (and recently revamped) *Canada's Food Guide.* Santé Publique France [Public Health France] established the *Programme national nutrition santé [Health and nutrition national programme]* in 2001, as part of an overarching plan to promote holistic health and healthy dietary habits. FAO states that more than 100 countries worldwide 'have developed or are currently developing food-based dietary guidelines' (2020). The FAO's website is available in Arabic, English, Chinese, Russian, French, and Spanish, and their data is classified regionally; as of 2018, seven countries in Africa reported having food-based dietary guidelines; 15 countries in the Asia Pacific region; 30 countries in Europe; 25 countries in Latin America and the Caribbean; four countries in the Near East; and two countries in North America (FAO 2020). It is worth noting that international public health and dietary experts have heralded Brazil's dietary guidelines as a gold standard. They are praised for overcoming some of the 'common limitations of [other] conventional dietary guidelines' by shifting from a sort of abstract nutritional prescriptivism to guidance that was relative to an individual's context and circumstance (Monteiro at al. 2015). The Brazilian guidelines are available in Portuguese, English and Spanish, and they are premised upon five overarching principles that include a broadening of food choice autonomy and a diversification of dietary advice (Monteiro *et al.* 2015). Perhaps the most significant component of these guidelines was the incorporation of the concept of sustainability in all dietary recommendations: a healthy diet should be simultaneously sustainable on a physical, emotional and environmental level. As we shall see, the Brazilian guidelines led to the revision of other guidelines thereafter, including Canada's *Food Guide*.

Narrative theory has been a useful framework in translation studies to understand how knowledge is constructed and circulated. Mona Baker examined the narrative theory/translation studies nexus in her book *Translation and Conflict* (2006); since then, narrative theory has been applied to other case studies examining narratives and translation. With regard to nutrition, many narratives co-exist to inform food behaviour. For instance, public health discourses function as public narratives (Somers and Gibson 1994; Baker 2006), as do nutritional guidelines. Both 'narrate' normative food behaviour, consumption, as well as beliefs on and about food/nutrition at national level. Because food also relates to family, community and the self, we can also examine how ontological narratives (Somers and Gibson, 1994; Baker 2006)[3] and public narratives related to nutrition/food intersect or diverge. The concept of knowledge translation is relevant here because it is this process that 'translates' public narratives on nutrition to individuals in order to inform behaviour. Experts who codify and transcribe scientific knowledge (e.g. medical or nutritional knowledge), participate in what Latour and Woolgar (1986: 245) have described as a '[...] material operation of creating order', which also relates to how food-related narratives are shaped. Food guidelines, public health recommendations, and prescribed diets are examples of this codified 'text-making' that interrelates with ontological narratives and public narratives:

> text-making goes beyond materializing or expressing something that already exists in the mind and goes hand in hand with sense-making. By communicating verbally and non-verbally, we constantly shape and reshape [...] the scientific concepts that we need for our purposes as well as the arguments in which they are embedded and the social interactions that we pursue.
>
> *Montalt-Resurrecció and Shuttleworth 2012: 12*

Part of successful nutritional knowledge translation, and by extension successful public health strategy, depends on all individuals of a given country to be able to access, understand, and implement this knowledge. Interlingual translation is one of the strategies public health authorities mobilise to successfully impart this knowledge. However, because public health communication also depends on symbols (signs) to represent and mediate knowledge, intersemiotic translation (cf. Jakobson 1959) is also relevant.

The translation, or rather the non-translation, of nutritional guidelines, has been part of the debate surrounding the need to update national guidelines to reflect increasingly multicultural and multilingual nations. Canada's *Food Guide* is an example of where and how translation has been mobilised to mediate nutritional guidelines. The original *Food Guide* was published in 1942 under the title *Canada's Official Food Rules* and it was supposed to help Canadians make judicious food choices. The title of the document changed a number of times: *Canada's Official Food Rules* (1942); *Canada's Food Rules* (1944, 1949); *Canada's Food Guide* (1961, 1977, 1982); *Canada's Food Guide to Healthy Eating* (1992); *Eating Well with Canada's Food Guide* (2007); *Canada's Food Guide* (2019). These successive editions of the *Food Guide* were published over the years to address an evolving food system (agrarian to more industrialised), shifting cultural norms (such as the role of women in households), and an increasingly diverse population (due to migration, but also due to the increasing interest in 'foreign' food cultures and traditions). In its early iterations, the *Food Guide* was only available in the country's official languages: English and French. This made it harder for those who did not speak these languages or who did not have the proficiency to understand some of the terminology in a second language. More importantly, it meant that lack of access to public health and nutritional guidance in one's own language created a barrier to managing one's health and wellbeing, which could have negative effects on health outcomes. But the lack of interlingual translation was not the only translation problem at hand: earlier editions of the *Food Guide* only had one iconographic rendering, meaning that regardless of language or culture, the foods represented visually illustrated only one dietary or nutritional narrative. For example, in the 1992 edition of the *Food Guide,* one can note certain packaged products. For most Canadians, these packages would be generally recognisable (e.g. a box of rice, a bag of frozen vegetables, a carton of milk). However, these items were not (and still are not) necessarily packaged in the same form in other countries. As a result, recent immigrants to Canada might have found this visual narrative confusing or misleading, not to mention that the *Guide*'s pictorial elements largely omitted food items or behaviours from other cultures. For instance, packaged cereals with milk for breakfast might represent a typical early morning meal in North American societies, but may strike some individuals from other locales as an odd meal choice if boxed cereals are not an accessible or a customary food item or if an intolerance to dairy milk is present. These earlier versions, therefore, did not necessarily reflect the food traditions or cultural preferences of *all* Canadians, nor did they reflect the shifting and evolving food behaviours of a country impacted by immigration and migration (given that travel also impacts food behaviours and trends).

In 2007, a new edition of the *Guide* was published, which sought to remedy some of the earlier shortcomings, including issues related to the lack of cultural diversity in terms of ingredients or food items. Moreover, the new iteration was translated into 10 languages, in addition to the French and English versions. The 2007 edition also included a version of the *Guide* adapted for Indigenous peoples in Canada, titled *Food Guide for First Nations, Inuit and Métis.* This latter version was translated into Cree, Ojibwe, Inuktitut as well as into French and English. Although the 2007 iterations of the *Guide* are now archived, it is worth noting that their original online presentation suggested a sort of subordination of the Indigenous guide to the English and French guide (cf. Desjardins, Cooke and Charron 2015). Curiously, the former iteration of the 2007 *Guide* or the 'standard' guide, was *not* translated into any of Canada's Indigenous languages. Though the idea was that the Indigenous guide catered specifically to Indigenous communities and food cultures, the non-translation of the 'standard' English/French guide into Indigenous languages nonetheless posed an issue: if all nutritional guidance should be available to all Canadians, then all versions of the Guide – be it the Indigenous or 'standard' version – should be available in an equal number of languages. In this food narrative, it was as though there were two different guides for two different groups, one secondary to the other – an issue that has been somewhat redressed in the guide's most recent edition (2019). Cultural communities have specific food norms and food behaviours; however, these communities do not exist in a vacuum and can be influenced by or overlap with others. The overt delineation between the two guides and implicit subordination of the Indigenous version did not reflect permeable and sometimes inter-dependent food communities.

In 2015, Health Canada published its *Evidence Review for Dietary Guidance: Summary of Results and Implications for Canada's Food Guide* (Health Canada 2016), which served to usher in the 2019 (and the most recent) version of the guidelines. The *Canada's Food Guide Snapshot* (Canada's Food Guide 2019) is now available in 17 multicultural languages (Arabic, Farsi, German, Hindi, Italian, Korean, Polish, Portuguese, Punjabi, Russian, Simplified Chinese (Mandarin), Spanish, Tagalog, Tamil, Traditional Chinese, Urdu and Vietnamese) and nine Indigenous languages (Dene, Inuinnaqtun, Inuktitut (Baffin), Inuktitut (Nunatsiavut), Inuktitut (Nunavik), Michif, Ojibwe, Oji-Cree and Plains Cree),[4] in addition to French and English (28 languages in total). The *Snapshot*'s visual content is the same across all language versions, addressing previous criticism about delineating food iconography 'neatly' according to different groups/language versions in other iterations. Ginette Petitpas Taylor, Canada's Minister of Health at the time of the 2019 release, notes how language and accessibility intersect in the new version:

> Canada's new *Food Guide* was developed to be relevant to and accessible by all Canadians. Today, I am pleased to announce the translation of *Canada's Food Guide Snapshot* into 17 multicultural languages – making it more accessible and easier to understand by Canadians whose first language is not English or French. Now, more Canadians will benefit from our healthy eating guidance.
>
> *Health Canada 2019*

In a similar vein, Jennifer Buccino, Regional Executive Director (Ontario) from the Dietitians of Canada alludes to the concept of linguistic justice in her assessment of the new *Snapshot*:

> When we can provide resources in the languages our patients and clients speak, we create a more positive and comfortable space to talk about food and nutrition. The translation of Canada's new *Food Guide Snapshot* into additional languages will help dietitians and health care professionals start more conversations about healthy eating with the patients, clients, and communities they serve.
>
> *Health Canada 2019*

The evolution of *Canada's Food Guide* shows the importance of creating nutritional guidance that is accessible. It also shows the power that institutional narratives can have in shaping food policy, food behaviour, and nutritional guidance. These narratives can create and perpetuate detrimental stereotypes or function as a gatekeeping mechanism, creating a barrier to health equity when they are not equally accessible to all. The newest version of the *Guide* is not without reproach, however. Some argue that the *Guide* still lacks representational diversity and does not sufficiently address the issue of food insecurity. For instance, Sarah Duignan, PhD candidate at McMaster University (Canada) and host of the podcast *Anthrodish*[5] laments the fact that the 2019 guidelines do not sufficiently incorporate Indigenous visuals or recipes:

> The guide does consider culture's role in maintaining a healthy diet, but falls short of incorporating this effectively into its visuals or recipes. The discussion on culture values eating in ways that help 'learn about cultural food traditions' or that 'keep your cultural roots and food traditions alive'. Yet this section frames culture as a part of 'enjoying your food' rather than as a critical part of overall well-being. Incorporating traditional Indigenous foods (for example game meat, corn soup or wild blueberries) or foods that would be recognizable to newcomers to Canada (such as plantains or cassava for Central American families) would have helped more communities recognize their own diverse histories and cultures.
>
> *Duignan 2019*

Another debate emerged around the addition of more plant-based recipes. The inclusion of plant-based recipes and food items was meant to encourage Canadians to implement more environmentally sustainable food habits and to represent vegetarian and vegan diets in the guidelines. It is worth noting that prior to the official release of the 2019 *Guide*, some voices in the agricultural industry, such as the Dairy Farmers of Canada, expressed concerns regarding this shift. They felt it indicated to Canadians that some meat and dairy products were less nutritious and that this would have deleterious effects for the farming sector (Kirkup 2019).[6] Although the scope of this entry does not allow for an in-depth analysis of these specific food narratives, what must be acknowledged are the many interrelated narratives that operate within national nutritional guidance and food policy. These narratives – whether verbal or visual – function to translate food-related and nutrition-related knowledge.

The *Canada's Food Guide* case study falls within product-oriented descriptive translation studies (DTS) (Saldanha and O'Brien 2013). For readers interested in studying institutional or public narratives on nutrition, a similar framework might be advisable. In addition, translation flow analysis (Brisset 2008) can illustrate the directional flow of information in the dissemination of food-related knowledge.

4 Nutrition, well-being, social media, apps and translation

Roland Barthes (1961), a French semiotician, argued that food functions as a system of communication. As such, 'people use food to differentiate themselves from others, to establish rules of behaviour [...] and as a form of classification' (Elliott 2016: 5). In transnational online spaces, like social media platforms (e.g. Instagram, Pinterest, YouTube, Reddit) food-related content has proliferated over the years. Users turn to food to create their online identities, to communicate social status, cultural heritage, culinary knowledge, as well as food ideologies (e.g. veganism). Food, then, is not just a matter of nutrition or sustenance; it is a 'language' that communicates our online and offline identities. We can also examine how the language of food and wellness (fitness; self-care) intersect online and offline. Indeed, consumers are increasingly going online to find information on proper nutrition, fitness, and wellbeing (Schumer, Amadi and Ashish 2018). While seeking good health and eating well are not inherently new pursuits, the self-care and 'fitspo' (fitness inspiration) revolutions of the 2010s have motivated many to take their nutritional health into their own hands (sometimes literally, with mobile devices and wearable technology like smart watches) in unprecedented ways. Eating and other food-related behaviours now intersect with the aspirational goal of finding holistic wellness. The pursuit of wellness through the language of food is performative (Cavanaugh 2015): on platforms like Instagram and Pinterest, users who post carefully curated feeds 'perform' (or, in Barthes terminology, communicate or translate through captions and iconographic content) ideals of wellness related to diet and nutrition. This performative content has an effect on other users who may either replicate similar posts, ignore the content, or refute/subvert it, all of which serve to define and maintain specific online identities. Social media ostensibly provides a space in which the Self is 'translated' (Desjardins, 2019). For instance, if a user creates an Instagram post featuring a photo of fresh, colourful vegetables, this image could be 'translated' any number of ways by the caption (see Desjardins 2017): it could be a statement on nutrition, as much as it could be about decrying socio-economic barriers around healthy eating. This would depend on how the user wishes to create and perform their online ontological narrative (see Somers and Gibson 1994; Baker 2006).

Food-related user-generated content also connects to larger narratives about wellness and self-care both offline and online. In this sense, food can also communicate some users' health behaviours. To illustrate, the *New York Times* (Carraway 2019) reports that in 2019 approximately 18 million[7] Instagram posts were tagged using the hashtag #selfcare, compared to 2 million for #selfhelp. Though #selfcare does not necessarily mean the content is food-specific, much of the online discourse surrounding #selfcare has to do with food-related behaviour: weight loss, healthy eating, espousing a plant-based diet, counting macro-nutrients (also known as 'counting macros'), snacking, etc. Mobile app developers have capitalised on this growing interest. From registered nutritionists looking to help clients manage disease, allergy, or food sensitivity through online counselling, to more insidious developers looking to capitalise on body insecurity and aspirational weight goals, many people have devised apps for the navigation and tracking of nutritional information (e.g. ingredients, recipes, food databases, macro calculators, 'diet diaries'). These apps can also track other health or wellness metrics (e.g. sleep, physical activity, prescription medications and their interactions). These apps are known as mobile health or 'mHealth' applications (Xu and Liu 2015; Schumer, Amadi and Ashish 2018). According to 2014 data (Research2Guidance 2014; Xu and Liu 2015), there were more than 100,000 apps classified under the categories of health, fitness, and medicine.

Schumer, Amadi and Ashish (2018) examined the features of 86 diet and nutrition apps available in the Google Play Store (a digital distribution service operated by and developed by Google that targets applications available for Android operating systems). Interestingly, the study does not mention the apps' linguistic or localised features at all. Elsewhere, in an earlier review of extant research on smartphone applications promoting healthy diets and nutrition, Coughlin *et al.* (2015) indicate that 'there are currently no culturally, research-tested smartphone apps suitable for non-English speakers or for persons with low health literacy', though it is worth noting their study focuses on research written in English only. However, mobile app development moves at a significantly faster pace than academic research and there has been some change in this situation since the publication of this research.

As of 2020, diet and nutrition apps do exist in languages other than English, although there is scant research on the languages involved, translation/localisation, uptake and effectiveness. Yuka, for instance, is an app that can operate on both iOS and Android devices and uses barcode (Scandit) technology to let users know about a 'product's impact on their health'.[8] The app currently supports English, French and Spanish. One could posit that localised apps or apps with multilingual features would probably reach a broader audience – a hypothesis that could supplement analyses focusing on app effectiveness and uptake. However, language support and translation features are often contingent on programming and user experience (UX) priorities. For instance, it took seven years for Instagram, one of the most dominant social platforms in the world in terms of global uptake and number of users, to enable right-to-left (RTL) languages, such as Farsi, Hebrew and Arabic (Tepper 2017). If it takes dominant players, such as Facebook Inc. (who owns Instagram), several years to offer this type of language support, it makes sense that smaller-scale nutrition apps would face similar issues or have similar development models. Then again, one might question whether this is a matter of priorities: since English is the most readily spoken second language on a worldwide scale, the English-as-default in software and application development is relatively unsurprising. One could ask why spend resources on multilingual development if most users can use the app in English anyway.

This recalls the idea of equitable knowledge translation discussed in the previous section. Technology meant to help users adopt healthier lifestyles and diets should be accessible, in the same way that nutritional guidelines developed by public health institutions are or should be. Encouraging the development of multilingual nutrition apps would also stand to address some of the issues related to what is commonly referred to as the 'digital divide': the uneven distribution of technology and/or the barriers to its access and use (Wikipedia 2020). Unequal technological access and distribution can lead to the uneven distribution of knowledge, further exacerbating the 'knowledge divide'. In a knowledge economy, lack of access can be a social determinant of health (CPHA 2020) and studies focusing on the development of mHealth apps should examine how localisation, translation, dubbing and subtitling (in the case of video counselling for dietitians and nutritionists) may serve to make these technologies more inclusive and accessible.

As for food-related content in transnational online spaces like social media, future research avenues could include examining the content indexed under hashtags in different languages referring to similar food practices or behaviours (e.g. #vegan / #végétalien / #vegano), the use of self-translation by food and wellness influencers (cf. Desjardins 2019), and how machine translation is leveraged in the mHealth arena.

5 Food production, translation and social determinants of health

The World Health Organisation is considered a leading health agency that has put multilingualism at the core of its mission statement.[9] The WHO conducts its advocacy for and promotion of health in six official languages: Arabic, Chinese, English, French, Russian, and Spanish. Its website was initially translated into all six languages in 2005 and much of its online content has since been translated into more languages. The WHO considers multilingualism a way to 'effectively guide public health practice, reach out to international audiences, and achieve better health outcomes worldwide. In this way, multilingual communication is an essential tool for improving global health' (WHO 2020a).

This section addresses translation, interpreting and multilingualism, as they inextricably connect to social determinants of health, but with a specific focus on the contexts of food production and processing. WHO defines the social determinants of health (SDH) as follows:

> The social determinants of health are the conditions in which people are born, grow, live, work and age. These circumstances are shaped by the distribution of money, power and resources at global, national and local levels. The social determinants of health are mostly responsible for health inequities – the unfair and avoidable difference in health status seen within and between countries.
>
> *2020b*

The main SDH include: income and social status, employment and working conditions, education and literacy, childhood experiences, physical environments, social supports and coping skills, healthy behaviours, access to health services, biology and genetic endowment, gender, culture, race/racism (cf. WHO 2020b; Government of Canada 2019). National public health agencies also generally recognise that specific marginalised groups (e.g. LGBTQIA communities; and Black, Indigenous, and Peoples of Colour) are affected by additional SDH based on systemic discrimination, racism, and historical trauma.

Translation, in all its forms, can intersect with all of the SDH listed above. For instance, one cannot advocate for their own health in a clinical setting if they cannot adequately communicate with their attending physician, a subject that has been extensively studied by researchers in translation and interpreting studies (Angelelli 2004; Antonini *et al.* 2017; Meyer *et al.* 2010; Montalt-Resurrecció and Shuttleworth 2012). Similarly, in situations of crisis, as with the recent COVID-19 pandemic, people rely on public health service announcements to stay informed, healthy and safe. This kind of messaging can take many forms: from online social media posts to pamphlets, websites, infographics and even workplace bulletin boards. Yet translation and multilingual access were in some cases neglected in COVID-19 public health communication. As Canadian linguist Gretchen McCulloch states in *Wired*, public health communication can be Anglocentric:

> It's easy to overlook how important language is for health if you're on the English-speaking internet, where "is this headache actually something to worry about"? is only a quick Wikipedia article or WebMD search away. For over half of the world's population, people can't expect to Google their symptoms, nor even necessarily get a pamphlet from their doctor explaining their diagnosis, because it's not available in a language they can understand.
>
> *McCulloch 2020*

The connection between language equity and healthcare, as in a healthcare consultation, is probably quite straightforward – at the very least, the connection between limited English proficiency (LEP) and healthcare provision has been addressed in a number of case studies examining the barriers that persons with LEP face in the English-speaking world (Kim *et al.* 2011). However, the links between translation/interpreting/multilingualism, SDH, food supply chains and production do not seem to have been readily examined in an interdisciplinary manner.

While companies have increasingly implemented equality, diversity, and inclusion plans (EDI), they have sometimes skirted the issue of translation and multilingualism – the assumption being that the workforce should have sufficient English proficiency in English-speaking countries. In administrative and managerial ranks, this assumption might be justified, but in the case of migrant and marginalised workers who may have LEP, translation becomes essential in navigating the workplace. Much like in healthcare settings, non-professional interpreters (Antonini *et al.* 2017) end up ensuring that information is shared in the languages spoken 'on the floor'. However, when a situation is rapidly evolving and where conflicting information is circulating, leaving non-professional interpreters responsible for mitigating and mediating a public health crisis places additional burden on this workforce.

Food supply chains and food processing rely heavily on a migrant and/or marginalised workforce (Lever and Milbourne 2017; Xu and Jordan 2016). Xu and Jordan state '[...] due to population aging and the absence of willing domestic workers, rich countries are increasingly looking outside their borders for low-skilled workers in agriculture, food processing, construction, manufacturing, and low-wage services such as domestic work and home health care' (Xu and Jordan 2016: 3–4, see also Münz 2008: 2). In the case of the COVID-19 pandemic, these workers were negatively and disproportionately impacted relative to the population that could safely work from home: in North America, for instance, governments declared food production and supply 'essential', meaning that food supply and food production/processing workers were obligated to continue work in the early stages of the pandemic. In late April 2020, it was reported that Canada's largest outbreak (at the time of writing) had occurred at a Cargill meat-processing plant in High River, Alberta. The plant employs 2,000 unionised workers, most of whom are immigrants, refugees or temporary foreign workers (Frangou 2020). By 5 May 2020, 945 workers had been infected, with another 600 cases elsewhere in the province associated to the same Cargill outbreak. Investigative reporting revealed a lack of translation was a contributing factor (Baum, Tait and Grant 2020).

The Cargill plant in High River employs temporary foreign workers, most of whom are Filipino and yet, reports indicated that 'bulletin-board postings and letters to employees were provided only in English, causing confusion about compensation, isolation protocols and eligibility for paid time off' (Baum, Tait and Grant 2020). To abate the lack of translation, workers would consult a Facebook group, where employees would help one another make sense of Cargill's English-only communications (*ibid.*), clearly illustrating the relevance of and recourse to bilingual co-workers in such situations.

The issue also went beyond linguistic translation; there was also a problem of *cultural translation*. Family configurations among migrant worker communities tend to take on many forms: to counter fragmentation, loss of identity, and to adapt to new surroundings as well as to share resources, the family structure may mean the blending of two or more families or a multigenerational configuration. Community members will carpool or leverage public transit (when available) to commute to work. In normal circumstances, these practices do not pose a specific health issue, but in the case of the COVID-19 pandemic, contagion was linked to close contact. Cargill said some of these practices (carpooling; living in close proximity) were likely responsible for the rise in cases (Baum, Tait and Grant 2020; Frangou 2020), but employees from these communities felt unduly vilified. Slaughterhouses and meat-processing plants are recognised as being 'dirty' and 'dangerous' where employees work long hours in cramped spaces with poor air circulation (Lever and Milbourne 2017). To suggest the rise in contagion was attributable only to family structures and/or commuting practices is to sidestep the issues posed by the work environment altogether. If carpooling or isolation from family members was a key concern, Cargill could have prioritised translated material on the subject. Instead of vilifying or scapegoating cultural practices that are part of survival and that overlap with SDH, Cargill could have invested in a form of cultural translation demonstrating more sensitivity and understanding, rather than forcing this responsibility onto migrant workers already facing compounding health risks.

Although difficult working conditions and labour issues are well-documented in research literature on agro-food migrant workers (though still inadequately addressed in policy), the COVID-19 pandemic added another layer of complexity. Not only did this context demand an examination of how language representation and translation are or could be incorporated in EDI plans, the pandemic also revealed the additional crises these groups can face when translation and interpreting services are not readily available. At a time when automatic machine translation could have proven to be an arguably cost-effective short-term solution, Cargill seems to have maintained an Anglocentric position as opposed to finding creative and viable ways to leverage technology. Further research could examine how machine translation could be used in the agro-food industry to help facilitate communication with and within migrant communities. Some may argue that migrant workers should simply 'upskill' and learn English. However, Lever and Milbourne (2017) indicate that plant workforces often comprise migrant workers from different cultural and linguistic communities within the same plant. Typically, these workers will group together according to the languages they speak or according to co-nationality. As a result, workers may not be inclined or feel the need to pivot to a dominant language, like English, since their immediate co-workers will speak their language. This, then, also constrains language skill improvement – not to suggest learning English inherently means 'improvement', but it does mean, to some degree, more language versatility and access. For those interested in further examination of machine translation in the agro-food arena it is important to consider additional parameters related to how machine translation functions. As McCulloch (2020) states:

> Machine translation disproportionately works for languages with lots of resources, with things like news sites and dictionaries that can be used as training data. Sometimes, like with French and Spanish, the well-resourced languages of former colonial powers also work as lingua francas for translation purposes. [...] Google Translate supports 109 languages, Bing Translate has 71, and even Wikipedia exists in only 309 languages-figures that pale in comparison to the 500-plus languages on the list from the Endangered Languages Project.

In sum, technology can be useful, but it is worth recalling that wealthier languages are usually better supported to begin with, as in the example of Instagram and RTL languages cited above. It is also important to understand the relationships migrant workers maintain in such contexts and to avoid simplistic solutions like learning English on the floor.

Since food supply and food production/processing is an inherently multilingual and multicultural space, it is incumbent upon researchers in translation and interpreting studies interested in power dynamics and translation ethics to add to the discussion. This work could then assist in more comprehensive EDI development in the agro-food industry.

6 Conclusion

While the intersection of food and translation is a relatively new area of interest, it is gaining momentum. Previous studies have examined food and translation in the context of literary studies, semiotics, tourism, menu and cookbook translation and examples of these have been given in the introductory section of this chapter. However, the subject of nutrition and translation remains relatively underdeveloped. Here, attention has been given to three areas that indicate a need for translation and for additional scholarly interest, be it in TS or FS or both. First, translation is an important part of public health communication, and, thus, nutritional guidance. As more nations and jurisdictions acknowledge this fact, it is likely that nutritional guidelines and guides will be increasingly translated into multiple languages as standard practice. However, the question of *how* warrants further scrutiny: is machine translation sufficient and ethical? What can be done with iconographic or contentious recommendations? Machine translation surely cannot resolve these questions without human intervention and reflection. Moreover, how do public health authorities develop nutritional guidelines that are at once adaptable to individual circumstance, but also applicable to national demographics that are increasingly heterogeneous? This chapter also explored people's increased desire to become more autonomous with their health and eating. Nutrition and food apps on mobile devices are one of the ways people are tracking and analysing their nutritional intake. For marketability and for better user experience, one can easily argue in favour of translation's value here again. Insights from TS can also serve to better develop multilingual strategy and advise developers in the programming of better UX, indicating a connection between web/app development and language-related research. Finally, in examining the links between social determinants of health and food production/processing, specifically with regard to meat-processing plants in Canada, we see that translation can be a question of health or sickness, and, in dire cases, life and death. Translation, then, seems all the more relevant at a time of rising concerns around pandemics, global migration, agro-food industrial practices, and zoonotic diseases.

Notes

1 When some food items are extolled for their health benefits, they often gain popularity quickly. Unfortunately, this has a downside: some of these food items – like avocado, but also quinoa and açai – require complex processes of exporting and importing, which can have detrimental environmental effects. So called 'superfoods', like the avocado, are also lucrative produce, which has attracted the attention of cartels looking to capitalise on 'green gold' (Linthicum 2019). Consumer marketing does not always address this 'darker side' of health food crazes.
2 It is worth noting that food studies, like translation studies, is considered a relative recent field. Charlene Elliott states that 'whereas food was once marginalised as a scholarly focus' (2016: 4) there has been a rapid and wide-ranging expansion of food studies scholarship.
3 The use of 'ontological' refers here to narratives that relate to the Self. Baker (2006) applies this category to occasionally signal disciplinary narratives about translation or TS (a sort of disciplinary self-reflexivity); I follow Somers and Gibson's definition (1994: 61): 'These are the stories that social actors use to make sense of – indeed, in order to act in – their lives. Ontological narratives are used to define who we are; this in turn is a precondition for knowing what to do'.
4 The distinction between multicultural languages and Indigenous languages is important: it signals recognition of the fact that Indigenous peoples and Indigenous languages were present prior to settler colonisation and not a product of latter waves of immigration.
5 www.anthrodish.com/.
6 https://nationalpost.com/health/diet-fitness/hot-potato-food-guide-makeover-creates-debate-as-health-canada-prepares-release.
7 As of February 2020, this number was 24 million and counting.
8 https://yuka.io/en/ (Accessed: 1 June 2020).
9 www.who.int/about/who-we-are/multilingualism.

Further reading

Chiaro, D. and Rossato, L. (eds) (2015) *Food and Translation, Translation and Food*. Special issue of *The Translator*, 3(21).

This special issue is the first dedicated entirely to examining the intersections between food and translation. The contributions tackle different aspects of this nexus, from the relationships between translation studies and food studies, food ecology, translation and food tourism, and food-related phraseology.

Cronin, M. (2016) *Eco-Translation: Translation and Ecology in the Age of Anthropocene*. London and New York: Routledge.

In the second chapter of his book, titled 'Eating our words', Cronin examines the 'translation consequences' of food movement across languages, cultures, spaces and places. One of the more probing questions lies with the increasing industrialisation of both professional translation and food production. Cronin invites us to think about applying principles from the Slow Food movement into our translation practice. He asks '[h]as there been a movement that has called into question the potential consequences for language ecology of the mass production of translated languages?' (2016: 59).

Related topics

Translating Global Epidémics, Quality, Accessibility and Readability in Medical Translation, Inter- and Intralingual Translation of Medical Information

References

Angelelli, C. (2004) *Revisiting the Interpreter's Role. A Study of Conference, Court, and Medical Interpreters in Canada, Mexico, and the United States.* Amsterdam and Philadelphia: John Benjamins.

Antonini, R., Cirillo, L., Rossato, L. and Torresi, I. (2017) 'Introducing NPIT studies', in Antonini, R., Cirillo, L., Rossato, L. and Torresi, I. (eds) *Non-Professional Interpreting and Translation: State of the Art and Future of an Emerging Field of Research.* Amsterdam and Philadelphia: John Benjamins, pp. 1–26.

Baker, M. (2006) *Translation and Conflict: A Narrative Account.* London and New York: Routledge.

Baker, M. and Saldanha, G. (2020) *Routledge Encyclopedia of Translation Studies*, 3rd ed. London and New York: Routledge.

Baños, R. (2019) 'Translating Reality TV Into Spanish: When Fast-Food TV Challenges AVT Conventions', *Perspectives*, 27(2), pp. 265–282.

Barthes R. (1961) 'Pour une psycho-sociologie de l'alimentation contemporaine', *Annales. Economies, sociétés, civilisations*, 16(5), pp. 977–986.

Baum, K. B., Tait, C. and Grant, T. (2020) 'How Cargill Became the Site of Canada's Largest Single Outbreak of COVID-19,' *The Globe and Mail.* Available at: www.theglobeandmail.com/business/article-how-cargill-became-the-site-of-canadas-largest-single-outbreak-of/ (Accessed: 1 June 2020).

Bender, D. A. (2014) *Dictionary of Food and Nutrition.* Available at: www.oxfordreference.com/view/10.1093/acref/9780191752391.001.0001/acref-9780191752391-e-3801?rskey=ZpuXrjandresult=5297 (Accessed: 10 March 2020).

Brisset, A. (2008) 'Frontières de la traduction', *ÉcArts d'identité*, *2*(113), pp. 30–37.

Canada's Food Guide (2019) *Food Guide Snapshot.* Available at: https://foodguide.canada.ca/en/food-guide-snapshot/ (Accessed: 10 March 2020).

Canadian Institutes of Health Research (2010) *Knowledge Translation.* Available at: https://cihr-irsc.gc.ca/e/41928.html (Accessed: 13 March 2020).

Carraway, K. (2019) 'When Did Self-Help Become Self-Care?' *The New York Times.* Available at: www.nytimes.com/2019/08/10/style/selfcare/when-did-self-help-become-self-care.html (Accessed: 20 May 2020).

Cavanaugh, J. R. (2015) *'Performativity', Anthropology.* Available at: www.oxfordbibliographies.com/view/document/obo-9780199766567/obo-9780199766567-0114.xml (Accessed: 19 April 2020).

Chiaro, D. (2004) 'Translational and Marketing Communication', *The Translator*, 10(2), pp. 313–328.

Chiaro, D. (2008) 'A Taste of Otherness Eating and Thinking Globally', *European Journal of English Studies*, 12(2), pp. 195–209.

Chiaro, D. and Rossato, L. (eds) (2015) *Food and Translation, Translation and Food.* Special issue of *The Translator*, 3(21).

Coughlin, S. S., Whitehead, M., Sheats, J. Q., Mastromonico, J., Hardy, D. and Smith, S. A. (2015) 'Smartphone Applications for Promoting Healthy Diet and Nutrition: A Literature Review', *Jacobs Journal of Food and Nutrition*, 2(3), p. 21.

CPHA (2020) 'What are the Social Determinants of Health?' *Canadian Public Health Association* (CPHA). Available at: www.cpha.ca/what-are-social-determinants-health. (Accessed: 1 June 2020).

Cronin, M. (2016) *Eco-Translation: Translation and Ecology in the Age of Anthropocene.* London and New York: Routledge.

Crowther, G. (2018) *Eating Culture: An Anthropological Guide to Food,* 2nd ed. Toronto: University of Toronto Press.

De Marco, A. (2015) 'Are Green-Lipped Mussels Really Green? Touring New Zealand Food in Translation', *The Translator* 21(3), pp. 310–326.

Desjardins, R. (2011) 'L'étude du menu comme representation de l'identité culinaire Québécoise: le cas des menus du Château Frontenac', *Cuizine*, 3(1). Available at: www.erudit.org/en/journals/cuizine/1900-v1-n1-cuizine1807820/1004729ar/ (Accessed: 6 January 2021).

Desjardins, R. (2017) *Translation and Social Media: In Theory, in Training and in Professional Practice.* Basingstoke and New York: Palgrave Macmillan.

Desjardins, R. (2019) 'A Preliminary Theoretical Investigation Into [Online] Social Self-Translation: The Real, the Illusory, and the Hyperreal', *Translation Studies*, special issue 'Online Social Translation: New Roles, New Actors?', 12(2), pp. 156–176.
Desjardins, R., Cooke, N. and Charron, M. (2015) 'Food and Translation on the Table: Exploring the Relationships Between Food Studies and Translation Studies in Canada', *The Translator*, 21(3), pp. 257–270.
Dragan, A. (2009) *The Importance of Addressing Linguistic Ethno-Cultural Diversity in the Delivery of Public Health Services a Literature Review*. Brampton, ON: Region of Peel Public Health.
Duignan, S. (2019) *Canada's New Food Guide: A Fail on Culture and Sustainability. the Conversation.* Available at: https://theconversation.com/canadas-new-food-guide-a-fail-on-culture-and-sustainability-109718 (Accessed: 1 June 2020).
Elliott, C. (2008) 'Consuming the Other: Packaged Representations of Foreignness in President's Choice', in Lebesco, K. and Naccarato, P. (eds) *Edible Ideologies*. Albany: SUNY Press, pp. 179–198.
Elliott, C. (2016) 'Introduction', in Elliott, C. (ed.) *How Canadians Communicate VI: Food Promotion, Consumption, and Controversy*. Edmonton: Athabasca University Press, pp. 3–18.
Ferrero, S. (2002) 'Comida Sin Par. Consumption of Mexican Food in Los Angeles: "Foodscapes" in Transnational Consumer Society', in Belasco, W. and Scranton, P. (eds) *Food Nations: Selling Taste in Consumer Societies*. New York and London: Routledge, pp. 194–219.
Food and Agriculture Organization of the United Nations (2020) *Food-Based Dietary Guidelines*. Available at: www.fao.org/nutrition/education/food-dietary-guidelines/en/ (Accessed: 1 June 2020).
Frangou, C. (2020) 'Lives on the Line: As Cargill Employees Return to the Site of Canada's Largest COVID-19 Outbreak, Fear Lingers Still,' *Maclean's*. Available at: www.macleans.ca/society/health/cargill-COVID-19-meat-plant/ (Accessed: 10 June 2020).
Fuentes-Luque, A. (2017) 'An Approach to Analysing the Quality of Menu Translation in Southern Spain Restaurants', *Journal of Multilingual and Multicultural Development*, 38(2), pp. 177–188.
Gaspari, F. (2015) 'Exploring Milani 2015: A Cross-Linguistic Comparison of Food-Related Phraseology in Translation Using a *Comparallel* Corpus Approach', *The Translator*, 21(3), pp. 327–349.
Ghafarian, M., Kafipour, R. and Soori, A. (2016) 'Domestication and Foreignisation Strategies in Restaurant Menu Translation', *Pertanika*, 24(4), pp. 1417–1429.
González-Vera, P. (2015) 'Food for Thought: The Translation of Culinary References in Animation', *Íkala: Revista de Lenguaje y Cultura*, 20(2), pp. 247–246.
Government of Canada (2019) *Social Determinants of Health and Health Inequalities*. Available at: www.canada.ca/en/public-health/services/health-promotion/population-health/what-determines-health.html (Accessed: 30 May 2020).
Handwerk, B. (2017) 'Holy Guacamole: How the Hass Avocado Conquered the World', *Smithsonian Magazine*. Available at: www.smithsonianmag.com/science-nature/holy-guacamole-how-hass-avocado-conquered-world-180964250/ (Accessed: 11 March 2020).
Health Canada (2019). *Health Canada Unveils Canada's Food Guide Snapshot in 17 Multicultural Languages.* www.canada.ca/en/health-canada/news/2019/06/health-canada-unveils-canadas-food-guide-snapshot-in-17-multicultural-languages.html (Accessed: 15 June 2020).
Health Canada (2016). *Evidence Review for Dietary Guidance: Summary of Results and Implications for Canada's Food Guide*. Available at: www.canada.ca/en/health-canada/services/publications/food-nutrition/evidence-review-dietary-guidance-summary-results-implications-canada-food-guide.html (Accessed: 10 June 2020).
Jakobson, R. (1959) 'On Linguistic Aspects of Translation', in Brower, R. A. (ed.) *On Translation*. Cambridge, MA: Harvard University Press, pp. 232–239.
Kim, G. *et al.* (2011) 'Vulnerability of Older Latino and Asian Immigrants with Limited English Proficiency', *Journal of the American Geriatrics Society*, 59, pp. 1246–1252.
Kirkup, K. (2019) *Farmers Fume Over Expected Focus on Plant-Based Proteins in Canada Food Guide Makeover*. Available at: nationalpost.com/health/diet-fitness/hot-potato-food-guide-makeover-creates-debate-as-health-canada-prepares-release (Accessed: 20 April 2020).
Latour, B. and Woolgar, S. (1986) *Laboratory Life: The Construction of Scientific Facts*. Princeton, NJ: Princeton University Press.

Lever, J. and Milbourne, P. (2017) 'The Structural Invisibility of Outsiders: The Role of Migrant Labour in the Meat-Processing Industry', *Sociology*, 51(2), pp. 306–322.
Linthicum, K. (2019) 'Inside the Bloody Cartel War for Mexico's Multibillion-Dollar Avocado Industry', *Los Angeles Times.* Available at: www.latimes.com/world-nation/story/2019-11-20/mexico-cartel-violence-avocados (Accessed: 29 June 2020).
McCulloch, G. (2020) 'COVID-19 is History's Biggest Translation Challenge', *Wired.* Available at: www.wired.com/story/covid-language-translation-problem/ (Accessed: 10 June 2020).
Meyer, B., Bührig, K., Ortrun, K. and Pawlack, B. (2010) 'Nurses as Interpreters? Aspects of Interpreter Training for Bilingual Medical Employees', in Meyer, B. and Apfelbaum, B. (eds) *Multilingualism at Work: From Policies to Practices in Public, Medical and Business Settings.* Amsterdam and Philadelphia: John Benjamins, pp. 163–184.
Montalt-Resurrecció, V. and Shuttleworth, M. (2012) 'Research in Translation and Knowledge Mediation in Medical and Healthcare Settings', *Linguistica Antverpiensia*, 11, pp. 9–29.
Monteiro, C. A. *et al.* (2015) 'Dietary Guidelines to Nourish Humanity and the Planet in the Twenty-First Century. a Blueprint from Brazil', *Public Health Nutrition*, 18(13), pp. 2311–2322.
Münz, R. (2008) 'Migration, Labor Markets, and Integration of Migrants: An Overview for Europe', *World Bank Social Protection and Labor*, SP Discussion Paper no. 0807.
Research2Guidance (2014) mHealth App Developer Economics 2014. Available at: https://research2guidance.com/product/mhealth-app-developer-economics-2014/ (Accessed: 14 June 2020).
Risku, H. (2013) 'Knowledge Management and Translation', in Gambier, Y. and van
Saldanha, G. and O'Brien, S. (2013) *Research Methodologies in Translation Studies.* London and New York: Routledge.
Schumer, H., Amadi, T. C. and Ashish, J. (2018) 'Evaluating the Dietary and Nutritional Apps in the Google Play Store', *Healthcare Informatics Research*, 24(1), pp. 38–45.
Somers, M. R. and Gibson, G. D. (1994) 'Reclaiming the Epistemological "Other": Narrative and the Social Constitution of Identity', *Social Theory and the Politics of Identity*, pp. 37–99.
Stano, S. (2016) 'Lost in Translation: Food, Identity and Otherness', *Semiotica*, 211, pp. 81–104.
Tepper, F. (2017) 'Instagram Now Supports Right-To-Left Languages Like Hebrew and Arabic', TechCrunch. Available at: https://techcrunch.com/2017/10/31/instagram-now-supports-right-to-left-languages-like-hebrew-and-arabic/ (Accessed: 30 March 2020).
Thaker. A. and Barton, A. (2012) *Multicultural Handbook of Food, Nutrition and Dietetics.* Chichester: Wiley-Blackwell.
Tolley, E. (2016) *Qualitative Methods in Public Health: A Field Guide for Applied Research,* 2nd ed. San Francisco, CA: Jossey-Bass.
Van Doorslaer, L. and Gambier, Y. (2010) *Handbook of Translation Studies.* Amsterdam and Philadelphia: John Benjamins.
Webster-Gandy, J., Madden, A. and Holdsworth, M. (2012) *Oxford Handbook of Nutrition and Dietetics,* 2nd ed. Oxford: Oxford University Press.
Wiedenmayer, A. (2016) 'The Translation of Food in Literature: A Culinary Journey Through Time and Genres', *Semiotica*, 211, pp. 27–43.
Wikipedia (2020) *Digital Divide.* Available at: https://en.wikipedia.org/wiki/Digital_divide (Accessed: 1 June 2020).
WHO (2020a) 'Multilingualism', *World Health Organization (WHO).* Available at: www.who.int/about/who-we-are/multilingualism (Accessed: 30 May 2020).
WHO (2020b) 'Social Determinants of Health', *World Health Organization (WHO)* Available at: www.who.int/social_determinants/sdh_definition/en/ (Accessed: 30 May 2020).
Xu, Q. and Jordan, L. (2016) 'Migration, Labor Market and Wellbeing: Theories, Policies and Practice', in Xu, Q. and Jordan, L. (eds) *Migrant Workers: Social Identity, Occupational Challenges and Health Practices*, New York: Nova Publishers, pp. 3–25.
Xu, W. and Liu, Y. (2015) 'mHealthApps: A Repository and Database of Mobile Health Apps', *JMIR MHealth UHealth*, 3(1). Available at: https://mhealth.jmir.org/2015/1/e28/ (Accessed: 1 June 2020).

Index

Note: Numbers in *italics* indicate a figure; those in **bold** refer to information in tables; those followed by 'n' indicate chapter note numbers

FSC
www.fsc.org
MIX
Papier | Fördert
gute Waldnutzung
FSC® C083411

Kolibri 360 GmbH
Ferdinand-Jühlke-Straße 7
99095 Erfurt, Deutschland
produktsicherheit@kolibri360.de